Autonomic Disorders in Clinical Practice

Giuseppe Micieli • Max Hilz • Pietro Cortelli
Editors

Autonomic Disorders in Clinical Practice

Springer

Editors
Giuseppe Micieli
Emergency Neurology
Fondazione Istituto Neurologico
Nazionale Mondino
Pavia, Italy

Max Hilz
Dept. of Neurology
University of Erlangen-Nuremberg
Erlangen, Germany

Pietro Cortelli
Neurology, Operative Director
IRCCS ISNB
University of Bologna
Bologna, Italy

ISBN 978-3-031-43035-0 ISBN 978-3-031-43036-7 (eBook)
https://doi.org/10.1007/978-3-031-43036-7

This Springer imprint is published by the registered company Springer Nature Switzerland AG
The registered company address is: Gewerbestrasse 11, 6330 Cham, Switzerland

Paper in this product is recyclable.

Foreword

In the last years, there has been an increased need to provide appropriate answers to requests for neurological assistance, due to the spread of diseases of the nervous system and the severity of clinical conditions. The complexity of the clinical landscape often requires an in-depth and selective preparation, which cannot be provided without knowledge of the pathophysiological mechanisms.

Dysfunctions of the Autonomic Nervous System are often significant in different clinical settings, both when they occur in isolation and in association with other symptoms of the disease. An improved knowledge of autonomic dysfunction is essential to assist clinical conditions which involve neurological damage.

Expanding the neurologist's skillset can be instrumental in dealing with the complexity of the nervous system disease, in which autonomic functions can be primarily compromised or following the body's response to damages affecting other functional systems. The assistance requested from the neurologist must therefore concern every aspect of the disease, regardless of the primary structure involved.

The volume edited by Micieli and Cortelli shows relevant applications in usual clinical practice; it paves the way for an improvement in the quality of care, which is often conditioned by the limited attention to autonomic aspects related to the nervous system lesions.

The approach to the diseases appears both impactful and comprehensive; the description of various conditions makes it easier to carry out a correct clinical diagnosis and therapy of the most common neurological conditions. It also allows neurologists to differentiate pathologies that share similar clinical aspects but have different causes and evolutions.

In many medical conditions, the presence of autonomic dysfunctions is clinically relevant; these situations are more important in chronic diseases due to a body's response to damage to an organ or functional system.

Sometimes autonomic disorders are considered infrequent events and treatable only in dedicated medical centers. This belief appears unfounded because very widespread diseases, such as headaches or hypertension, often display vegetative aspects. For this reason, knowledge of autonomic disorders is crucial in clinical practice, with specific focus on the methods of evaluation, control, and treatment.

During their daily practice, neurologists can refer to tables of this book, which summarize both the causes and therapeutic approaches to different pathological conditions, to aid their decision-making.

Some chapters outline the correct approach to clinical problems that are shared between the neurologist and other medical specialists; the chapter regarding the neuropathic pain, for example, illustrates a blueprint for defining the correct way to manage the condition. The neurological approach is supported by a pathophysiological evaluation of all parameters influencing the pain occurrence and its clinical relevance, strengthening the impact of the symptomatic treatment offered by other medical specializations.

The autonomic syndromes require both a correct identification and an evaluation of all conditions influencing the occurrence of symptoms; the approach is clearly explained in many chapters which highlight all risk factors causing the vegetative impairment.

The description of detailed conditions and the broad spectrum of diseases make the book instrumental to the improvement of the neurological practice; every neurologist can benefit from the synthesis between principles of pathophysiology and clinical/instrumental evaluation to ensure an appropriate treatment.

Given this, both students and specialists will find the book to be a valid tool for improving both quality and completeness of the neurological care.

Neurology
Polytechnic University of Marche
Ancona, Italy
April 12, 2023

Leandro Provinciali

Contents

Chapter 1
Introductive Chapter of the Autonomic Nervous System

Pietro Cortelli

1.1 ANS Definition

The Autonomic Nervous System (ANS) represents a neuronal network that collects internal, both hormonal and visceral, along with external information (afferents), to integrate them and promote coordinated biological responses (efferents). Notably, this complex interplay is minimal if not influenced by human willingness and has the purpose of preserving the human body's homeostasis in rest and stressful conditions. To carry out this duty, the ANS has to be closely interconnected with each human organ, orchestrate autonomic responses, and modulate behavioural, neuroendocrine, and neuro-immunological responses. This dense network of relationships with peripheral organs makes the ANS a pivotal contributor to every physiological and pathological human process. Therefore, the study of ANS should be a matter of interest shared by every branch of medicine.

1.2 Anatomical and Physiological Basis of ANS

Detailed knowledge of ANS's anatomical, physiological, and pathological basics is paramount to comprehending the clinical evaluation and management of the manifestations related to ANS disorders. The ANS is composed of a vast neuronal network

P. Cortelli (✉)
Department of Biomedical and NeuroMotor Sciences (DIBINEM), University of Bologna, Bologna, Italy

IRCCS Istituto delle Scienze Neurologiche di Bologna, Bologna, Italy
e-mail: pietro.cortelli@unibo.it

G. Micieli et al. (eds.), *Autonomic Disorders in Clinical Practice*,
https://doi.org/10.1007/978-3-031-43036-7_1

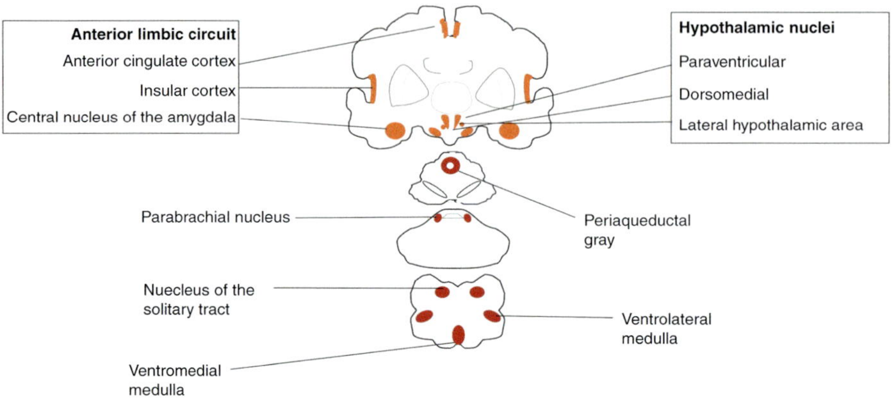

Fig. 1.1 Graphical representation of the Central Autonomic Network (CAN) anatomy

topographically distributed in different regions of the central nervous system, defined as the *Central Autonomic Network (CAN),* and the peripheral nervous system [1]. The CAN is responsible for integrating afferents and modulating tonic, phasic, and state-dependent autonomic functions. It comprises multiple nervous structures localised within deep cerebral areas, the brainstem, and the spinal cord (Fig. 1.1). From an organisational and functional perspective, the CAN could be subdivided into multiple hierarchical levels with increasing modulation complexity moving rostrally. Accordingly, spinal cord autonomic neurons mediate simple autonomic reflexes with a segmental organisation, in the medulla and the pons, the solitary tract nucleus, the rostral ventrolateral and ventromedial medulla, and the parabrachial nucleus control cardiovascular, respiratory, gastrointestinal, and urogenital reflexes.

Within the midbrain, the periaqueductal grey integrates pain modulation, stress-driven behavioural responses, sleep function, and autonomic control. More rostrally, the hypothalamus orchestrates endocrine, sleep, and autonomic responses, while the anterior limbic circuit (anterior cingulate cortex, amygdala, and insular cortex) coordinates corporeal sensations with the autonomic-behavioural responses. Additionally, functional brain MRI studies have revealed that many other brain structures controlling different biological mechanisms also contribute to homeostatic autonomic regulations. Collectively, these landmark studies substantiate the concept that the CAN is not a static network yet somewhat integrated with all other cerebral networks [2].

The observation that the ANS does not merely operate based on "autonomic" reflexes yet belongs to an overarching complex architecture of modulation and integration with somatic and emotive systems has convinced some Authors to prefer the term "vegetative" compared to the historical "autonomic."

In the peripheral nervous system, the autonomic afferents are composed of visceral receptors that transduce specific information, such as the blood electrochemical composition or arterial pressure, into electrical signals that reach the CAN to inform about the internal body status constantly. Conversely, the autonomic efferents are mediated by the sympathetic and parasympathetic systems, which operate complementary functions. Both these systems are composed of the brainstem and spinal cord pre-ganglia neurons, as well as neurons that reside outside the central nervous systems, which innervate the target organs directly. The former use acetylcholine as a neurotransmitter, whereas the latter use noradrenaline (sympathetic system) or acetylcholine (parasympathetic system).

Arterial pressure and thermoregulation are mainly under the control of the sympathetic system. Therefore, sympathetic dysfunction may result in clinical manifestations of orthostatic arterial hypotension (sympathetic adrenergic failure) and anhidrosis (sympathetic cholinergic failure). Conversely, the parasympathetic system coordinates local organ reflexes. Therefore, its dysfunction may result in photophobia, xerostomia, xerophthalmia, gastrointestinal dysmotility, micturition disorders, and erectile dysfunction. A third peripheral autonomic nervous system exists, the so-called enteric nervous system (ENS), yet it has been historically more neglected. The ENS is wholly located within the gastrointestinal walls and acts as an independent regulator of gastrointestinal functions, where the overarching control of the CAN mediates only limited modulations.

1.3 Diagnostic Methodology (Medical History, Examination, Instrumental Investigations)

Autonomic manifestations are ubiquitous in daily clinical practice, yet they are often neglected. A systematic evaluation is, therefore, necessary to recognise and diagnose these disorders [3, 4]. An accurate medical history that assesses the presence, temporal evolution, and clinical features of dysautonomic manifestations remains paramount. Furthermore, the presence of predisposing disorders (such as diabetes or Parkinson's disease) and drugs (such as alpha-antagonists or anticholinergic drugs) should also be investigated.

The neurological clinical examination should be comprehensive of the evaluation of arterial pressure in orthostat and clinostat positions, pupillary reflex, vasomotor signs (i.e., pallor, flushing, and cold hands or feet), secretomotor signs (i.e., xerostomia and xerophthalmia), and sudomotor signs (i.e., skin lesions).

After that, ancillary diagnostic tests that investigate the ANS's morphological and/or functional features may be required to support the diagnosis.

In order to explore the functions of the ANS, the patients are exposed to stressful conditions to register the transitory physiological modifications mediated by the homeostatic activity of the ANS. These autonomic responses may be investigated by either non-neurologist or neurologist physicians and include urodynamic tests, gastrointestinal transit time, lacrimal secretion tests, sudomotor tests, or catecholamines levels. However, cardiovascular reflexes are the most frequent autonomic responses assessed in clinical practice [5].

Conversely, the morphological integrity of the peripheral and central ANS could be assessed with skin biopsy and neuroimaging studies, respectively. The ultimate goal of this systematic, comprehensive evaluation (medical history, physical examination, and ancillary tests) is to define the potential presence and localisation of an autonomic disorder that can either result from a hyper- or hypo-stimulation of the ANS and to quantify its magnitude.

Even though every human body organ is innervated, hence regulated, by the ANS, it may be broadly categorised into seven macro clinic-anatomical systems for practical purposes: (i) cardiovascular, (ii) gastrointestinal, (iii) secretomotor, (iv) sudomotor, (v) genitourinary, (vi) sexual, and (vii) respiratory.

1.4 A Clinical Perspective on ANS Manifestations

Many neurological (e.g., multiple sclerosis, epilepsy, headache, etc.) and non-neurological (e.g., diabetes, obstructive sleep apnoea syndrome, rheumatological disorders, etc.) conditions comprise ANS manifestations among a constellation of different clinical symptoms and signs. Nonetheless, there are a few disorders where ANS dysfunction has a critical role, and the comprehensive examination of ANS reflexes is pivotal for diagnosis. These conditions include non-traumatic transitory loss of consciousness, neurodegenerative disorders related to pathological synuclein accumulation, and autonomic neuropathies [3].

1.5 Conclusions and Presentation of the Following Chapters

In this book, all relevant ANS topics will be discussed to enable the readers to (i) comprehend the ANS's elegant function through the study of its anatomical-physiological basics, (ii) explain the clinical manifestations related to its dysfunctions, (iii) diagnose the underlying aetiology, and (iv) master available pharmacological and non-pharmacological therapies.

References

1. Benarroch EE. Physiology and pathophysiology of the autonomic nervous system. Continuum (Minneap Minn). 2020;26:12–24.
2. Sklerov M, Dayan E, Browner N. Functional neuroimaging of the central autonomic network: recent developments and clinical implications. Clin Auton Res. 2019;29:555–66.
3. Benarroch EE. The clinical approach to autonomic failure in neurological disorders. Nat Rev Neurol. 2014;10:396–407.
4. Cheshire WP Jr. Autonomic history, examination, and laboratory evaluation. Continuum (Minneap Minn). 2020;26:25–43.
5. Kaufmann H, Norcliffe-Kaufmann L, Palma JA. Baroreflex dysfunction. N Engl J Med. 2020;382:163–78.

Chapter 2
Orthostatic Hypotension

Pietro Guaraldi and Giovanna Calandra-Buonaura

2.1 Definition

Orthostatic hypotension (OH) is defined as a sustained decrease in systolic blood pressure (SBP) of at least 20 mmHg and/or diastolic blood pressure (DBP) of at least 10 mmHg within 3 min of standing or head-up tilt to at least 60° on a tilt table compared to the supine position [1].

In patients presenting with supine hypertension (SH), a reduction in SBP of at least 30 mmHg is suggested for the diagnosis of OH since the magnitude of the BP drop depends on the baseline BP value.

In addition to the classical form, the following are defined (Table 2.1):

Table 2.1 OH: diagnostic criteria

Classic OH	A sustained reduction of SBP of at least 20 mmHg and/or DBP of 10 mmHg within 3 min of standing or head-up tilt to at least 60° on a tilt table
Delayed OH	A sustained reduction of SBP of at least 20 mmHg and/or DBP of 10 mmHg after 3 min and within 10 min of standing or head-up tilt to at least 60° on a tilt table
Initial OH	A transient BP decrease (>40 mmHg SBP and/or >20 mmHg DBP) within 15 s of standing

OH orthostatic hypotension, *SBP* systolic blood pressure, *DBP* diastolic blood pressure

P. Guaraldi (✉)
IRCCS Istituto Delle Scienze Neurologiche di Bologna, Bologna, Italy
e-mail: p.guaraldi@isnb.it

G. Calandra-Buonaura
IRCCS Istituto Delle Scienze Neurologiche di Bologna, Bologna, Italy

Department of Biomedical and NeuroMotor Sciences (DiBiNeM), Alma Mater Studiorum University of Bologna, Bologna, Italy
e-mail: giovanna.calandra@unibo.it

G. Micieli et al. (eds.), *Autonomic Disorders in Clinical Practice*,
https://doi.org/10.1007/978-3-031-43036-7_2

Initial orthostatic hypotension: A transient decrease in SBP >40 mmHg and/or DBP >20 mmHg that occurs within 15 sec after standing. Diagnosis requires continuous beat-to-beat monitoring of blood pressure values. Blood pressure reduction is frequently associated with symptoms of cerebral hypoperfusion.

Delayed orthostatic hypotension: An OH that occurs after a 3-min and within 10 min standing or tilt test. This variant could represent a mild and early form of vegetative sympathetic insufficiency [1, 2].

2.2 Pathogenesis

The transition from supine to standing (Fig. 2.1) determines the redistribution of 300–800 ml of blood volume to the lower limbs and the splanchnic circulation [3]. This results in a reduction in venous return to the heart and in the left ventricular filling pressure with a consequent decrease in stroke volume and cardiac output. In response to these modifications, in physiological conditions, the baroreceptor reflex determines the activation of the sympathetic vasoconstrictor efferents and the reduction of the vagal tone of the heart. These responses lead to an increase in vascular tone, heart rate (HR), and contractility, and restore blood pressure values within seconds.

In the presence of impaired functioning of the baroreceptor reflex arc, cardiac or vascular dysfunctions, or reduced circulating volume, it is not possible to compensate for orthostatic stress, with consequent development of OH and tissue hypoperfusion.

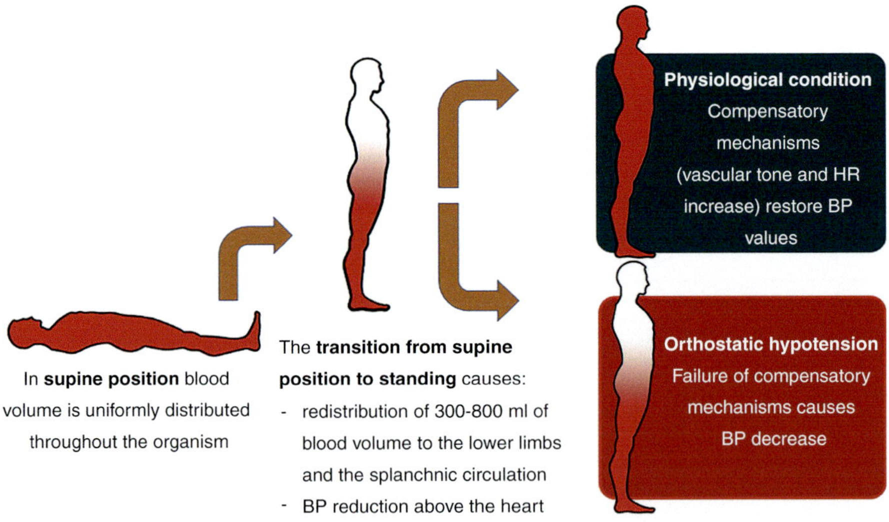

Fig. 2.1 Hemodynamic changes during the orthostatic challenge

2.3 Clinic

OH is a clinical sign and can occur symptomatic or asymptomatic. When symptomatic OH is manifested by symptoms of hypoperfusion that appear on transition from supine to standing or during prolonged standing (Table 2.2). These symptoms recover promptly upon acquisition of the sitting or lying position.

Cerebral hypoperfusion causes symptoms of "dizziness," "light-headedness," "blurred vision," slowing of cognitive performance, up to syncope. Hypoperfusion of the neck muscles manifests with a painful contracture defined "coat-hanger" pain; cardiac hypoperfusion may cause symptoms similar to angina. The reduced blood flow to the kidneys leads to oliguria during standing, often associated with nocturnal polyuria favored by increased renal perfusion in the supine position. The patient will hardly spontaneously report these symptoms, which must therefore be sought with specific questions:

- Have you had fainting spells recently?
- Do you feel dizzy or light-headed when you stand up?
- Do you have visual disturbances when standing?
- Do your legs feel weak when standing?
- Do you have neck/shoulder pain when standing?
- Do symptoms improve/recover when sitting/lying down?
- Are symptoms worse in the morning or after meals?

The onset of symptoms does not correlate with the extent of the blood pressure drop but with the blood pressure value reached during orthostatism. Patients typically become symptomatic with mean BP <75 mmHg (SBP/DBP <90/70 mmHg) [4].

However, patients with chronic orthostatic hypotension may be asymptomatic even with very low blood pressure values due to the gradual development of cerebral autoregulatory mechanisms.

In 50% of cases, the OH is asymptomatic, and it is therefore necessary to actively search for it during the visit.

Table 2.2 Symptoms resulting from orthostatic hypotension

Site of hypoperfusion	Symptom
Brain	Dizziness, light-headedness Visual disturbances (blurred vision, tunnel vision, scotoma, color defects, blacking out) Slowing of cognitive performance Syncope
Muscles	Paracervical and suboccipital ache ("coat-hanger" pain) Low back pain
Heart	Angina
Kidney	Oliguria
Nonspecific	Weakness, fatigue, falls

2.4 Diagnostic Process

OH can be easily diagnosed in an outpatient clinic or ward by measuring BP after 5 min of supine position and within 3 min of upright position, preferably using an automatic sphygmomanometer capable of providing heart HR value [5].

In specialized centers, it can be detected by tilt table testing performed at 60 degrees (at least), with continuous beat-to-beat measurement of BP and HR. It may be necessary to retest the presence of OH in the morning when the blood pressure drop is most pronounced or after meals (postprandial OH).

Twenty-four-hour home blood pressure monitoring may be useful as diagnostic support.

OH can be due to neurogenic (nOH) or non-neurogenic causes (Table 2.3, Fig. 2.2).

Table 2.3 Causes of OH

Non neurogenic causes
Cardiac pump failure
Myocardial infarction
Myxoma
Myocarditis
Pericarditis
Tachyarrhythmia
Bradyarrhythmia
Hypovolemia
Dehydration (chronic vomiting, diarrhea)
Hemorrhage
Salt-losing nephropathy
Hemodialysis
Adrenal insufficiency
Venous pooling
Alcohol
Heat exposure
Fever
Prolonged standing
Prolonged recumbency
Severe varicosities
Drugs
Antihypertensive drugs
Diuretics
Nitric oxide-mediated vasodilator (nitrates, 5-phosphodiesterase inhibitor)
Adrenoceptor blockers (especially α1-adrenoceptor)
α2-adrenoceptor agonist
Levodopa, dopamine agonist
Tricyclic antidepressants

Table 2.3 (continued)

Neurological causes
With signs of CNS involvement
Neurodegenerative disorders
Multiple system atrophy
Parkinson's disease
Lewy body dementia
Lesions of CNS
Cervical spinal cord injury
Syringomyelia
Multiple sclerosis
Without signs of CNS involvement
Pure autonomic failure
Peripheral neuropathies
Small fibers neuropathy
Diabetes mellitus
Renal failure/posthemodialysis
Paraneoplastic
Amyloidosis
Porphyria
Guillain-Barré syndrome
Familial dysautonomia (Riley-day)

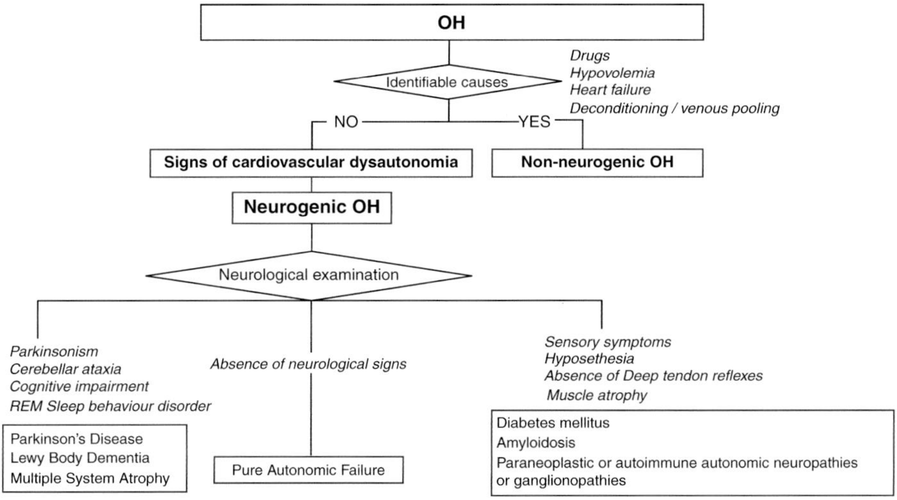

Fig. 2.2 Flow chart showing the diagnostic approach to patient with orthostatic hypotension

A detailed anamnesis is crucial for the exclusion of secondary causes of OH, such as concomitant cardiac pathologies or hypovolemia or venous insufficiency. A complete list of all the medications taken by the patient should be collected to rule out an iatrogenic cause.

The nOH depends on an alteration of the autonomic nervous system, which controls the cardiovascular function, in particular, an alteration of the sympathetic component.

An easy tool that can lead to early identification of nOH is the calculation of the ratio between the increase in HR and decrease in SBP at the third minute of the orthostatic test compared to the values in the supine position (DeltaFC/DeltaPAS index) [6]. When the ratio is less than 0.5 (therefore, if a drop in SBP of at least 20 mmHg does not correspond to a compensatory increase in HR of at least 10 bpm) it can be hypothesized with a sensitivity of 91.3% and a specificity of 88 0.4% that the OH is neurogenic. This index was validated both for the tilt test [6, 7] and standing [8].

The direct method for the assessment of sympathetic function is represented by the dosage of plasma catecholamines during supine rest and the tilt test. Under physiological conditions, noradrenaline values double in the transition from supine to upright position; if this does not occur, OH is considered neurogenic [9].

An alternative method is represented by the Valsalva maneuver (Fig. 2.3), which allows us to investigate the entire baroreceptor reflex arc.

The maneuver requires continuous monitoring of the cardiovascular parameters and is performed in the reclined position (in order to avoid the interference of gravitational force). The subject is asked to blow in a mouthpiece connected to a sphygmomanometer, maintaining a pressure of 40 mmHg for 15 s [10]. In physiological conditions, the maneuver evokes variations of BP and HR, which can be divided into four phases (Fig. 2.3). In patients with nOH there is a progressive fall in BP in phase II without recovery and the absence of the typical pressure increase ("overshoot") at the end of the expiration.

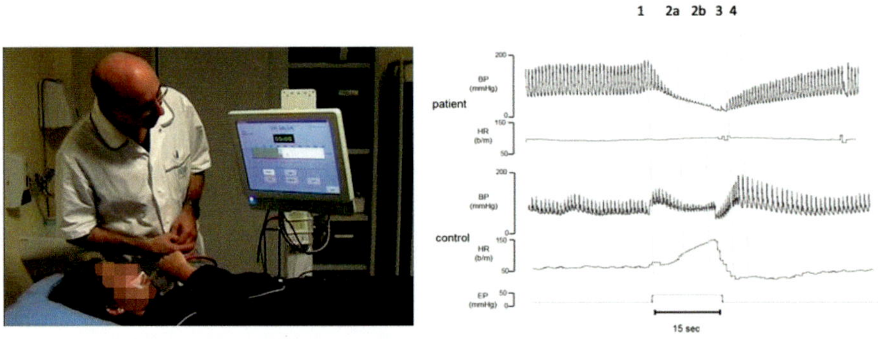

Fig. 2.3 The Valsalva maneuver. The box on the left shows a patient performing the Valsalva maneuver. The box on the right shows a continuous recording of arterial pressure (BP), heart rate (HR), and expiratory pressure (Exp Pre) during the Valsalva maneuver in a healthy control and in a patient with vegetative insufficiency. The various phases in which the cardiac parameters are modified during the examination are shown; in particular, it can be noted the absence of pressure "overshoot" at the end of expiration and the absence of changes in HR

Once the diagnosis of nOH is established, the neurological physical examination should search for the presence or absence of signs of central nervous system (CNS) or peripheral (PNS) involvement to guide the possible origin of the disorder (Table 2.3, Fig. 2.2).

nOH can be found in all α-synucleinopathies (Parkinson's disease, multiple system atrophy, dementia with Lewy bodies). nOH is earlier, more frequent, and severe in multiple system atrophy. Previous studies in Parkinson's disease indicate a 30% prevalence of patients affected by OH throughout the course of the disease [11]. However, it was not always specified whether it was neurogenic or non-neurogenic OH. In the early Parkinson's disease stages (within 3 years of onset), nOH has been detected with a much lower frequency [12]. Therefore, the detection of nOH in a patient with Parkinsonian syndrome at onset demands the exclusion of iatrogenic causes or an accurate investigation to exclude atypical parkinsonism.

nOH is the cardinal sign of Pure Autonomic Failure (PAF), a rare synucleinopathy characterized by cardiovascular dysautonomia associated or not with generalized dysautonomia in the absence of other neurological deficits. However, it should be remembered that about 30% of PAF patients evolve toward other forms of synucleinopathy even 5 years after the onset of symptoms, and an appropriate follow-up is mandatory [13, 14].

Furthermore, nOH can complicate various forms of polyneuropathy (diabetic, autoimmune, paraneoplastic) and is also a characteristic element of some rare peripheral nervous system pathologies such as amyloidosis.

Finally, the nOH can be secondary to lesions affecting the areas responsible for the autonomic control of the cardiovascular system (i.e., in spinal cord injuries or multiple sclerosis).

2.5 Supine Hypertension

Approximately 50% of patients with nOH display supine hypertension (SH), defined as the occurrence of SBP ≥ 140 mmHg and/or DBP ≥90 mmHg after at least 5 min of rest in the supine position in a patient with nOH [15]. SH, as OH, is an expression of altered baroreceptor control.

SH is classified as mild, moderate, or severe according to the range of blood pressure values (Table 2.4).

It is important to recognize SH because:

Table 2.4 Ranges of the Severity of SH

	Mild	Moderate	Severe
SBP (mmHg)	140–159	160–179	≥180
DBP (mmHg)	90–99	100–109	≥110

SH supine hypertension, *SBP* systolic blood pressure, *DBP* diastolic blood pressure

- Causing natriuresis at night, it can lead to an increase in diuresis with consequent dehydration and worsening of morning OH.
- May contribute to organ damage (ventricular hypertrophy, cerebral vasculopathy, chronic renal failure) [16].
- The presence of SH contraindicates some treatments for nOH (i.e., fludrocortisone).

In addition to SH, a reduction in the physiological drop in mean nocturnal BP compared to mean daytime BP (nondipper pattern, <10% reduction) or an increase in mean nocturnal BP compared to mean daytime BP (reverse dipper pattern) may be found. Therefore, in patients with SH, it is advisable to perform 24-h blood pressure monitoring.

2.6 Treatment

2.6.1 Treatment of OH

- Varies depending on whether the OH is symptomatic or not and must be tailored to the severity of the disorder.
- The goal of the treatment is the improvement of symptoms, not the normalization of blood pressure values.
- It must consider the possible presence of SH.

The treatment of OH is based on a four-step process (Fig. 2.4) [17]:

1. *Review of current therapy*: consider reducing the dose or discontinuing medications that could cause/aggravate the OH (Table 2.3).
2. *Nonpharmacological treatments* aimed at expanding the volume, reducing natriuresis, and counteract deconditioning such as:

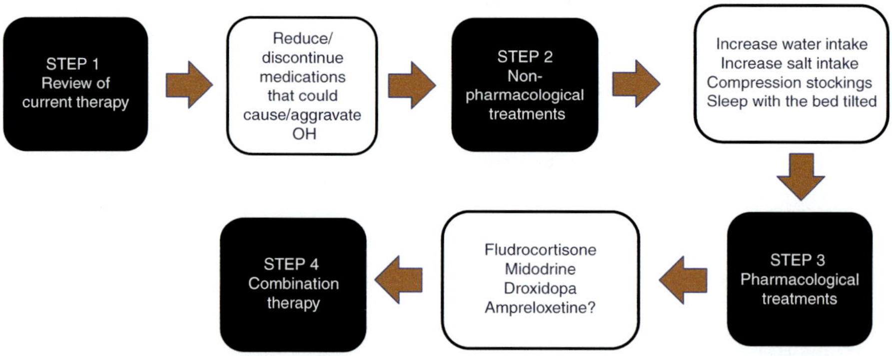

Fig. 2.4 Treatment flowchart

- Increase water intake to 2–3 L/day.
- Increase the consumption of salt (8 g per day).
- Use compression stockings and abdominal bands to reduce venous pooling.
- Practice regular aerobic physical activity.
- Sleep with the bed tilted keeping the head raised about 30° with respect to the feet.
- Instruct patients on possible aggravating factors that must be avoided (rapid postural changes, large and carbohydrate-rich meals, alcohol intake, excessive straining during defecation, and exposure to high temperatures)
- Teach the patient some physical counter maneuvers aimed at acutely contrasting the drop in BP (e.g., crossing the legs, or squatting down) [18].

3. If nonpharmacological measures are not effective in countering the symptoms of OH, *pharmacological treatment* is indicated. To date, only two drugs have been recognized for the treatment of OH:

   - *Midodrine (Gutron)*: is a peripheral α-1 adrenergic receptor agonist that acts as a vasoconstrictor. It has a short half-life (about 3 h) and it is usually used before meals to counteract postprandial hypotension [19]. It is used at a dosage of 2.5 mg 2–3 times a day, which can be increased up to a maximum of 10 mg 3 times a day. The last daily intake should not be taken after 6 PM to avoid SH. Possible side effects are SH, urinary retention, headache, and piloerection [20].
   - *Droxidopa (Dops)* [21]: is a precursor of norepinephrine that acts as a vasoconstrictor, and its use is like that of midodrine – It should be tapered starting from 100 mg 3 times a day, which can be increased up to 600 mg 3 times a day. This drug appears to have fewer side effects than the others, especially for SH [22]. The drug is not available in Europe but can be imported from abroad (USA, Japan) in many European countries according to specific procedures.
     Off-label treatments:
   - *Fludrocortisone (Florinef, Astonin)*: is a mineralocorticoid that increases the reabsorption of sodium from the renal tubules and the renal excretion of potassium. Its intravascular volume expansion action is dose dependent: the starting dose of 0.1 mg/day can be increased weekly by 0.1 mg, up to a maximum of 0.3 mg/day. Possible side effects are SH, hypokalemia, ankle edema, worsening heart failure, and weight gain [23]. This drug is also not available in some countries but can be imported from abroad with a specific procedure.
   - *Pyridostigmine (Mestinon)*: is an acetylcholinesterase inhibitor which, by amplifying the neurotransmission at the level of the peripheral cholinergic synapses between the pre- and postganglionic neurons, could enhance the sympathetic tone in response to standing. Evidence to support its efficacy in the treatment of OH is scarce, but it may be useful as an add-on therapy, especially in patients with gastrointestinal manifestations such as gastroparesis and severe constipation. It is used at a dosage of 30–60 mg one to three times

a day. Possible side effects are abdominal cramps, diarrhea, drooling, excessive sweating, urinary incontinence.

4. Since these drugs act by different mechanisms, if monotherapy is not effective, *combination therapy* can be used.

2.7 Treatment of Supine Hypertension

The treatment of SH should be tailored to the severity of the disorder and is based on a graduated approach [24]. The fundamental principle is to prioritize the treatment of OH while considering possible exacerbations of SH.

2.7.1 Nonpharmacological Treatments Aimed at Reducing SH

- Avoid lying supine during the day and sleep with the bed tilted at about 30° (head higher than feet) [25].
- Exploit the hypotensive effect of carbohydrate and alcohol intake, recommending the consumption of a sweet snack or small quantities of alcohol before bedtime [26].

2.7.2 Pharmacological Treatment of SH

When nonpharmacological treatment is not sufficient to counteract the nocturnal blood pressure rise, the use of antihypertensive drugs with a short half-life and at reduced dosage can be considered. Among the most commonly used are:

- Short-acting sartans such as losartan 50 mg, 1 cp at bedtime.
- ACE inhibitors with a short half-life such as captopril 25 mg, 1 cp before going to bed;
- Phosphodiesterase inhibitors (sildenafil) [27];
- Transdermal nitroglycerin patch (nitroderm 5 mg applied at bedtime and removed about 30–60 min before getting up in the morning) [28].

2.8 Conclusions

- OH is a frequent sign in neurological and internal medicine pathologies.
- OH is easily diagnosed.
- nOH significantly affects the quality of life and the activities of daily living.

- nOH can be treated with pharmacological and nonpharmacological measures.
- The goal is the improvement of symptoms and not the normalization of pressure values.
- nOH is often associated with supine hypertension.

References

1. Freeman R, et al. Consensus statement on the definition of orthostatic hypotension, neurally mediated syncope and the postural tachycardia syndrome. Clin Auton Res. 2011;21(2):69–72.
2. Gibbons CH, Freeman R. Delayed orthostatic hypotension: a frequent cause of orthostatic intolerance. Neurology. 2006;67(1):28–32.
3. Cheshire WP, et al. Electrodiagnostic assessment of the autonomic nervous system: a consensus statement endorsed by the American Autonomic Society, American Academy of Neurology, and the International Federation of Clinical Neurophysiology. Clin Neurophysiol. 2021;132(2):666–82.
4. Palma JA, et al. Orthostatic hypotension in Parkinson disease: how much you fall or how low you go? Mov Disord. 2015;30(5):639–45.
5. Palma JA, Kaufmann H. Management of orthostatic hypotension. Continuum (Minneap Minn). 2020;26(1):154–77.
6. Norcliffe-Kaufmann L, et al. Orthostatic heart rate changes in patients with autonomic failure caused by neurodegenerative synucleinopathies. Ann Neurol. 2018;83(3):522–31.
7. Guaraldi P, et al. Validation of the new index of baroreflex function to identify neurogenic orthostatic hypotension. Auton Neurosci. 2020;229:102744.
8. Fanciulli A, et al. Validation of the neurogenic orthostatic hypotension ratio with active standing. Ann Neurol. 2020;88(3):643–5.
9. Goldstein DS, Sharabi Y. Neurogenic orthostatic hypotension: a pathophysiological approach. Circulation. 2009;119(1):139–46.
10. Cheshire WP, et al. Corrigendum to "Electrodiagnostic assessment of the autonomic nervous system: A consensus statement endorsed by the American Autonomic Society, American Academy of Neurology, and the International Federation of Clinical Neurophysiology" [Clin. Neurophysiol. 132(2) (2021) 666–682]. Clin Neurophysiol. 2021;132(5):1194.
11. Velseboer DC, et al. Prevalence of orthostatic hypotension in Parkinson's disease: a systematic review and meta-analysis. Parkinsonism Relat Disord. 2011;17(10):724–9.
12. Baschieri F, et al. Neurogenic orthostatic hypotension in early stage Parkinson's disease: new insights from the first 105 patients of the BoProPark study. Parkinsonism Relat Disord. 2021;93:12–8.
13. Kaufmann H, et al. Natural history of pure autonomic failure: a United States prospective cohort. Ann Neurol. 2017;81(2):287–97.
14. Giannini G, et al. The natural history of idiopathic autonomic failure: the IAF-BO cohort study. Neurology. 2018;91(13):e1245–54.
15. Fanciulli A, et al. Consensus statement on the definition of neurogenic supine hypertension in cardiovascular autonomic failure by the American Autonomic Society (AAS) and the European Federation of Autonomic Societies (EFAS) : Endorsed by the European Academy of Neurology (EAN) and the European Society of Hypertension (ESH). Clin Auton Res. 2018;28(4):355–62.
16. Palma JA, et al. The impact of supine hypertension on target organ damage and survival in patients with synucleinopathies and neurogenic orthostatic hypotension. Parkinsonism Relat Disord. 2020;75:97–104.

17. Gibbons CH, et al. The recommendations of a consensus panel for the screening, diagnosis, and treatment of neurogenic orthostatic hypotension and associated supine hypertension. J Neurol. 2017;264(8):1567–82.
18. Wieling W, et al. Physical countermeasures to increase orthostatic tolerance. J Intern Med. 2015;277(1):69–82.
19. Wright RA, et al. A double-blind, dose-response study of midodrine in neurogenic orthostatic hypotension. Neurology. 1998;51(1):120–4.
20. McClellan KJ, Wiseman LR, Wilde MI, Midodrine. A review of its therapeutic use in the management of orthostatic hypotension. Drugs Aging. 1998;12(1):76–86.
21. Kaufmann H, et al. Norepinephrine precursor therapy in neurogenic orthostatic hypotension. Circulation. 2003;108(6):724–8.
22. Kaufmann H, et al. Droxidopa for neurogenic orthostatic hypotension: a randomized, placebo-controlled, phase 3 trial. Neurology. 2014;83(4):328–35.
23. van Lieshout JJ, ten Harkel AD, Wieling W. Fludrocortisone and sleeping in the head-up position limit the postural decrease in cardiac output in autonomic failure. Clin Auton Res. 2000;10(1):35–42.
24. Jordan J, et al. Management of supine hypertension in patients with neurogenic orthostatic hypotension: scientific statement of the American Autonomic Society, European Federation of Autonomic Societies, and the European Society of Hypertension. J Hypertens. 2019;37(8):1541–6.
25. Freeman R, et al. Orthostatic hypotension: JACC state-of-the-art review. J Am Coll Cardiol. 2018;72(11):1294–309.
26. Young TM, Mathias CJ. Treatment of supine hypertension in autonomic failure with gastrostomy feeding at night. Auton Neurosci. 2008;143(1–2):77–8.
27. Gamboa A, et al. Excessive nitric oxide function and blood pressure regulation in patients with autonomic failure. Hypertension. 2008;51(6):1531–6.
28. Shannon J, et al. The hypertension of autonomic failure and its treatment. Hypertension. 1997;30(5):1062–7.

Chapter 3
Autonomic Dysfunction in Hypertension

Gianfranco Parati and Juan Eugenio Ochoa

3.1 Introduction

Autonomic dysfunction is a crucial component in the development and progression of hypertension. It results from alterations in a variety of reflex and non-reflex mechanisms of cardiovascular modulation. Given the reciprocal interactions between sympathetic and parasympathetic cardiovascular regulation, the reduced cardiac parasympathetic modulation frequently observed in essential hypertension is associated with persistent activation of sympathetic outflows to the heart, the kidneys and the peripheral vessels. Sustained impairment in autonomic cardiovascular modulation and the associated adrenergic overdrive lead to haemodynamic and cardiometabolic alterations and to elevation of blood pressure (BP) levels. Such a persistent BP increase in turn promotes development of hypertension-mediated organ damage (HMOD), ultimately leading to an increased risk of cardiovascular events. However, although a wide choice of effective antihypertensive drugs is available, about half of hypertensive patients present with uncontrolled hypertension, either because of poor adherence to prescribed treatment or due to inadequate correction of the responsible alterations in cardiovascular control mechanisms. On such a background, given the important role played by autonomic dysfunction in the pathogenesis of arterial hypertension, over the last decades, several device-based approaches aimed at reducing the enhanced sympathetic activation of hypertensive patients have been introduced. They have been proposed as an additional tool to

G. Parati (✉)
Department of Cardiology, Istituto Auxologico Italiano, IRCCS, Milan, Italy

Department of Medicine and Surgery, University of Milano-Bicocca, Milan, Italy
e-mail: gianfranco.parati@unimib.it

J. E. Ochoa
Department of Cardiology, Istituto Auxologico Italiano, IRCCS, Milan, Italy

G. Micieli et al. (eds.), *Autonomic Disorders in Clinical Practice*,
https://doi.org/10.1007/978-3-031-43036-7_3

lower BP in difficult-to-control and in resistant hypertension. Renal sympathetic denervation (RDN) and electrical stimulation of carotid baroreceptors are the most extensively investigated device-based therapies in this context. This chapter is aimed at reviewing: 1 – the main techniques for evaluating autonomic cardiovascular regulation in hypertension, 2 – the role of autonomic dysfunction in favouring the development and progression of hypertension, 3 – the mechanisms by which autonomic dysfunction promotes BP elevation, 4 – the impact of autonomic dysfunction on HMOD and cardiovascular prognosis and 5 – the impact of pharmacological or device-based treatment strategies, aimed at improving autonomic nervous system (ANS) function, on BP values and on cardiovascular prognosis in hypertension.

3.2 Techniques for Evaluating Autonomic Cardiovascular Regulation in Hypertension

3.2.1 Methods for Evaluation of Adrenergic Drive

The pathophysiological role of enhanced sympathetic activity in hypertension has been confirmed by a relevant number of studies which assessed adrenergic drive. This was done indirectly by measuring circulating blood levels of the adrenergic neurotransmitters epinephrine and norepinephrine or by evaluating via the power spectral approach frequency components of BP variability (BPV) and heart rate (HR) variability (V) reflecting vagal and sympathetic cardiovascular modulation. Sympathetic activity was also measured directly by quantifying efferent postganglionic muscle sympathetic nerve traffic in peroneal nerves as well as regional norepinephrine release and reuptake by adrenergic nerves via the norepinephrine radiolabelled spillover technique [1, 2].

An assumption underlying the use of the early neurochemical tests exploring the whole sympathetic nervous system (SNS) activity was that the SNS acts in a global, undifferentiated fashion. However, SNS responses are often regionalized, activation of sympathetic outflow in one district commonly being accompanied by no change, or a reduction, in other districts [3, 4]. For instance, the hypertension-related increase in adrenergic outflow is specific for some cardiovascular districts, such as the heart, the kidneys, and the skeletal muscle vasculature, and is characteristic of primary and not secondary hypertension [2, 5, 6]. Quantification of individual regional SNS outflows can be achieved by using sympathetic nerve recording technique, and by radiotracer-derived measurements of regional norepinephrine spillover to plasma, from individual organs (Fig. 3.1).

These methods are complementary; neither is ‘best’.

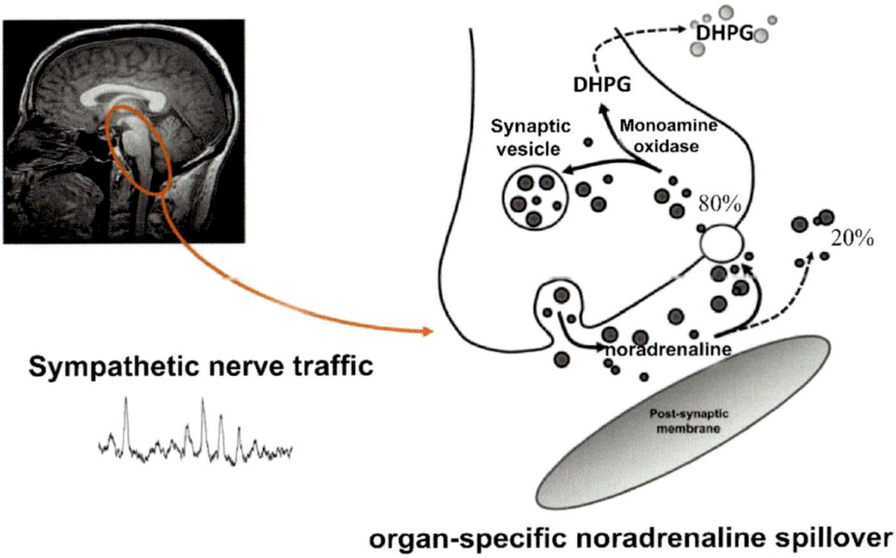

Fig. 3.1 Sympathetic nervous system responses are often regionalized, activation in sympathetic outflow of one district commonly being accompanied by no change, or a reduction, in other districts. Precise quantification of individual regional sympathetic nervous outflows can be achieved with clinical microneurography, a nerve recording technique measuring firing in sympathetic nerves directed to the skeletal muscle vasculature, and by radiotracer-derived measurements of regional norepinephrine spillover to plasma from individual organs not accessible to nerve recording, including the heart and kidneys. Taken from Parati and Esler [7] by permission

3.2.1.1 Microneurography

Hagbarth and Vallbo [8] 1968 reported a method for measuring efferent multi-fibre traffic in sympathetic nerves. This technique, defined as microneurography, provides a method for studying firing in subcutaneous sympathetic nerves directed to skin and the skeletal muscle vasculature. Multi fibre recordings of 'bursts' of nerve activity, synchronous with the heartbeat, are generated and can be recorded thanks to microelectrodes introduced into skin. More recently, single-fibre sympathetic recording has also been successfully performed in humans [9, 10]. The microneurography method provides instantaneous data on electrical efferent transmission in sympathetic nerves, with multi-unit or single-fibre recordings, but may be open to an investigator bias in case of studies based on manual and not blinded analysis of recordings obtained in small groups of subjects.

3.2.1.2 Noradrenaline Spillover

Development of other techniques for estimating the rates of overflow of noradrenaline to the circulation was stimulated by a lack of clinical methods for studying sympathetic nervous outflow in humans to otherwise inaccessible organs, such as the heart and kidneys, where the nerve recording technique is not applicable. Measurement of regional, organ-specific, norepinephrine spillover to plasma from sympathetic terminals [3, 4, 11] became the gold standard for this aim because it provides objective information on sympathetic neurotransmitter release in individual organs. During constant rate infusion of tritiated norepinephrine, the outward flux of endogenous norepinephrine from an organ (regional norepinephrine 'spillover') can be measured by isotope dilution:

$$\text{Regional norepinephrine spillover} = \left[\left(\text{CV} - \text{CA}\right) + \text{CAE}\right]\text{PF},$$

where CV and CA are the plasma concentrations of norepinephrine in regional venous and arterial plasma, E is the fractional extraction from blood of tritiated noradrenaline in transit through the organ, and PF is the organ plasma flow. A routine application of this approach, however, has been prevented by the safety procedures required to handle radioactive material.

3.2.2 Methods for Evaluation of Alterations in Sympathetic/ Parasympathetic Balance in Autonomic Cardiovascular Modulation. The Role of Heart Rate and Blood Pressure Variability Analysis and Arterial Baroreflex Sensitivity Assessment

Another commonly used method to explore autonomic cardiovascular modulation is based on computer analysis of heart rate variability (HRV) and BPV. Variability in these cardiovascular parameters has been shown to reflect the activity of cardiovascular control mechanisms, including sympathetic and parasympathetic cardiovascular modulation, both in health and disease [12–14]. Several methodological approaches are available to this aim. A number of techniques focus on estimates of BP or HR variance, on their spectral powers [12–14], or on HR turbulence [15], entropy, self-similarity and symbolic logic [16]. Other techniques assess BP–HR interactions to quantify the spontaneous sensitivity of baroreflex control of HR (BRS) [17, 18]. Evidence that cardiovascular variability does represent an index of autonomic control of circulation comes from either animal or human studies, and the latter performed both in normal individuals and in patients affected by diseases where the autonomic nervous system was primarily or indirectly affected [19]. While HRV largely reflects selective autonomic control of the heart, BP fluctuations are the result of complex interactions between multiple mechanisms, including cardiac and vascular neural regulation, mechanical influences of ventilation, humoral and endothelial factors, large arteries stiffening and genetic factors. Nevertheless, when properly applied, methods based on time or frequency domain analysis of either BPV or HRV can provide valuable insight into integrated cardiovascular regulation. The advantages of this approach, in spite of a possible limited specificity in some circumstances, consist in its easy applicability also in daily practice and in the avoidance of any external intervention on individuals under evaluation [19].

3.2.2.1 Heart Rate Variability Analysis

Vagal and sympathetic cardiac influences operate on HRV in different frequency bands. While vagal regulation has a relatively high cut-off frequency, modulating HR both at low frequencies (LF) and high frequencies (HF), up to 1.0 Hz, sympathetic cardiac control operates only at frequencies <0.15 Hz [12, 20, 21]. It has to be acknowledged, however, that although HRV is certainly affected by sympathetic cardiac modulation, no individual HR spectral component is a specific marker of sympathetic cardiac modulation because of the interference by other participating factors, including the accompanying parasympathetic modulation, humoral mechanisms, gender, age, respiration and resonance in the baroreflex loop ~0.1 Hz [22]. Normalization of LF powers by total variance, or computation of the LF/HF power ratio, may help to increase the reliability of spectral parameters in reflecting sympathetic cardiac modulation [12, 13]. Recent evidence suggests that also non-linear models for cardiovascular variability analysis, such as heart-rate self-similarity [23], or the multi-fractal multi-scale approach [24–26], may reflect autonomic cardiovascular regulation.

3.2.2.2 Blood Pressure Variability Analysis

Blood pressure variability increases in conditions characterized by sympathetic activation. Indeed, increased daytime ambulatory BPV in humans is associated with an increase in sympathetic efferent traffic in the peroneal nerve [27]. When considering BP spectral powers, however, their pathophysiological interpretation is more complex. While HF fluctuations largely depend on the mechanical effects of respiration, LF and very LF (VLF) powers are predominantly caused by fluctuations in the vasomotor tone and systemic vascular resistance and are influenced by complex interactions between neural, humoral, genetic and endothelial factors, by myogenic tone and by thermoregulation [12]. Thus, although BP and HR LF powers have been repeatedly suggested as markers of sympathetic cardiovascular control [14], their specificity in this regard is limited [12].

3.2.2.3 Arterial Baroreflex Sensitivity Assessment

The arterial baroreflex represents a fundamental mechanism of autonomic cardiovascular modulation to avoid excessive BP oscillations and to maintain its values within a range that preserves organ perfusion while at the same time avoiding the risk associated with excessive BP peaks.

Arterial baroreflex sensitivity (BRS) can be assessed by delivering an external stimulus to baroreceptors and measuring the baroreflex mediated response. An example is the 'Oxford' method, based on the intravenous injection of vasoactive drugs that induce reflex HR changes in response to drug-induced increases or reductions of systolic BP (SBP) [28]. Another example is the 'neck-chamber' method that stimulates or deactivates the carotid baroreceptors by respectively increasing or reducing carotid transmural pressure through changes in air pressure within a tight collar [29, 30]. Other more recent approaches are based on the analysis of baroreflex modulation of HR in response to the spontaneous fluctuations in BP, which physiologically occur in daily life. At variance from the 'Oxford' and 'neck chamber' methods, such approaches avoid the inconveniences related to the need to deliver external stimuli in the context of artificial laboratory settings and allow monitoring 'spontaneous' baroreflex function in ambulant subjects over long recording periods [31], without significantly interfering with their activities [18, 32, 33]. In fact, the ability of cardiovascular variability to reflect autonomic cardiovascular control is improved by use of multivariate models for its assessment. The simplest ones consider the relationship between spontaneous fluctuations in BP and HR, either in the time (sequence technique) [17, 18] or in the frequency domain (alpha-coefficient, transfer function analysis) to assess BRS and its modulation in daily life [17, 34, 35] (Fig. 3.2).

Both the laboratory and the 'spontaneous' methods to study the arterial baroreflex estimate the feedback effects of SBP changes on pulse interval (PI, reciprocal of HR), neglecting the simultaneously occurring feedforward effects of PI on SBP, induced through changes in cardiac output. This can be acceptable under the 'open-loop' assumption that these feedforward effects do not significantly influence the estimation of the gain of the feedback arc from SBP to PI. If the feedforward effects are not considered to be negligible, the open-loop assumption cannot be made and the feedforward effects of PI on SBP should be quantified simultaneously with the reflex feedback effects of SBP on PI, in the frame of a 'close-loop' model. To date, 'spontaneous' methods for evaluating the baroreflex function by simultaneously assessing feedback and feedforward effects have been developed by mathematically modelling the beat-by-beat reciprocal interactions of these cardiovascular variables through a closed-loop analysis of the time SBP and PI series [36, 37]. Simplified closed-loop models were based on bivariate autoregressive representations of the interactions between couples of cardiovascular time series or on trivariate autoregressive models that also include respiratory signals [38]. Closed-loop autoregressive moving average (ARMA) models of the SBP and PI beat-by-beat interactions

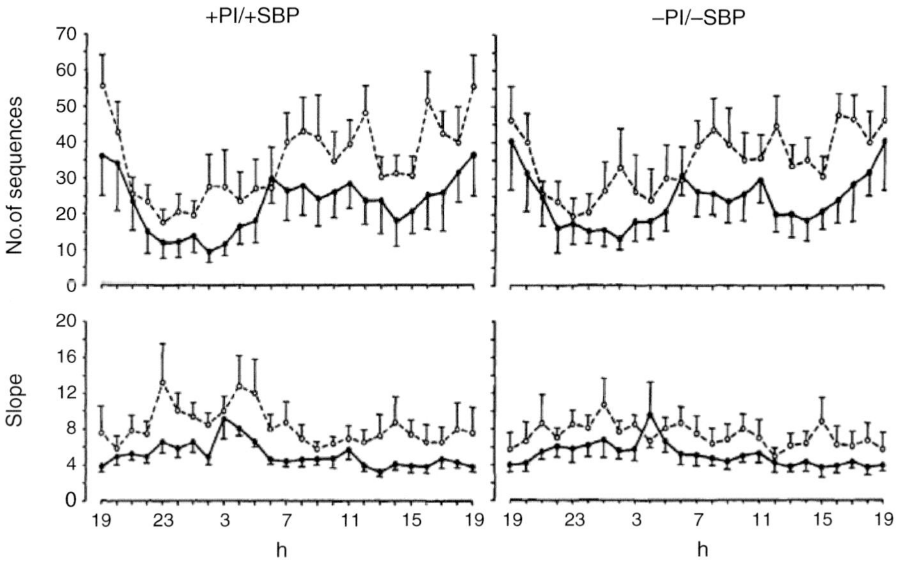

Fig. 3.2 Number and slope of +PI/+SBP and −PI/-SBP sequences during each hour of a 24-h intra-arterial ambulatory blood pressure recording (means+ SE) for 10 normotensive (open circle) and 10 hypertensive (closed circle) subjects. The slope of these sequences is taken as an estimate of spontaneous sensitivity of barorefelx control of heart rate. Taken from Parati et al. [18] by permission. *PI* pulse interval, *SBP* systolic blood pressure

were also proposed [39, 40]. Applications of these models, however, have been limited to the laboratory environment only.

Recent studies have been conducted to characterize both the feedback and feedforward components of the SBP-PI coupling over 24-h in ambulant subjects, including the assessment of their modulation at the time of the various activities which characterize the day and night. These studies have also compared the results obtained in normotensive and hypertensive individuals, respectively, aimed at detecting differences in their autonomic closed-loop cardiovascular modulation [41].

The removal of the open-loop assumption when modelling the interaction between BP and HR fluctuations offers a deeper insight into the mechanisms involved in daily life cardiovascular regulation. In particular, it allows the detection of specific patterns characterizing the altered cardiovascular regulation reported in essential hypertension separately for feedback and feedforward gains (Fig. 3.3).

Such closed-loop evaluation might improve the clinical relevance of SBP-PI coupling assessment over the 24-h. Indeed, it may allow us to separately quantify the contribution of the baroreflex feedback gain and of the mechanical feedforward coupling between SBP and PI in relation to target organ damage, the incidence of cardiovascular events and efficacy of treatments in hypertension, a possibility which deserves to be specifically explored in future studies [41].

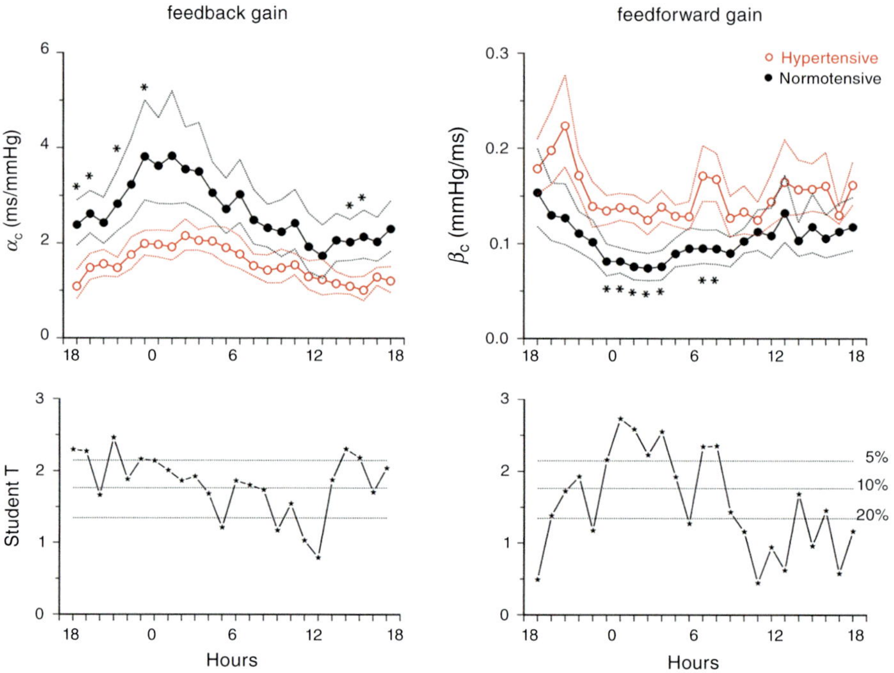

Fig. 3.3 24-h closed-loop profiles. (Upper) Feedback and feedforward gains in normotensive (solid black circle) and hypertensive (open red circle) subjects: geometric mean ± geometric standard error, with * indicating significant differences ($p < 0.05$) between normotensive and hypertensive groups (unpaired *t*-test). (Lower) Student's t-test statistics for the difference between groups, with dotted horizontal lines representing the thresholds at 20, 10, and 5% significance. (From Parati G et al. [41] by permission)

3.3 Role of Autonomic Dysfunction in the Development and Progression of Hypertension

A large body of evidence over more than a century has consistently supported the contribution of the ANS in the pathogenesis of hypertension. However, over the past three decades, clinical research in hypertension has extensively emphasized the pathogenetic role of the renin–angiotensin system (RAS), sometimes leading to underestimating the contribution of other pathophysiological mechanisms, including the sympathetic nervous system (SNS). In spite of this, undisputable evidence supports the concept that ANS dysfunction and chronic activation of the SNS are major contributors to essential and renal hypertension, also based on the evidence that renal sympathetic nerves are intrinsically related to the RAS.

3.3.1 Role of Autonomic Dysfunction in the Development of Hypertension

The extent to which alterations in ANS function are causally involved in the development of essential hypertension has been a matter of intense investigation in the past decades. Early stages of hypertension (i.e. high normal BP levels or 'prehypertensive' state) are often associated with a 'hyperkinetic' circulatory state characterized by a reduced parasympathetic cardiac modulation and by an increased adrenergic activity [1, 42]. Evidence in this regard was provided by a study in which a group of young patients with borderline hypertension and hyperkinetic circulation were compared to a group of healthy controls [43]. After propranolol infusion, compared to healthy controls, individuals with borderline hypertension and high cardiac output (hyperkinetic circulation) showed higher reductions in HR and cardiac output, even if these parameters remained significantly elevated. After atropine administration (i.e. which blocks the effects of the parasympathetic neurotransmitter acetylcholine on muscarinic receptors) the difference in cardiac output and HR between the two groups disappeared [43]. Based on these results, authors concluded that patients with borderline hypertension and hyperkinetic circulation simultaneously exhibit a decrease of parasympathetic tone and an increase in sympathetic activity [43]. This evidence indicates that impairment in the autonomic control of HR occurring in hypertension is not limited to the parasympathetic function but also affects sympathetic cardiovascular regulation. Further evidence supporting this concept comes from a meta-analysis of 78 studies comparatively evaluating values of plasma norepinephrine (i.e. an indirect marker of sympathetic activity) between patients with essential hypertension and normotensive controls [44]. Although there was high variability in catecholamine values within and across studies, virtually all studies assessing norepinephrine levels in young individuals, consistently reported elevated values of norepinephrine in hypertensive patients, which is consistent with a pathophysiologic role of increased sympathetic neural activity in this subgroup [44].

Studies implementing radiotracer tests for evaluation of norepinephrine plasma kinetics have provided evidence that even in the early phases of hypertension sympathetic nervous outflow to the heart and kidneys is strikingly increased [5]. In one of these studies, overall and regional rates of norepinephrine spillover from the neuroeffector junctions to plasma were comparatively measured in 55 untreated patients with essential hypertension and in 40 healthy controls [5]. Total norepinephrine spillover was increased in primary hypertension, particularly in patients aged less than 40 years, largely due to higher rates of renal and cardiac norepinephrine overflow. Renal renin release and arterial plasma renin activity were highest in these younger patients with increased renal sympathetic nervous activity. In older patients, sympathetic activity and norepinephrine release were typically normal. The selective increase in the sympathetic nervous outflow to the heart and kidneys (i.e. two organs of key importance in BP homeostatic control) observed in young patients with primary hypertension led authors to conclude that SNS dysfunction plays an important role in the early pathogenesis of essential hypertension [5].

Studies have also been conducted in order to determine whether elevated plasma catecholamine levels in borderline hypertension are associated with greater sympathetic neural outflow. In one of these reports, muscle sympathetic nerve activity (MSNA, directly recorded by microneurography) was comparatively evaluated in a group of borderline hypertensives and in a group of age-matched normotensive controls. Compared to normotensive controls, borderline hypertensive individuals showed higher values of MSNA, and higher values of systolic and diastolic BP. A significant interaction between sympathetic cardiovascular modulation and sodium intake was also observed. Specifically, compared with the normotensive group, plasma norepinephrine levels in the borderline hypertensive group tended to be higher on low sodium diet and lower on high sodium diet. Based on these results, authors concluded that borderline hypertension is associated not only with elevated values of plasma catecholamines but also with an increased central sympathetic neural outflow [45].

A number of conditions such as obesity and cardiometabolic syndrome as well as its components (i.e. hyperinsulinemia, insulin resistance, dyslipidaemia and hypercholesterolaemia) are frequently associated with autonomic dysfunction and adrenergic overdrive, which in turn may promote the development and progression of a hypertensive state. Several studies implementing microneurography or the norepinephrine spillover technique have indeed shown that the metabolic syndrome is characterized by sympathetic activation and that this abnormality is also detectable even when BP values are still within the normal range [46, 47].

3.3.2 Role of Autonomic Dysfunction in Established Hypertension

Some degree of autonomic dysfunction can be seen in more than 50% of all cases of arterial hypertension. This estimate is based on both the proportion of untreated patients with essential hypertension who have a demonstrable increase in sympathetic activity, and on the number of patients in whom substantial BP lowering is achieved with anti-adrenergic drugs. Box 3.1 resumes the main characteristics of autonomic dysfunction in hypertension.

Box 3.1: Main Characteristics of Autonomic Dysfunction in Hypertension

- Activation of the sympathetic nervous outflow.
  - Increase in cardiac norepinephrine spillover,
  - Increase in renal norepinephrine spillover,
  - Increase in muscle sympathetic nerve activity,
- Reduced parasympathetic modulation.
  - Impaired parasympathetic cardiac control,

    Reduced sensitivity of arterial baroreflex control of the heart rate.
- Sympatho-vagal imbalance in cardiovascular modulation.

3.3.2.1 Sympathetic Nervous System Activation in Essential Hypertension

Studies in hypertension implementing the norepinephrine spillover methodology have demonstrated activation of the sympathetic nervous outflows to the kidneys and heart [3]. Renal norepinephrine spillover, on average, is elevated two- to three-fold in both normal weight patients with essential hypertension and in obesity-related hypertension [3]. Multi-unit recordings from sympathetic nerve fibres directed to the skeletal muscle vasculature similarly show a doubling or tripling of the sympathetic outflow [10, 48–50]. Single-fibre sympathetic recording demonstrates increased fibre firing frequencies, and multiple firings within a cardiac cycle not seen in healthy individuals [10, 49].

The application of sympathetic nerve recording and norepinephrine spillover methodologies, in multiple studies from different research groups [10, 48–50] has identified activated sympathetic outflow to the skeletal muscle vasculature and kidneys in ~50% of hypertensive patients (Fig. 3.4).

3.3.2.2 Reduced Parasympathetic Tone and Baroreflex Dysfunction in Hypertension

Clinical studies, have provided evidence that baroreflex dysfunction may unveil the early occurrence of autonomic impairment in conditions such as arterial hypertension, diabetes, sleep apnoea syndrome and ageing. Even with the limitations

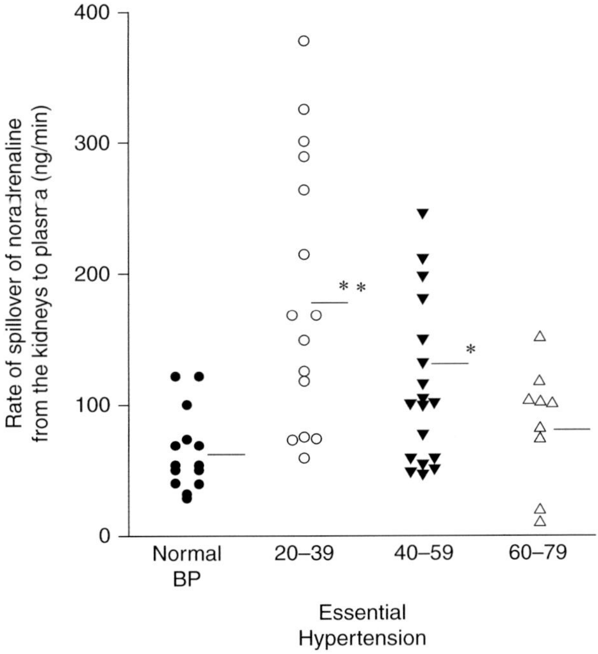

Fig. 3.4 Renal noradrenaline spillover to plasma in patients with untreated essential hypertension, in relation to their age (numbers on the horizontal axis), compared with measurements in healthy volunteers. Taken from Parati and Esler [7] by permission. Individual and mean values are shown. Renal sympathetic activation is evident in patients under 60 years of age. *P, 0.05 **P, 0.01

mentioned above, an overall measure of autonomic cardiac modulation such as the sensitivity of arterial baroreflex control of the HR (estimated either with laboratory or with 'spontaneous' methods for arterial baroreflex sensitivity analysis) provides consistent evidence of reduced cardiac BRS in hypertension, mainly due to impaired parasympathetic cardiac control [17, 18]. Given the reciprocal interactions between sympathetic and parasympathetic cardiovascular regulation, reduced cardiac parasympathetic activity implies an increase in the activity of the SNS to the heart. The occurrence of such a systematic imbalance between parasympathetic and sympathetic cardiac modulation in hypertensive patients was demonstrated not only in the laboratory, but also over the 24-h in ambulatory conditions [18] (see Fig. 3.2).

It should be emphasized, however that autonomic cardiovascular modulation in hypertension undergoes complex changes. As an example, studies using either the neck chamber technique or the injection of vasoactive drugs have shown that arterial hypertension is associated with a clearcut impairment of the baroreflex control of HR and with a preserved and reset baroreflex control of BP and efferent sympathetic nerve activity [51, 52].

Both clinical and experimental studies in hypertension have provided evidence that alterations in autonomic cardiovascular control not only contribute to development but also to the progression of the hypertensive state, being more pronounced with an increased severity of the hypertensive state. While Parasympathetic and baroreflex dysfunction remain relatively stable in the course of the hypertensive state, the sympathetic activation undergoes a progressive potentiation which parallels the increase in BP levels over time i.e. from normotensive to borderline hypertension and to progressively more severe increases in BP levels, including resistant hypertension [6, 45, 53–55].

3.4 Role of Autonomic Dysfunction in the Pathophysiology of Hypertension: Mechanisms by Which Autonomic Dysfunction Promotes Blood Pressure Elevation

The ANS plays an important role in the pathogenesis of primary hypertension and in certain secondary forms of hypertension. Although hypertension is a disease of multifactorial aetiology, the pathophysiological role of ANS dysfunction has been supported by a large body of evidence. The question on whether sympathetic activation causes BP elevation has been addressed by several studies. Once, it was thought that the SNS is involved in short-term cardiovascular regulation only and is not important in the pathogenesis of sustained hypertension. Other studies, however, have disproved this hypothesis. Evidence is available that sympathetic activation is associated with chronic BP elevation. Moreover, evidence is available that the renal sympathetic nerves are pivotal in the pathogenesis of experimental hypertension through influences on renin release, glomerular filtration rate and renal tubular reabsorption of sodium [56, 57]. Experimental studies also showed that sub-vasoconstrictor levels of renal sympathetic activity can increase renin secretion and renal sodium retention without changing renal haemodynamics [56]. Similar features seem to characterize essential hypertension. Younger patients with mild essential hypertension very commonly have 'high renin essential hypertension', where renal sympathetic activity is sufficiently elevated to increase renal secretion of renin but not to reduce renal blood flow. On the other hand, in patients with resistant hypertension responding inadequately to concurrent treatment with multiple antihypertensive drug classes, including angiotensin-converting enzyme inhibitors (ACEIs), angiotensin receptor blockers (ARBs), dihydropyridine calcium channel blockers (CCBs), and diuretics, radiofrequency ablation of the renal sympathetic nerves lowers BP remarkably, thus emphasizing the role played by the SNS [58, 59].

3.4.1 Autonomic Nervous System Influences on Blood Pressure Regulation

Neural influences have a significant impact on two major determinants of BP levels, namely cardiac output and systemic vascular resistance. Influences of the SNS on the arteriolar tone (which is determined by the balance between vasoconstrictor and vasodilatory stimuli) are mainly mediated by neurotransmitters such as epinephrine, norepinephrine, and dopamine, which exert their actions on adrenergic receptors [60]. Adrenergic and dopaminergic receptors are the main target sites through which neurotransmitters exert their effects on vasomotor tone. Regional differences in the distribution and density of α-, β-, and dopaminergic receptors have been reported, which determine differences in the degree of response to adrenergic stimulus in different tissues. While the main effect of a stimulation of the α-adrenergic receptors is vasoconstriction, stimulation of α2-adrenergic receptors leads to vasodilation. At variance from α-adrenergic receptors, both β1 and β2-adrenergic receptors have a prevalent influence on HR and cardiac output but not so much on vascular resistance, although β2-adrenergic receptor stimulation at the skeletal muscle level leads to peripheral vasodilation. The net effects of a stimulation of the β-adrenergic receptors at the heart levels result in increases in HR and cardiac output. Although dopamine receptors also play an important role in hormonal signalling and in the regulation of renal sodium and blood flow, evidence is still needed to better understand the precise physiological role of dopaminergic receptor stimulation in BP regulation [61].

Of note, neural control of BP levels is exerted not only in the short-term (i.e. beat-by-beat) by the central vasomotor centre [62] but also in the long-term with the participation of several mechanisms of autonomic cardiovascular modulation [63]. For instance, arterial baroreceptors, which provide a tonic restraint on sympathetic drive on a beat-by-beat basis, contribute not only to short-term but also to long-term regulation of sympathetic activity, fluid/volume homeostasis, and BP levels [64–66].

Blood pressure and blood volume regulation closely depend on the interaction among the SNS, the RAS and renal sodium excretion [67, 68]. In support of this concept, a series of studies in animals have provided evidence that electrical stimulation of renal sympathetic nerves increases renin release from juxtaglomerular cells either directly through the stimulation of β-adrenergic receptors located in the juxtaglomerular cells or indirectly through changes in renal blood flow [67–69]. Renal sympathetic nerve stimulation has also been reported to have anti-natriuretic effects by direct action on tubular renal sodium reabsorption thus further supporting the role of the SNS on sodium regulation [67].

3.5 Impact of Autonomic Dysfunction on Hypertension Mediated Organ Damage and Cardiovascular Prognosis

3.5.1 Impact of Autonomic Dysfunction on Hypertension Mediated Organ Damage

Autonomic dysfunction is not only involved in the initiation and progression of hypertension but also in promoting HMOD such as left ventricular (LV) hypertrophy (LVH) or renal dysfunction [1, 2, 42].

Although the precise mechanisms leading to LVH remain unclear, they include haemodynamic and humoral factors. Autonomic alterations and sympathetic overdrive may be important, particularly because catecholamines not only have important effects on systemic haemodynamics but also recognize trophic properties. Indeed, in the case of LVH, a marked increase in sympathetic nerve traffic values and in cardiac norepinephrine spillover rate compared with the uncomplicated hypertensive state have been reported [50, 70]. A study comparatively evaluating peripheral MSNA in patients with hypertension with or without the presence of LVH showed significantly higher values of sympathetic discharge in subjects with moderate to severe hypertension with LVH compared to those without LVH [70]. Further evidence in this regard was provided by a study comparatively evaluating total systemic and regional sympathetic activity by radiotracer dilution methods and microneurography in untreated hypertensive subjects with LVH, in hypertensive subjects with similar BP but without LVH, and in a group of age-matched normotensive controls [50]. Although cardiac norepinephrine spillover correlated positively with LV mass index in all subjects, it was significantly higher in subjects with LVH, suggesting that increased cardiac norepinephrine release is related to the development of LVH [50].

Evidence has also been provided that activation of the SNS may contribute to the development of LV dysfunction and heart failure [71]. In hypertension, LVH has also been shown to be an independent predictor of increased morbidity and mortality.

Another complication of untreated (and/or uncontrolled) high BP is represented by the deterioration in renal function that may promote the occurrence of an overt renal insufficiency state over time [72]. Also, in this case, sympathetic activity appears to be involved in the pathogenesis of kidney damage, given the evidence that adrenergic activation is detectable even in the initial forms of renal dysfunction when the estimated glomerular filtration rate is only mildly impaired [73].

It has also been shown that sympathetic nerve hyperactivity present in the metabolic syndrome is further intensified by the additional presence of hypertension, which in turn may contribute to the higher cardiovascular risk and metabolic abnormalities seen in subjects who have both metabolic syndrome and hypertension [47].

Autonomic dysfunction has also been associated with hypertension-related vascular alterations, such as reduced arterial compliance, impaired endothelial function, vascular remodelling and hypertrophy, which, particularly when present together, favour the development of the atherogenic plaque [42, 74].

3.5.2 Impact of Autonomic Dysfunction on Cardiovascular Prognosis

The adverse haemodynamic and humoral alterations resulting from ANS dysfunction in hypertension represent the pathophysiological background for the development and progression of several clinical conditions (i.e. congestive heart failure, ischaemic stroke, obstructive pulmonary disease, chronic kidney disease), the severity of which is correlated with the degree of ANS dysfunction and adrenergic overdrive. For instance, increases in HR and myocardial contractility in the presence of reduced coronary perfusion favour the occurrence of myocardial ischaemia [75]. Arteriolar vasoconstriction increases both cardiac afterload and preload, augmenting cardiac work and myocardial oxygen consumption in the context of reduced oxygen supply to the myocardium [75]. Moreover, an increase in adrenergic drive reduces the arrhythmogenic threshold predisposing to arrhythmias. Indeed, a number of clinical studies have provided evidence that sympathetic activation and alterations in autonomic cardiovascular modulation in hypertension are associated with an increased risk of cardiovascular morbidity and mortality and with aggravation of the preexisting clinical conditions [76–78].

For instance, in patients with congestive heart failure, increased values of cardiac sympathetic activity (assessed through cardiac noradrenaline spillover) were shown to be a risk factor for sudden death, particularly in the presence of intact cardiac sympathetic innervation [77]. Conversely, the progression of myocardial disease and heart failure was closely associated with the depletion of sympathetic nerves in the heart, especially if rates of noradrenaline release paradoxically remain high [77]. Additional evidence has also linked norepinephrine spillover from adrenergic nerve terminals in the myocardium with the development of life-threatening cardiac rhythm disturbances, such as ventricular fibrillation and sudden cardiac death [79].

In post-stroke patients, increased values of serum norepinephrine (i.e. >300 pg/mL) were independently associated with poor prognosis at 1 year after the first stroke event (i.e. mortality rate, cardiovascular and cerebrovascular events, and activities of daily living assessed with the Barthel index and Rankin score) [78].

Also, in end-stage renal disease (ESRD) patients, elevated plasma concentrations of norepinephrine (i.e. >75th percentile) were associated with an increased risk of mortality and cardiovascular outcomes [80].

The information on autonomic cardiac control provided by HRV and BPV parameters has clinical relevance, too. Evidence is available that reduced HRV and reduced BRS are associated with increased mortality after myocardial infarction as well as in heart failure patients and with increased risk of sudden arrhythmic death [81].

3.6 Impact of Pharmacological or Device-Based Treatment Strategies, Aimed at Improving Autonomic Nervous System Function, on BP Values and on Cardiovascular Prognosis in Hypertension

Despite the general importance of the SNS in BP regulation and the specific demonstration that the BP elevation in essential hypertension is commonly initiated and sustained by SNS activation, pharmacological and non-pharmacological strategies known to improve cardiovascular autonomic modulation are often underutilized in the care of patients with hypertension.

3.6.1 Effects of Non-pharmacological Strategies on Autonomic Function

Two commonly applied non-pharmacological therapies for hypertension, aerobic exercise training and calories restriction, reduce SNS activity. These non-pharmacological interventions are particularly effective in improving metabolic syndrome and obesity-related hypertension, supported by the evidence that sympathetic inhibition may reduce both BP and insulin resistance [82]. Another non-pharmacological approach with an anti-adrenergic component is the regular application at night of continuous positive air pressure (CPAP) ventilation in patients with obstructive sleep-apnoea-related resistant hypertension. This therapeutic approach has been shown to prevent nocturnal obstruction of upper airways, abolish the concomitant intermittent hypoxia, reduce sympathetic activity and favour BP reduction [83, 84].

3.6.2 *Current Place of Anti-adrenergic Therapies in the Treatment of Hypertension*

Antihypertensive drugs are available to specifically target the SNS activation of essential and renal hypertension. Centrally acting sympathetic suppressants, such as imidazoline-binding agents (i.e. moxonidine and rilmenidine), could be specifically prescribed in patients with essential hypertension. Both drugs reduce sympathetic outflows to the heart, kidneys, and skeletal muscle vasculature and are largely free of the side effects of their progenitor, clonidine (such as rebound hypertension when doses were missed). Alpha-adrenergic blockers have also shown to be effective in reducing both SNS activation and BP levels; however, their use has declined due to common side effects of postural and exercise hypotension and their presumptive link with heart failure risk in patients with hypertension. In consideration of their safety profiles, these drugs are currently recommended by hypertension guidelines as the third or fourth choice, and sometimes, they do not make the list at all.

Along the same line, the use of beta-adrenergic blocking drugs has declined in recent decades, given the propensity of this drug class to have adverse metabolic effects including predisposition to diabetes development. In the 2018 ESC/ESH Hypertension guidelines, beta-blockers are not recommended as a first-line choice for the treatment of uncomplicated hypertension, their use being allowed when there are specific indications [i.e. angina, post-myocardial infarction, heart failure with reduced ejection fraction (HFrEF), or when HR control is required in the case of atrial fibrillation] [85]. Along the same line, the American Heart Association and British NICE guidelines do not recommend beta-blockers as first-line therapy for the treatment of uncomplicated hypertension. Although most BP-lowering classes are equally effective in preventing the risk of fatal and non-fatal cardiovascular events both in older and younger patients, recent meta-analyses have indicated that beta-blockers, lose some of their effectiveness in subjects older than 65 years [86]. Compared with other antihypertensive agents, beta-blockers have been shown to be substantially less protective against stroke and overall mortality. However, they exhibited a substantial risk-reducing ability for all events when prescribed to lower BP in patients with modest or more pronounced BP elevations and, therefore, can be used as additional agents in hypertensive patients [87]. Based on recent studies and on recent and better conducted meta analyses of available trials, however, the very recent 2023 ESH Hypertension guidelines have placed beta-blockers back again among drugs to be considered for first line hypertension treatment. This was done because of the evidence that, in addition to their compelling use as guidelines driven medical treatment in specific diseases, beta blockers exhibit favorable effects in about 50 clinical conditions including various cardiac diseases less or not related to hypertension, other vascular conditions and non-cardiovascular diseases [88].

3.6.3 Interventional Device-Based Strategies Aimed at Improving Autonomic Nervous System Function

In the last decades, several device-based approaches have been introduced to lower BP levels, most of which are aimed at modulating ANS activity [89]. Renal sympathetic denervation and electrical stimulation of the area of carotid baroreceptors are the most extensively investigated device-based therapies. A series of studies have provided evidence that these techniques are effective in reducing SNS activity and BP levels in resistant hypertensives.

3.6.3.1 Baroreflex Activation Therapy (BAT)

A surgically implantable arterial barostimulator operates by continuous electrical stimulation of the carotid sinus buffer nerves [90]. Baroreflex activation therapy (BAT) has been shown to reduce office BP values in patients with resistant hypertension either in the short- and in the long-term [91]. In a recent meta-analysis of available literature, significant reductions in office SBP/DBP after BAT treatment of −24.01/−12.53, were reported [91].

Additional studies have also shown BAT to be effective in also reducing ambulatory BP (i.e. 24 h, day and nighttime BP values) in patients with resistant hypertension [92, 93]. In one of these studies, in a group of subjects with uncontrolled resistant hypertension, ambulatory BP monitoring (ABPM) was performed before BAT implantation and after initiation of BAT. After 6 months, significant reductions in 24-h ambulatory SBP/DBP were observed from 148/82 mmHg to 140/77 mmHg, respectively. Significant reductions were also observed in day and nighttime systolic and diastolic BP values, separately considered [93]. In a more recent report by the same group, in which office and ambulatory BP measurements were performed at 12 and 24 months after initiation of BAT, there was a significant reduction of −25/−9 mmHg in office SBP/DBP and −8/−5 mmHg in 24-h ambulatory SBP/DBP after 24 months of follow-up. Despite the reported significant effects of BAT in lowering both office and ambulatory BP values, the available evidence is limited by the risk of bias, small sample size and small number of randomized controlled trials. Thus, further investigation on a larger scale and over prolonged follow-up time is still needed to fully conclude the efficacy and safety of BAT for patients with resistant hypertension.

3.6.3.2 Renal Sympathetic Denervation (RDN)

Renal sympathetic denervation is the most extensively investigated device-based therapy for hypertension, and randomized, sham-controlled trials have provided proof-of-concept data for its BP-lowering efficacy. It involves ablation of the renal sympathetic nerves with a radiofrequency emitting catheter inserted percutaneously

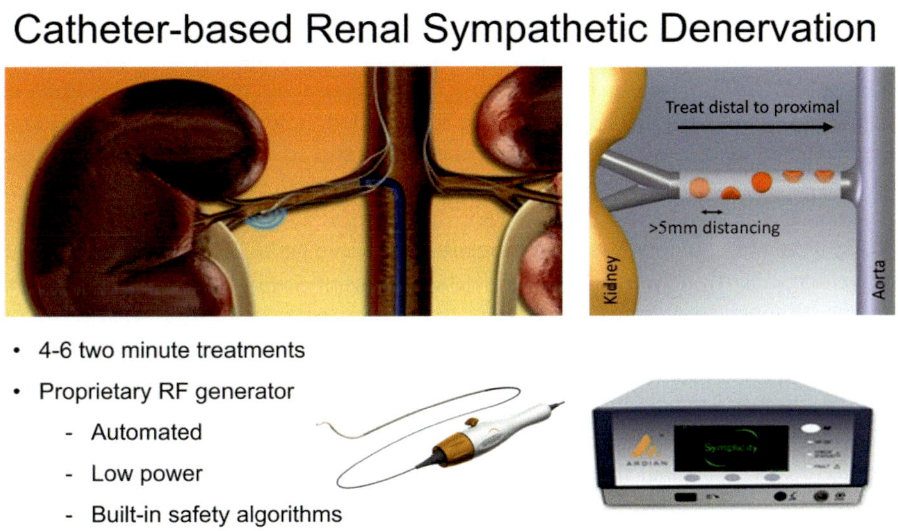

Fig. 3.5 The renal sympathetic nerves pass to the kidney in the wall of the renal arteries, within reach of radiofrequency energy delivered by a catheter placed in the artery lumen. The radiofrequency energy is transmitted through the catheter from an external generator, delivered at four to six sites in both arteries, aimed at achieving a full circumference of dosing coverage to ablate all nerves in the passage. This procedure is not limited to a single point on the artery wall because such an approach might, in principle, predispose to stenosis or aneurysm formation. (From Parati and Esler [7] by permission)

into the femoral artery in the groin and advanced to lie, in turn, in the lumen of both renal arteries [58] (Fig. 3.5).

Development of RDN was based on the observation that renal sympathetic outflow to the kidneys is activated in essential hypertension [3] and that renal sympathectomy typically prevents the development of hypertension [56] (see Fig. 3.4).

While the Simplicity 3 trial [94] raised serious doubts about the effectiveness of RDN in reducing BP levels, recent meta-analyses of randomized sham controlled trials have shown that RDN provides significant reductions in both conventional office and ambulatory BP levels, either in medicated or unmedicated patients with hypertension [95, 96]. In one of these meta-analyses, after 2–6 months of the intervention, compared to the sham procedure, RDN significantly reduced 24-h ambulatory SBP by 3.31 mmHg, daytime SBP by 3.53 mmHg, nighttime SBP by 3.20 mmHg, and office SBP by 5.25 mmHg. There were no significant differences in the magnitude of BP reduction between first- and second-generation trials, between devices, or between studies with or without medication, including those addressing resistant/uncontrolled hypertension [95].

In another meta-analysis including 7 eligible trials and 1368 patients, compared to placebo, RDN significantly reduced ambulatory SBP/DBP by 3.61/1.85 mmHg; and office SBP/DBP by 5.86/3.63 mmHg, respectively. Although the magnitude of benefit, about 4/2 mm Hg, was modest, it was similar between patients who were on background antihypertensive medications and those who were not. Therefore, RDN could be a useful strategy not only in resistant hypertension but also in patients who are not willing to add antihypertensive agents or who are intolerant to several antihypertensive drugs [96]. Evidence is still needed, however, regarding the long-term efficacy and safety of RDN. Another issue still to be investigated by future studies is whether the benefits of RDN are translated into improved cardiovascular prognosis. While reducing BP using antihypertensive drugs is associated with risk reductions of major CV events, it remains unclear whether RDN confers similar beneficial effects. The recent 2023 ESH Hypertension Guidelines have taken more recent evidence into account, provided by studies using either radiofrequency or ultrasound -based renal denervation, now acknowledge that RDN can be considered as a treatment option in patients with an eGFR >40 ml/min/1.73m2 who have uncontrolled BP despite the use of antihypertensive drug combination therapy, or if drug treatment elicits serious side effects and poor quality of life. RDN can be considered as an additional treatment option also in patients with true resistant hypertension if eGFR is >40 ml/min/1.73m2. Selection of patients to whom RDN is offered should be done in a shared decision-making process after objective and complete patient's information. Finally, the ESH 2023 guidelines recommend that RDN should only be performed in experienced specialized centers to guarantee appropriate selection of eligible patients and completeness of the denervation procedure [97].

3.7 Conclusions

Alterations in autonomic cardiovascular regulation characterize arterial hypertension. Specifically, an increased sympatho-vagal balance in cardiac neural modulation, and an increased SNS activity are associated with elevated BP levels. These alterations have a pathophysiologic relevance and may represent a suitable target for therapy, either when focusing on lifestyle changes, on pharmacological therapy or on device-based therapy. More evidence is needed, however, to clarify the actual impact of interventions aimed at normalizing autonomic cardiovascular modulation in hypertension on cardiovascular prognosis.

References

1. Esler M. The sympathetic nervous system through the ages: from Thomas Willis to resistant hypertension. Exp Physiol. 2011;96(7):611–22.
2. DiBona GF. Sympathetic nervous system and hypertension. Hypertension. 2013;61(3):556–60.
3. Esler M, Jennings G, Korner P, Willett I, Dudley F, Hasking G, et al. Assessment of human sympathetic nervous system activity from measurements of norepinephrine turnover. Hypertension. 1988;11(1):3–20.

4. Friberg P, Meredith I, Jennings G, Lambert G, Fazio V, Esler M. Evidence for increased renal norepinephrine overflow during sodium restriction in humans. Hypertension. 1990;16(2):121–30.
5. Esler M, Lambert G, Jennings G. Regional norepinephrine turnover in human hypertension. Clin Exp Hypertens A. 1989;11(Suppl 1):75–89.
6. Grassi G, Cattaneo BM, Seravalle G, Lanfranchi A, Mancia G. Baroreflex control of sympathetic nerve activity in essential and secondary hypertension. Hypertension. 1998;31(1):68–72.
7. Parati G, Esler M. The human sympathetic nervous system: its relevance in hypertension and heart failure. Eur Heart J. 2012;33(9):1058–66.
8. Hagbarth KE, Vallbo AB. Pulse and respiratory grouping of sympathetic impulses in human muscle-nerves. Acta Physiol Scand. 1968;74(1):96–108.
9. Macefield VG, Wallin BG, Vallbo AB. The discharge behaviour of single vasoconstrictor motoneurones in human muscle nerves. J Physiol. 1994;481(Pt 3):799–809.
10. Lambert E, Straznicky N, Schlaich M, Esler M, Dawood T, Hotchkin E, et al. Differing pattern of sympathoexcitation in normal-weight and obesity-related hypertension. Hypertension. 2007;50(5):862–8.
11. Hasking GJ, Esler MD, Jennings GL, Burton D, Johns JA, Korner PI. Norepinephrine spillover to plasma in patients with congestive heart failure: evidence of increased overall and cardiorenal sympathetic nervous activity. Circulation. 1986;73(4):615–21.
12. Parati G, Saul JP, Di Rienzo M, Mancia G. Spectral analysis of blood pressure and heart rate variability in evaluating cardiovascular regulation. A critical appraisal. Hypertension. 1995;25(6):1276–86.
13. Heart Rate Variability. Standards of measurement, physiological interpretation, and clinical use. Task force of the European Society of Cardiology and the North American Society of Pacing and Electrophysiology. Eur Heart J. 1996;17(3):354–81.
14. Malliani A, Pagani M, Lombardi F, Cerutti S. Cardiovascular neural regulation explored in the frequency domain. Circulation. 1991;84(2):482–92.
15. Bauer A, Malik M, Barthel P, Schneider R, Watanabe MA, Camm AJ, et al. Turbulence dynamics: an independent predictor of late mortality after acute myocardial infarction. Int J Cardiol. 2006;107(1):42–7.
16. Voss A, Kurths J, Kleiner HJ, Witt A, Wessel N, Saparin P, et al. The application of methods of non-linear dynamics for the improved and predictive recognition of patients threatened by sudden cardiac death. Cardiovasc Res. 1996;31(3):419–33.
17. Parati G, Di Rienzo M, Mancia G. How to measure baroreflex sensitivity: from the cardiovascular laboratory to daily life. J Hypertens. 2000;18(1):7–19.
18. Parati G, Di Rienzo M, Bertinieri G, Pomidossi G, Casadei R, Groppelli A, et al. Evaluation of the baroreceptor-heart rate reflex by 24-hour intra-arterial blood pressure monitoring in humans. Hypertension. 1988;12(2):214–22.
19. Parati G, Mancia G, Di Rienzo M, Castiglioni P. Point: cardiovascular variability is/is not an index of autonomic control of circulation. J Appl Physiol (1985). 2006;101(2):676–8; discussion 81–2
20. Saul JP, Berger RD, Albrecht P, Stein SP, Chen MH, Cohen RJ. Transfer function analysis of the circulation: unique insights into cardiovascular regulation. Am J Phys. 1991;261(4 Pt 2):H1231–45.
21. van de Borne P, Rahnama M, Mezzetti S, Montano N, Porta A, Degaute JP, et al. Contrasting effects of phentolamine and nitroprusside on neural and cardiovascular variability. Am J Physiol Heart Circ Physiol. 2001;281(2):H559–65.
22. Julien C, Chapuis B, Cheng Y, Barres C. Dynamic interactions between arterial pressure and sympathetic nerve activity: role of arterial baroreceptors. Am J Physiol Regul Integr Comp Physiol. 2003;285(4):R834–41.
23. Castiglioni P, Merati G, Veicsteinas A, Parati G, Di Rienzo M. Influence of sympathetic vascular regulation on heart-rate scaling structure: spinal cord lesion as a model of progressively impaired autonomic control. Biomed Tech (Berl). 2006;51(4):240–3.

24. Castiglioni P, Merati G, Parati G, Faini A. Decomposing the complexity of heart-rate variability by the multifractal-multiscale approach to detrended fluctuation analysis: an application to low-level spinal cord injury. Physiol Meas. 2019;40(8):084003.
25. Castiglioni P, Omboni S, Parati G, Faini A. Day and night changes of cardiovascular complexity: a multi-fractal multi-scale analysis. Entropy (Basel). 2020;22(4)
26. Castiglioni P, Parati G, Faini A. Multifractal and multiscale detrended fluctuation analysis of cardiovascular signals: how the estimation bias affects ShortTerm coefficients and a way to mitigate this error. Annu Int Conf IEEE Eng Med Biol Soc. 2021;2021:257–60.
27. Narkiewicz K, Winnicki M, Schroeder K, Phillips BG, Kato M, Cwalina E, et al. Relationship between muscle sympathetic nerve activity and diurnal blood pressure profile. Hypertension. 2002;39(1):168–72.
28. Smyth HS, Sleight P, Pickering GW. Reflex regulation of arterial pressure during sleep in man. A quantitative method of assessing baroreflex sensitivity. Circ Res. 1969;24(1):109–21.
29. Eckberg DL, Cavanaugh MS, Mark AL, Abboud FM. A simplified neck suction device for activation of carotid baroreceptors. J Lab Clin Med. 1975;85(1):167–73.
30. Mancia G, Ferrari A, Gregorini L, Parati G, Ferrari MC, Pomidossi G, et al. Control of blood pressure by carotid sinus baroreceptors in human beings. Am J Cardiol. 1979;44(5):895–902.
31. Mancia G, Ferrari A, Gregorini L, Parati G, Pomidossi G, Bertinieri G, et al. Blood pressure and heart rate variabilities in normotensive and hypertensive human beings. Circ Res. 1983;53(1):96–104.
32. Laude D, Elghozi JL, Girard A, Bellard E, Bouhaddi M, Castiglioni P, et al. Comparison of various techniques used to estimate spontaneous baroreflex sensitivity (the EuroBaVar study). Am J Physiol Regul Integr Comp Physiol. 2004;286(1):R226–31.
33. Parati G, Saul JP, Castiglioni P. Assessing arterial baroreflex control of heart rate: new perspectives. J Hypertens. 2004;22(7):1259–63.
34. Pagani M, Somers V, Furlan R, Dell'Orto S, Conway J, Baselli G, et al. Changes in autonomic regulation induced by physical training in mild hypertension. Hypertension. 1988;12(6):600–10.
35. Robbe HW, Mulder LJ, Ruddel H, Langewitz WA, Veldman JB, Mulder G. Assessment of baroreceptor reflex sensitivity by means of spectral analysis. Hypertension. 1987;10(5):538–43.
36. Barbieri R, Bianchi AM, Triedman JK, Mainardi LT, Cerutti S, Saul JP. Model dependency of multivariate autoregressive spectral analysis. IEEE Eng Med Biol Mag. 1997;16(5):74–85.
37. Barbieri R, Parati G, Saul JP. Closed- versus open-loop assessment of heart rate baroreflex. IEEE Eng Med Biol Mag. 2001;20(2):33–42.
38. Baselli G, Cerutti S, Civardi S, Malliani A, Pagani M. Cardiovascular variability signals: towards the identification of a closed-loop model of the neural control mechanisms. IEEE Trans Biomed Eng. 1988;35(12):1033–46.
39. Patton DJ, Triedman JK, Perrott MH, Vidian AA, Saul JP. Baroreflex gain: characterization using autoregressive moving average analysis. Am J Phys. 1996;270(4 Pt 2):H1240–9.
40. Wyller VB, Barbieri R, Saul JP. Blood pressure variability and closed-loop baroreflex assessment in adolescent chronic fatigue syndrome during supine rest and orthostatic stress. Eur J Appl Physiol. 2011;111(3):497–507.
41. Parati G, Castiglioni P, Faini A, Di Rienzo M, Mancia G, Barbieri R, et al. Closed-loop cardiovascular interactions and the baroreflex cardiac arm: modulations over the 24 h and the effect of hypertension. Front Physiol. 2019;10:477.
42. Grassi G, Mark A, Esler M. The sympathetic nervous system alterations in human hypertension. Circ Res. 2015;116(6):976–90.
43. Julius S, Pascual AV, London R. Role of parasympathetic inhibition in the hyperkinetic type of borderline hypertension. Circulation. 1971;44(3):413–8.
44. Goldstein DS. Plasma catecholamines and essential hypertension. An analytical review. Hypertension. 1983;5(1):86–99.

45. Anderson EA, Sinkey CA, Lawton WJ, Mark AL. Elevated sympathetic nerve activity in borderline hypertensive humans. Evidence from direct intraneural recordings. Hypertension. 1989;14(2):177–83.
46. Grassi G, Dell'Oro R, Quarti-Trevano F, Scopelliti F, Seravalle G, Paleari F, et al. Neuroadrenergic and reflex abnormalities in patients with metabolic syndrome. Diabetologia. 2005;48(7):1359–65.
47. Huggett RJ, Burns J, Mackintosh AF, Mary DA. Sympathetic neural activation in non-diabetic metabolic syndrome and its further augmentation by hypertension. Hypertension. 2004;44(6):847–52.
48. Grassi G, Colombo M, Seravalle G, Spaziani D, Mancia G. Dissociation between muscle and skin sympathetic nerve activity in essential hypertension, obesity, and congestive heart failure. Hypertension. 1998;31(1):64–7.
49. Greenwood JP, Stoker JB, Mary DA. Single-unit sympathetic discharge : quantitative assessment in human hypertensive disease. Circulation. 1999;100(12):1305–10.
50. Schlaich MP, Kaye DM, Lambert E, Sommerville M, Socratous F, Esler MD. Relation between cardiac sympathetic activity and hypertensive left ventricular hypertrophy. Circulation. 2003;108(5):560–5.
51. Mancia G, Grassi G, Parati G, Pomidossi G, Saino A, Malaspina D, et al. Control of circulation by arterial baroreceptors and cardiopulmonary receptors in hypertension. J Cardiovasc Pharmacol. 1986;8(Suppl 5):S82–8.
52. Mancia G, Leonetti G, Picotti GB, Ferrari A, Galva MD, Gregorini L, et al. Plasma catecholamines and blood pressure responses to the carotid baroreceptor reflex in essential hypertension. Clin Sci (Lond). 1979;57(Suppl 5):165s–7s.
53. Seravalle G, Lonati L, Buzzi S, Cairo M, Quarti Trevano F, Dell'Oro R, et al. Sympathetic nerve traffic and baroreflex function in optimal, normal, and high-normal blood pressure states. J Hypertens. 2015;33(7):1411–7.
54. Grassi G, Seravalle G, Brambilla G, Pini C, Alimento M, Facchetti R, et al. Marked sympathetic activation and baroreflex dysfunction in true resistant hypertension. Int J Cardiol. 2014;177(3):1020–5.
55. Grassi G, Ram VS. Evidence for a critical role of the sympathetic nervous system in hypertension. J Am Soc Hypertens. 2016;10(5):457–66.
56. DiBona GF, Kopp UC. Neural control of renal function. Physiol Rev. 1997;77(1):75–197.
57. DiBona GF, Esler M. Translational medicine: the antihypertensive effect of renal denervation. Am J Physiol Regul Integr Comp Physiol. 2010;298(2):R245–53.
58. Krum H, Schlaich M, Whitbourn R, Sobotka PA, Sadowski J, Bartus K, et al. Catheter-based renal sympathetic denervation for resistant hypertension: a multicentre safety and proof-of-principle cohort study. Lancet. 2009;373(9671):1275–81.
59. Schlaich MP, Sobotka PA, Krum H, Lambert E, Esler MD. Renal sympathetic-nerve ablation for uncontrolled hypertension. N Engl J Med. 2009;361(9):932–4.
60. Guyenet PG. The sympathetic control of blood pressure. Nat Rev Neurosci. 2006;7(5):335–46.
61. Jose PA, Eisner GM, Felder RA. Role of dopamine receptors in the kidney in the regulation of blood pressure. Curr Opin Nephrol Hypertens. 2002;11(1):87–92.
62. Dampney RA, Coleman MJ, Fontes MA, Hirooka Y, Horiuchi J, Li YW, et al. Central mechanisms underlying short- and long-term regulation of the cardiovascular system. Clin Exp Pharmacol Physiol. 2002;29(4):261–8.
63. Osborn JW. Hypothesis: set-points and long-term control of arterial pressure. A theoretical argument for a long-term arterial pressure control system in the brain rather than the kidney. Clin Exp Pharmacol Physiol. 2005;32(5–6):384–93.
64. Krieger EM. Arterial baroreceptor resetting in hypertension (the J. W. McCubbin memorial lecture). Clin Exp Pharmacol Physiol Suppl. 1989;15:3–17.
65. Thrasher TN. Arterial baroreceptor input contributes to long-term control of blood pressure. Curr Hypertens Rep. 2006;8(3):249–54.

66. Lohmeier TE, Iliescu R. The baroreflex as a long-term controller of arterial pressure. Physiology (Bethesda). 2015;30(2):148–58.
67. Kopp UC, DiBona GF. Neural regulation of renin secretion. Semin Nephrol. 1993;13(6):543–51.
68. Johns EJ, Kopp UC, DiBona GF. Neural control of renal function. Compr Physiol. 2011;1(2):731–67.
69. Iliescu R, Irwin ED, Georgakopoulos D, Lohmeier TE. Renal responses to chronic suppression of central sympathetic outflow. Hypertension. 2012;60(3):749–56.
70. Greenwood JP, Scott EM, Stoker JB, Mary DA. Hypertensive left ventricular hypertrophy: relation to peripheral sympathetic drive. J Am Coll Cardiol. 2001;38(6):1711–7.
71. Grassi G, Seravalle G, Quarti-Trevano F, Dell'Oro R, Arenare F, Spaziani D, et al. Sympathetic and baroreflex cardiovascular control in hypertension-related left ventricular dysfunction. Hypertension. 2009;53(2):205–9.
72. Converse RL Jr, Jacobsen TN, Toto RD, Jost CM, Cosentino F, Fouad-Tarazi F, et al. Sympathetic overactivity in patients with chronic renal failure. N Engl J Med. 1992;327(27):1912–8.
73. Grassi G, Quarti-Trevano F, Seravalle G, Arenare F, Volpe M, Furiani S, et al. Early sympathetic activation in the initial clinical stages of chronic renal failure. Hypertension. 2011;57(4):846–51.
74. Mancia G, Grassi G. The autonomic nervous system and hypertension. Circ Res. 2014;114(11):1804–14.
75. Florea VG, Cohn JN. The autonomic nervous system and heart failure. Circ Res. 2014;114(11):1815–26.
76. Cohn JN, Levine TB, Olivari MT, Garberg V, Lura D, Francis GS, et al. Plasma norepinephrine as a guide to prognosis in patients with chronic congestive heart failure. N Engl J Med. 1984;311(13):819–23.
77. Brunner-La Rocca HP, Esler MD, Jennings GL, Kaye DM. Effect of cardiac sympathetic nervous activity on mode of death in congestive heart failure. Eur Heart J. 2001;22(13):1136–43.
78. Sander D, Winbeck K, Klingelhofer J, Etgen T, Conrad B. Prognostic relevance of pathological sympathetic activation after acute thromboembolic stroke. Neurology. 2001;57(5):833–8.
79. Shen MJ, Zipes DP. Role of the autonomic nervous system in modulating cardiac arrhythmias. Circ Res. 2014;114(6):1004–21.
80. Zoccali C, Mallamaci F, Parlongo S, Cutrupi S, Benedetto FA, Tripepi G, et al. Plasma norepinephrine predicts survival and incident cardiovascular events in patients with end-stage renal disease. Circulation. 2002;105(11):1354–9.
81. La Rovere MT, Bigger JT Jr, Marcus FI, Mortara A, Schwartz PJ. Baroreflex sensitivity and heart-rate variability in prediction of total cardiac mortality after myocardial infarction. ATRAMI (autonomic tone and reflexes after myocardial infarction) investigators. Lancet. 1998;351(9101):478–84.
82. Esler M, Straznicky N, Eikelis N, Masuo K, Lambert G, Lambert E. Mechanisms of sympathetic activation in obesity-related hypertension. Hypertension. 2006;48(5):787–96.
83. Parati G, Lombardi C, Narkiewicz K. Sleep apnea: epidemiology, pathophysiology, and relation to cardiovascular risk. Am J Physiol Regul Integr Comp Physiol. 2007;293(4):R1671–83.
84. Pepperell JC, Ramdassingh-Dow S, Crosthwaite N, Mullins R, Jenkinson C, Stradling JR, et al. Ambulatory blood pressure after therapeutic and subtherapeutic nasal continuous positive airway pressure for obstructive sleep apnoea: a randomised parallel trial. Lancet. 2002;359(9302):204–10.
85. Williams B, Mancia G, Spiering W, Agabiti Rosei E, Azizi M, Burnier M, et al. 2018 practice guidelines for the management of arterial hypertension of the European Society of Hypertension and the European Society of Cardiology: ESH/ESC Task Force for the Management of Arterial Hypertension. J Hypertens. 2018;36(12):2284–309.
86. Thomopoulos C, Parati G, Zanchetti A. Effects of blood pressure-lowering treatment on cardiovascular outcomes and mortality: 14 - effects of different classes of antihypertensive drugs in older and younger patients: overview and meta-analysis. J Hypertens. 2018;36(8):1637–47.

87. Thomopoulos C, Bazoukis G, Tsioufis C, Mancia G. Beta-blockers in hypertension: overview and meta-analysis of randomized outcome trials. J Hypertens. 2020;38(9):1669–81.
88. Mancia G, Kreutz R, Brunström M, Burnier M, Grassi G, et al. Authors/Task Force Members:. 2023 ESH Guidelines for the management of arterial hypertension The Task Force for the management of arterial hypertension of the European Society of Hypertension Endorsed by the International Society of Hypertension (ISH) and the European Renal Association (ERA). J Hypertens. 2023 Jun 21. https://doi.org/10.1097/HJH.0000000000003480. Epub ahead of print. PMID: 37345492.]
89. Lauder L, Azizi M, Kirtane AJ, Bohm M, Mahfoud F. Device-based therapies for arterial hypertension. Nat Rev Cardiol. 2020;17(10):614–28.
90. Mohaupt MG, Schmidli J, Luft FC. Management of uncontrollable hypertension with a carotid sinus stimulation device. Hypertension. 2007;50(5):825–8.
91. Chunbin W, Fu S, Jing H. Efficacy and safety of baroreflex activation therapy for treatment of resistant hypertension: a systematic review and meta-analysis. Clin Exp Hypertens. 2018;40(6):501–8.
92. Heusser K, Tank J, Engeli S, Diedrich A, Menne J, Eckert S, et al. Carotid baroreceptor stimulation, sympathetic activity, baroreflex function, and blood pressure in hypertensive patients. Hypertension. 2010;55(3):619–26.
93. Wallbach M, Lehnig LY, Schroer C, Luders S, Bohning E, Muller GA, et al. Effects of baroreflex activation therapy on ambulatory blood pressure in patients with resistant hypertension. Hypertension. 2016;67(4):701–9.
94. Bhatt DL, Kandzari DE, O'Neill WW, D'Agostino R, Flack JM, Katzen BT, et al. A controlled trial of renal denervation for resistant hypertension. N Engl J Med. 2014;370(15):1393–401.
95. Ogoyama Y, Tada K, Abe M, Nanto S, Shibata H, Mukoyama M, et al. Effects of renal denervation on blood pressures in patients with hypertension: a systematic review and meta-analysis of randomized sham-controlled trials. Hypertens Res. 2022;45(2):210–20.
96. Ahmad Y, Francis DP, Bhatt DL, Howard JP. Renal denervation for hypertension: a systematic review and meta-analysis of randomized, blinded, placebo-controlled trials. JACC Cardiovasc Interv. 2021;14(23):2614–24.
97. Mancia et al. ESH 2023 Hypertension Guidelines, J. Hypertension 2023.

Chapter 4
Autonomic Nervous System and Cardiac Arrhythmias

Alessio Menditto, Lucia Mancinelli, and Roberto Antonicelli

4.1 Sympathetic and Parasympathetic System: Their Role in Cardiovascular Physiopathology

4.1.1 Anatomy of Autonomic Nervous System

The Autonomic Cardiac Nervous System (ACNS) is a complex neural network responsible for autonomic cardiac control and organised in various and multilevel parts of the nervous system: afferent neural impulses are transmitted from the heart to the intrinsic neurons of the heart, to extracardiac intrathoracic ganglia, to the spinal cord and to the brain stem. Thereafter, these afferent neural signals are processed by different parts of the nervous system in order to generate a cardiomotor neural output to the heart: the transmission of afferent and efferent impulses is achieved by the sympathetic and parasympathetic nerves [1]. This autonomic control results in four final effects:

- **Dromotropic effect**: It modifies the conduction's velocity of electrical impulses at the atria, at the ventricles and at the atrioventricular node.
- **Chronotropic effect**: It changes the cardiac rate.
- **Lusitropic effect**: It depends on the myocardial relaxation and describes the filling capacity for every diastolic pressure; it is influenced by the elastic properties of the cardiac wall and the interaction of contractile proteins.
- **Inotropic effect**: It is the variation of cardiac contractility.

At the level of the heart, the intrinsic cardiac nervous system (ICNS) consists of interconnecting nerves that form the ganglionated plexi (GPs): a subset of these

A. Menditto · L. Mancinelli · R. Antonicelli (✉)
Cardiology Unit, IRCCS INRCA, Ancona, Italy
e-mail: A.MENDITTO@inrca.it; L.MANCINELLI@inrca.it; r.antonicelli@inrca.it

G. Micieli et al. (eds.), *Autonomic Disorders in Clinical Practice*,
https://doi.org/10.1007/978-3-031-43036-7_4

intrinsic cardiac neurons (25%) receives direct inputs from extracardiac parasympathetic and sympathetic neurons, and the rest are local circuit neurons (LCN), that dependent on sensory inputs and local circuit interconnections. The LCN are not directly transducing cardiac indices (cardiac afferent neurons) or having direct motor function, but clearly play a role in integrating local sensory inputs along with inputs from the central nervous system. These neurons are located throughout all intrathoracic ganglia, including those distributed in the heart and receive sensory feedback from the heart and intrathoracic veins and arteries. The GPs are mainly placed in the superior and posterior regions of atrial and ventricular fat pads (around the heart); a minor part of them is located in other areas between atrial and ventricular muscle fascicles. Previous studies have suggested that there is an inter-human variability of the ICNS anatomy because the distribution, the sizes and the anatomical configuration of GPs vary from specimen and specimen [2, 3]. Specific aggregates of intrinsic cardiac ganglia are preferentially associated with sectorial controls in the different cardiac regions: for example, neural control of dromotropic function is primarily associated with the inferior vena cava-inferior atrial ganglionated plexus, the ventral right atrial ganglionated plexus is mainly responsible for the atrial rate (mediating direct parasympathetic inhibition of sinoatrial nodal rhythm) [4], the posterior atrial ganglionated plexus contributes to the regulation of chronotropic function [5]. The ICNS connects with intrathoracic extracardiac ganglia, the extrathoracic cardiac ganglia and the central nervous system. Interactions between the central nervous system, intrathoracic extracardiac ganglia and intrinsic cardiac ganglia in normal cardiac control add even more complexity because, at each level, neurons act both individually and in concert with others. In fact, intrathoracic extracardiac ganglia contain efferent sympathetic post-ganglionic, afferent and local circuit neuronal somata, but there are also neurons projecting axons solely to adjacent neurons, called interneurons, that mediate cardiac reflexes [6]. The various intrathoracic reflexes represent cardio-centric short-loop reflexes that regulate cardiodynamics on a beat-to-beat basis. They continue to do so even when the intrathoracic nervous system is disconnected from the central nervous system [7, 8].

The somata of afferent neurons associated with cardiac or great thoracic vascular mechanoreceptors and chemoreceptors are located in nodose ganglia, C6-T6 dorsal root ganglia, intrathoracic extracardiac ganglia and intrinsic cardiac ganglia. In the heart, the sensory neurites associated with these afferent somata are located throughout both atria and ventricles, being concentrated in the sinoatrial nodal region and in the outflow tracts of each ventricle. These somata transduce mechanical distortion, chemical signals or both to second-order neurons, and cardiac sensory information are the primary input to generate a response to different levels of neuro-axis [9]. Cardiac parasympathetic efferent preganglionic somata are placed primarily in the ventral-lateral region of the nucleus ambiguous, and a small amount of them in the medullary dorsal motor nucleus and in the intermediate zone between these two medullary nuclei [10]. Via bilateral vagus sympathetic trunks and multiple intrathoracic cardiopulmonary nerves, the parasympathetic neurons project signals to post-ganglionic neurons, located in atrial and ventricular GPs: widely distributed in epicardial fat pads; they provide direct innervation to the sinus node, atrioventricular node as well as both atria and ventricles. The parasympathetic motor control of the heart influences both atrial and ventricular tissues [11]. The cardiac sympathetic preganglionic neurons originate in the brainstem and are modulated by higher centres such as the subthalamic, the periaqueductal grey and the rostral ventrolateral medulla. Cardiac-related sympathetic efferent preganglionic neurons are located in the intermedio-lateral cell column of the spinal cord (C6–T6) and, via C6–T6 rami, project axons to the cardiac post-ganglionic neuronal somata located in superior cervical, middle cervical and stellate ganglia [12]. In particular, the sympathetic innervation fibres originate mainly in the right and left stellate ganglia, via multiple cardiopulmonary nerves and arrive at the heart, where they travel along the epicardial vascular structures of the heart and, as well as coronary vessels, penetrate into the underlying myocardium, reaching the endocardium. The sympathetic post-ganglionic neurons are distributed in all cardiac regions, but a difference exists in sympathetic innervation from the atria to the ventricles and from base to apex of the heart: the atria are most densely innervated, but the ventricles are also supplied with a sympathetic network, most densely at the base. In contrast to sympathetic neurons, after parasympathetic fibres cross the atrioventricular (AV) groove along the surface of the heart, they get into the ventricular wall into the subendocardium before projecting their individual terminal axons intramurally. Parasympathetic neurons are distributed more heterogeneously throughout the heart: the density of parasympathetic innervation in the sinoatrial (SA) and AV nodes is considerably higher than the surrounding atrial or ventricular tissue [13]. Figures 4.1 and 4.2 give

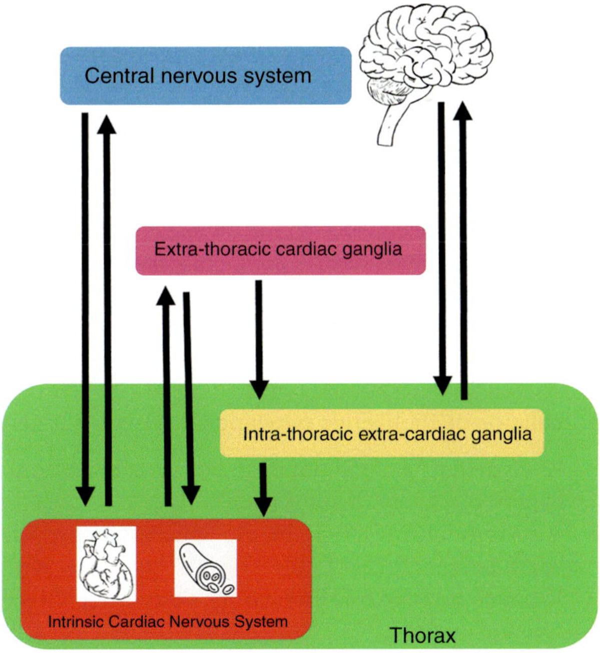

Fig. 4.1 A schematic representation of cardiac autonomic nervous system

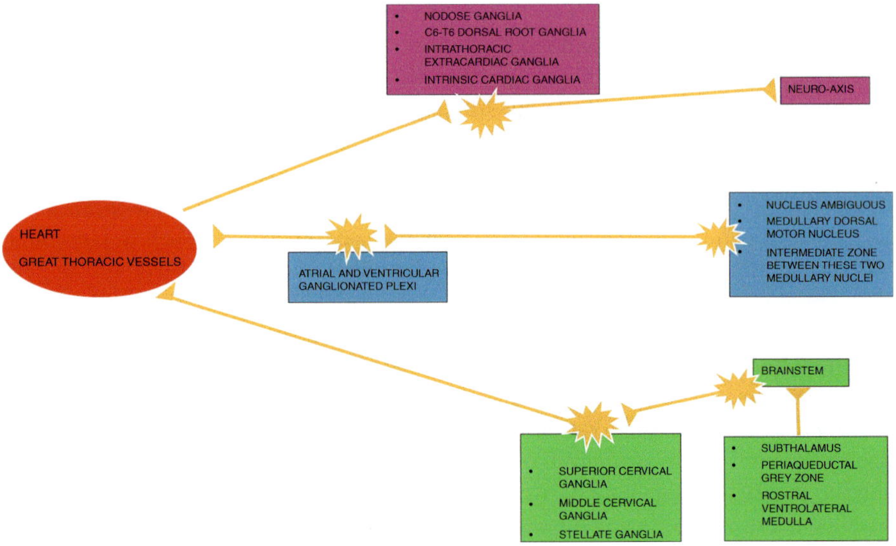

Fig. 4.2 A representation of afferent and efferent systems: in purple afferent system, in blue efferent parasympathetic system and in green sympathetic system

a schematic representation of the complex neural network of the cardiac autonomic nervous system.

4.1.2 Physiopathology of Sympathetic and Parasympathetic System: Their Role in Cardiac Arrhythmias, Heart Failure and Myocardial Infarction

The major neurotransmitters released by nervous terminals of autonomic nervous system are the acetylcholine for the parasympathetic nervous system, whereas the sympathetic neurons release principally noradrenaline: these two categories of neurotransmitters generally exert opposing effects. There are then other neurotransmitters, such as neuropeptide Y, nitric oxide, galanin, which are summarised in Table 4.1.

Acetylcholine is the major parasympathetic neurotransmitter of the heart and the stimulation of cholinergic muscarinic receptors (largely M2-type) results in:

- Bradycardia, by inhibition of the sympathetic nervous system and by direct hyperpolarisation of sinus nodal cells;
- Atrioventricular (AV) block, mediated predominantly through the left vagus nerve;
- Reduced myocardial contractility, decreasing intracellular cAMP production and calcium currents.

Table 4.1 Neurotransmitters of ANS and their receptors

Neurotransmitters	Receptor	Principal actions in cardiovascular system
Noradrenaline	α_1	Stimulate the arterial muscle contraction
	α_2	Pre-synaptic inhibition of the release of the neurotransmitter from the orthosympathic and parasympathetic nerve endings; stimulates the contraction of the smooth muscles of some arteries
	β_1	Increase heart rate and contractility, increase conduction speed via the atrioventricular node
	β_2	Increase heart rate and contractility, increase conduction speed via the atrioventricular node (more less present in the heart)
	β_3	Decrease heart contractility and vasodilation (high doses)
Acetylcholine	M_1	Dilation of blood vessels by NO release
	M_2	Decrease heart rate and contractility, decrease conduction speed via the atrioventricular node
	M_3	Dilation of blood vessels by NO release
Neuropeptide Y	Y_1, Y_2	Stimulates contraction of arteries and boosts responses mediated by adrenergic α_1 receptors; pre-synaptic inhibition of neurotransmitter release from some post-ganglionic orthosympathic nerve endings
Nitric Oxide	Diffused throughout the membranes	Vasodilation

Other co-transmitters released with vagus nerve stimulation include nitric oxide and vasoactive intestinal peptide, that dilate coronary arteries, increasing coronary artery blood flow, and vasorelaxation of blood vessel walls [14].

Sympathetic stimulation instead:

- Increases the outflowing of SA node (tachycardia);
- Raises AV nodal conduction;
- Increases the atrial and ventricular myocardial contractility.

The most important mechanism underlying sympathetic-mediated arrhythmogenesis is the activation of the β-adrenergic receptors and stimulatory Gs proteins, which leads to an increase calcium release from the sarcoplasmic reticulum (SR) and a stimulation of several other ventricular currents, including inflow sodium current, the delayed rectifier potassium current (IKs), the chloride current, and the pacemaker current: the overall effect in humans results in shortening of ventricular action potential duration (APD) and refractory period [15].

These effects are mediated by postsynaptic myocardial β-adrenergic receptors: both β1 and β2 subtypes are present with a ratio of approximately 5:1 in the healthy human heart. A third cardiac β-adrenergic receptor, β3, is described, and the stimulation of this receptor results in a decrease in cardiac contractility and vasodilation, likely through the nitric oxide synthase pathway. β3 receptors are stimulated by catecholamines only at high doses [16, 17].

During parasympathetic activation there is a quicker response of the heart and the influence of parasympathetic system stops much more rapidly. This is because norepinephrine, which is highly conserved, is taken up by neurons after release, whereas acetylcholine is rapidly hydrolysed by acetylcholinesterase. No acetylcholine transporter exists, and only choline is taken back up into the neuron to be resynthesised into new acetylcholine molecules [18].

Interaction between sympathetic and parasympathetic nervous systems is complex: a dynamic interaction, modulated partially by secondary messengers (cAMP and cyclic guanosine monophosphate, cGMP), occurs between them. Parasympathetic activation can inhibit sympathetic nerve traffic presynaptically and, likewise, sympathetic system can inhibit parasympathetic activation presynaptically. Vagal tone predominates over sympathetic tone at rest and under normal physiological conditions, sudden parasympathetic stimulation will inhibit tonic sympathetic activation and its effects at rest and during exercise. This response is known as "accentuated antagonism." Intracoronary acetylcholine inhibits a β-adrenergic-stimulated increase in the first derivative of left ventricular pressure over time. β-adrenergic stimulation causes apoptosis of cardiac myocytes, and this effect, mediated by protein kinase A and requiring calcium entry via voltage-dependent calcium channels, contributes to the progression of myocardial failure: muscarinic receptor stimulation opposes this action by a G(i)-mediated signalling pathway that opposes actions of adenylyl cyclase. Carbachol, a muscarinic agonist, can prevent β-adrenergic receptor-stimulated apoptosis [14].

Excessive calcium influx and sarcoplasmic reticulum calcium release have arrhythmogenic effects because calcium homeostasis is crucial in maintaining normal cardiomyocyte functions, excitability and mitochondrial stability. Additionally, increased intracellular calcium concentration activates the sodium-calcium exchanger to extrude intracellular calcium to the extracellular space and extruding one calcium ion occurs at the expense of importing three sodium ions, which is electrogenic and can lead to early or delayed *after-depolarisation*: abnormal depolarisation of cellular membrane dependent on cycle-length and repolarisation lengthens. Disturbed calcium homeostasis caused by high sympathetic outflow-induced ventricular tachyarrhythmias (VAs) such as catecholaminergic polymorphic ventricular tachycardia, long QT syndrome and sudden cardiac death [19]. Mechanisms of cardiac arrhythmias are categorised into two groups: abnormal focal activity and triggered activity. Increased sympathetic tone can lead to enhanced automaticity in pacemaker cells in both atria and ventricles, but can also modulate triggered activities, including both early (EAD) and delayed (DAD) afterdepolarisation: instead, β-adrenergic stimulation leads to the increased occurrence and magnitude of EAD whereas cholinergic stimulation suppresses EAD activity. In addition, genetic mutations in subunits of delayed rectifier potassium current can underlie long QT syndromes and predispose carriers to polymorphic ventricular tachycardia in the face of increased sympathetic stimulation [20].

Transmural myocardial infarction (MI) causes denervation and death of sympathetic fibres within the scar, likely due to disruption of sympathetic fibres that run along the coronaries, and also produced loss of efferent sympathetic innervation in non-infarcted apical sites as early as 5–20 min after coronary occlusion, significantly increasing over the following 3 h. Therefore, disruption of neurotransmission can lead to a heterogenous response in an effective refractory period even in areas of viable non-infarcted myocardium situated apical to the necrosis, leading to a non-uniform electrophysiologic response early in the stages of acute ischaemia. The denervated sites, although no longer responsive to nerve stimulation, demonstrated an elevated sensitivity to infusion of β agonists. Consequently, the heterogeneous response to left or right sympathetic nerve stimulation, an exaggerated response to circulating catecholamines, and reduced protection from vagal denervation all contribute to the genesis of ventricular arrhythmias in both acute and chronic MI [21]. There is evidence that in heart failure (HF) vagal tone decreased, often preceding the enhancement of sympathetic activity, activity of the arterial chemoreceptors and cardiac sympathetic afferent fibres is increased, in part, to drive the increase in sympathetic outflow: the elevated cardiac norepinephrine spillover results from both increased neuronal release (augmented nerve firing) and impaired neuronal uptake of norepinephrine. Enhanced sympathetic activation occurs before the development of symptoms in patients with left ventricular dysfunction, and reduced parasympathetic drive is present early in patients with symptomatic heart failure resulting from even mild left ventricular impairment [22]. In HF, vagal ganglionic transmission is reduced, muscarinic receptor density and composition are altered, and acetylcholinesterase activity is decreased [14].

4.2 Non-pathological ANS Mediated Heart Rhythm Disturb

4.2.1 Inappropriate Sinus Tachycardia (IST)

4.2.1.1 Definition and Epidemiology

Sinus rhythm is the normal cardiac rhythm, and normal heart rate (HR) has a range between 60 beats per minute (bpm) and 100 bpm. Sinus tachycardia (ST) is characterised by a rhythm that normally originates from the sinus node but has an HR of more than 100 bpm (typical 100–180 bpm). This condition is the normal heart response to a stressed physiological or pathological situation (emotion, exercise, pregnancy, fever, anaemia, hyperthyroidism, drugs, etc.). HR returns to normal range when the cause is eliminated [23, 24].

When there is a resting sinus rate more than 100 bpm without a trigger or with an out-of-proportion trigger then it is an IST. IST affects more frequent young female patients, but it is not limited to this category [23–25]. The underlying mechanism is not perfectly clear. It is not known if IST is secondary to an intrinsic high heart rate or secondary to an autonomic imbalance (with an increase of sympathetic tone) or it is secondary to both causes. Ptaszynski, in his study, which uses pharmacological denervation to compare ITS patients and healthy people, shows an intrinsic high heart rate in IST patients with respect to healthy control as well as abnormal or borderline results in cardiovascular autonomic tests [26]. Nwazue colleagues claim that there is a stronger autonomic influence in the pathophysiology of IST without significant abnormalities in sinus node automaticity, in fact, they do not find the difference in intrinsic heart rate between IST patients and healthy control after a pharmacological protocol with administration of propranolol and atropine. Instead, they find an increased sympathetic tone and a decreased parasympathetic tone in IST patients than in control [27]. Probably, the pathophysiology depends both on sinus node automaticity and on autonomic tone balance [26, 28].

4.2.1.2 Clinical Presentation and Diagnosis

Patients affected by IST may be asymptomatic or have a spectrum of symptoms ranging from palpitation to dyspnoea, from exercise intolerance to dizziness.

Diagnosis is made by resting electrocardiogram (ECG) that shows an ST (typical sinus P waves morphology and HR more than 100 bpm) and with trigger exclusion. Differential diagnosis can be made with postural orthostatic tachycardia syndrome (POTS) that is characterised by a heart rate increasing with orthostatic position, with sinus reentrant tachycardia and with atrial tachycardia origin from superior part of atrium (crista terminalis or upper right pulmonary vein).

Holter-ECG is useful for diagnosis because it excludes the white-coat effect in resting ECG ST registration and generally documented 24 h mean HR of more than 90 bpm and a daily HR of more than 100 bpm.

Head-up tilt test is useful to differentiate IST from POTS. With a passive orthostatic position in POTS patient can be observed an increase of HR greater than 30 bpm and the absence of orthostatic hypotension [23].

4.2.1.3 Therapy

IST have a benign prognosis and are usually not associated with tachycardia-induced cardiomyopathy, in fact, treatments are indicated only for symptom control [23–25]. Beta-blockers are often used to treat IST but require high dosage with the consequent appearance of undesirable side effects like fatigue. Non-dihydropyridine calcium channel blockers (NDHP-CCB) can be used but can often cause hypotension. Ivabradine, a selective I_f-blocker in sinus nodes, is effective to reduce sinus rate, but if chronically used, it can be pro-arrhythmic because it up-regulates sympathetic activity to the heart. This side effect can be reduced using ivabradine in association with beta-blockers [23, 24]. Cardiac ablation is the extreme ratio in IST. The results generally are not good because, although a good technical result, symptoms often persist for recurrence of sinus high rate or for rapid junctional rhythm due probably to a high sympathetic sensitivity of patient pacemaker cells [24].

4.2.2 *Nocturnal Bradyarrhythmias*

4.2.2.1 Definition and Epidemiology

Bradyarrhythmia is any heart rhythm with a rate of less than 60 bpm. Nocturnal bradyarrhythmias are common in both healthy and unhealthy people. These nocturnal bradyarrhythmias are more common in young and sportive people and reduce in frequency in middle-aged and older people. Sinus bradycardia is the most frequent bradyarrhythmia during sleep, but sinus arrest, sinus block, atrioventricular block and junctional rhythm can occur [29, 30].

These nocturnal arrhythmias are more often vagally mediated, in fact during sleep parasympathetic tone is prevalent over sympathetic tone, and the effect is the reduction of heart rate. Another mechanism is sleep apnoea. In people affected by sleep apnoea syndrome, bradyarrhythmias can occur in apnoeic periods (hypoxemia mechanism) [29–31].

4.2.2.2 Clinical Presentation and Diagnosis

During sleep, the heart rate physiologically decreases. In some people, the high vagal tone can reduce heart rate significantly (sinus bradycardia with HR <40 bpm or pauses with RR interval >5 s). In most cases, all of these bradyarrhythmias remain asymptomatic and not-diagnosed [29, 30].

Heart rhythm monitor systems (Holter-ECG, hospital vital parameter monitor, loop-recorder, etc.) allow for diagnosing nocturnal bradyarrhythmias [29].

It is important to differentiate between vagally-mediated (physiological) and sleep disorder-mediated (pathological) nocturnal bradyarrhythmias. Polysomnography helps clinicians to diagnose sleep disorders, especially sleep apnoea syndrome. Also, a careful analysis of nocturnal ECG registration can help to differentiate vagally mediated from sleep apnoea-mediated bradyarrhythmias. In vagally mediated events, there is a progressive slowing of heart rhythm with basal sinus bradycardia to which atrioventricular block or pauses can be associated. In sleep apnoea-mediated, instead, bradyarrhythmias occur during apnoea time and are often followed by tachycardia during arousal [29, 31, 32].

4.2.2.3 Therapy

Usually, nocturnal bradycardia does not need therapy and, especially vagally mediated bradyarrhythmias, are not an indication of pacemaker implant. Some problems occur in hospitalised patients when heart rhythm is continuously monitored, and the presence of severe bradycardia or of asystolic pauses scares the carers. In this case, it is necessary to differentiate between physiological bradycardia and pathological bradycardia (e.g. hypoxemia, drug overdose, stroke, etc.). In case of sleep apnoea syndrome, specific treatment (e.g. continuous positive airway pressure ventilation and weight loss) is recommended because it reduces bradycardia events and improves cardiovascular outcomes [29, 31, 32].

4.3 Bradyarrhythmias

4.3.1 Sinus Node Dysfunction

4.3.1.1 Definition, Epidemiology

The sinus node dysfunction (SND) is a chronic condition in which the deterioration of sinoatrial nodal function results in abnormalities such as sinus bradycardia, sinus pauses, sinus arrest, sinoatrial nodal exit block and chronotropic incompetence, defined as inappropriate responses to physiological demands during exercise or stress (Table 4.2). SND is most often related to age-dependent progressive fibrosis of the sinus nodal tissue and surrounding atrial myocardium, leading to abnormalities of atrial impulse formation and propagation and will therefore result in various bradycardic or pause-related syndromes [33].

The epidemiology of SND is difficult to estimate because of its varying manifestations, including non-specific symptoms and electrocardiographic findings. The incidence of SND is approximately 1 in 600 cardiac patients older than 65 years, and the prevalence is 1 per 1000 person-years in adults >45 years of age. The incidence increases with age. The natural history of SND is characterised by progressive rhythm disturbances and adverse cardiovascular events, and the time course can

Table 4.2 Sinus node dysfunction

Sinus node dysfunction	Electrocardiographic findings
Sinus bradycardia	Sinus rate < 50 bpm
Ectopic atrial bradycardia	Atrial depolarization attributable to an atrial pacemaker other than the sinus node with a rate < 50 bpm
Sinoatrial exit block	Sinus pauses and atrial depolarization (blocked conduction between the sinus node and adjacent atrial tissue)
Sinus pause	Sinus node depolarizes > 3 s after the last atrial depolarization
Sinus node arrest	No evidence of sinus node depolarization
Tachycardia-Bradycardia syndrome (Tachy-Brady)	Bradyarrhythmia (such as sinus bradycardia, ectopic atrial bradycardia or sinus pause) alternating with abnormal atrial tachycardia, atrial flutter or fibrillation
Chronotropic incompetence	Inability of the heart to increase its rate commensurate with the increased demand
Isorrhythmic dissociation	Atrial depolarization (from sinus node or ectopic atrial site) is slower than ventricular depolarization (from atrioventricular nodal, His Bundle or ventricular site)

be lengthy and unpredictable: the progression from bradycardia to sinoatrial block or sinus arrest can extend over an average of 13 years (range, 7–29 years) [34].

4.3.1.2 Clinical Presentation and Diagnosis

The SND recognises intrinsic causes, such as degenerative fibrosis, ion channel dysfunction and remodelling of the sinoatrial node, and extrinsic causes, that can be pharmacologic (e.g., beta-blockers and other antiarrhythmic drugs), metabolic (such as disionium, hypothyroidism, infectious processes) or autonomic. Signs and symptoms are absent or subtle in the early disease course and become more obvious as the disease progresses. They are commonly related to end-organ hypoperfusion, and cerebral hypoperfusion is the most common, with syncope or near-fainting in half of patients. Other less common symptoms are transient light-headedness, confusion, fatigue, palpitations, angina, congestive heart failure, stroke, transient ischaemic attacks, vague gastrointestinal symptoms and oliguria [35].

The diagnosis may be challenging because it must correlate symptoms of end-organ hypoperfusion with the occurrence of electrocardiographic findings of bradyarrhythmia, such as sinus bradycardia, sinoatrial pause of 3 s or more, sinoatrial exit block or sinus arrest, with or without accompanying tachyarrhythmias (the most common is the atrial fibrillation and the disease is called tachy-brady syndrome). Nevertheless, if the electrocardiogram is often normal, then prolonged cardiac monitoring may be used: for example, inpatient telemetry monitoring, outpatient Holter monitoring, event monitoring or loop recorder [36]. Electrophysiologic studies also may be used but are not routinely needed.

4.3.1.3 Therapy

The first therapy of SND is the removal of extrinsic causes when present. The only effective treatment for chronic symptomatic SND, that is not caused by correctable extrinsic factors, is the permanent pacemaker placement and it is recommended in patients with symptomatic SND and documented bradyarrhythmia [37]. Pacemaker therapy has not been shown to increase survival rates in this population and the primary goal of this treatment is to relieve symptoms and improve quality of life [38].

4.3.2 Atrioventricular Node Dysfunction

4.3.2.1 Definition, Epidemiology

Ageing results in varying degrees of calcification of the cardiac skeleton, particularly in the region including the central fibrous body and the left-sided valves (aortic and mitral valve rings): the Atrioventricular (AV) node, the AV bifurcation and the proximal left and right bundle branches are located near the central fibrous body and are thus vulnerable to slowed signal transmission with increasing age-related changes. It can result in a progressive prolongation of the PR interval with advancing age, and an overstatement of this phenomenon can manifest as, incomplete or complete, AV nodal block. The AV nodal block exists in three degrees: the electrocardiographic findings are summarised in Table 4.3.

- **First-degree AV block** is defined as a PR interval of >200 ms, representing a delay in AV conduction within the AV junction, usually within the AV node (Fig. 4.3). Studies show that the increase in mean PR interval occurred between the third and ninth decades of life, both in men and women, but the prevalence of PR prolongation is uncommon among younger population aged <60 years (1%) and it becomes more prevalent among the older population aged over 60 years, reaching up to 6% [39].
- **Second-degree AV block** that is distinguished in
  - **Mobitz type 1 second-degree AV block** that is characterised by a progressively lengthening of PR interval until complete block occurs in the AV node, resulting in a non-conducted P wave. This conduction disorder is often asymptomatic and clinically silent.
  - **Mobitz type 2 second-degree AV block** is a form of "incomplete" heart block, in which some, but not all, atrial beats are blocked before reaching the ventricles.

Table 4.3 AV nodal block degrees and electrocardiographic findings

	Electrocardiographic findings
First degree AV block	PR interval of >200 ms. PR interval has always the same duration
Mobitz type 1 second-degree AV block	PR interval progressively increase, until a P wave is not conducted (there's no QRS complex after the P wave, but a pause)
Mobitz type 2 second-degree AV block	Some P wave, but not all are blocked: after P wave there's not a QRS complex, but a pause. PR interval has always the same duration
2:1 AV block	One P wave is conducted and the following is blocked in a repetitive way
Second-degree AV block, type 2 advanced	More than two P wave are blocked and one of is conducted in a repetitive way
High degree AV block	Complete dissociation between P wave and QRS complex

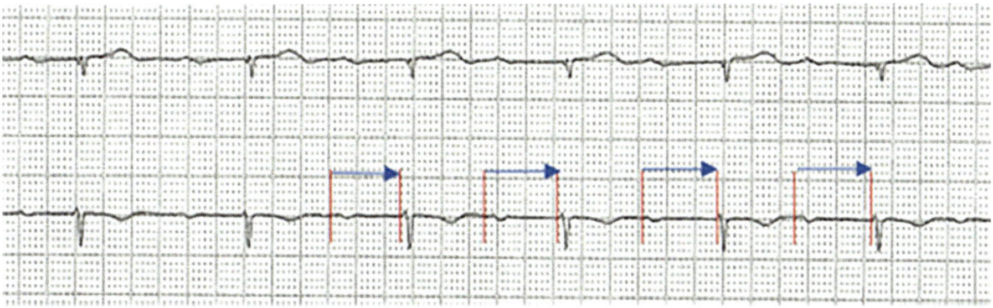

Fig. 4.3 First-degree AV block: the PR intervals (blue arrows) are >200 ms, and they have the same duration

- **2:1 AV block** is a form of "incomplete" heart block, in which the P waves are alternately conducted and blocked.
- **Second-degree AV block, type II advanced** is a form of "incomplete" heart block, in which more than two P waves are consecutively blocked.

There have not been large population-based studies on the prevalence of Mobitz type 1 or 2 atrioventricular blocks. At this time, there is no associated age, racial or gender correlation. AV block is sometimes seen in athletes and in patients with congenital heart disorders.

- **High-degree AV block** (HAVB) is the most severe because in this type of block, electrical signals do not pass from atria to ventricles at all for periods of time, and there is a complete failure of electrical conduction (Fig. 4.4). This results in a complete dissociation between atrial rhythm and ventricular rhythm with severe bradyarrhythmia. The prevalence of third-degree atrioventricular block in this population is low, but this disease accounts for approximately 40% of all implanted pacemakers [40].

His-Purkinje conduction abnormalities can result in two forms of bundle branch block: **Right bundle branch block**, often without concurrent clinical heart disease, and **Left bundle branch block**, that is more specific for the presence of cardiovascular disease, such as hypertension, cardiac enlargement, cardiomyopathy, or coronary heart disease [41].

4.3.2.2 Clinical Presentation and Diagnosis

The most part of the atrioventricular node dysfunctions are asymptomatic. Symptoms are related to end-organ hypoperfusion, and they are evident in advanced form of AV block (HAVB and Mobitz type 2 second-degree): syncope, near-fainting, transient light-headedness, confusion, fatigue, palpitations, angina, congestive heart failure, stroke, transient ischaemic attacks, vague gastrointestinal symptoms and oliguria. HAVB may occur either as an isolated diagnosis in the elderly, often in the setting of hypertension and/or diabetes mellitus, or as a complication following

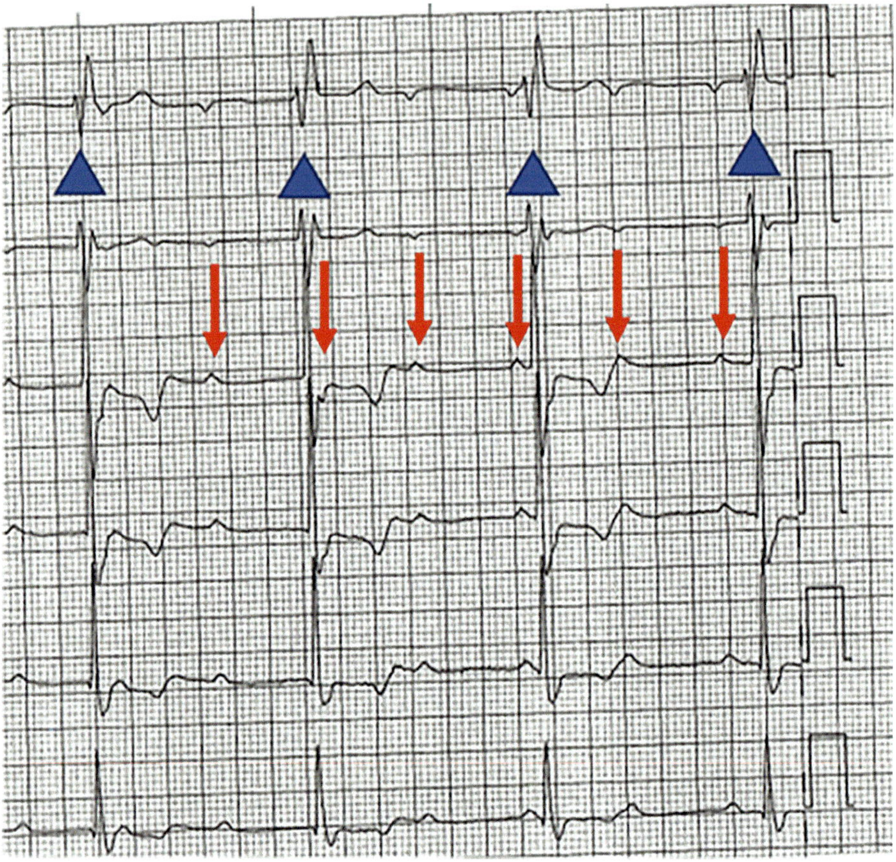

Fig. 4.4 A High-degree AV block: there is a dissociation between atrial rhythm (red arrows) and ventricular rhythm (blue triangles)

acute myocardial infarction, cardiac surgery, endocarditis or other cardiac injury. Atrioventricular node dysfunctions are diagnosed recording the heart's electrical activity through an electrocardiogram or a prolonged cardiac monitoring should be considered in patients with symptoms of peripheral hypoperfusion [42].

In 50% of patients, the AV nodal block is caused by fibrosis ageing-related, but in other cases, they have other causes, such as ischaemic coronary heart disease, drugs (beta-blockers, calcium channel blockers, amiodarone, digoxin), valvular disease, electrolytes disorders. Therefore, possible and removable causes must be investigated. Laboratory tests, such as thyroid function tests, potassium, calcium, renal function and high-sensitive Troponin, are useful to exclude myocardial infarction or electrolyte's disorders. Transthoracic Echocardiography (TTE) is important in order to detect myocardial contraction, the pericardium, and the presence and severity of valvular pathology and endocarditis. Screening for sleep apnoea syndrome (SAS) is recommended in patients with symptoms of SAS and in the presence of severe bradycardia or advanced AV block during sleep.

4.3.2.3 Therapy

The first therapy of AV nodal blocks is the treatment of removable causes, if present. Patients with asymptomatic first-degree AV block require no further treatment. Usually, the prognosis is good in the absence of structural heart disease, and progression to a high-degree block is uncommon.

Mobitz Type 1 second-degree AV block has a benign course, and the risk of progression to type II or a higher degree of AV block is low. Generally, it does not need therapy; permanent pacemaker placement should be considered in patients with symptoms AV block-related.

Permanent pacemaker placement is indicated in patients with permanent or paroxysmal HAVB or Mobitz Type 2 second-degree AV block or second-degree AV block type 2 advanced, that are not caused by correctable extrinsic factors, irrespective of symptoms [42].

4.4 Tachyarrhythmias

4.4.1 Atrial Fibrillation

4.4.1.1 Definition, Epidemiology

Atrial fibrillation (AF) is an atrial arrhythmia characterised by a high rate of irregular activation of atria (with ineffective atrial contraction) and a variable conduction to ventricle with typical irregularity of R-R interval.

AF is the most frequently arrhythmia diagnosed in clinical practice, and it is an important cause of hospitalisation. The prevalence is about 2–4% of the adult population, with an increase of incidence with older age (age is the principal risk factor for AF with a hazard ratio that rises from 4.98 to 9.33, passing from 60 to 80 years) [43].

4.4.1.2 Clinical Presentation and Diagnosis

AF generally cause symptoms like palpitations, dyspnoea and fatigue, in some cases, can be asymptomatic and accidentally diagnosed.

AF can be supposed by a clinical visit that documented irregular cardiac activity, but a definite diagnosis is made with ECG, which documents irregular R-R interval and absence of P waves (Fig. 4.5).

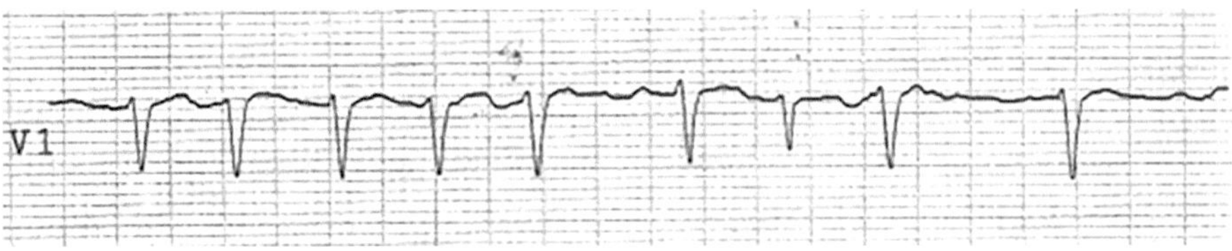

Fig. 4.5 Atrial fibrillation

Considering the socio-sanitary impact of AF, several tools have been developed to discover this arrhythmia specially in asymptomatic patients (silent AF). These tools vary from the "classic" Holter-ECG (24–48 h of heart rhythm monitoring), event recorder (from 1 week to 1 month of heart rhythm monitoring) and internal loop recorder (ILR) (until 5 years of heart rhythm monitoring) to the new "smart-tools" integrated in patients smart-phone or smart-watch (photoplethysmogram or single lead ECG technology).

Other diagnostic tools are important not to diagnose AF but to characterise AF patients. Transthoracic Echocardiography (TTE) is indispensable to detect myocardial contraction, chamber size (specially left atrial (LA) volume) and the presence and severity of valvular pathology. Transesophageal Echocardiography (TEE) is used to assess the presence of left atrial (LA) or left atrial appendage (LAA) thrombi before a non-datable AF cardioversion. Polysomnography can be used to diagnose sleep apnoea syndrome triggering AF in some patients [43–45].

4.4.1.3 Therapy

Therapy of AF is based on two objectives: (1) cardio-embolic prevention and (2) symptom control.

AF is an arrhythmia characterised by ineffective atrial contraction and the increased risk of thrombus formation especially in LAA, where blood flow is slower. CHA_2DS_2VASc score [Congestive heart failure (1 point), Hypertension (1 point), Age more than 75 (2 points), Diabetes (1 point), previous Stroke or TIA (2 points), vascular disease (1 point), Age more than 65 (1 point), Sex category female (1 point)] is the point system used to estimate cardio-embolic risk. The cardio-embolic rate in AF patients increases progressively from 1.3%/year ($CHA_2DS_2VASc = 1$) to 15.2%/year ($CHA_2DS_2VASc = 9$). If the CHA_2DS_2VASc score is greater than or equal to 2 (or 3 for female patients), there is a strong indication to long-life oral anticoagulant therapy (Class I, level of evidence A). If the CHA_2DS_2VASc score is 0 (or 1 for female patients), there is no indication of oral anticoagulant therapy (I, A). If the CHA_2DS_2VASc score is 1 (or 2 for female patients), there is a less strong indication to oral anticoagulation therapy (IIa, B) and therapy should be individualised. Direct oral anticoagulation (DOAc) drugs can be used in patients with non-valvular AF (no mechanical valvular prosthesis or mitral stenosis more than moderate) and without severe renal impairment. There are four drugs available:

three drugs are Xa factor direct inhibitors (Apixaban, Rivaroxaban and Edoxaban) and one drug is a direct thrombin inhibitor (Dabigatran). For patients with valvular AF or severe renal impairment, oral anticoagulation therapy is made by vitamin K antagonist (VKA). When possible, the use of DOAc is preferred to VKA for a better risk-benefit ratio. LAA occlusion (surgical or percutaneous) is an alternative way to reduce stroke risk when long-term anticoagulant therapy is contraindicated.

Symptom control can be achieved by a rhythm control strategy or by a rate control strategy. Rhythm control strategy is superior to the rate control strategy only in symptom relief, but not in mortality [43].

Rhythm control strategy provides the sinus rhythm by electrical or pharmacological cardioversion and the sinus rhythm maintenance by antiarrhythmic drugs (AAD) or AF ablation. In hemodynamically unstable patients, AF electrical cardioversion can be done as soon as possible regardless of anticoagulation state (emergency cardioversion). In hemodynamically stable patients, AF cardioversion (pharmacological or electrical) can be done if AF is recent onset (<48 h) or after 3 weeks of optimal anticoagulant therapy or after a TEE that excludes the presence of LA or LAA thrombi. After cardioversion, 1 month of anticoagulation therapy is recommended in patients without cardio-embolic risk factors. For maintenance, sinus rhythm can be used in AAD (see Table 4.4) or AF ablation [43, 45].

Rate control strategies have the only objective to control HR during AF. The principal class of drugs used are beta-blockers, NDHP-CCB and digoxin. Beta-blockers and NDHP-CCB are the most effective drugs; digoxin alone has no effect in high sympathetic tone patients and is usually used in association with the other drug classes. Beta-blockers are preferred in patients with left ventricular systolic dysfunction; instead, NDHP-CCB is preferred in patients with asthma or chronic obstructive pulmonary disease. The target of the rate control strategy is an HR of less than 110 bpm (lenient strategy) or less than 80 bpm (strict strategy) if symptoms persist [43].

Table 4.4 Antiarrhythmic drugs

	Mild or absent structural heart disease	**Structural heart disease**		
		• *Significant left ventricular hypertrophy*	*Heart failure with reduced ejection fraction (HFrEF)*	
		• *Significant heart valve disease*	*NYHA I o II*	*NYHA III o IV o unstable*
		• *Heart failure with preserved ejection fraction (HFpEF)*		
		• *Ischemic cardiopathy*		
Antiarrhythmic drugs	Flecainide Propafenone Dronedarone Sotalol	Amiodarone Dronedarone Sotalol	Dronedarone Amiodarone	Amiodarone

4.4.2 *Ventricular Tachycardias*

4.4.2.1 Definition, Epidemiology

Ventricular tachycardia (VT) is a tachyarrhythmia that originates from ventricular myocardium cells or from the conduction system distal to His bundle bifurcation. VT is a series of three or more ventricular beats [46].

Sudden cardiac death (the extreme consequence of VT) is approximately 25% of total cardiovascular death. It is more frequent in men than in women (6.68 vs. 1.40 per 100,000 person-years) [47].

VT can be associated with structural heart disease (myocardial infarction, myocarditis, cardiomyopathies, valvular heart disease and heart failure), with channelopathies (long QT syndrome, short QT syndrome, Brugada syndrome, catecholaminergic polymorphic ventricular tachycardia) or in healthy heart (idiopathic VT) [46, 47].

4.4.2.2 Clinical Presentation and Diagnosis

Palpitations, presyncope/syncope or cardiac arrest are the more frequent clinical presentation of VT.

Diagnosis is based on ECG that shows a tachyarrhythmia with a wide QRS complex (more than 120 ms) (Fig. 4.6). QRS morphology can be constant (monomorphic VT) or variable (polymorphic VT). Duration less or more than 30 s distinguishes between non-sustained or sustained VT. Differential diagnosis must be done with supraventricular tachycardias (SVT) with conduction aberrance (ECG difference between VT and SVT with conduction aberrance is not the aim of this chapter). ECG without VT is important to find specific heart disease signs, for example, Q waves or ST-T ischaemic alteration can suggest an ischaemic heart disease, ECG signs of left ventricular hypertrophy can suggest a cardiomyopathy or a valvular heart disease, alteration of QT duration can suggest long QT or short QT syndrome or a coved ST elevation in right precordial leads can suggest a Brugada pattern.

Other diagnostic tools to diagnose VT are all ECG recording systems: Holter-ECG (24–48 h), event recorder (7–30 days) and ILR (until 5 years). These diagnostic tools are generally used in patients with syncope to find, if present, an arrhythmic cause.

Echocardiography, cardiac magnetic resonance, single photon emission computed tomography (SPECT-TC), and coronary angiography are important diagnostic tools for studying heart structure and function. Electrophysiological study with electro-anatomical mapping can help to diagnose VT mechanism and, in some cases, it can also be used to try VT ablation [46].

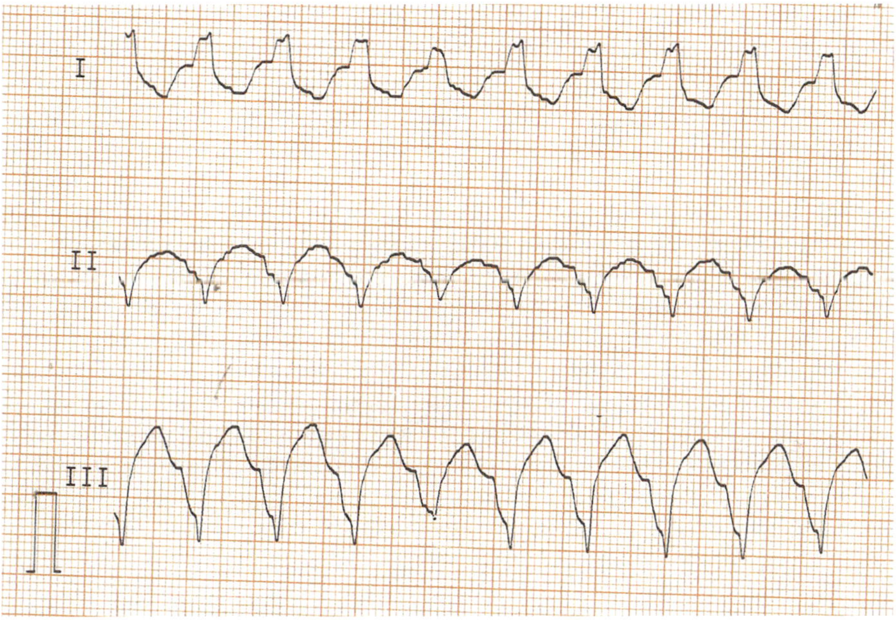

Fig. 4.6 Ventricular tachycardias

4.4.2.3 Therapy

Acute therapy: in hemodynamically stable VT, the first line of treatment is patient sedation and direct electrical cardioversion. Therapy with AAD can be tried to interrupt arrhythmia. Drugs used are procainamide or flecainide in patients without heart failure or myocardial infarction, amiodarone or lidocaine in heart failure or myocardial infarction patients and beta-blockers or NDHP-CCBs only in fascicular VT. Magnesium sulphate is useful in case of polymorphic VT (torsades de pointes). In hemodynamically unstable VT or in pulseless VT, patients are treated by cardiopulmonary resuscitation protocol with cardiac massage and early defibrillation. Patients with an electrical storm (more than three episodes in 1 day) find benefit with sedation therapy, probably due to reduced adrenergic tone [47].

Chronic therapy: The most important therapy that shows survival improvement is the implantable cardioverter defibrillator (ICD). ICD is indicated in secondary prevention (patient survived a previous cardiac arrest or at a sustained VT) or in primary prevention in a specific high-risk setting (very low ejection fraction or specific high-risk heart disease) when ICD benefit exceeds the risks (implant complications, device infection, inappropriate shock). ICD protects patients from sudden cardiac death but does not prevent arrhythmic events [47]. To reduce arrhythmic episodes, drug therapy can be used. Beta-blockers are the only AAD class that show a reduction in mortality. The effect of beta-blockers is mediated by the reduction sympathetically mediated trigger, possible reduction of intracellular calcium released by ryanodine receptor channels and reduced sinus rate. Beta-blockers are used in patients with or without heart failure, in ischaemic heart disease and in specific heart pathology like arrhythmogenic cardiomyopathies, long QT syndrome and catecholaminergic polymorphic ventricular tachycardia. This antiadrenergic therapy is particularly effective in ischaemic heart disease and in long QT syndrome. Beta-blockers therapy or left cardiac sympathetic denervation (LCSD) reduces sudden cardiac death risk from 22 to 3%. LCDS is a surgical method to decrease adrenergic heart stimulus and is used specially in long QT syndrome and catecholaminergic polymorphic ventricular tachycardia when beta-blockers are ineffective or not tolerated or when ICD is refused [47, 48]. Amiodarone is a class III AAD that reduces arrhythmic episodes by influencing automaticity and re-entry. Amiodarone can be used safely in patients with structural heart disease. Other AADs that can be used in specific settings are sotalol, mexiletine and flecainide. VT catheter ablation can be a good alternative to eliminate arrhythmic substrate, especially in patients with structural heart disease and fibrotic myocardial areas who sustained a re-entry mechanism. Ablation can be made in endocardium or in epicardium or both sites [47].

References

1. Goldberger JJ, Arora R, Buckley U, Shivkumar K. Autonomic nervous system dysfunction: JACC focus seminar. J Am Coll Cardiol. 2019;73(10):1189–206.
2. Armour JA, Murphy DA, Yuan BX, MacDonald S, Hopkins DA. Gross and microscopic anatomy of the human intrinsic cardiac nervous system. Anat Rec. 1997;247:289–98.
3. Randll DC, Brown DR, McGuirt AS, Thompson GW, Armour JA, Ardell JL. Interaction within the intrinsic cardiac nervous system contribute to chronotropic regulation. Am J Physiol Regul Integr Comp Physiol. 2003;285:R1066–75.
4. Bluemel KM, Wurster RD, Randall WC, Duff MJ, O'Toole MF. Parasympathetic postganglionic pathways to the sinoatrial node. Am J Physiol Heart Circ Physiol. 1990;259:H1504–10.
5. Mick JD, Wurster RD, Duff MJ, Weber M, Randall WC, Randall DC. Epicardial sites for vagal mediation of sinoatrial function. Am J Physiol Heart Circ Physiol. 1992;262:H1401–6.
6. Malliani A, Recordati G, Schwartz PJ. Nervous activity of afferent cardiac sympathetic fibres with atrial and ventricular endings. J Physiol. 1973;229:457–69.
7. Shivkumar K, et al. Clinical neurocardiology defining the value of neuroscience-based cardiovascular therapeutics. J Physiol. 2016;594(14):3911–54.
8. Kember G, Armour JA, Zamir M. Neural control hierarchy of the heart has not evolved to deal with myocardial ischemia. Physiol Genomics. 2013;45:638–44.
9. Armour JA. Cardiac neuronal hierarchy in health and disease. Am J Physiol Regul Integr Comp Physiol. 2004;287:R262–71.
10. Hopkins DA, Bieger D, deVente J, Steinbusch WM. Vagal efferent projections: viscerotopy, neurochemistry and effects of vagotomy. Prog Brain Res. 1996;107:79–96.
11. Ardell JL, Rajendran PS, Nier HA, KenKnight BH, Armour JA. Central-peripheral neural network interactions evoked by vagus nerve stimulation: functional consequences on control of cardiac function. Am J Physiol Heart Circ Physiol. 2015;309:H1740–52.
12. Norris JE, Lippincott D, Wurster RD. Responses of canine endocardium to stimulation of the upper thoracic roots. Am J Physiol Heart Circ Physiol. 1977;233:H655–9.

13. Angelakos E, King M, Millard R. Regional distribution of catecholamines in the heart of various species. Ann N Y Acad Sci. 1969;156:219–40.
14. Olshansky B, Sabbah HN, Hauptman PJ, Colucci WS. Parasympathetic nervous system and heart failure: pathophysiology and potential implications for therapy. Circulation. 2008;118(8):863–71.
15. Rubart M, Zipes DP. Mechanisms of sudden cardiac death. J Clin Invest. 2005;115:2305–15.
16. Bristow M. Changes in myocardial and vascular receptors in heart failure. J Am Coll Cardiol. 1993;22:61A–71A.
17. Gauthier C, Leblais V, Kobzik L, et al. The negative inotropic effect of beta3-adrenoceptor stimulation is mediated by activation of a nitric oxide synthase pathway in human ventricle. J Clin Invest. 1998;102:1377–84.
18. Raffel DM, Wieland DM. Assessment of cardiac sympathetic nerve integrity with positron emission tomography. Nucl Med Biol. 2001;28:541–59.
19. Shen MJ, Zipes DP. Role of the autonomic nervous system in modulating cardiac arrhythmias. Circ Res. 2014;114:1004–21.
20. Lingjin M, Kalyanam S, Olujimi A. Autonomic regulation and ventricular arrhythmias. Curr Treat Options Cardio Med. 2018;20:38.
21. Vaseghi M, Shivkumar K. The role of the autonomic nervous system in sudden cardiac death. Prog Cardiovasc Dis. 2008;50(6):404–19.
22. Rundqvist B, Elam M, Bergman-Sverrisdottir Y, Eisenhofer G, Friberg P. Increased cardiac adrenergic drive precedes generalized sympathetic activation in human heart failure. Circulation. 1997;95:169–75.
23. Brugada J, Katritsis DG, Arbelo E, et al. 2019 ESC guidelines for the management of patients with supraventricular tachycardia. Eur Heart J. 2020;41(5):655–720.
24. Mann DL, Zipes DP, Libby P, Bonow RO, Braunwald E. Braunwald's heart disease: a textbook of cardiovascular medicine. Philadelphia, PA: Elsevier/Saunders; 2015. p. 751–2.
25. Still AM, Raatikainen P, Ylitalo A, et al. Prevalence, characteristics and natural course of inappropriate sinus tachycardia. Europace. 2005;7:104–12.
26. Ptaszynski P, Kaczmarek K, Klingenheben T, et al. Noninvasive assessment of autonomic cardiovascular activity in patients with inappropriate sinus tachycardia. Am J Cardiol. 2013;112:811e815.
27. Nwazue VC, Paranjape SY, Black BK, et al. Postural tachycardia syndrome and inappropriate sinus tachycardia: role of autonomic modulation and sinus node automaticity. J Am Heart Assoc. 2014;3:e000700.
28. Morill CA, Klein GJ, Thakur RK, et al. Mechanism of 'inappropriate' sinus tachycardia. Role of sympathovagal balance. Circulation. 1994;90:873–7.
29. Kusumoto FM, Schoenfeld MH, Coletta B, et al. 2018 ACC/AHA/HRS guideline on the evaluation and management of patients with bradycardia and cardiac conduction delay. J Am Coll Cardiol. 2019;74(7):e51–156.
30. Clarke JM, Hamer J, Shelton JR, et al. The rhythm of the normal human heart. Lancet. 1976;1:508–12.
31. Guilleminault C, Connolly SJ, Winkle RA. Cardiac arrhythmia and conduction disturbances during sleep in 400 patients with sleep apnea syndrome. Am J Cardiol. 1983;52:490–4.
32. Stegman SS, Burroughs JM, Henthorn RW. Asymptomatic bradyarrhythmias as a marker for sleep apnea: appropriate recognition and treatment may reduce the need for pacemaker therapy. Pacing Clin Electrophysiol. 1996;19:899–904.
33. Jensen PN, Gronroos NN, Chen LY, Folsom AR, deFilippi C, Heckbert SR, Alonso A. Incidence of and risk factors for sick sinus syndrome in the general population. J Am Coll Cardiol. 2014;64:531–8.
34. Semelka M, Gera J, Usman S. Sick sinus syndrome: a review. Am Fam Physician. 2013;87(10):691–6.
35. Adán V, Crown LA. Diagnosis and treatment of sick sinus syndrome. Am Fam Physician. 2003;67(8):1725–32.

36. Zimetbaum P, Goldman A. Ambulatory arrhythmia monitoring: choosing the right device. Circulation. 2010;122(16):1629–36.
37. Stockburger M, Trautmann F, Nitardy A, et al. Pacemaker-based analysis of atrioventricular conduction and atrial tachyarrhythmias in patients with primary sinus node dysfunction. Pacing Clin Electrophysiol. 2009;32(5):604–13.
38. Masumoto H, Ueda Y, Kato R, et al. Long-term clinical performance of AAI pacing in patients with sick sinus syndrome: a comparison with dual-chamber pacing. Europace. 2004;6(5):444–50.
39. Perlman LV, Ostrander LD, Keller JB, Chiang BN. An epidemiologic study of first degree atrioventricular block in Tecumseh, Michigan. Chest. 1971;59:40–6.
40. Kojic EM, Hardarson T, Sigfusson N, Sigvaldason H. The prevalence and prognosis of third-degree atrioventricular conduction block: The Reykjavik study. J Intern Med. 1999;246(1):81–6.
41. Chow GV, Marine JE, Fleg JL. Epidemiology of arrhythmias and conduction disorders in older adults. Clin Geriatr Med. 2012;28(4):539–53.
42. Glikson M, et al. ESC Guidelines on cardiac pacing and cardiac resynchronization therapy (2021). Eur Heart J. 2021;42(35):3427–520.
43. Hindricks G, Potpara T, Dagres N, et al. 2020 ESC Guidelines for the diagnosis and management of atrial fibrillation developed in collaboration with the European Association for Cardio-Thoracic Surgery (EACTS). Eur Heart J. 2020;42:373–498.
44. Mann DL, Zipes DP, Libby P, Bonow RO, Braunwald E. Braunwald's heart disease: a textbook of cardiovascular medicine. Philadelphia, PA: Elsevier/Saunders; 2015. p. 798–812.
45. Ricciotti J, Menditto A. Atrial fibrillation and related disorders. In: Capucci A, editor. Clinical cases in cardiology. Cham: Springer; 2015. p. 227–39.
46. Mann DL, Zipes DP, Libby P, Bonow RO, Braunwald E. Braunwald's heart disease: a textbook of cardiovascular medicine. Philadelphia, PA: Elsevier/Saunders; 2015. p. 773–90.
47. Priori SG, Blomstrom-Lundqvist C, Mazzanti A, et al. 2015 ESC guidelines for the management of patients with ventricular arrhythmias and the prevention of sudden cardiac death. Eur Heart J. 2015;36(41):2757–9.
48. Schwartz PJ, Verrier RL. Autonomic nervous system: emerging concepts and clinical applications. In: Priori SG, Zipes DP, editors. Sudden cardiac death: a handbook for clinical practice. Malden, MA: Blackwell Publishing; 2006. p. 62–70.

Chapter 5
Autonomic Nervous System and Cerebrovascular Diseases

Giuseppe Micieli, Isabella Canavero, Federico Mazzacane, and Anna Cavallini

5.1 Introduction

Autonomic nervous system and cerebrovascular pathology are closely interconnected topics, and from different perspectives: from anatomic and physiological bases to diagnostic and management implications, to therapeutic potential in pathological conditions. Autonomic functions underlie a coordinated but complex organization that is often difficult to study, especially in the presence of concomitant acute or chronic 'disturbing' factors that can often occusr in patients with cerebrovascular diseases [1–6].

5.2 Cerebral Autoregulation

When examining the relationship between autonomic nervous system and cerebrovascular pathology, it is essential to take into account the physiological peculiarities of the cerebral circulation, which in particular is characterized by the phenomenon of cerebral autoregulation (AR), i.e., the mechanism by which the *cerebral blood flow* (CBF) is kept constant when systemic arterial blood pressure remains in the range between 50 and 150 mmHg [7], and also for values above or below this range in some populations (e.g. patients with chronic hypo- or hypertension) [7–11]. CBF

G. Micieli (✉)
Department of Emergency Neurology, C. Mondino Neurological Institute, Pavia, Italy

I. Canavero
Cerebrovascular Unit, Fondazione IRCCS Istituto Neurologico Carlo Besta, Milan, Italy
e-mail: isabella.canavero@istituto-besta.it

F. Mazzacane · A. Cavallini
Stroke Unit, C. Mondino Neurological Institute and Policlinico San Matteo, Pavia, Italy
e-mail: federico.mazzacane01@universitadipavia.it; anna.cavallini@mondino.it

G. Micieli et al. (eds.), *Autonomic Disorders in Clinical Practice*,
https://doi.org/10.1007/978-3-031-43036-7_5

depends on *arterial blood pressure* (ABP), cerebral venous pressure (tends to coincide with *intracranial pressure (*ICP)) and *cerebrovascular resistance* (CVR), according to the formula CBF = (ABP − ICP) / CVR [7, 11, 12].

These criteria, however, essentially define a “static” model of autoregulation as described by Lassen [7], that subsequently has been furtherly characterized and now is known to be a more “dynamic” mechanism, potentially modified by several factors influencing the CBF during rapid changes in BP (seconds or minutes) [13] (Table 5.1).

In fact, a dynamic model of AR has the capacity to buffer changes in CBF, but it is strongly dependent on the speed of BP changes [14].

The slower the change in BP, the smaller the impact on CBF, up to a point after which CBF becomes almost unaffected. However, for more rapid changes in BP, the buffering capacity is progressively reduced, and changes in CBF become larger, up to a point after which changes in CBF become as large as the change in BP, so that CBF “passively” follows BP.

To skip a more detailed description of cerebral AR, that is not the principle aim of this text, let’s just state that the control that AR plays on CBF values to ensure an adequate functioning of brain structures is evident, together with the regulation of blood pressure at the microvascular level and the protection of the blood-brain barrier (BBB), targeted to protecting, by adequate self-regulation, both cognitive and noncognitive functions.

On the contrary, an alteration of AR (acute or chronic) can be observed in different pathological conditions, such as hypoperfusion or stroke, syncope, hyperperfusion syndromes, pressure alteration at the microvascular level, loss of BBB integrity with the appearance of edema, hemorrhage and/or micro bleedings.

The cerebrovascular system is richly innervated by adrenergic and cholinergic fibers, with a complex organization that can be simplified by subdividing the extrinsic innervation of the extraparenchymal arteries (from the cervical, otic, sphenopalatine, and trigeminal ganglia) from the intrinsic innervation of the

Table 5.1 Main modifiers of cerebral autoregulation

• Hemodynamics
• O_2, CO_2, pH
• Endothelium
• Neurons
• Metabolism
• Vascular stiffness
• Vascular structure
• Behavior
• Posture
• Genetics
• Temperature
• Vascular risk factors
• Vascular disease

Table 5.2 Extrinsic innervation of the cerebral circulation [15, 16]

	Autonomic innervation	
System	Ganglion	Transmitter
Sympathetic	Superior cervical	Epinephrine, norepinephrine, dopamine Neuropeptide Y
Parasympathetic	Otic, sphenopalatine	Acetylcholine, vasoactive intestinal polypeptide
Sensory (trigeminal)	Trigeminal	Calcitonin gene-related peptide, substance P, pituitary adenylate cyclase-activity peptide

intraparenchymal arterioles (from the truncus encephalic nuclei: locus coeruleus, nucleus of the fastigial, nucleus of the dorsal raphe).

The main sympathetic neurotransmitter is norepinephrine (NA): in the cerebral circulation, α1-adrenergic receptors are the most represented at the postsynaptic level, while α2-adrenoceptors are mainly located at the presynaptic terminal. NA release causes vasoconstriction through vascular smooth muscle contraction mediated by α1-adrenergic receptors, whereas activation of α2-adrenoceptors inhibits further NA release from the presynaptic neuron [17], creating local negative feedback that is useful in regulating NA release. The reactivity of α-adrenergic receptors proportionally decreases with the reduction in caliber of cerebral afferent vessels, being greatest at the level of large-caliber extracranial arteries, progressively decreasing through intracranial arteries, then lowest for small pial arterioles. The β-adrenergic receptors are also located post (β-1) and presynaptically (β-2), and are mainly involved in vasodilatory mechanisms (Table 5.2) [18–22].

A contemporary model of autoregulation, derived from the intra-patient reanalysis of 41 studies, shows essentially a reduction of the plateau and a substantial increase in the passive pressure-CBF ratio, i.e. a more effective buffering property against pressure increases or decreases [23].

Beyond acting on the control of vascular caliber, cerebral blood flow, and cerebrovascular resistance, autonomic fibers determine changes in arterial and venous pressure parameters, thus acting also indirectly on CBF regulation. Although the contribution of the sympathetic nervous system to the resting state is estimated to be modest, its role during rapid and/or acute increases in arterial BP is very important. Several studies seem to confirm that it contributes to CBF autoregulation [24], and during acute hypertension, its vasoconstrictor effect buffers surges in microvascular pressure, thus contributing to CBF, and ideally BBB, preservation of CBF [25, 26]. Other studies suggest that intracerebral vascular response induced by cold pressor test (i.e., a marked pressure reduction obtained by pretreatment with clonidine, that is a central alpha2-agonist) may rely on a central noradrenergic mechanism, which is possibly modulated at the locus coeruleus level [27] (Fig. 5.1). The generalized sympathetic discharge determines increases in ABP and can prevent concomitant increases in CBF by acting on both small and large vessels' resistance and compliance [28].

Transient systemic hypotension is accompanied in experimental models by a sympathetic-mediated response leading to vasoconstriction of cerebral afferent

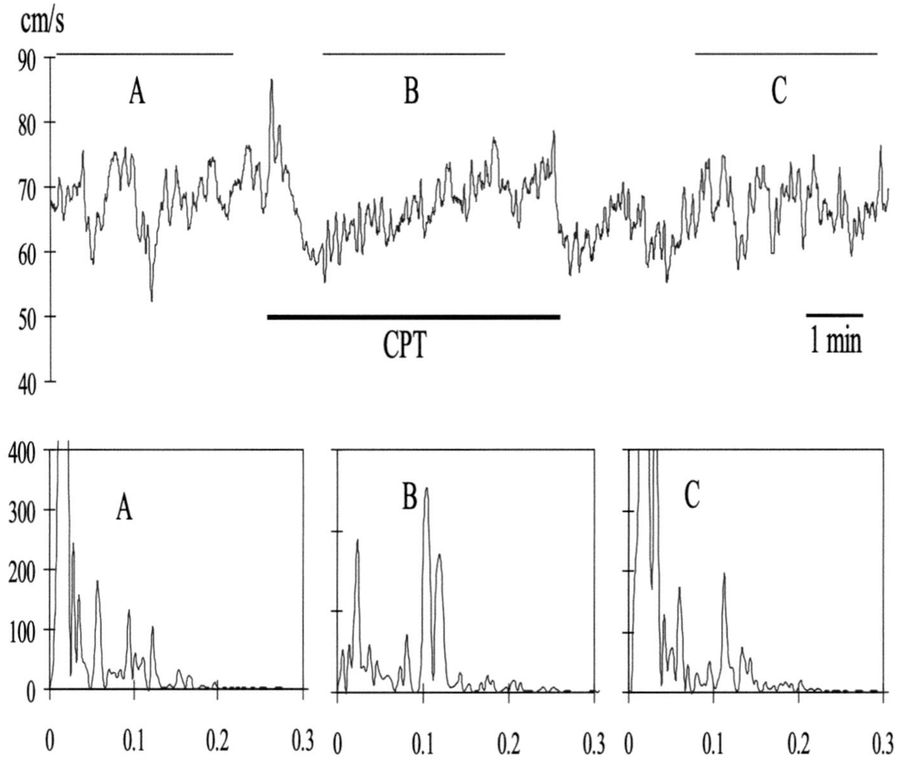

Fig. 5.1 Effect of cold pressor test on blood flow velocity in Middle Cerebral Artery (MCA): time course and power spectra [G Micieli, 1994, personal communication]. In the figure, Middle Cerebral Artery (MCA) blood flow velocity, registered by means of Transcranial Doppler ultrasounds, shows a marked reduction during (prolonged: 5 min) cold pressor test, whereas the frequent oscillations in flow velocity can be attributable to rapid change induced in AR during the exercise

arteries [29, 30]. Of note, AR appears to be better adapted to transient increases in BP rather than reduction, a phenomenon also known as hysteresis [31].

Despite the anatomical presence of cholinergic nerve terminals throughout intracranial vessels, located proximal to Virchow-Robin spaces, the exact role of parasympathetic nervous system in the regulation of CBF in not clear [32, 33]. It seems to influence parenchymal neurons and the vasculature by releasing their neurotransmitters, whereas cholinergic projections induce the local release of NO [34] and the intrinsic system can be influenced by cholinergic or anticholinergic drugs.

In addition, the trigeminal sensory system represents an emerging subject in CBF autoregulation, mainly through the release of the potent Calcitonin gene-related neuropeptide (CGRP), which is currently thought to mediate most of the effects of the trigeminal nerve on vascular tone. However, despite the emerging role of trigeminal sensory nerves in acute conditions like severe hypertension, the influence of this neural system on resting CBF is estimated to be minimal [35].

In addition to neurogenic control, several other factors may affect AR and, thus, CBF: myogenic vasomotor response, arterial partial pressures of oxygen and carbon dioxide, and cerebral metabolism [23]. More specifically, partial pressures of gasses determine changes mainly in the arterial vessels with larger caliber, while the pial and cortical vessels appear to be more sensitive to variations in systemic pressure parameters and local neural stimuli.

Several pathological conditions are associated with CBF alterations because of various dysregulation phenomena, such as cerebral ischemia, both acute and "chronic" (due to atherosclerosis with hemodynamic repercussions, or small vessel disease) [9, 36–38], and late ischemic damage after subarachnoid hemorrhage [39, 40]. While the myogenic tone is the predominant component of AR under physiological conditions, it may be overridden by other factors promoting increased vascular tone under pathological conditions, such as cerebral vasospasm [1, 40, 41]. In these specific contexts, therapeutic intervention could aim to impede sympathetic tone.

The study of AR in response to vasoactive stimuli and, in particular, clinical contexts beyond the traditional neurosonological methods (Transcranial Doppler) could also take advantage of high-resolution magnetic resonance imaging techniques dedicated to the study of tissue perfusion parameters [1, 39].

5.3 Autonomic Nervous System and Cerebrovascular Diseases: Anatomical Peculiarities

Often, the interconnection between autonomic dysfunction and cerebrovascular pathology is also a direct consequence of close anatomic-functional contiguity [41]. In fact, in addition to the centers located within the neuraxis [41], several autonomic structures are characteristically located close to the course of the cerebral afferent vessels, thus being potentially susceptible to damage in the event of pathological phenomena affecting the latter, giving rise to some characteristic clinical syndromes whose early diagnostic recognition is crucial to set up their proper management [1–6, 42].

Indeed, in some cases, signs of autonomic dysfunction may be the only clinical expression of potentially dangerous cerebrovascular pathologies, such as aneurysms and arterial dissections [43–45].

Oculo-sympathetic fibers run along the walls of the internal carotid artery, forming the internal pericarotic plexus, and then distributing to the deep structures of the eye (superior tarsal muscle and pupil dilator muscle), interconnecting with the trigeminal ganglion, the abducens nerve, the sphenopalatine ganglion, and the tympanic branch of the glossopharyngeal nerve. The vaso- and sudomotor fibers separate at the carotid bifurcation. The sympathetic fibers directed to innervate the ipsilateral arterial vessels and the sweat glands of the medial portion of the forehead and nose run along the internal carotid artery, while the fibers directed to the remaining facial areas run along the external carotid artery.

Horner's syndrome includes a combination of dysautonomic signs due to damage to the ipsilateral oculosympathetic trunk. In its full expression, it is characterized by the presence of miosis (due to inactivation of the pupil dilator muscle), eyelid ptosis with enophthalmos (due to inactivation of the superior tarsal muscle), and anhidrosis (due to inactivation of the sudomotor fibers). Sometimes, ipsilateral flushing is present, due to vasodilation of the skin vessels by interruption of the vasomotor sympathetic fibers [44]. Pathologies such as cavernous sinus thrombosis and carotid dissection may produce disruption of the peri-carotid sympathetic pathway, leading to the appearance of incomplete Horner's syndrome without anhidrosis. In addition to neurological examination findings, anamnestic data and accompanying symptoms (mode of onset, associated symptoms such as headache, neck pain and cranial nerve palsy) may help guide the diagnostic pathway.

The *harlequin sign* is characterized by flushing with unilateral facial hyperhidrosis. It may be a consequence of both pre- and postganglionic damage to the vaso- and sudomotor fibers, resulting in pallor and anhydrous hemiface, and has been reported for example in association with carotid dissections, although less frequently than Horner's syndrome [45].

On the parasympathetic side, of cerebrovascular interest is the case of the third cranial or oculomotor nerve, whose Edinger-Westphal nucleus provides parasympathetic fibers directed to the eye to control the pupil sphincter muscle (which controls pupillary constriction) and the ciliary muscle (which controls accommodation). After emergence from the brainstem, the oculomotor passes between the superior cerebellar artery and the posterior cerebral artery, near the posterior communicating artery; it then crosses the cavernous sinus, receives sympathetic fibers from the peri-carotid plexus and a communicating branch of the ophthalmic branch of the trigeminal nerve. Since the parasympathetic fibers run in the outer portion of the nerve, any extrinsic compressive element would first damage the parasympathetic component of the motor fibers. The proximity of the nerve to certain vessels of the Willis circle may therefore explain the finding of pupillary abnormalities in the case of aneurysmal dilatations (aneurysm of the apex of the internal carotid artery, aneurysm of the posterior communicating artery) [43].

5.4 Autonomic Nervous System and Cerebrovascular Diseases: Management and Therapeutic Perspectives

The profound interconnection between the autonomic nervous system and cerebrovascular pathology, particularly if acute, has been effectively described with the expression "striking reciprocity" [42, 46]. In fact, if on the one hand the cerebral damage following the cerebrovascular event can determine secondary dysautonomia with important repercussions on the prognosis, during the hyperacute phase, on the other hand the dysfunction of the ANS can play a decisive role in the development of pathological conditions that determine the occurrence of the event itself (Fig. 5.2).

Chronic risk factors, which act in the long term, and acute risk factors (*triggers*), which rapidly increase the risk of an ischemic event and often determine the timing of its presentation, are involved in the etiopathogenesis of stroke. Both chronic risk factors and triggers are susceptible to modulation by the ANS. Different autonomic responses are associated with different etiopathogenetic mechanisms of cerebrovascular pathology: atherosclerotic (large or small vessel occlusion, athero-arterial embolization), cardioembolism and vasospasm. A careful assessment of the activity of the SNA, although complex, could allow the identify the effects of chronic stress/ risk factors and acute triggers in the different subtypes of ischemic stroke, contributing to outline a personalized risk profile useful for modulating the necessary management and pharmacological interventions.

As is well known, the NES and its various components have the task of maintaining homeostasis, which can be defined as the state of physiological equilibrium, since it is susceptible to various perturbing elements, both intrinsic and extrinsic.

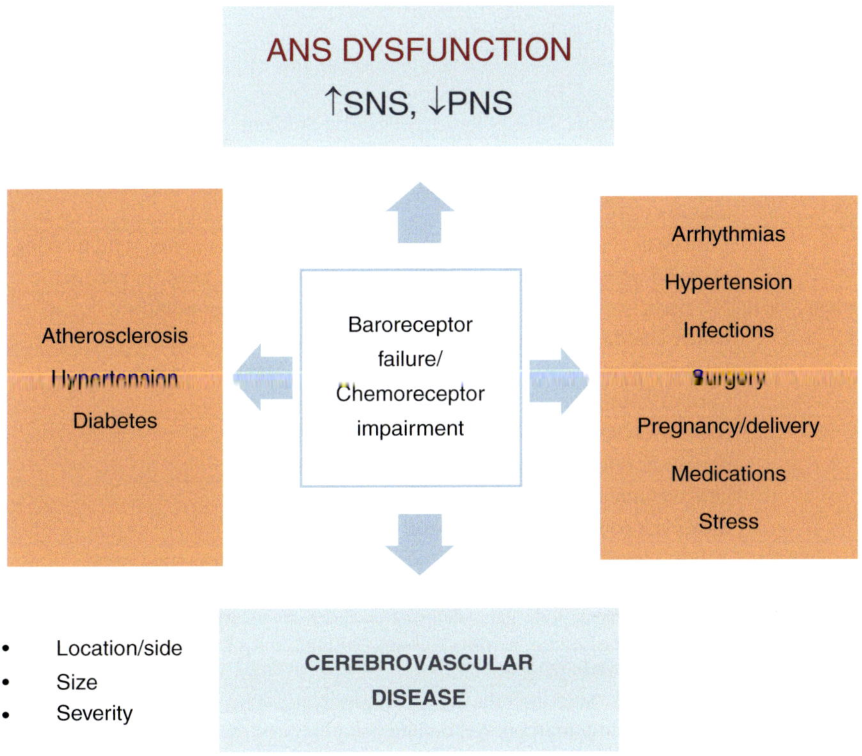

Fig. 5.2 The 'striking reciprocity' between the autonomic nervous system and cerebrovascular pathology [42, 46]

The term ‘stress’ was coined to describe a state, whether transient or chronic, of altered homeostasis induced by various factors (stressors), listed in Table 5.3, which in turn may be acute, episodic, or chronic.

The role of the ANS is to respond to acute stressful events by implementing countermeasures to maintain homeostasis through the activity of both its sympathetic and parasympathetic branches, which in turn act on the target organs. Although this process is physiological and aimed at maintaining the proper functioning of the organism, under conditions of chronic/acute recurrent stress its response may become maladaptive. In chronic stress, in fact, the ability of the parasympathetic nervous system to keep the stress response under control is particularly impaired, with possible anticipatory or dysregulated activation phenomena. Adaptation to stress can lead to stress-related disorders. The maladaptive phenomena of the ANS lead to secondary effects on the target organs with the consequent development of dysfunctional/dysmetabolic conditions such as hyperglycemia, dyslipidemia, and

Table 5.3 Possible stressors

Stressors	Examples
Exteriors	Physical-environmental: Noise, excessive brightness, heat, confined spaces
	Social: Roughness, bullying, aggression by others
	Organizational: Rules, deadlines
	Major life-events: Death of a family member, loss of job, promotion, birth of a child
	Daily annoyances: Loss of keys, mechanical problem
Interiors	Lifestyle choice: Not enough sleep, excessive commitments
	Negative self: Pessimistic thinking/speaking, excessive self-criticism, excessive analysis
	Unrealistic expectations, taking things personally, exaggeration, rigid thinking
	Stressful personality traits: Perfectionism, workaholism, need for pleasure
Occupational	Not participating in decisions concerning one’s own responsibilities
	Unreasonable demands on performance
	Lack of effective communication and conflict between colleagues
	Lack of safety at work
	Excessively long working hours
	Too much time spent away from home and family
	Office politics and worker conflicts
	Salary not commensurate with level of responsibility
Development	Young adults: Marriage, leaving home, managing home, starting work, continuing school, having children
	Middle age: Accepting age-related physical changes, maintaining social status and standard of living, helping teenage children to become independent, managing elderly parents
	Older people: Accepting the decline in physical and health capacities, changing home, accepting retirement and reduction of income, accepting the death of spouse and friends
Situational	Death of a family member, marriage or divorce, birth of a child, new job, illnesses

arterial hypertension, which in turn cause further damage to the ANS. The resulting vicious cycle may culminate in the occurrence of an acute cerebrovascular event [47–49].

As patients grow older, comorbidity in the form of multiple concurrent chronic conditions is the norm rather than the exception. One attempt to provide an answer to this phenomenon has been the introduction of the concept of allostatic load as a measure of the cumulative physiological load imposed on the body through attempts to adapt to the demands of life. Allostasis is in fact understood as the ability to adapt to challenges [50]. The concept of allostasis emphasizes the physiological imperative that, to survive, "an organism must vary the parameters of its internal environment and adapt appropriately to environmental demands". When adaptive responses to challenge are chronically outside normal operating ranges, wear, and tear on regular systems, primarily the SNA, occurs, and allostasis accumulates, leading to progressive wear and tear on physiological systems [51] (Fig. 5.3).

5.4.1 Chronic Risk Factors

Chronic stress has been proposed as a factor favoring the occurrence of a metabolic syndrome. The metabolic syndrome, an important risk factor for ischemic stroke, cardiovascular diseases, and diabetes, is made up of a cluster of disorders (Table 5.4) which recognize a dysfunction of the sympathetic nervous system as the *primum movens* of cardiovascular and metabolic changes.

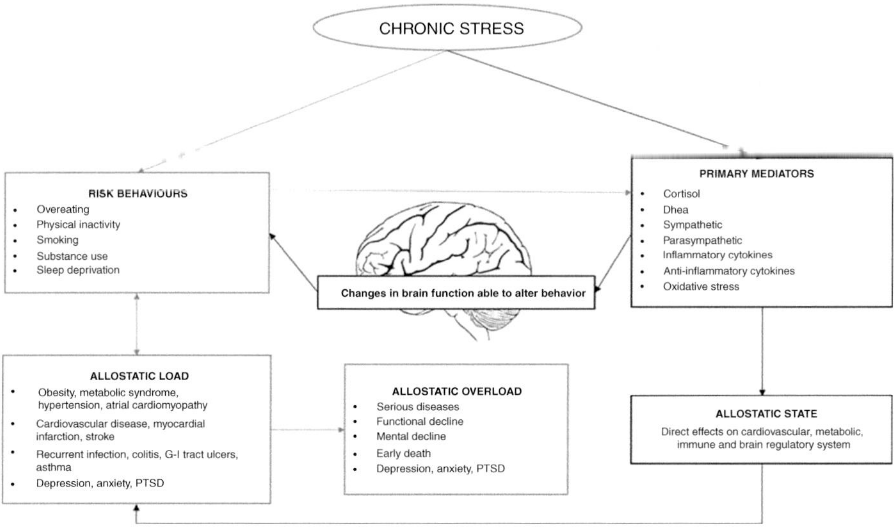

Fig. 5.3 Biological mechanisms of allostatic loading

Table 5.4 Diagnostic criteria for Metabolic Syndrome [52]

Presence of at least three of the following criteria
• Abdominal circumference: > = 88 cm for women and > = 102 cm for men
• Trigliceride: > = 150 mg/dL
• HDL cholesterol: <40 mg/dL in men and < 50 mg/dL in women
• Blood pressure: Systolic BP > = 130 mm hg and/or diastolic BP > = 85 mm hg
• Fasting blood glucose > = 100 mg/dL

On the other hand, severe SNA dysregulation can lead to insulin resistance, altered lipid metabolism, and increased blood pressure. An increase in HR and a reduction in respiratory sinus arrhythmia, indicators of reduced parasympathetic activity, and a reduction in the cardiac preejection period, indicative of elevated sympathetic activity, were correlated with elevated blood pressure, hypertriglyceridemia, hyperglycemia, and increased abdominal circumference. In patients with metabolic syndrome, sympathetic overactivity and reduced parasympathetic activity have been documented. Moreover, sympathetic hyperactivity seems to be predictive, in a 2-year follow-up of an increase in the number of metabolic alterations, suggesting its role as a predictor for the development of cardiovascular disease and diabetes through dysregulation of lipid metabolism and blood pressure over time [53].

The sympathetic nervous system (SNS) plays a role in the genesis or progression of the metabolic syndrome as it can reduce insulin sensitivity by both hemodynamic mechanisms and direct cellular effects (arteriolar vasoconstriction induced by the release of noradrenaline reduces glucose re-uptake by altering the ability of cells to transport glucose across their membranes, a hallmark of insulin resistance). Insulin resistance, a metabolic disorder characterized by reduced tissue sensitivity to insulin that originates from the effect of a sedentary lifestyle and central obesity, among other environmental factors, in individuals with a significant genetic predisposition, has been proposed as a common pathophysiological mechanism underlying the metabolic syndrome. It is less clear whether it is insulin resistance that leads to a condition of sympathetic overactivity or vice versa. The work of Anderson et al. [54] has documented that systemic infusion of insulin while maintaining constant plasma glucose concentrations results in a marked increase in outflow from sympathetic endings to skeletal muscle vessels. This ability of the SNS to determine or worsen insulin resistance resulted in a further increase in plasma insulin levels, which in turn triggered further sympathetic activation. Furthermore, the work of Masuo et al. [55] documented that in young, nonobese subjects who were normotensive at study inclusion but had a significant increase in BP over 10 years, sympathetic overactivity preceded the onset of hyperinsulinemia; at the onset of the first stages of hypertension, on the other hand, both sympathetic hyperactivity and hyperinsulinemia were present, suggesting that sympathetic hyperactivity may be the *primum movens* capable of triggering both hypertension and insulin resistance [56].

In fact, in subjects with a family history of hypertension or with white-coat hypertension, an abnormal increase in serum adrenaline and noradrenaline has been shown to be caused by an increased release from the sympathetic nerve endings. Sympathetic overactivity has also been found in different subtypes of hypertensive patients, irrespective of age group, and in particular groups of patients, e.g., in pregnancy hypertension. This suggests that autonomic dysfunction may be a process involved in the genesis of hypertension regardless of the specific context in which the disease develops. In these patients a progressive parasympathetic dysfunction accompanies sympathetic hyperactivity, as evidenced by a gradual reduction in responses to arterial baroreceptor stimulation, leading to reduced vagal modulation and an altered cardiac vagal response, resulting in reduced Heart Rate Variability (HRV), particularly low-frequency fluctuations [57]. A possible substrate for the relationship between autonomic dysfunction and the development and maintenance of hypertension is provided by some evidence in favor of the importance of arterial baroreceptors not only in the short-term control of blood pressure but also in its long-term control. In particular, the resetting of these baroreceptors to higher pressure levels appears to be an important element, and involves hypothalamic regions located antero-ventral to the third ventricle, structures that are sensitive to arterial pressure and volemic changes [58]. As evidence of this autonomic dysfunction in hypertensive patients a reduction in HRV has been shown and in normotensive patients a lower HRV has been correlated with an increased risk of developing hypertension [59]. Furthermore, autonomic dysfunction with sympathetic hyperactivation correlates not only with the development of hypertension but also with the severity of vascular and cardiac damage in hypertensive patients, independent of blood pressure values [57].

Insulin resistance, through the vicious circle triggered by the SNS, can in turn lead to:

- Impaired glucose metabolism with the development of diabetes mellitus.
- Alterations in the metabolism of plasma triglycerides and free fatty acids resulting in atherogenic dyslipidemia.
- Increased blood pressure.
- Alterations in vascular reactivity.
- Endothelial dysfunction.
- Chronic subclinical inflammation.
- Prothrombotic phenotype.

Thus, insulin resistance is a key pathophysiological factor in the development of vascular risk. Epidemiological data support its role in cerebrovascular pathology, reporting that metabolic syndrome is an independent risk factor for stroke in all ethnic groups and in both sexes, particularly for atherothrombotic stroke. In prospective studies, metabolic syndrome increases the risk of ischemic stroke by about fivefold [60].

The persistence of a condition of sympathetic overactivity is decisive not only in the appearance but also in the progression of atherosclerosis. The evolution of the atherosclerotic plaque and its vulnerability to rupture is determined by several factors that can be modulated by the ANS. A vulnerable plaque is characterized by the presence of a lipid-rich core, a thin fibrous cap, the presence of active inflammatory processes, and active remodeling processes. On the other hand, the vulnerability of a plaque is not predictable when based on its size and degree of stenosis. An autonomic dysfunction, in particular a predominance of SNS activity, can favor the evolution towards plaque instability, facilitating the occurrence of chronic inflammatory processes at the level of the atherosclerotic plaque [61]. In addition, sympathetic hyperactivity can induce an increase in the uptake of LDL cholesterol by endothelial cells, a pivotal process in the induction and progression of atherosclerosis [62, 63]. Carotid atherosclerosis can also enhance autonomic dysfunction secondary to the atherosclerotic process by interfering with carotid baroreceptors and chemoreceptors, directly promoting sympathetic-vagal dysregulation with a prevalence of sympathetic activity and a reduction in vagal tone [59].

In addition to arterial vessels, another target organ of sympathetic overactivity is the heart (as will be discussed later in this chapter).

The role of SNA in the emergence and maintenance of risk factors for ischemic stroke is summarized in Fig. 5.4.

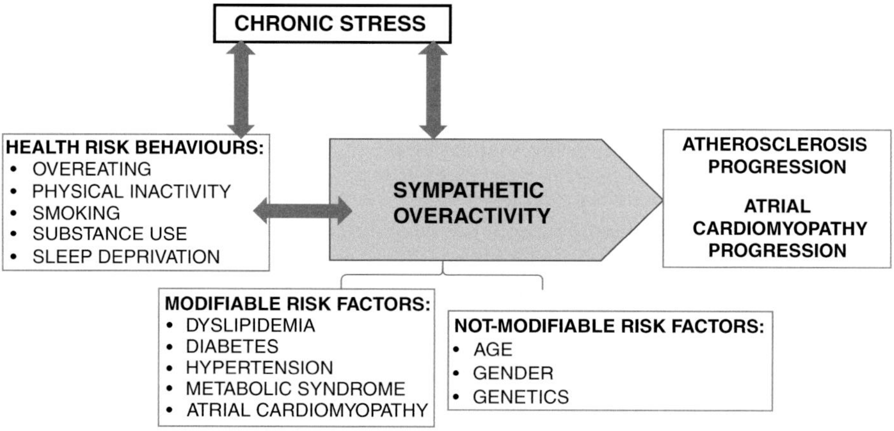

Fig. 5.4 Interrelationships between the Autonomic Nervous System and chronic risk factors for ischemic stroke

5.4.2 *Acute Risk Factors or Triggers*

To determine the occurrence of an acute cerebrovascular event on a terrain predisposed to the presence of chronic risk factors, it is necessary that acute risk factors or triggers capable of determining an abrupt increase in short-term risk (days, hours) intervene to be able to explain the occurrence of a cerebral ischemic event at a specific time. The ANS, already chronically unbalanced towards a state of sympathetic hyperactivity due to the presence of chronic risk factors, responds in a dysfunctional manner with a further accentuation of the sympathetic response, which in turn can trigger phenomena such as vasoconstriction, acute prothrombotic state, sudden increase in blood pressure and heart rate, arrhythmias, and endothelial dysfunction capable of triggering the cerebral ischemic event.

The main acute risk factors for ischemic stroke and their relationship to SNA are shown in Table 5.5.

Circadian Rhythm: Several studies have reported a circadian rhythm in the incidence of stroke, both ischemic and hemorrhagic, characterized by a peak between 6 a.m. and noon, and a less evident one between 2 p.m. and 4 p.m. The circadian distribution is not influenced by the etiopathogenetic category of the stroke [64]. Circadian rhythms, generated centrally, are influenced by the activity of the ANS, whose activity is in turn modulated by the CNS according to the different phases of the circadian rhythm. By assessing the variation in HRV at different times of the day, we can see a peak in HRV during the night (prevalence of parasympathetic activity during nighttime rest) and a maximum reduction in the early morning hours, at the transition between sleep and wakefulness. This reduction reflects greater sympathetic activity in this phase, which is reflected in the cardiovascular system. The imbalance towards sympathetic activity, as previously highlighted, leads to unfavorable changes in the cardiovascular system, in blood pressure and

Table 5.5 Main triggers of the acute ischemic event

Trigger	Influence on the autonomic nervous system
Circadian rhythm (morning hours)	Reduction in parasympathetic activity
Intense physical exertion/activity	Acute increase in sympathetic activity
Acute psychological stress	Acute increase in sympathetic activity
Acute and excessive alcohol intake	Sympathetic hyperactivity and decreased parasympathetic activity
Low-moderate dose cannabis	Increased sympathetic activity and decreased parasympathetic activity
Exposure to excessively cold temperatures	Increased sympathetic and renin-angiotensin system activity
Exposure to excessively warm temperatures	Increased sympathetic activity in the sweat glands and cutaneous vasodilation sympathetic activity
Infections	Amplify the pro-inflammatory and prothrombotic response induced by chronic sympathetic hyperactivity

heart rate values, as well as in the hormonal profile and inflammatory activation, promoting the development of acute cerebrovascular events [65].

Exercise/Physical Activity: Regular physical activity has been widely shown to be a protective factor for stroke. However, isolated episodes of intense physical activity may lead to an acute increase in sympathetic nervous system activity, resulting in a transient increase in heart rate, blood pressure, and an alteration of the coagulation balance towards a prothrombotic profile [66]. In the hour following intense physical exertion, a significant increase in the risk of stroke, up to 2.3 times greater, has been demonstrated, particularly in subjects who do not habitually practice physical activity [67]. Similar data have emerged about hemorrhagic stroke, and intense physical activity can also be considered a trigger event for this type of event [68].

Acute Psychological Stress: The occurrence of particularly stressful life-events has been recognized as a possible trigger for acute cerebrovascular events through activation of the hypothalamic-pituitary-adrenal axis and the autonomic nervous system. It has been shown that this activation in response to stressful psychological events can lead to an increase in heart rate and blood pressure, release of catecholamines and procoagulant factors, and even transient endothelial dysfunction. Overall, this alteration in homeostasis creates a substrate favoring the occurrence of stroke [69]. In some cases, it is possible to document an acute, nonischemic but stress-induced myocardial dysfunction, probably as expression of an acute and tendentially reversible organ damage caused by a massive release of catecholamines as a result of stressful events: this condition is called Takotsubo syndrome, after the original name of a Japanese octopus trap whose shape resembles the appearance of the left ventricle on ultrasound investigations performed in such cases (this appearance is also known as 'apical ballooning'). Takotsubo syndrome is a cause of cardioembolism as it is associated with the formation of thrombotic apposition in the left ventricle due to contraction dyssynergy; a 1–5% risk of developing ischemic stroke after a diagnosis of Takotsubo has been reported [70, 71].

Substances: Acute intake of an excessive amount of alcohol induces sympathetic hyperresponsiveness and a decrease in parasympathetic activity. This autonomic dysregulation may lead to an acute alcohol-induced arrhythmogenic substrate and be an exogenous trigger for an acute cerebrovascular event [72]. Cocaine, amphetamine and its derivatives result in indirect stimulation of the ANS through the release of norepinephrine, dopamine and serotonin. Cannabis is also capable of causing a sympathetic-vagal imbalance. The effect of marijuana and its active component THC on the cardiovascular system varies depending on the dose taken, the frequency and duration of intake, and the route of administration. In low to moderate doses, smoked marijuana increases sympathetic activity and reduces parasympathetic activity, leading to tachycardia and hypertension. It may also trigger atrial fibrillation [73]. High doses cause bradycardia and hypotension [74].

Environmental Temperature: Global warming produces not only hotter summers and more frequent heatwaves but also colder winters, especially in more temperate areas where populations are not used to extreme weather conditions. Exposure to excessively cold or warm temperatures can increase the risk of stroke through different mechanisms. In cold weather, the increased risk has been linked mainly to increased blood pressure, peripheral vasoconstriction, increased platelet count and increased blood viscosity caused mainly by increased sympathetic activity. However, the data are still contradictory. In contrast, elevated room temperature may increase the risk of stroke through increased sweating and skin blood flow, dehydration, increased blood viscosity, hemoconcentration and increased plasma cholesterol levels [75].

Infections: Numerous case-control studies have demonstrated an association between a previous systemic – mostly viral—infection, and the occurrence of a stroke, often with a time interval of several days from the onset of the infectious symptoms. The mechanisms by which viral infection can promote the occurrence of a cerebral ischemic event are manifold: activation of the immune system, hypercoagulability, hemodynamic alterations secondary to myocardial involvement, endothelial damage, and destabilization of atherosclerotic plaque [76].

5.4.3 After the Cerebrovascular Event

There is a great deal of evidence of interactions between SNA and stroke, both in the acute phase and in the outcome. The acute attack is known to be associated with a central autonomic alteration responsible for a marked increase in BP and heart rate, also associated with a reduction in parasympathetic activity compared to controls (increase in HF at the frequency spectrum) both in patients with pathology of the large vessel (Large Artery Atherosclerosis—LAA) and in those with lacunar infarction (LAC or SVO, from Small Vessel Occlusion, symptomatic of pathology of the small cerebral vessel). At 7 days, this reduction in parasympathetic function is present only in the first group (LAA), while lacunar ischemia seems to be especially pronounced if the ischemia is at the level of the putamen or thalamus, key structures of the central autonomic network (CAN). Therefore, it can be said that it is, above all, the ischemic (or hemorrhagic) lesion at the supratentorial site that determines a more relevant and lasting reduction in parasympathetic activity and a concomitant increase in sympathetic activity [77]. In turn, the severity of neurological impairment (NIHSS) directly correlates with the degree of impairment of cardiovascular autonomic function, with the fall in parasympathetic tone and baroreceptor sensitivity, as well as the progressive shift towards sympathetic dominance. The resulting autonomic dysfunction increases the risk of cardiovascular complications and worsens the outcome [78]. The parasympathetic deficit, also assessed by Ewing tests and HRV spectral analysis, is always greater in LAA patients (82% of patients) than in LAC patients (63%), who together have a greater parasympathetic deficit than control subjects [79]. Outdated studies show that it is mainly ischemic lesions of the trunk-brain that present a greater functional impairment (HRV) than supratentorial lesions, which show a higher level of plasma catecholamines than the former [80].

It is interesting to underline how the impairment of the SNA, and in particular of the pressor response to the Valsalva test (with a reduced increase in systolic pressure in phase IV), has been shown to characterize the greater evolutivity of the pathology linked to the lacunar lesions or the progression, sometimes observed during hospitalization, of subjects with cerebral small-vessel disease, even at an outcome of 3 months [81].

Autonomic dysfunction is also associated with an increase in the pathological changes observed in the disease of the small cerebral vessels, and in lesions of the white matter, regardless of the form of cognitive impairment. This suggests that dysfunction is a risk factor for cerebral hypoperfusion, which may contribute, in different ways among the various forms of dementia, to induce pathology in the advanced phase of the disease [82].

Demonstrating the role of altered cerebral autoregulation in determining autonomic dysfunction, recent studies seem to show that, after a lacunar infarction, while no significant differences are found in the "overall" vegetative function of patients and control subjects, there is a reduction in cerebral blood flow in the middle cerebral artery (mCBFV) and in systolic blood pressure before, during and after a breath-holding test. The positive correlation found between systolic pressure and mCBFV in patients compared to controls suggests an alteration of parasympathetic drive in this pathology, especially of autonomic control over CBF in the pathophysiological mechanisms of vasodilation induced by hypercapnia caused by deep breathing. Cerebral vascular reactivity is indeed reduced in patients with lacunar infarction due to reduced parasympathetic activity [83].

The pathological sympathetic activation associated with acute cerebral vascular injury (both ischemic and hemorrhagic) has repercussions on autonomic functions, with an increased risk of cardiac arrhythmias, increased levels of circulating catecholamines, myocardial damage, and heart failure (even in the absence of cardiac pathologies), pressure instability and neurogenic pulmonary edema. In fact, the main autonomic dysfunction in the post-stroke period involves the *baroreflex dysfunction (BRS)* as the probable mechanism underlying the almost invariable occurrence of arterial hypertension (hypertensive crises, pressure lability, altered circadian variability of blood pressure, altered dipping) during the acute phase of stroke (more than 80% in several cases) [84–86].

Post-stroke impairment of BRS is associated with worse clinical outcomes and is directly proportional to mortality and morbidity. The site and extent of vascular injury are major determinants of the duration, extent and reversibility of autonomic dysfunction. The anatomo-functional central connections of the baroreceptors include the nucleus of the solitary tract, the ventrolateral bulbar portion, the insula, the medial prefrontal cortex, the cingulate cortex, and finally, the amygdala, hypothalamus and thalamus, and the cerebellum. In particular, the insula is a strategic area for autonomic control of the heart, with parasympathetic regulation located in the left insula and sympathetic regulation located contralaterally.

Significant alteration of BRS has been documented in acute stroke patients with insular lesion, with greater impairment in patients with bilateral insular involvement. Especially lesions in the left insular cortex seem to be associated with sympathetic hyperactivation, and, consequently, with increased circulating levels of catecholamines, baroreceptor dysfunction, cardiac arrhythmias, catecholamine-mediated myocardial damage (myocytolysis), immune dysregulation, and hyperglycemia. In contrast, right insular damage is associated with marked bradycardia and asystole because of reduced sympathetic tone and subsequent predominance of parasympathetic tone [1, 85, 87, 88].

Interindividual differences also depend on hemispheric dominance; an advantage has been observed for left-handed and ambidextrous people, who have a lower rate of sudden death than right-handed people. Functional lateralization is more frequent in men, whereas in women, a pattern of physiological bihemispheric activation is described. In rats, stimulation of the posterior rostral region of the left insula causes an increase in heart rate, while stimulation of the caudal region of the insula causes bradycardia; stimulation of the left insular cortex during the T wave of the cardiac cycle causes arrhythmias, QT prolongation, ST-segment elevation, and asystole. These evidence, based on preclinical research experiences, is, however, complicated by several factors in the clinical setting: first of all, ischemic or hemorrhagic lesions are very rarely limited to the insular region. Moreover, as already mentioned, other brain areas are involved in autonomic control. In general, however, it can be asserted that hemispheric stroke carries an increased risk of cardiac arrhythmias such as atrial fibrillation and sudden death [89, 90].

As mentioned, a massive release of circulating catecholamines, which is possible in conditions of acute stress of any kind, can lead to an acute cardiomyopathy known as Takotsubo syndrome or "apical ballooning," which has significant hemodynamic repercussions as well as a potential cardioembolism due to the possible formation of intraventricular thrombotic apposition. Of note, Takotsubo can be triggered by the occurrence of a stroke, as a "stressor," but because of the emboligenic potential, it determines it can also be the cause of a cerebral ischemic event [70].

The arterial hypertension frequently observed during the acute phase of stroke is thought to be an expression of increased sympathetic tone resulting in renin release and arteriolar vasoconstriction. It may result from direct damage to inhibitory/modulatory brain regions or indirect damage from reduced parasympathetic activation, which in turn leads to dysregulation of the baroreceptor reflex. Other contributory factors may be nitric oxide release during ischemic injury, increased intracranial pressure, and compression on the brain stem. In addition, the increase in pressure may be an attempt to compensate for the perfusion deficit that occurs in ischemic conditions, especially when the etiopathogenesis of the stroke is atherothrombotic or lacunar, whereas in cases of cardioembolism, pressures tend to be lower [91–93].

Sympathetic hyperactivation is also hypothesized to be the cause of neurogenic pulmonary edema, which is associated with lesions in certain 'trigger' areas: the hypothalamus, the bulb, cortical areas A1 and A5, the nucleus of the solitary tract and the postrema area, which are closely linked to the central control of respiration [94].

Vascular lesions in the insula have also been correlated with the immunosuppression that accompanies acute stroke in about a third of cases, and which is characterized by a systemic anti-inflammatory response with increased susceptibility to infections, especially in the respiratory and urinary systems, with a significant impact on 30-day mortality. Stroke in fact alters the balance between sympathetic and parasympathetic connections that regulate the immune system and endocrine organs, part of the hypothalamic-pituitary axis. The early occurrence of infections after acute stroke is in fact associated with hyperactivation of the adrenomedullin axis, documented by elevated circulating levels of catecholamines during the first day after stroke. Clinical severity and extent of the lesion do not seem to determine an increased risk of infection, which would be favored in the case of lesions in the territory of the anterior circulation [95].

Another form of autonomic dysfunction associated with acute stroke is urinary disorders, which affect about one-third of patients and include various forms of incontinence, either transient or persistent. The gastrointestinal tract may also show post-stroke functional alterations, with constipation, fecal incontinence, dysphagia and sialorrhea. Finally, thermoregulation is often altered in the acute phase of stroke, due to damage to both vaso- and sudomotor autonomic fibers, leading mainly to contralateral hyperhidrosis and asymmetry of thermal sensitivity [96–98].

5.4.4 Evaluation of Dysautonomia in Patients with Cerebrovascular Risk

In clinical practice, various invasive and noninvasive techniques are used to assess SNA. In fact, it has been carried out with the study of orthostatic PA and HR changes [99], the head-up tilt test [100], the baroreceptor sensitivity study [101], the Valsalva maneuver [100], the complete Ewing battery [102], the plasma catecholamine assay [103], and the SNA assessment [101].

Their in-depth description is beyond the scope of this chapter and is amply illustrated in the reference ones. Here, we will focus on the role of the Heart Rate Variability (HRV) assessment as the most widely used in the evaluation of SNA in patients with cerebrovascular disease. It is in fact a noninvasive test, which can be performed in patients with cerebrovascular risk factors, with stroke in both acute and chronic phases as it does not require the cooperation of the patient. It only requires the recording of an ECG trace. This allows for continuous monitoring in both hospital and outpatient settings using wearable devices. Further advantages of the method are its high reliability and reproducibility as well as its low cost; however, it cannot be applied in patients with heart rhythm disorders such as AF and frequent extrasystoles.

HRV is the variation in time of the interval between two consecutive beats; the regulation is mainly extrinsic, dependent on the activity of the SNA. Specifically, the sympathetic nervous system (SNS) causes an acceleration and the parasympathetic nervous system (SNP) a deceleration of the heartbeat, the result being the balance of the two activities.

The measurement can be easily obtained using pulse oximetry or photoplethysmography, even over long periods of time using wearable devices; however, acquisition of an ECG trace provides more accurate results.

The rhythmic contribution to heart rate variability made by the two systems, SNS and SNP, occurs at different frequencies. In particular, the SNS is associated with low frequencies (0.04–0.15 Hz), and the SNP with high frequencies (0.15–0.4 Hz). This difference makes it possible, by means of an HRV analysis, to distinguish the activity of the two branches of the SNS [104].

Two main categories of variables are obtained from the ECG recording, *time domain* and *frequency domain*. The time domain variables can be divided into short-time variability and longtime variability (less than 6/min), both calculated from the RR intervals in the recording. Several parameters can be calculated from the duration of the RR intervals in the recording (Table 5.6). Among the time domain variables, the evaluation of RMSSD is preferable because it is more sensitive and less influenced by respiratory rate, heart rate and duration of recording, and largely reflects parasympathetic activity [105].

Table 5.6 Main measures of the HR—time domain

	Variable	Definition	Meaning
Frequency domain	Total power (ms^2)	The variance of NN intervals in a time segment or in 24 h (≤0.4 Hz)	Overall SNA activity
	ULF (ms^2)	Ultra-low-frequency power (≤0.003 Hz)	Reflects the influence of many uncontrollable factors; only on records of at least 24 h
	VLF (ms^2)	Very low-frequency power (0.003–0.04 Hz)	It reflects the influence of the renin-angiotensin system and peripheral vasomotor mechanisms plus other uncontrollable factors
	LF (ms^2)	Low-frequency power (0.04–0.15 Hz)	Mediated by complex interactions between sympathetic and parasympathetic activity
	LF norm (n.u.)	LF power normalized units: LF/(LF + HF) × 100%	Relative value of LF in relation to sum of LF and HF; represents balance between the two branches of SNA
	HF (ms^2)	High-frequency power (0.15–0.4 Hz)	Regulated only by the parasympathetic; an increase in value reflects an increase in parasympathetic activity
	HF norm (n.u.)	HF power in normalized units: HF/(LF + HF) × 100%	Relative value of HF in relation to sum of LF and HF; represents balance between the two branches of the SNA
	LF/HF	Ratio of LF to HF power	Reflects the balance between sympathetic and parasympathetic activity
	HF + LF (ms^2)	Sum of HF and LF power (0.04–0.4 Hz)	More accurate indicator of overall NES activity (higher values correspond to higher activity)

The frequency domain variables (Table 5.7) require more complex analyses; however, they allow better discrimination between SNS and SNP activity by identifying activity in the low and high frequencies, which are related to the SNS and SNP, respectively. The LF/HF ratio expresses this relationship. However, the respiratory rate can influence these measurements and should therefore be considered in the interpretation [105].

From a clinical point of view, it should be remembered that a reduction in HRV correlates with the degree of carotid stenosis. In these patients, the real impact of carotid atherosclerotic lesions on SNA is evidenced by the partial recovery of HRV values after long-term treatment with statins [63].

In addition, a reduction in HRV has been associated with an increased risk of AF and in diabetic patients, a reduction in the LF/HF ratio, a marker of predominant sympathetic activity, has been associated with an increase in AF episodes [59].

Although lacking definitive evidence, HRV assessment shows promise in both identifying patients at increased risk of cerebrovascular events in selected populations and in post-event monitoring. Indeed, reduced values of the time and frequency domain parameters are associated with an increased risk of ischemic stroke, particularly in diabetic patients [106]. In addition, low nocturnal SDNN values seem to be predictive of a first ischemic event, independently of traditional vascular risk factors, and therefore their integration into individual patient risk assessment could allow a more personalized therapeutic approach [107]. Low HRV values have been associated with the occurrence of early complications such as in-hospital mortality, post-stroke infections and motor function recovery [108].

From the point of view of the risk of early recurrence, TIA, and minor stroke patients with low SDNN values showed an increased risk of ischemic recurrence at 90 days. These data might suggest the integration of HRV measurement into risk stratification models, allowing a better identification of high-risk patients, both to modulate secondary prevention therapy and to identify a possible target population for new therapeutic trials. High post-event SDNN values have been associated with improved functional recovery at 90 days in patients with ischemic stroke, suggesting a possible contribution of post-stroke dysautonomia in the development of an unfavorable functional outcome [109].

Table 5.7 Main measures of HRV—frequency domain

Time domain	**SDNN (ms)**	**Standard deviation of the NN intervals**	**Corresponds to total power**
	SDANN (ms)	SD of the average of the NN intervals in all 5-min intervals of the recording	Corresponds to ULF
	RMSSD (ms)	The square root of the mean of the sum of the squares of the differences between adjacent NN intervals	Corresponds to HF
	SDNN index (ms)	Average of the SDs of all NN intervals for all 5 min segments of the recording	5-min total power average, similar significance

5.4.5 Therapeutic Perspectives

It follows that in the quantification of cerebrovascular risk both the metabolic syndrome and indicators of the state of activation of the sympathetic nervous system such as HRV should be introduced to better define the long-term and short-term risk profile and consequently adjust the type and timing of therapeutic interventions. For example, at HRV assessment, a reduction in the values of the time and frequency domain parameters has been associated with an increased risk of ischemic stroke, particularly in diabetic patients [106]. In addition, low nocturnal SDNN values have been found to be associated with the development of a first ischemic event, independent of traditional vascular risk factors and therefore could be integrated with this in individual patient risk assessment [107]. From the point of view of the risk of early recurrence, patients with TIA and minor stroke with low SDNN values showed an increased risk of ischemic recurrence at 90 days. These data might suggest the integration of HRV measurement into risk stratification models, allowing a better identification of high-risk patients, both to modulate secondary prevention therapy and to identify a possible target population for new therapeutic trials. High values of post-stroke SDNN have been associated with better functional recovery at 90 days in patients with ischemic stroke, suggesting a possible contribution of post-stroke dysautonomia in the development of an unfavorable functional outcome [109]. Low HRV values have also been associated with early complications such as intra-hospital mortality, post-stroke infections and motor function recovery [108].

Although, to date, there is no conclusive data on therapies aimed at modulating the autonomic nervous system, the evidence in favor of a contribution of dysautonomia, with sympathetic hyperactivity, in the development and worsening of vascular risk factors, as well as the deleterious effects of sympathetic hyperreactivity in the acute phase, makes SNP stimulation and SNS blockade interesting therapeutic possibilities.

The effect of SNP stimulation can lead to CNS neuroplasticity, anti-inflammatory, antioxidant and anti-apoptotic effects through activation of the α7nAchR cholinergic receptor. In animal models, both invasive and noninvasive stimulation of the vagus nerve (VNS) has been shown to [59, 110]:

- Reduce systemic inflammation.
- Reducing appetite and body weight.
- Significantly reduce the volume of the ischemic core.

If these are confirmed in humans, vagal stimulation may be an interesting therapeutic strategy for both the prevention and acute treatment of ischemic stroke.

Two randomized pilot studies showed the benefit of VNS combined with rehabilitation in the recovery of moderate to severe upper limb motor deficits. The same favorable effect on motor recovery was obtained by transcutaneous stimulation, making the procedure easier and more tolerable [111]. However, evidence on efficacy is preliminary and needs to be confirmed, as does the safety of stimulation, particularly regarding possible cardiological side effects [110].

References

1. Al-Qudah ZA, Yacoub HA, Souayah N. Disorders of the autonomic nervous system after hemispheric cerebrovascular disorders: an update. J Vasc Interv Neurol. 2015;8(4):43–52.
2. Benarroch E, Biaggioni I. Central autonomic control primer on the autonomic nervous system. San Diego, CA: Academic Press; 2012. p. 9–12.
3. CB Knowledge. The central autonomic nervous system: conscious visceral perception and autonomic pattern generation. Ann Rev Neurosci. 2002;25:433–69.
4. Cechetto DF. Central representation of visceral function. Fed Proc. 1987;46:17–23.
5. Verberne AJ, Owens NC. Cortical modulation of the cardiovascular system. Prog Neurobiol. 1998;54:149.
6. Cheyuo C, Jacob A, Wu R, Zhou M, Coppa GF, Wang P. The parasympathetic nervous system in the quest for stroke therapeutics. J Cereb Blood Flow Metab. 2011;31:1187–95.
7. Lassen NA. Cerebral blood flow and oxygen consumption in man. Physiol Rev. 1959;39:183–238.
8. Kaplan NM. Management of hypertensive emergencies. Lancet. 1994;344:1335.
9. Strandgaard S, Olesen J, Skinhoj E, Lassen NA. Autoregulation of brain circulation in severe arterial hypertension. Br Med J. 1973;1:507–10.
10. Pires PW, Dams Ramos CM, Matin N, Dorrance AM. The effects of hypertension on the cerebral circulation. Am J Physiol Heart Circ Physiol. 2013;304:1598–614.
11. Paulson OB, Strandgaard S, Edvinsson L. Cerebral autoregulation. Cerebrovasc Brain Metab Rev. 1990;2:161–92.
12. Wagner EM, Traystman RJ. Hydrostatic determinants of cerebral perfusion. Crit Care Med. 1986;14:484–90.
13. Tiecks FP, Lam AM, Aaslid R, Newell DW. Comparison of static and dynamic cerebral autoregulation measurements. Stroke. 1995;26:1014–9. https://doi.org/10.1161/01.STR.26.6.1014.
14. Birch AA, Dirnhuber MJ, Hartley-Davies R, Iannotti F, Neil-Dwyer G. Assessment of autoregulation by means of periodic changes in blood pressure. Stroke. 1995;26:834–7. https://doi.org/10.1161/01.STR.26.5.834.
15. Claassen JAHR, et al. Regulation of cerebral blood flow in humans: physiology and clinical implications and autoregulation. Physiol Rev. 2021;101:1487–559.
16. Goadsby PJ. Autonomic nervous system control of the cerebral circulation. In: Buijs RM, Swaab DF, editors. Handbook of Clinical Neurology, Vol. 117 (3rd series) Autonomic Nervous System. Elsevier B.V.: Amsterdam; 2013.
17. Giovannitti JA Jr, Thoms SM, Crawford. Alpha-2 adrenergic receptor agonists: a review of current clinical applications. Anesth Prog. 2015;62(1):31–8.
18. Dacey RG, Duling BR. Effect of norepinephrine on penetrating arterioles of rat cerebral cortex. Am J Phys. 1984;246:H380–5.
19. Rosendorff C, Mitchell G, Mitchell D. Adrenergic innervation affecting local cerebral blood flow. In: Owman C, Edvinsson L, editors. Neurogenic control of brain circulation: Werner-Gren center international symposium series, vol. 30. Oxford: Pergamon; 1977. p. 455–64.
20. Sandor P. Nervous control of the cerebrovascular system: doubts and facts. Neurochem Int. 1999;35:237–59.
21. Sercombe R, Hardebo JE, Kahrstrom J, Seylaz J. Amine-induced responses of pial and penetrating cerebral arteries: evidence for heterogeneous responses. J Cereb Blood Flow Metab. 1990;10:808–18.
22. Edvinsson L, Owman C, Sjoberg NO. Autonomic nerves, mast cells, and amine receptors in human brain vessels. A histochemical and pharmacological study. Brain Res. 1976;115:377–93.
23. Willie CK, Tzeng Y-C, Fisher JA, Ainsli PN. Integrative regulation of human brain blood flow. J Physiol. 2014;592(5):841–59.

24. ter Laan M, et al. Sympathetic regulation of cerebral blood flow in humans: a review. Br J Anaesth. 2013;111:361–7. https://doi.org/10.1093/bja/aet122.
25. Faraci FM, et al. Cerebral circulation: effects of sympathetic nerves and protective mechanisms during hypertension. Circ Res. 1987;61:102–6.
26. Marcus ML, Heistad DD. Effects of sympathetic nerves on cerebral blood flow in awake dogs. Am J Physiol Heart Circ Physiol. 1979;236:H549–53. https://doi.org/10.1152/ajpheart.1979.236.4.H549).
27. Micieli G, et al. Intracerebral vascular changes induced by cold pressor test: a model of sympathetic activation. Neurol Res. 1994;15:163–7.
28. Roatta S, et al. Effect of generalised sympathetic activation by cold pressor test on cerebral haemodynamics in healthy humans. J Auton Nerv Syst. 1998;71:159–66.
29. Lewis NC, Smith KJ, Bain AR, Wildfong KW, Numan T, Ainslie PN. Impact of transient hypotension on regional cerebral blood flow in humans. Clin Sci (Lond). 2015;129:169–78.
30. Tymko MM, Richards CA, Skow RJ, Ingram-Cotton NC, Howatt MK, Day TA. The effects odf superimposed tilt and lower body negative pressure on anterior and posterior cerebral circulation. Physiol Rep. 2016;4(17):e12957. https://doi.org/10.14814/phy2.12957.
31. Tzeng YC, Willie CK, Atkinson G, Lucas SJ, Wong A, Ainslie PN. Cerebrovascular regulation during transient hypotension and hypertension in humans. Hypertension. 2010;56(2):268–73.
32. D'Alecy LG, Rose CJ. Parasympathetic cholinergic control of cerebral blood flow in dogs. Circ Res. 1977;41:324–31. https://doi.org/10.1161/01.res.41.3.324.
33. Hamner JW, et al. Cholinergic control of the cerebral vasculature in humans. J Physiol. 2012;590:6343–52. https://doi.org/10.1113/jphysiol.2012.245100.
34. Faraci FM, Brian JE Jr. Nitric oxide and the cerebral circulation. Stroke. 1994;25:692–703. https://doi.org/10.1161/01.STR.25.3.692.
35. Sakas DE, et al. Trigeminovascular fibers increase blood flow in cortical gray matter by axon reflex-like mechanisms during acute severe hypertension or seizures. Proc Natl Acad Sci U S A. 1989;86:1401–5. https://doi.org/10.1073/pnas.86.4.1401.
36. Lammie GA. Hypertensive cerebral small vessel disease and stroke. Brain Pathol. 2002;12:358–70.
37. Iadecola C. Hypertension and dementia. Hypertension. 2014;64:03–5.
38. Federico A, Di Donato I, Bianchi S, Di Palma C, Taglia I, et al. Hereditary cerebral small vessel diseases: a review. J Neurol Sci. 2012;322:25–30.
39. Brassard P, Tymko MM, Ainslie PN. Sympathetic control of the brain circulation: appreciating the complexities to better understand the controversy. Auton Neurosci Bas Clin. 2017;207:37–47. https://doi.org/10.1016/j.autneu.2017.05.003.
40. Uryga A, Nasr N, Kasprowicz M, Budohoski K, Sykora M, Smielewski P, Burzyńska M, Czosnyka M. Relationship between baroreflex and cerebral autoregulation in patients with cerebral vasospasm after aneurysmal subarachnoid hemorrhage. Front Neurol. 2022;12:740338.
41. Benarroch EE. The central autonomic network: functional organization, dysfunction, and perspective. Mayo Clin Proc. 1993;68:988–1001.
42. Micieli G, Cavallini A. The autonomic nervous system and ischemic stroke: a reciprocal interdependence. Clin Auton Res. 2008;18:308–17.
43. Jefferson G. Isolated oculomotor palsy caused by intra- cranial aneurysm. Proc R Soc Med. 1947;40(8):419–32.
44. Martin TJ. Horner syndrome: a clinical review. ACS Chem Neurosci. 2018;9(2):177–86.
45. Drexler I, Traenka C, von Hessling A, Gensicke H. Internal carotid artery dissection and asymmetrical facial flushing: the harlequin sign. Stroke. 2014;45(5):e78–80.
46. Oppenheimer S. Striking reciprocity. Clin Auton Res. 2008;18(6):296–7.
47. Guan L, Collet J-P, Mazowita G, Claydon VE. Autonomic nervous system and stress to predict secondary ischemic events after transient ischemic attack or minor Stroke: possible implications of heart rate variability. Front Neurol. 2018;9:90.

48. Curtis BM, O'Keefe JH. Autonomic tone as a cardiovascular risk factor: the dangers of chronic fight or flight. Mayo Clin Proc. 2002;77(1):45–54.
49. Black PH. The inflammatory response is an integral part of the stress response: implications for atherosclerosis, insulin resistance, type II diabetes and metabolic syndrome X. Brain Behav Immun. 2003;17(5):350–64.
50. Sterling P, Eyer J. Allostasis: a new paradigm to explain arousal pathology. In: Fisher S, Reason J, editors. Handbook of life stress, cognition, and health. J. Wiley: Chichester; 1988. p. 629–49.
51. Suvarnaa B, Suvarnaa A, Phillips R, Justerc R-P, McDermott B, Sarnyaia Z. Health risk behaviours and allostatic load: a systematic review. Neurosci Biobehav Rev. 2020;108:694–711.
52. Alberti KGMM, Eckel RH, Grundy SM, Zimmet PZ, Cleeman JI, Donato KA, Fruchart J-C, James WPT, Loria CM, Smith SC Jr. Harmonizing the metabolic syndrome. Circulation. 2009;120:1640–5.
53. Licht CMM, de Geus EJC, Penninx BWJH. Dysregulation of the autonomic nervous system predicts the development of the metabolic syndrome. J Clin Endocrinol Metab. 2013;98(6):2484–93.
54. Anderson EA, Hoffmann RP, Balon TW, Sinkey CA, Mark AL. Hyperinsulinemia produces both sympathetic neural activation and vasodilation in normal humans. J Clin Invest. 1991;87:2246–52.
55. Masuo K, Mikami H, Ogihara T, Tuck ML. Sympathetic nerve hyperactivity precedes hyperinsulinemia and blood pressure elevation in a young, nonobese Japanese population. Am J Hypertens. 1997;10:77–83.
56. Mancia G, Bousquet P, Elghozi JL, Esler M, Grassi G, Julius S, Reid J, Van Zwieten PA. The sympathetic nervous system and the metabolic syndrome. J Hypertens. 2007;25:909–20.
57. Mancia G, Grassi G. The autonomic nervous system and hypertension. Circ Res. 2014;114(11):1804–14.
58. Grassi G, Ram VS. Evidence for a critical role of the sympathetic nervous system in hypertension. J Am Soc Hypertens. 2016;10(5):457–66.
59. Carandina A, Lazzeri G, Villa D, et al. Targeting the autonomic nervous system for risk stratification, outcome prediction and neuromodulation in ischemic Stroke. Int J Mol Sci. 2021;22(5):2357.
60. Zhang F, Liu L, Zhang C, Ji S, Mei Z, Li T. Association of metabolic syndrome and its components with risk of stroke recurrence and mortality: a meta-analysis. Neurology. 2021;97(7):e695–705.
61. Ulleryd MA, Prahl U, Bö Rsbo J, et al. The association between autonomic dysfunction, inflammation and atherosclerosis in men under investigation for carotid plaques. PLoS One. 2017;12(4):e0174974.
62. Chistiakov DA, Ashwell KW, Orekhov AN, Bobryshev YV. Innervation of the arterial wall and its modification in atherosclerosis. Auton Neurosci Basic Clin. 2015;193:7–11.
63. Rupprecht S, Finn S, Hoyer D, Guether A, Witte OW, Schultze T, Schwab M. Association between systemic inflammation, carotid arteriosclerosis, and autonomic dysfunction. Transl Stroke Res. 2020;11(1):50–9.
64. Fodor DM, Marta MM, Perju-Dumbravă L. Implications of circadian rhythm in Stroke occurrence: certainties and possibilities. Brain Sci. 2021;11(7):865.
65. Riganello F, Prada V, Soddu A, di Perri C, Sannita WG. Circadian rhythms and measures of CNS/autonomic interaction. Int J Environ Res Public Health. 2019;16(13):2336.
66. Do LC, Folsom AR, Blair SN. Physical activity and stroke risk: a meta-analysis. Stroke. 2003;34(10):2475–81.
67. Mostofsky E, Laier E, Levitan EB, Rosamond WD, Schlaug G, Mittleman MA. Physical activity and onset of acute ischemic stroke: the stroke onset study. Am J Epidemiol. 2011;173(3):330–6.

68. Anderson C, Ni Mhurchu C, Scott D, Bennett D, Jamrozik K, Hankey G. Triggers of subarachnoid hemorrhage: role of physical exertion, smoking, and alcohol in the Australasian cooperative research on subarachnoid hemorrhage study (ACROSS). Stroke. 2003;34(7):1771–6.
69. Guiraud V, Touzé E, Rouillon F, Godefroy O, Mas J-L. Stressful life events as triggers of ischemic stroke: a case-crossover study. Int J Stroke. 2013;8(5):300–7.
70. Ranieri M, Finsterer J, Bedini G, Parati EA, Bersano A. Takotsubo syndrome: clinical features, pathogenesis, treatment, and relationship with cerebrovascular diseases. Curr Neurol Neurosci Rep. 2018;18(5):20. https://doi.org/10.1007/s11910-018-0833-7.
71. Templin C, Ghadri J, Diekmann J, Napp C, Bataiosu D, Jaguszewski M, Cammann V, Sarcon A, Geyer V, Neuman C, Seifert B, Hellermann J. Clinical features and outcomes of takotsubo (stress) cardiomyopathy. NEJM. 2015;373(10):929–38.
72. Brunner S, Winter R, Werzer C, von Stülpnagel L, Clasen I, Hameder A, Stöver A, Graw M, Bauer A, Sinner MF. Impact of acute ethanol intake on cardiac autonomic regulation. Sci Rep. 2021;11(1):13255.
73. Singh A, Saluja S, Kumar A, et al. Cardiovascular complications of marijuana and related substances: a review. Cardiol Ther. 2018;7(1):45–59.
74. Fisher BAC, Ghuran A, Vadamalai V, Antonios TF. Cardiovascular complications induced by cannabis smoking: a case report and review of the literature. Emerg Med J. 2005;22(9):679–80.
75. Lavados PM, Olavarría VV, Hoffmeister L, Ambient Temperature and Stroke Risk. Evidence supporting a short-term effect at a population level from acute environmental exposures. Stroke. 2018;49:255–61.
76. Bahouth MN, Venkatesan A. Acute viral illnesses and ischemic Stroke pathophysiological considerations in the era of the COVID-19 pandemic. Stroke. 2021;52:1885–94.
77. Chen P-L, Kuo TBJ, Hang CCH. Parasymapthetic activity correlates with early outcome in patients with large artery atherosclerotic stroke. J Neurol Sci. 2012;314(1–2):57–61.
78. Hilz MJ, Moeller S, Akhundova A, Marthol H, Pauli E, De Fina P, Schwab S. High NIHSS values predict impairment of cardiovascular autonomic control. Stroke. 2011;42(6):1528–33.
79. Xiong L, Leung HW, Chen XY, Leung WH, Soo OY, Wong KS. Autonomic dysfunction in different subtypes of post-acute ischemic stroke. J Neurol Sci. 2014;337(1-2):141–6.
80. Meglic B, Kobal J, Psredkar J, Pogacnik T. Autonomic nervous system function in patients with acute brainstem stroke. Cerebrovasc Dis. 2001;11(1):2–8.
81. Ha SY, Park KM, Kim SE, Lee BI, Shin KJ. Autonomic function in progressive lacunar infarction. Acta Neurol Scand. 2018;138:1–9.
82. Hase Y, Polvikoski TM, Firbank MJ, Craggs LJL, Hawthorne E, Platten C, Stevenson W, Deramecourt V, Ballard C, Kenny RA, Perry RH, Ince P, Carare RO, Allan LM, Hosburgh L, Kalaria RN. Small vessel disease pathological changes in neurodegenerative and vascular dementias concomitant with autonomic dysfunction. Brain Pathol. 2020;30(1):191–202.
83. Intarhakham K, Suwanpraset K, Muengtaweepongsa S. Correlation between parasymnathetic activity and reduced cerebrovascular reactivity in patients with lacunar infarct. Curr Neurovasc Res. 2017;14(1):65–70.
84. Zygmunt A, Stanczyk J. Methods of evaluation of auto- nomic nervous system function. Arch Med Sci. 2010;6(1):11–8.
85. Sykora M, Diedler J, Rupp A, Turcani P, Steiner T. Impaired baroreceptor reflex sensitivity in acute stroke is associated with insular involvement, but not with carotid atherosclerosis. Stroke. 2009;40:737–42.
86. Acampa M, Lazzerini PE, Martini G. Atrial cardiopathy and sympatho-vagal imbalance in cryptogenic stroke: pathogenic mechanisms and effects on electrocardiographic markers. Front Neurol. 2018;9:1–10.
87. Korpelainen JT, Sotaniemi KA, Huikuri HV, Myllyä VV. Abnormal heart rate variability as a manifestation of autonomic dysfunction in hemispheric brain infarction. Stroke1996;27:2059–2063.
88. Kolin A, Norris JW. Myocardial damage from acute cerebral lesions. Stroke. 1984;15:990–3.

89. Togha M, Sjarifpour A, Asharf H, Moghadam M, Sahraian MA. Electrocardiographic abnormalities in acute cerebrovascular events in patients with/without cardiovascular disease. Ann Indian Acad Neurol. 2013;16:66–71.
90. Abboud H, Berroir S, Labreuche J, et al. On behalf of the GENIC investigators. Insular involvement in brain infarction increases risk for cardiac arrhythmias and death. Ann Neurol. 2006;59:691–9.
91. Meyer S, Strittmatter M, Fischer C, Georg T, Schmitz B. Lateralization in autonomic dysfunction in ischemic stroke involving the insular cortex. Neuroreport. 2004;15:357–61.
92. Orlandi G, Fanucchi S, Strata G, Pataleo L, Landucci Pellegrini L, Prontera C, Martini A, Murri L. Transient autonomic nervous system dysfunction during hyper- acute stroke. Acta Neurol Scand. 2000;102:317–21.
93. Marcheselli S, Cavallini A, Tosi P, Quaglini S, Micieli G. Impaired blood pressure increase in acute cardioembolic stroke. J Hypertens. 2006;24(9):1849–56.
94. Davison DL, Terek M, Chawla LS. Neurogenic pulmonary edema. Crit Care. 2012;16(2):212.
95. Chamorro A, Urra X, Planas AM. Infection after acute ischemic stroke: a manifestation of brain-induced immunodepression. Stroke. 2007;38:1097–103.
96. Fowler CJ, Griffiths D, de Groat WC. The neural control of micturition. Nat Rev Neurosci. 2008;9:453–66.
97. Gelber DA, Good DC, Laven LJ, Verhulst SJ. Causes of urinary incontinence after acute hemispheric strokes. Stroke. 1993;24:378–82.
98. Ullman T, Reding M. Gastrointestinal dysfunction in stroke. Semin Neurol. 1996;16:269–75.
99. Naver HK, Blomstrand C, Wallin BG. Reduced heart rate variability after right-sided stroke. Stroke. 1996;27(2):247–51.
100. Ha SY, Park KM, Park J, Kim SE, Lee BI, Shin KJ. Autonomic function testing in progressive lacunar infarction et al. Acta Neurol Scand 2018;138(1):32–40.
101. Tang S, Xiong L, Fan Y, Mok VCT, Wong KS, Leung TW. Stroke outcome prediction by blood pressure variability, heart rate variability, and baroreflex sensitivity. Stroke. 2020;51(4):1317–20.
102. Xiong L, Leung HHW, Chen XY, Han JH, Leung TWH, Soo YOY, Chan AYY, Lau AYL, Wong LKS, et al. Int J Stroke. 2013;8(8):645–51.
103. Feibel JH, Hardy PM, Campbell RG, Goldstein MN, Joynt RJ. Prognostic value of the stress response following stroke. JAMA. 1977;238(13):1374–6.
104. Acharya RU, Joseph PK, Kannathal N, Lim CM, Suri JS. Heart rate variability: a review. Med Biol Eng Comput. 2006;44(12):1031–51.
105. Singh N, Moneghetti KJ, Christle JW, Hadley D, Plews D, Froelicher V. Heart rate variability: an old metric with new meaning in the era of using mHealth technologies for health and exercise training guidance. part one: physiology and methods. Arrhythm Electrophysiol Rev. 2018;7(3):193–8.
106. Fyfe-Johnson AL, Muller CJ, Alonso A, et al. Heart rate variability and incident Stroke: the atherosclerosis Risk in communities study. Stroke. 2016;47(6):1452–8.
107. Binici Z, Mouridsen MR, Køber L, Sajadieh A. Decreased nighttime heart rate variability is associated with increased stroke risk. Stroke. 2011;42(11):3196–201.
108. Lees T, Shad-Kaneez F, Simpson AM, Nassif NT, Lin Y, Lal S. Heart rate variability as a biomarker for predicting stroke, post-stroke complications and functionality. Biomark Insights. 2018;13:1177271918786931.
109. Li C, Meng X, Pan Y, Li Z, Wang M, Wang Y. The association between heart rate variability and 90-Day prognosis in patients with transient ischemic attack and minor Stroke. Front Neurol. 2021;12:861.
110. Zhao M, Gun L, Wang Y. The association of autonomic nervous system function with ischemic stroke and treatment strategies. Front Neurol. 2020;10:141.
111. Capone F, Miccinilli S, Pellegrino G, et al. Transcutaneous Vagus nerve stimulation combined with robotic rehabilitation improves upper limb function after Stroke. Neural Plast. 2017;2017:1–6.

Chapter 6
Atrial Fibrillation and Stroke

Jaime Eduardo Rodríguez and Luciano A. Sposato

6.1 Epidemiology

Atrial fibrillation is a supraventricular tachyarrhythmia characterized by an uncoordinated atrial electrical activation that produces an ineffective atrial contraction. It is a highly prevalent cardiac arrhythmia affecting 2–4% of global population [1]. In 2017, the global incidence and prevalence were 403 new cases and 4977 cases per million inhabitants, respectively, a significant increase relative to 1997 (309 new cases and 3751 cases per million) [2]. The incidence of AF is expected to continue growing in future years [1–3]. Population studies from the USA and Europe have estimated a 2.3-fold increase in the prevalence of the disease in the next few decades [3, 4].

The most prominent risk factor for AF is age, with a yearly prevalence increase of approximately 5% after the age of 65 [5], and older cohort studies indicate an OR of 2.1 for every extra decade of life [6]. The risk of developing AF depends on genetic predisposition and clinical risk factor's burden [7–10]. Males have a slightly

J. E. Rodríguez (✉)
Stroke Center, Neurology Department, Hospital Universitario Fundación Santa Fe de Bogotá, Bogotá, Colombia

L. A. Sposato
Department of Clinical Neurological Sciences, Schulich School of Medicine and Dentistry, Western University, London, ON, Canada

Heart and Brain Laboratory, Western University, London, ON, Canada

Departments of Epidemiology and Biostatistics and Anatomy and Cell Biology, Schulich School of Medicine and Dentistry, Western University, London, ON, Canada

Robarts Research Institute, Western University, London, ON, Canada

Lawson Health Research Institute, London, ON, Canada
e-mail: luciano.sposato@lhsc.on.ca

G. Micieli et al. (eds.), *Autonomic Disorders in Clinical Practice*,
https://doi.org/10.1007/978-3-031-43036-7_6

increased risk of developing AF compared to females, with a ratio of 1.11 [2]. There are also racial differences on prevalence, with being AF less frequent in non-Caucasians compared with Caucasians [11–13]. The lifetime risk of AF in the European ancestry population is 1 out of 3 (37%), and 1 out of 5 in the black and Asian population [14–17]. Genetic polymorphisms have shown an association with incidence of AF after adjusting for other factors [7, 18].

Modifiable risk factors typically associated with cardiovascular disease have demonstrated association with AF in several different studies: smoking, alcohol abuse, obesity, and inappropriate nutritional behaviour. Physical activity has a bimodal association, since both, a sedentary lifestyle and intense physical activity, are associated with the disease [17, 19–21]. There is interest in the reduction of these risk factors to help reduce the burden of the disease [22]. Additionally, diseases like hypertension, diabetes, coronary artery disease (CAD), heart failure, valvular heart disease, chronic kidney disease, chronic obstructive pulmonary disease (COPD), and sleep-disordered breathing (SDB), and acute illnesses or surgery have been associated with AF [17, 20, 23–28].

Estimating death rates for AF-related mortality is challenging, given that patients usually do not die from the arrythmia itself, but from associated complications. AF is associated with an increased risk of death [29]. The mortality risk from AF seems to be higher in women than in men [30], and in patients with comorbidities such as CAD, heart failure, end-stage renal disease (ESRD), diabetes, sepsis, among others [7].

AF-related costs range from 1% of the UK's health budget [31] to 26 billion dollars per year in the USA, equivalent to 10% of all cardiovascular disease expenses [32]. Yearly AF-related patient-based costs for high-income, upper-middle-income, and lower-middle-income countries are 41.420, 12.895, and 8.184 international dollars [33].

The association between AF and stroke has been clearly established, with early studies showing a 3 to 5 times higher risk of stroke in patients with AF, and the presence of AF in around 1 in 3 patients with stroke [6, 34, 35]. Contemporary studies have shown AF-associated stroke (known or newly detected) in 28% of stroke patients, with higher prevalence in North American and European populations and lower prevalence in Latin America (35%, 33%, and 17%, respectively) [36].

6.2 Pathophysiology

The association between AF and stroke is currently considered to have three explanations [37]:

- AF is a direct cause of stroke.
- Stroke can trigger AF.
- AF and stroke share risk factors.

AF pathogenesis in stroke patients can be considered as two distinct entities: AF as a consequence of an abnormal atrial substrate, also known as cardiogenic AF, that could be later on associated with a cardioembolic stroke; or AF as a consequence of stroke-induced heart injury (SIHI), also known as neurogenic AF. Additionally, stroke and AF can co-exist without being etiologically related in two contexts: a non-cardioembolic stroke in a patient with AF, known as a bystander AF; and stroke and AF both as the consequence of an abnormal atrial substrate, known as atrial cardiopathy.

In the next sections, we are going to expand these ideas and clarify some of the evidence behind these concepts.

6.2.1 Cardiogenic AF

The left atrium (LA) has many functions in the cardiovascular system. It initiates and transmit the electric stimulus for myocardial contractions employing the pacemaker cells in the sinus node, intra atrial conduction pathway and the AV node. It also acts as a blood reservoir that is filled during ventricular systole, and then is emptied into the left ventricle during ventricular diastole. There are also atrial homeostatic functions mediated by the secretion of atrial natriuretic peptides (**ANP**) and brain natriuretic peptides (**BPN**), which contribute to systemic volume regulation [38]. The atrium is very sensitive to both intrinsic and extrinsic injury, which can affect its normal functioning with subsequent irregular beating and loss of contractile function [39, 40].

AF is an electrophysiological state characterized by poor contractility, increased automaticity, decreased refractoriness, and re-entry activity [18, 39, 41]. The physiopathology involves a complex interplay of several contributors, facilitators, and perpetuators that lead to atrial remodelling and, eventually abnormal atrial substrate. It has been previously resumed with four interconnected loops, all producing positive feedback to each other [41]:

1. Electrical loop.
2. Triger loop.
3. Hemodynamic loop.
4. Structural loop.

There are important mechanisms that are central to these loops and deserve additional explanation

- Ion channel dysfunction via K+ and Ca2+ currents produce a facilitated depolarization and a decreased refractoriness, facilitating re-entry [42, 43].
- Ectopic activity with rapid focal firing can act on vulnerable tissue creating re-entry circuits or discrete rotors that help maintain the rapid firing activity [39, 43]. This is the most frequent mechanism initiating AF.
- Structural remodelling, primarily fibrosis but also changes in cellular ultrastructure, alter the electrophysiological characteristics of the LA, producing hypocon-

tractility, dilatation, and conduction disturbances; which facilitates unidirectional blocks and re-entry circuits [39, 44–47].

- Atrial myocardial stretch secondary to atrial overload is considered a main contributor to the structural remodelling [48].
- Autonomic dysfunction via vagal and adrenergic dysregulation produces shortening of action potential duration and promotes delayed afterdepolarizations mostly via Ca++ currents, levels and sensitivities (both in transmembrane and sarcoplasmic reticulum channels and pumps) [39, 42, 49].

The development and perpetuation of AF constitutes a dynamic process over time: atrial remodelling secondary to age, underlying heart disease and the AF itself are associated with increasing arrhythmia burden [38, 50–52], and the abnormal rhythm potentiates all pathological mechanisms, increasing the abnormal atrial substrate and producing a positive loop between both entities [38, 41].

Finally, genetics have been recently recognized as having a significant role in AF pathogenesis. A series of genes implicated in ion channels, transporters, myocytes structural components, and others factors have been associated with the disease (PITX2, TTN, MYL4, HCN4, ZFHX3, KCNN3) [18, 53–57]. There is familial aggregation even in the absence of risk factors, and the calculated heritability from a study in twins was 62% [58, 59] (Fig. 6.1).

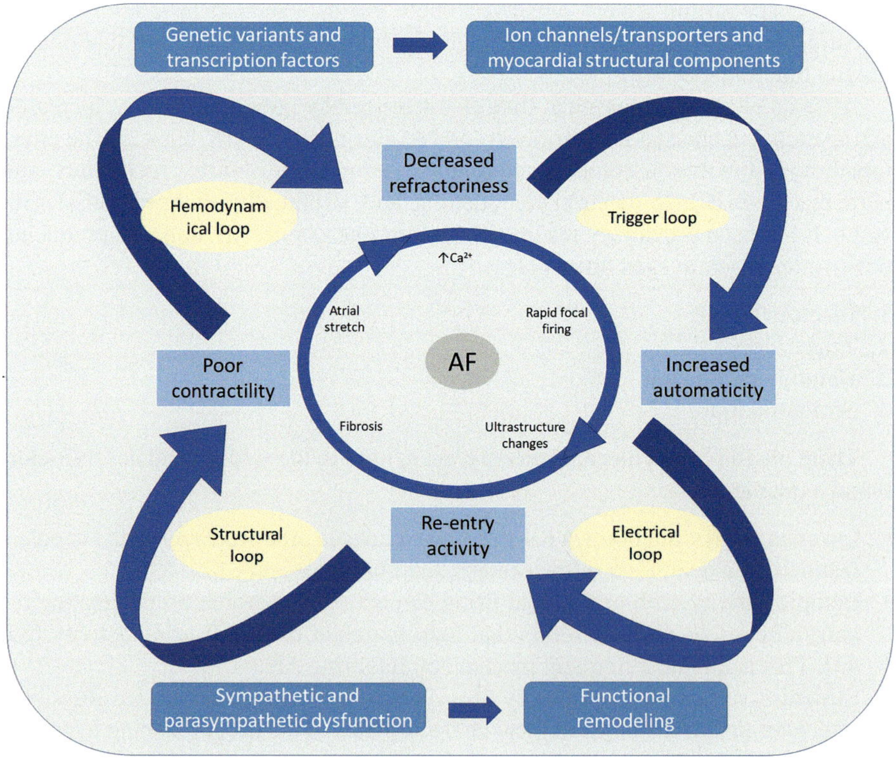

Fig. 6.1 Resumed AF loops

Subject to genetic predisposition, autonomic dysfunction and atrial cardiopathy, four distinct pathophysiological loops act synchronously and interdependently in the onset and maintenance of AF.

6.2.2 *Neurogenic AF*

In some cases, AF can be a manifestation of neurogenic myocardial damage on the context of the recently described stroke-heart syndrome [60–62]. This kind of AF is called neurogenic AF [63]. Based on population-based data showing a time-varying risk of cardiovascular complications post-stroke in patients without known heart disease, current timeframe for heart-brain syndrome is 30 days after the stroke, with the peak on the first 72 hours, so only AF first detected in this period of time could fix into this category [61, 63, 64].

There are three described mediators in the stroke-heart syndrome:

- Immunological: increased systemic inflammatory response, myocardial proinflammatory cytokines and macrophage infiltration [65].
- Humoral: increased systemic norepinephrine and cardiac catecholamine production [66].
- Neuronal: lesions in the insula or the broadly distributed central autonomic network have been described to produce autonomic tone disbalance and secondary cardiogenic damage [67, 68].

The neuronal mechanism and the so-called cardiac neuronal network have been widely studied in recent decades. The heart has important autonomic innervation via the vagus nerve, the cervicothoracic ganglia and the cardiac ganglionated plexus. Brain damage in certain regions such as a stroke in the insular cortex has been associated with increased sympathetic and reduced parasympathetic function [69], but increase in both sympathetic and parasympathetic outflow has also been linked to arrhythmias [70]. Studies in humans and animals have found evidence of autonomic dysregulation after a stroke including increased serum norepinephrine, increased heart catecholamine-driven transcription, and abnormal autonomic reflexes [71–75]. This autonomic disbalance is considered associated with development and propagation of AF via increased calcium in presynaptic neurons and subsequent increased action potential frequency, shortening of action potential duration via potassium channel modulation, and vagal induced conduction delays [76]. In this context, the use of autonomic modulation with betablockers have been proposed to prevent SIHI and stroke-heart syndrome, but clinical evidence this is needed [61].

6.2.3 The AFDAS Concept

Atrial fibrillation detected after stroke (AFDAS) is a unique type of AF, with different characteristics and prognosis compared to AF known before stroke occurrence (KAF).

- Age: AFDAS patients may be younger than KAF patients [77].
- Heart disease: AFDAS patients have less frequently LA enlargement, prior myocardial infarction, coronary artery disease or heart failure than KAF patients [77–79].
- Stroke location: AFDAS patients have stroke in the insular territory more frequently [77].
- Stroke severity: AFDAS is found more frequently on stroke than on transient ischaemic attack (TIA) patients [80, 81]. AFDAS related stroke has higher NIHSS and LVO than KAF [82].
- Risk of stroke recurrence: AFDAS risk of recurrent stroke is lower than that of KAF [78].
- AF burden: AFDAS patients have lower AF burden, lower rates of sustained AF and higher rates of spontaneous conversion to sinus rhythm [82–84].

While KAF is understood as mediated primarily by intrinsic cardiac factors (hypertension, structural heart disease, ischaemic heart disease, etc.), AFDAS can be triggered by the same cardiac mechanisms (cardiogenic AFDAS) or stroke-related neurogenic mechanisms (e.g., autonomic dysfunction or inflammation). However, it is challenging to differentiate if an AF episode after a stroke is neurogenic, or if it is a previously unrecognized cardiogenic AF. The pathogenesis of these two entities is clearly different, and so seem to be patients' characteristics and stroke risk profiles [77]. Moreover, a dichotomous classification is probably wrong in most patients. The concept of AF detected after stroke (AFDAS) has been proposed with the aim of acknowledging and better characterizing the pathophysiological and prognostic differences related to the timing of AF diagnosis in patients with ischaemic stroke and transient ischaemic attack (TIA).

AFDAS phenotypes constitute a spectrum of AF-related risk, with each patient representing a specific combination of multiple factors, including but not limited to (a) the severity of atrial substrate, (b) the basic underlying mechanism (cardiogenic vs. neurogenic), (c) the burden of AF, and (d) the overall demographic and risk factor profile (age, sex, hypertension, etc.). The risk of subsequent stroke depends on the interplay of these characteristics [37, 78, 83].

Extensive research has identified reliable markers of atrial cardiopathy. These markers have also been associated with the risk of AFDAS. The most consistent makers are left atrial (LA) strain, LA size, p-wave terminal force in V1, natriuretic peptides, and cardiac troponin [63, 85, 86]. The severity of atrial cardiopathy seems to be related to the risk of cardiogenic AFDAS, similarly to what has been found in patients without stroke. Also, a "rise and fall" pattern of cardiac troponin (acute myocardial injury) instead of chronically increased troponin (chronic myocardial injury) is a candidate biomarker to differentiate neurogenic vs cardiogenic AFDAS [83].

6.2.4 AFDAS as an Incidental Finding and Its Potential Bystander Role

A multitude of cardiovascular risk factors are independently associated with both AF and stroke [39, 87]. Patients with AF can have non-cardioembolic strokes, for example secondary to small vessel disease or carotid atherosclerosis, so AF would be a bystander [88]. These patients could have a stroke without temporal relationship to AF episodes [89–92]. This is supported by the findings of the Stroke of Known Cause and Underlying Atrial Fibrillation (STROKE-AF) study, in which patients with strokes attributed to small or large vessel disease undergoing implantable loop recording (ILR) had a strikingly high AFDAS detection rate [93].

On the other hand, atrial cardiopathy, a potential cause and consequence of AF, can also be a source of atrial embolic strokes independently of AF rhythm; hence, AF and stroke could potentially share a common precursor [94]. This abnormal atrial substrate could be secondary to AF, ageing, cardiovascular disease, metabolic risk factors, or other systemic comorbidities [37]. Patients with both AF and atrial cardiopathy have an even higher risk of ischaemic stroke compared with patients with just one of them [37, 95]. Evidence supporting this concept comes from several different studies, for example:

- Rhythm control does not eliminate the risk of stroke in AF patients [96].
- There is no temporal relationship between AF episodes and incident ESUS [97, 98] (Table 6.1).

Table 6.1 Risk factors for AF. Risk factors for AF can be classified as modifiable and non-modifiable. Many of the risk factors are also risk factors for cardiovascular disease

Non-modifiable	Modifiable		
Age	Valve disease	Obesity	Endurance exercise or sedentarism
Male sex	Heart failure	Smoking	Diabetes
White/European race	Coronary artery disease	Obstructive sleep apnoea	Thyroid disease
Genetics	Hypertension	Alcohol consumption	Diet

6.3 AF and Thrombus Formation

Thrombogenesis in AF is no longer though to be secondary only to blood stasis, and it is now considered that it follows the same three principles Virchow described more than a century ago: hypercoagulability, blood stasis, and prothrombotic endothelial (in this case endocardial) changes [99].

6.3.1 Prothrombotic Endocardial Remodelling

In atrial cells of patients with AF, the excess of cytosolic calcium produces a chain reaction [100]:

- Increased generation of reactive oxygen species (ROS).
- Proinflammatory effect on the endocardium.
- Increased synthesis of prothrombotic molecules.
  - Plasminogen activator inhibitor 1 (PAI1).
  - Von-Willebrand factor (vWF).
  - ICAM, VCAM, selectins.

This endocardial remodelling is not exclusive to AF but is also independently associated with the same cardiovascular risk factors that produce the AF [100].

6.3.2 Blood Stasis

The atrial dilation in the context of AF, and the ineffective atrial contraction during AF rhythm, contribute to incomplete atrial voiding and blood stasis. It has also been described that even in sinus rhythm, the atrial contraction of AF patients is impaired, so this mechanism is enduring even in paroxysmic AF [100–103]. The blood pooling happens preferentially at the left atrial appendage (LAA), a 1.2–4.5 cm pouch-like structure with great size and shape variability. The LAA is the most common location of atrial thrombus formation both in AF and non-AF patients [38, 104]. Indeed, 90% of thrombi in AF patients are found in the LAA.

There have been several prothrombotic LAA markers described: pulse wave doppler phenotype, lower LAA flow velocity, non-'chicken-wing' morphology (especially 'cauliflower' morphology), larger orifice area, fibrosis, and spontaneous echocardiographic contrast [105–107]. LAA and LA can also have a discordance in rhythm (LAA pulse wave despite sinus rhythm in ECG) [105]. A high-risk LAA phenotype may explain a portion of the embolic events in AF patients with otherwise low stroke risk [104].

6.3.3 *Hypercoagulability*

There is increasing evidence for hypercoagulability in AF. The finding of spontaneous echo contrast (SEC) on LA or LAA during an AF paroxysm is a marker of blood stasis, but it is also considered a marker of fibrinogen-erythrocytes interaction and is associated with stroke risk [99, 108]. Prothrombin fragment 1 + 2 is a marker of active coagulation and is higher on stroke patients with AF than in other stroke patients [109]. Other coagulation and endothelial markers such as fibrinogen, Von-Willebrand factor or soluble P-selectin, have a linear correlation with FA burden markers such as LA volume and permanent instead of paroxysmal AF [110, 111]. Nitric Oxide Synthetase (NOS) levels are downregulated and oxidative stress is higher, and the thrombogenic Plasminogen Activator Inhibitor-1 (PAI-1) is upregulated in cardiomyocytes of AF patients [112, 113]. Finally, platelet activation and thrombin generation are increased in patients with rapid atrial rate or AF [99, 114, 115].

6.4 Diagnosis of AF

There are multiple definitions that need to be stablished first:

- AF rhythm: Supraventricular tachyarrhythmia with irregular R-R intervals, absence of distinct repeating P waves and irregular atrial activations.
- Atrial high-rate episodes (AHRE): Event of atrial beating at ≥175 bpm for ≥5 min detected with a cardiac implantable electronic device (CIED) with an atrial lead or sensor (cut-off values are not standardized).
- Subclinical AF (SCAF): Event of AHRE or device-detected AF (implantable cardiac monitor (ICM) or wearable) that has been confirmed by a physician's review of the recorded intracardiac electrogram or ECG-recorded rhythm.
- Clinical AF: AF rhythm documented for at least the entire duration of a 12-lead ECG, or 30 s of an ECG tracing (telemetry, Holter, wearable monitor with a recorded ECG…).
- Excessive supraventricular ectopic activity (ESVEA): Holter-detected premature supraventricular contractions (PSC) ≥30/h or an episode of PSC longer than ≥20 beats. Usually considered a surrogate of AF.

AHRE/SCAF events (AHRE and SCAF are not the same but in the literature are often use together or even interchangeable) require that the patient remains asymptomatic during the episode and that a diagnosis of AF has not been previously made. A clinical AF diagnosis can be made in either symptomatic or asymptomatic patients. An asymptomatic AF event that found in a patient with a previous stroke is not asymptomatic anymore [116] and should not be named SCAF.

6.4.1 Screening for AF

There are many different options available for screening for AF. They can be classified depending on how invasive vs non-invasive the strategy is and on whether intermittent vs permanent monitoring is intended. There is not a consensus on how intense or which methods we should be used for screening for AF in stroke patients. Longer monitoring will also detect patients with a lower AF burden [117–119].

If an asymptomatic patient is detected to have an AHRE, a SCAF, or an irregular rhythm on pulse palpation, oscillometry or photoplethysmography, then a 12-lead ECG or at least a single-lead ECG tracing longer than 30 s should be done in order to make a definitive diagnosis of clinical AF [1, 120].

In post-stroke patients, early start of continuous cardiac monitoring improves the detection of AF (in this case: AFDAS) and increases the rate of anticoagulation [121–123]. In this population, a staircase approach can result in an overall detection rate of approximately 24 [124]. However, it remains unknown if this approach is timelier, more clinically effective, or more cost-effective than skipping Phases 2 and 3 by applying an ILR immediately after stroke with a less stringent selection process.

- Phase 1: emergency room ECG.
- Phase 2: serial ECG, continuous inpatient ECG monitoring, continuous inpatient cardiac telemetry, and in-hospital Holter monitoring.
- Phase 3: Ambulatory Holter.
- Phase 4: Mobile cardiac outpatient telemetry, external loop recording, and implantable loop recording.

Some wearable monitors such as smartwatches, belts or smartphones have proven efficacy for detecting AF patients and are new option for screening [1]. There are clinical risk cores that could help identify patients with high probability of AF such as C2HEST score that has been validated in cohorts with stroke history [125] (Table 6.2).

6.4.2 The Burden Of AF

The burden of the arrythmia is a measure of how often and for how long a patient has the abnormal rhythm. It can be measured or reported in several different ways: number of episodes per day, amount of time with an abnormal rhythm over a period, longest arrhythmia event during monitoring... Continuous monitoring devices allow for a precise determination of the arrythmia burden, while intermittent monitoring tend to underestimate it.

There is a classification based on the temporal pattern of abnormal rhythm in AF has been historically used [1].

- First diagnosed: AF not diagnosed before, irrespective of duration or symptoms.

Table 6.2 Screening methods for AF. Many different screening methods can be used to detect possible AF. The sensitivity increases with more prolonged and continuous screening time, and specificity increases with more invasive techniques

	Least invasive		More invasive
Intermittent	• Pulse palpation • Oscillometric pressure cuff	Wearable belt In-hospital telemetry monitoring	
	Photoplethysmogram or Intermittent ECG rhythm strip on smartphone or device	• Long-term holter •1-2 week continuous ECG patches	
Continuous	Photoplethysmogram on smartwatch/wearable		• Implantable cardiac monitor • Cardiac implanted electronic devices

ICM: single-lead bipolar surface ECG
CIED: atrial lead can monitor atrial rhythm and store the tracings (pacemakers, implantable cardioverter defibrillator (ICD), biventricular pacemakers, and cardiac loop recorders)

- Paroxysmal: episodes terminating within 7 days of onset.
- Persistent: AF continuously sustained beyond 7 days but less than 12 months.
- Long-standing persistent: AF continuously sustained beyond 12 months.
- Permanent: Continuous AF without any further attempts of rhythm control.

The method of the AF episode termination (after medical treatment or spontaneous) is not relevant for the classification.

The AF burden is supposed to be related to the stroke risk, but it remains unclear if this relationship is linear and what the AF burden threshold to warrant anticoagulation is, especially in subclinical patients. The risk of stroke is smaller in AHRE/SCAF than in paroxysmal AF, and is smaller in paroxysmal AF than in non-paroxysmal AF (persistent, long-standing or permanent) [50, 91, 126–129]. Non-paroxysmal AF patients tend to have higher risk profiles than patients with paroxysmal AF [130], but the increased stroke risk persists even after adjusting for risk factors. Paroxysmal AF is more often associated with stroke because its more prevalent than non-paroxysmal AF and its more frequently undiagnosed [131]. It has been proposed that AF newly detected with a short monitoring technique such as a 12-lead ECG is generally considered as high burden [132]. Lastly, SCAF is a strong predictor of clinical AF, the burden of both clinical and subclinical AF tend to increase over time, and high initial burden is a stronger predictor of subsequent burden increase [133–135].

Studies with implantable devices have found a cutoff value of >1 h/day of AF burden as a predictor of stroke, with increasing risk as the burden increases [127]. It has been proposed that AF burden is especially predictive of the stroke risk in patients with low cardiovascular risk [91, 136].

AF rhythm events shorter than 30 s are a matter of controversy; these episodes represent more than half of AF rhythm episodes detected in monitoring after a stroke, and it is not clear if they entail a significant risk of stroke. Stroke neurologists are twice as likely to consider these short events as clinical AF [116, 137–139].

The role of low-burden AHRE/SCAF in stroke is also controversial as the temporal association of these events with an incident stroke is not always clear, and several studies have shown no association of short events (<20 s) with stroke [98, 140]. Some authors argue that these episodes should be considered as stroke risk markers instead of a direct cause of stroke [97, 141]. Recent studies have shown that high-intensity screening of AF with implantable devices increases the rate of AF detection and the rate of treatment with anticoagulation, but there is no impact on reducing stroke incidence [142, 143]. This reflects the fact that AF detected only after long monitoring is probably low burden, and as such, the risk of stroke is not as high [117, 118]. High intensity screening should be reserved for high-risk patients, for which there is evidence of benefit of prolonged cardiac monitoring for the reduction of ischaemic stroke [144].

6.4.3 Neuroimaging in AF

There are distinctive patterns of stroke distribution in patients with cardioembolism: bilateral, multiple vascular territories, larger size. Other characteristics such as lesion shape or anterior/posterior distribution has not been proven different from non-cardioembolic stroke [145, 146]. About 1 in 6 patients with classic lacunar syndromes have been found to have cardioembolic looking strokes in MRI [147]. Other differential etiologies of multiple territory infarcts such as hypercoagulability, cancer, vasculitis, and multiple arterial dissections should be kept in mind.

6.5 Approach to Treatment of AF

Multiple guidelines recommend the 'Atrial fibrillation Better Care Pathway (ABC)' to treat AF patients: **A**nticoagulation/**A**void stroke, **B**etter symptom management, **C**ardiovascular and **C**omorbidity optimization. This approach has evidence for better results than standard care [148, 149].

6.5.1 Stroke Prevention

6.5.1.1 Oral Anticoagulation

Current recommendations for preventing thromboembolism with oral anticoagulation (OAC) in clinical AF are not based on the AF burden but on the calculated stroke risk [126, 150–152]. This stroke risk assessment can be made with different tools such as GARFIELD-AD, ATRIA, or ABC-stroke, but the most widely recommended and used is the CHA2DS2-VASc score [1, 153].

The CHA2DS2-VASc score is based exclusively on clinical data (age, sex, and comorbidities), but it does not include any measures of AF burden or atrial cardiopathy biomarkers [126, 154]. Patients with high-risk CHA2DS2-VASc scores have an overall high risk of cardiovascular events, not only secondary to AF episodes [89]. In general, the higher the thrombotic risk, the higher the benefit or OAC [155]. Real-world studies have shown that each item of the CHA2DS2-VASc score imply a different weight for stroke risk [156]. Patients with low scores (CHA2DS2-VASc score of 0 for males or 1 for females) have a low thromboembolic risk that is no different from that of people without AF, and the recommendation is to not use OAC [38, 157]. In male patients with CHA2DS2-VASc scores ≥1 or females with scores ≥2 most guidelines recommend OAC to prevent stroke [1, 150, 151]. Another important aspect of using the CHA2DS2-VASc score is that it can increase over time, as patients age and develop new risk factors or comorbidities.

In the context of AFDAS, even though it carries a lower burden of AF, fewer comorbidities and fewer rate of complications than KAF, it is clear that it implies a higher stroke risk compared with non-AF patients [83], so the current recommendation is to treat AFDAS the same as KAF, and they should receive OAC unless contraindicated [1, 150, 151, 158]. Future research may find a way to identify lower-risk individuals with AFDAS, such as low-burden self-limited neurogenic AFDAS, that may not need life-long anticoagulation [124]. Careful monitoring of AF burden and determination of atrial cardiopathy probably will be helpful to establish the subsequent risk of stroke in these patients [132, 152]. It is recommended that FA detected on admission ECG should not be considered AFDAS, as it is probably a previously undiagnosed AF [83].

In patients without diagnosis of clinical AF, but a diagnosis of AHRE/SCAF, the decision to start anticoagulation is more difficult. It is clear that the burden of both AHRE and SCAF is associated with the risk of stroke and death [94, 116, 159–161], but the amount of burden where the risks of stroke are large enough to warrant anticoagulation is not clearly established because the studies have used different cut off values (>5 min, >1 h, >5.5 h, >24 h). Current guidelines and expert consensus recommend an individualized approach based on the burden of AHRE/SCAF and the individual's calculated stroke risk based on CHA2DS2-VASc score to make the decision for anticoagulation [1, 135, 162, 163] (Table 6.3).

Warfarin was the standard of treatment for stroke prevention in AF for decades until the direct oral anticoagulants (DOACs) entered the market. These newer anticoagulants not only prevent strokes, with a risk reduction of around 2/3 [164], but they also diminish the severity of incident strokes [165, 166]. DOACs: rivaroxaban, dabigatran, apixaban, edoxaban; have a similar efficacy than warfarin for stroke prevention (slightly better reduction of ischaemic stroke or systemic embolism), but the risk of ICH is lower with DOACs than with warfarin [167]. There main results of pivotal randomized clinical trials suggest the following:

Table 6.3 When to start OAC dependent on AF burden and stroke risk score. AF burden and clinical risk factors for stroke can be used to determine the threshold of benefit for anticoagulation in AF. The exact threshold is not fully elucidated, and more research is needed

	Burden				
CHA2DS2-VASc	AHRE/SCAF			AF	
	<1 h/day	1–24 h/day	>24 h/day	Neurogenic AFDAS	Cardiogenic AFDAS or KAF
Low risk: 0(m), 1 (f)	NO	NO	NO	NO	NO
Intermediate risk 1(m), 2(f)	NO	NO	MAYBE	YES (maybe self-limited)	YES
High risk ≥2 (m), ≥3(f)	NO	MAYBE	YES	YES	YES
Consider atrial cardiopathy markers (imaging, biomarkers, etc.)					
In AHRE/SCAF: Always review electrograms to exclude false positives					

Source: Based on ESC 2020 guideline on AF diagnosis and treatment

- Warfarin safety and efficacy rely on a good INR control (time in therapeutic range > 70%) [168].
- Dabigatran 150 mg has a higher risk of gastrointestinal bleeding than warfarin [169].
- Rivaroxaban 20 mg has a higher risk of gastrointestinal bleeding than warfarin [170].
- Apixaban 5 mg was superior to warfarin in preventing ischaemic stroke or systemic embolism [171].
- Reduced-dose regimens of DOACs have worst efficacy and safety results than full-dose regimens, but reduced- and full-dose regimens have consistent results compared to warfarin [172].
- In patients with AF and any mechanical heart valve or mitral moderate or severe stenosis, warfarin is the only OAC recommended as DOACs have not shown clear benefit in these patients [173].

It is clear that both single antiplatelet therapy (SAPT) with AAS, and dual antiplatelet therapy (DAPT) with AAS and clopidogrel, are inferior in the prevention of thromboembolic events in patients with AF compared to anticoagulation [174]. It should be noted that the level of protection is around 22% with SAPT compared with no antithrombotic medication [175].

6.5.1.2 LAA Occlusion

In patients with AF, device-occlusion of the LAA seems to be non-inferior for ischaemic stroke prevention and have a lower risk of haemorrhagic stroke compared to warfarin [104, 176–178], although some considerations need to be made regarding the inclusion criteria and outcomes used in some randomized clinical trials. This discussion is beyond the scope of this chapter. No studies have been conducted comparing this technique versus DOACs [104]. It is usually reserved for patients with high bleeding risk or contraindications for OAC use. There is no randomized evidence for the selection of antithrombotic treatment after LAA occlusion, long-term SAPT or temporary OAC are commonly used [1, 179, 180].

6.5.1.3 Assessment of Bleeding Risk

The best tool for the prediction of bleeding risk in AF patients is the HASBLED score [181]. Guidelines recommend using this score to identify modifiable risk factors for bleeding, and also, depending on the risk level, the clinician should establish the frequency of follow-ups. This score should not be used to hold back anticoagulation, as patients with high bleeding risk based on HASBLED usually also have high thrombotic risk based on CHA2DS2-VASc [182], and unless there is an absolute contraindication, patients should receive OAC. Both scores should be reassessed regularly as the risks of patients are not static and could prompt adjustment in treatments [183–185].

6.5.1.4 Rhythm Control

Based on current evidence [96], most guidelines consider symptom control to be the only indication of rhythm management in AF patients, as it seems to be of no benefit in preventing thromboembolic events. Guidelines usually recommend rate-control measures as first line of treatment, and others antiarrhythmic medication in patients with residual symptoms, leaving ablation of the arrhythmogenic loci for refractory patients. Detailed rate or rhythm management and cardioversion in AF is beyond the scope of this chapter [1, 150, 151].

Some trials have shown that rhythm control may be beneficial compared to rate-control in slowing AF progression [186]. Recently, a subgroup analysis of a large, randomized trial on patients with recently diagnosed AF (<12 months) showed that early rhythm control was superior to usual care for the prevention of cardiovascular death, stroke, and hospitalization in patients with a history of stroke. It is yet to be seen if this will change current guidelines [187, 188].

6.5.1.5 Cardiovascular Comorbidities

All cardiovascular comorbidities and risk factors should be treated, controlled, or optimized to improve outcomes in AF patients. There should be a focus on metabolic control, avoidance of alcohol, weight loss, cardiovascular fitness, SAHOS and hypertension treatment [189–192].

6.5.2 *Special Interest Circumstances*

6.5.2.1 Haemorrhagic Stroke

Patients with AF and an intracranial haemorrhage (ICH) have a high risk of ischaemic stroke if antithrombotics are withheld. Observational evidence in this population has shown that OAC (including warfarin) protects against ischaemic stroke compared to antiplatelets or no treatment without a significant increase in ICH recurrence [193–195]. The safer risk profile of DOACs has been proven in this scenario in randomized trials and should be the OAC of choice over warfarin [167, 196]. Patients with traumatic ICH or ICH without evidence of cerebral amyloid angiopathy are the subgroups that benefit the most from OAC [197]. Reversible risk factors for bleeding such as high blood pressure or problematic drug interactions, should be controlled.

There is no clear evidence on the optimal time to (re-)start OAC after ICH and patient selection should be made on a personalized basis after a thorough discussion with them or their substitute decision-makers. Guidelines usually suggest waiting 4 to 8 weeks, but in patients with high thrombotic risk (for example, with a mechanical heart valve), starting as early as after 2 weeks or LAA occlusion could be considered [1, 198, 199]. Observational evidence on patients with ICH and mechanical heart valve found that OACs increase the haemorrhagic risk when initiated before day 14, but balancing the ischaemic and haemorrhagic risks suggests that the earliest possible OAC resumption is in day 6 [200]. Small randomized controlled trials have not provided definite evidence yet.

6.5.2.2 AF and Concurrent Acute or Chronic Coronary Syndrome

Coronary artery disease is present in 1/3 of patients with AF, and it is not infrequent that these patients require percutaneous coronary intervention (PCI) and stenting, for which antiplatelets are required to prevent stent thrombosis [201]. Current guidelines recommend the use of triple therapy (ASS + clopidogrel + DOAC) for 1 to 4 weeks, then dual therapy (preferable clopidogrel + DOAC) until 6 to 12 months after the PCI, and then continue monotherapy with a DOAC unless there's a new coronary event. Full-dose regimens should be used unless patient weight and renal function do not allow it [202–206].

6.5.2.3 Recent TIA or Ischaemic Stroke

Patients with recent brain ischaemia are considered to have a transient increased risk of haemorrhagic transformation, so OAC is usually withheld temporally. The risk is considered to be related to the stroke size, so this is usually the marker used to decide when to (re-) start OAC [206]. Evidence in this matter is lacking. Some guidelines recommend (re-)starting OAC in the 4–14 days after the stroke based on prospective observational data [207, 208]. Other guidelines recommend a 1–3–6-12-days rule according to the initial stroke severity (TIA, NIHSS <8, NIHSS 8–15, and NIHSS >15, respectively) based on expert recommendations [209].

Recent trials are trying to update these recommendations in the context of DOACs, probably allowing an earlier start than with warfarin. A non-randomized trial using database information formulated the 1–2–3–4-day rule using the same NIHSS cutoffs as for the 1–3–6–12 rule. It showed increased efficacy without increasing the haemorrhagic risk [210]. A more recent randomized trial showed no difference in early (<4 days) vs late (5–10 days) OAC initiation in a population of mostly low and moderate severity strokes [211]. However, this was a small trial and we await the results of other ongoing randomized controlled trials.

Bridging with low-molecular-weight heparin is associated with more bleeding and more ischaemic strokes, so it should not be used [212]. Antiplatelet bridging is recommended in some guidelines and could be used based on the small protection against ischaemic stroke in AF conferred by these medications [213].

6.5.2.4 Kidney and Liver Disease

The efficacy and safety of DOACs in AF patients with CrCl 30–49 mL/min is similar compared with patients with normal renal function [214, 215]. Apixaban safety profile compared to warfarin is even greater in patients with CrCl 25–30 mL/min than in patients with CrCl >30 mL/min [216]. Different guidelines disagree on the management of patients with AF and CrCl <15 mL/min or in dialysis, some recommend apixaban or warfarin, and other recommend no antithrombotic treatment (considering that patients on dialysis receive anticoagulation for the procedure) [150, 151, 217]. A randomized trial comparing apixaban to warfarin in AF patients on haemodialysis could not find differences between groups, but bleeding events were tenfold more frequent than ischaemic events [218]. Depending on the bleeding and thrombotic risks LAA closure may be an option for these patients [218].

Cirrhotic patients have high risk of devolving AF and of haemorrhagic complications. DOACs have shown consistent benefit and safety in patients with active liver disease [219], but evidence in severely impaired liver function is poor as they were not included in the pivotal trials. Based on mostly retrospective data, DOACs has shown safety superiority compared to warfarin in cirrhotic patients with AF [220].

6.5.2.5 Postoperative AF

Even though the risk of stroke in postoperative AF (OPAF) is not as high as other forms of AF, it is still associated with an increased risk of late AF and with both early and late stroke. In this patients OAC is protective against embolic stroke and should be used [221, 222].

6.5.2.6 Atrial Flutter

Auricular flutter (AFL) patients have higher risk of stroke compared with sinus rhythm patients, but lower compared with AF patients. AFL patients can also progress to have AF. All recommendations for management of patients with AF also apply for AFL patients [1, 151, 223].

6.5.2.7 Atrial Cardiopathy

There are many proposed markers of atrial cardiopathy that are currently under extensive research to establish if they could be used to detect patients that could benefit from anticoagulation even in the absence of confirmed AF. They could also help increase the accuracy of stroke risk estimation in AF, the risk of progression to AF in AHRE/SCAF or the risk of stroke in neurogenic AFDAS [128, 132, 154, 224–227].

- Indexed LA volume.
- Spontaneous LA contrast.
- Reduced LA strain.
- Low peak LAA velocity.
- LA fibrosis.
- Troponin I.
- P-wave terminal force in lead V1.
- Premature atrial complexes.
- Supraventricular tachycardia.
- Clinical scores.

The ARCADIA trial has been recently stopped and we are awaiting the presentation of its results.

References

1. Hindricks G, Potpara T, Dagres N, Arbelo E, Bax JJ, Blomström-Lundqvist C, et al. 2020 ESC Guidelines for the diagnosis and management of atrial fibrillation developed in collaboration with the European Association for Cardio-Thoracic Surgery (EACTS). Eur Heart J. 2021;42(5):373–498.
2. Lippi G, Sanchis-Gomar F, Cervellin G. Global epidemiology of atrial fibrillation: An increasing epidemic and public health challenge. Int J Stroke. 2021;16(2):217–21.
3. Krijthe BP, Kunst A, Benjamin EJ, Lip GYH, Franco OH, Hofman A, et al. Projections on the number of individuals with atrial fibrillation in the European Union, from 2000 to 2060. Eur Heart J. 2013;34(35):2746–51.
4. Colilla S, Crow A, Petkun W, Singer DE, Simon T, Liu X. Estimates of current and future incidence and prevalence of atrial fibrillation in the U.S. adult population. Am J Cardiol. 2013;112(8):1142–7.

5. Piccini JP, Hammill BG, Sinner MF, Jensen PN, Hernandez AF, Heckbert SR, et al. Incidence and prevalence of atrial fibrillation and associated mortality among Medicare beneficiaries, 1993-2007. Circ Cardiovasc Qual Outcomes. 2012;5(1):85–93.
6. Benjamin EJ, Levy D, Vaziri SM, D'Agostino RB, Belanger AJ, Wolf PA. Independent risk factors for atrial fibrillation in a population-based cohort. The Framingham Heart Study. JAMA. 1994;271(11):840–4.
7. Weng LC, Preis SR, Hulme OL, Larson MG, Choi SH, Wang B, et al. Genetic predisposition, clinical risk factor burden, and lifetime risk of atrial fibrillation. Circulation. 2018;137(10):1027–38.
8. Lloyd-Jones DM, Wang TJ, Leip EP, Larson MG, Levy D, Vasan RS, et al. Lifetime risk for development of atrial fibrillation: the Framingham Heart Study. Circulation. 2004;110(9):1042–6.
9. Heeringa J, van der Kuip DAM, Hofman A, Kors JA, van Herpen G, Stricker BHC, et al. Prevalence, incidence and lifetime risk of atrial fibrillation: the Rotterdam study. Eur Heart J. 2006;27(8):949–53.
10. Shen AYJ, Contreras R, Sobnosky S, Shah AI, Ichiuji AM, Jorgensen MB, et al. Racial/ethnic differences in the prevalence of atrial fibrillation among older adults—a cross-sectional study. J Natl Med Assoc. 2010;102(10):906–13.
11. Dewland TA, Olgin JE, Vittinghoff E, Marcus GM. Incident atrial fibrillation among asians, hispanics, blacks, and whites. Circulation. 2013;128(23):2470–7.
12. Martinez C, Katholing A, Wallenhorst C, Granziera S, Cohen AT, Freedman SB. Increasing incidence of non-valvular atrial fibrillation in the UK from 2001 to 2013. Heart Br Card Soc. 2015;101(21):1748–54.
13. Magnussen C, Niiranen TJ, Ojeda FM, Gianfagna F, Blankenberg S, Njølstad I, et al. Sex differences and similarities in atrial fibrillation epidemiology, risk factors, and mortality in community cohorts: results from the BiomarCaRE Consortium (Biomarker for Cardiovascular Risk Assessment in Europe). Circulation. 2017;136(17):1588–97.
14. Guo Y, Tian Y, Wang H, Si Q, Wang Y, Lip GYH. Prevalence, incidence, and lifetime risk of atrial fibrillation in China: new insights into the global burden of atrial fibrillation. Chest. 2015;147(1):109–19.
15. Chao TF, Liu CJ, Tuan TC, Chen TJ, Hsieh MH, Lip GYH, et al. Lifetime risks, projected numbers, and adverse outcomes in Asian patients with atrial fibrillation: a report from the Taiwan nationwide AF cohort study. Chest. 2018;153(2):453–66.
16. Mou L, Norby FL, Chen LY, O'Neal WT, Lewis TT, Loehr LR, et al. Lifetime risk of atrial fibrillation by race and socioeconomic status: ARIC Study (atherosclerosis risk in communities). Circ Arrhythm Electrophysiol. 2018;11(7):e006350.
17. Benjamin EJ, Muntner P, Alonso A, Bittencourt MS, Callaway CW, Carson AP, et al. Heart disease and stroke statistics-2019 update: a report from the American Heart Association. Circulation. 2019;139(10):e56–528.
18. Andersen JH, Andreasen L, Olesen MS. Atrial fibrillation-a complex polygenetic disease. Eur J Hum Genet EJHG. 2021;29(7):1051–60.
19. Gorenek B, Pelliccia A, Benjamin EJ, Boriani G, Crijns HJ, Fogel RI, et al. European Heart Rhythm Association (EHRA)/European Association of Cardiovascular Prevention and Rehabilitation (EACPR) position paper on how to prevent atrial fibrillation endorsed by the Heart Rhythm Society (HRS) and Asia Pacific Heart Rhythm Society (APHRS). Europace. 2017;19(2):190–225.
20. Allan V, Honarbakhsh S, Casas JP, Wallace J, Hunter R, Schilling R, et al. Are cardiovascular risk factors also associated with the incidence of atrial fibrillation? A systematic review and field synopsis of 23 factors in 32 population-based cohorts of 20 million participants. Thromb Haemost. 2017;117(5):837–50.
21. Magnani JW, Hylek EM, Apovian CM. Obesity begets atrial fibrillation: a contemporary summary. Circulation. 2013;128(4):401–5.

22. Huxley RR, Lopez FL, Folsom AR, Agarwal SK, Loehr LR, Soliman EZ, et al. Absolute and attributable risks of atrial fibrillation in relation to optimal and borderline risk factors: the Atherosclerosis Risk in Communities (ARIC) study. Circulation. 2011;123(14):1501–8.
23. Conen D, Tedrow UB, Koplan BA, Glynn RJ, Buring JE, Albert CM. Influence of systolic and diastolic blood pressure on the risk of incident atrial fibrillation in women. Circulation. 2009;119(16):2146–52.
24. Mitchell GF, Vasan RS, Keyes MJ, Parise H, Wang TJ, Larson MG, et al. Pulse pressure and risk of new-onset atrial fibrillation. JAMA. 2007;297(7):709–15.
25. Chatterjee S, Bavishi C, Sardar P, Agarwal V, Krishnamoorthy P, Grodzicki T, et al. Meta-analysis of left ventricular hypertrophy and sustained arrhythmias. Am J Cardiol. 2014;114(7):1049–52.
26. Manolis AJ, Kallistratos MS, Poulimenos LE. Recent clinical trials in atrial fibrillation in hypertensive patients. Curr Hypertens Rep. 2012;14(4):350–9.
27. Greve AM, Gerdts E, Boman K, Gohlke-Baerwolf C, Rossebø AB, Nienaber CA, et al. Prognostic importance of atrial fibrillation in asymptomatic aortic stenosis: the Simvastatin and Ezetimibe in Aortic Stenosis study. Int J Cardiol. 2013;166(1):72–6.
28. Kannel WB, Wolf PA, Benjamin EJ, Levy D. Prevalence, incidence, prognosis, and predisposing conditions for atrial fibrillation: population-based estimates. Am J Cardiol. 1998;82(8A):2N–9N.
29. Chamberlain AM, Gersh BJ, Alonso A, Chen LY, Berardi C, Manemann SM, et al. Decade-long trends in atrial fibrillation incidence and survival: a community study. Am J Med. 2015;128(3):260–267.e1.
30. Emdin CA, Wong CX, Hsiao AJ, Altman DG, Peters SA, Woodward M, et al. Atrial fibrillation as risk factor for cardiovascular disease and death in women compared with men: systematic review and meta-analysis of cohort studies. BMJ. 2016;532:h7013.
31. Stewart S, Murphy NF, Murphy N, Walker A, McGuire A, McMurray JJV. Cost of an emerging epidemic: an economic analysis of atrial fibrillation in the UK. Heart Br Card Soc. 2004;90(3):286–92.
32. Coyne KS, Paramore C, Grandy S, Mercader M, Reynolds M, Zimetbaum P. Assessing the direct costs of treating nonvalvular atrial fibrillation in the United States. Value Health. 2006;9(5):348–56.
33. Li X, Tse VC, Au-Doung LW, Wong ICK, Chan EW. The impact of ischaemic stroke on atrial fibrillation-related healthcare cost: a systematic review. Europace. 2017;19(6):937–47.
34. Wolf PA, Dawber TR, Thomas HE, Kannel WB. Epidemiologic assessment of chronic atrial fibrillation and risk of stroke: the Framingham study. Neurology. 1978;28(10):973–7.
35. Freedman B, Potpara TS, Lip GYH. Stroke prevention in atrial fibrillation. Lancet. 2016;388(10046):806–17.
36. Perera KS, Vanassche T, Bosch J, Swaminathan B, Mundl H, Giruparajah M, et al. Global survey of the frequency of atrial fibrillation–associated stroke. Stroke. 2016;47(9):2197–202.
37. Kamel H, Okin PM, Elkind MSV, Iadecola C. Atrial fibrillation and mechanisms of stroke: time for a new model. Stroke. 2016;47(3):895–900.
38. Goette A, Kalman JM, Aguinaga L, Akar J, Cabrera JA, Chen SA, et al. EHRA/HRS/APHRS/SOLAECE expert consensus on atrial cardiomyopathies: definition, characterization, and clinical implication. Europace. 2016;18(10):1455–90.
39. Andrade J, Khairy P, Dobrev D, Nattel S. The clinical profile and pathophysiology of atrial fibrillation: relationships among clinical features, epidemiology, and mechanisms. Circ Res. 2014;114(9):1453–68.
40. Corradi D. Atrial fibrillation from the pathologist's perspective. Cardiovasc Pathol. 2014;23(2):71–84.
41. Schotten U, Verheule S, Kirchhof P, Goette A. Pathophysiological mechanisms of atrial fibrillation: a translational appraisal. Physiol Rev. 2011;91(1):265–325.
42. Wakili R, Voigt N, Kääb S, Dobrev D, Nattel S. Recent advances in the molecular pathophysiology of atrial fibrillation. J Clin Invest. 2011;121(8):2955–68.

43. Nattel S. New ideas about atrial fibrillation 50 years on. Nature. 2002;415(6868):219–26.
44. Yue L, Xie J, Nattel S. Molecular determinants of cardiac fibroblast electrical function and therapeutic implications for atrial fibrillation. Cardiovasc Res. 2011;89(4):744–53.
45. Burstein B, Nattel S. Atrial fibrosis: mechanisms and clinical relevance in atrial fibrillation. J Am Coll Cardiol. 2008;51(8):802–9.
46. Burstein B, Comtois P, Michael G, Nishida K, Villeneuve L, Yeh YH, et al. Changes in connexin expression and the atrial fibrillation substrate in congestive heart failure. Circ Res. 2009;105(12):1213–22.
47. Frustaci A, Chimenti C, Bellocci F, Morgante E, Russo MA, Maseri A. Histological substrate of atrial biopsies in patients with lone atrial fibrillation. Circulation. 1997;96(4):1180–4.
48. De Jong AM, Maass AH, Oberdorf-Maass SU, Van Veldhuisen DJ, Van Gilst WH, Van Gelder IC. Mechanisms of atrial structural changes caused by stretch occurring before and during early atrial fibrillation. Cardiovasc Res. 2011;89(4):754–65.
49. Chen PS, Chen LS, Fishbein MC, Lin SF, Nattel S. Role of the autonomic nervous system in atrial fibrillation: pathophysiology and therapy. Circ Res. 2014;114(9):1500–15.
50. de Vos CB, Pisters R, Nieuwlaat R, Prins MH, Tieleman RG, Coelen RJS, et al. Progression from paroxysmal to persistent atrial fibrillation clinical correlates and prognosis. J Am Coll Cardiol. 2010;55(8):725–31.
51. Padfield GJ, Steinberg C, Swampillai J, Qian H, Connolly SJ, Dorian P, et al. Progression of paroxysmal to persistent atrial fibrillation: 10-year follow-up in the Canadian Registry of Atrial Fibrillation. Heart Rhythm. 2017;14(6):801–7.
52. Kerr CR, Humphries KH, Talajic M, Klein GJ, Connolly SJ, Green M, et al. Progression to chronic atrial fibrillation after the initial diagnosis of paroxysmal atrial fibrillation: results from the Canadian Registry of Atrial Fibrillation. Am Heart J. 2005;149(3):489–96.
53. Chinchilla A, Daimi H, Lozano-Velasco E, Dominguez JN, Caballero R, Delpón E, et al. PITX2 insufficiency leads to atrial electrical and structural remodeling linked to arrhythmogenesis. Circ Cardiovasc Genet. 2011;4(3):269–79.
54. Benjamin EJ, Rice KM, Arking DE, Pfeufer A, van Noord C, Smith AV, et al. Variants in ZFHX3 are associated with atrial fibrillation in individuals of European ancestry. Nat Genet. 2009;41(8):879–81.
55. Nielsen JB, Fritsche LG, Zhou W, Teslovich TM, Holmen OL, Gustafsson S, et al. Genome-wide study of atrial fibrillation identifies seven risk loci and highlights biological pathways and regulatory elements involved in cardiac development. Am J Hum Genet. 2018;102(1):103–15.
56. Peng W, Li M, Li H, Tang K, Zhuang J, Zhang J, et al. Dysfunction of myosin light-chain 4 (MYL4) leads to heritable atrial cardiomyopathy with electrical, contractile, and structural components: evidence from genetically engineered rats. J Am Heart Assoc. 6(11):e007030.
57. Ellinor PT, Lunetta KL, Albert CM, Glazer NL, Ritchie MD, Smith AV, et al. Meta-analysis identifies six new susceptibility loci for atrial fibrillation. Nat Genet. 2012;44(6):670–5.
58. Christophersen IE, Ravn LS, Budtz-Joergensen E, Skytthe A, Haunsoe S, Svendsen JH, et al. Familial aggregation of atrial fibrillation: a study in Danish twins. Circ Arrhythm Electrophysiol. 2009;2(4):378–83.
59. Oyen N, Ranthe MF, Carstensen L, Boyd HA, Olesen MS, Olesen SP, et al. Familial aggregation of lone atrial fibrillation in young persons. J Am Coll Cardiol. 2012;60(10):917–21.
60. Scheitz JF, Nolte CH, Doehner W, Hachinski V, Endres M. Stroke–heart syndrome: clinical presentation and underlying mechanisms. Lancet Neurol. 2018;17(12):1109–20.
61. Scheitz JF, Sposato LA, Schulz-Menger J, Nolte CH, Backs J, Endres M. Stroke–heart syndrome: recent advances and challenges. J Am Heart Assoc. 2022;11(17):e026528.
62. Sposato LA, Hilz MJ, Aspberg S, Murthy SB, Bahit MC, Hsieh CY, et al. Post-stroke cardiovascular complications and neurogenic cardiac injury. J Am Coll Cardiol. 2020;76(23):2768–85.
63. Sposato LA, Riccio PM, Hachinski V. Poststroke atrial fibrillation: cause or consequence? Critical review of current views. Neurology. 2014;82(13):1180–6.

64. Sposato LA, Lam M, Allen B, Shariff SZ, Saposnik G, PARADISE Study Group. First-ever ischemic stroke and incident major adverse cardiovascular events in 93 627 older women and men. Stroke. 2020;51(2):387–94.
65. Yan T, Chen Z, Chopp M, Venkat P, Zacharek A, Li W, Shen Y, Wu R, Li L, Landschoot-Ward J, Lu M, Hank K-H, Zhang J, Chen J. Inflammatory responses mediate brain–heart interaction after ischemic stroke in adult mice. J Cereb Blood Flow Metab. 2020;40(6):1213–29. https://doi.org/10.1177/0271678X18813317.
66. Meloux A, Rigal E, Rochette L, Cottin Y, Bejot Y, Vergely C. Ischemic stroke increases heart vulnerability to ischemia-reperfusion and alters myocardial cardioprotective pathways. Stroke. 2018;49(11):2752–60.
67. Krause T, Werner K, Fiebach JB, Villringer K, Piper SK, Haeusler KG, et al. Stroke in right dorsal anterior insular cortex Is related to myocardial injury. Ann Neurol. 2017;81(4):502–11.
68. Prats-Sánchez L, Guisado-Alonso D, Painous C, Fayos F, Pascual-Goñi E, Delgado-Mederos R, et al. Insular damage, new-onset atrial fibrillation and outcome after acute intracerebral hemorrhage. Eur J Neurol. 2018;25(3):491–6.
69. Dorrance AM, Fink G. Effects of stroke on the autonomic nervous system. Compr Physiol. 2015;5(3):1241–63.
70. Pfenniger A, Geist GE, Arora R. Autonomic dysfunction and neurohormonal disorders in atrial fibrillation. Card Electrophysiol Clin. 2021;13(1):183–90.
71. Bieber M, Werner RA, Tanai E, Hofmann U, Higuchi T, Schuh K, et al. Stroke-induced chronic systolic dysfunction driven by sympathetic overactivity. Ann Neurol. 2017;82(5):729–43.
72. Myers MG, Norris JW, Hachinski VC, Weingert ME, Sole MJ. Cardiac sequelae of acute stroke. Stroke. 1982;13(6):838–42.
73. Veltkamp R, Uhlmann S, Marinescu M, Sticht C, Finke D, Gretz N, et al. Experimental ischaemic stroke induces transient cardiac atrophy and dysfunction. J Cachexia Sarcopenia Muscle. 2019;10(1):54–62.
74. Tang S, Xiong L, Fan Y, Mok VCT, Wong KS, Leung TW. Stroke outcome prediction by blood pressure variability, heart rate variability, and baroreflex sensitivity. Stroke. 2020;51(4):1317–20.
75. Jimenez-Ruiz A, Racosta JM, Kimpinski K, Hilz MJ, Sposato LA. Cardiovascular autonomic dysfunction after stroke. Neurol Sci. 2021;42(5):1751–8.
76. Khan AA, Lip GYH, Shantsila A. Heart rate variability in atrial fibrillation: The balance between sympathetic and parasympathetic nervous system. Eur J Clin Investig. 2019;49(11):e13174.
77. González Toledo ME, Klein FR, Riccio PM, Cassará FP, Muñoz Giacomelli F, Racosta JM, et al. Atrial fibrillation detected after acute ischemic stroke: evidence supporting the neurogenic hypothesis. J Stroke Cerebrovasc Dis. 2013;22(8):e486–91.
78. Sposato LA, Cerasuolo JO, Cipriano LE, Fang J, Fridman S, Paquet M, et al. Atrial fibrillation detected after stroke is related to a low risk of ischemic stroke recurrence. Neurology. 2018;90(11):e924–31.
79. Fridman S, Jimenez-Ruiz A, Vargas-Gonzalez JC, Sposato LA. Differences between atrial fibrillation detected before and after stroke and TIA: a systematic review and meta-analysis. Cerebrovasc Dis Basel Switz. 2022;51(2):152–7.
80. Buchwald F, Norrving B, Petersson J. Atrial fibrillation in transient ischemic attack versus ischemic stroke: a Swedish stroke register (Riksstroke) study. Stroke. 2016;47(10):2456–61.
81. Korompoki E, Del Giudice A, Hillmann S, Malzahn U, Gladstone DJ, Heuschmann P, et al. Cardiac monitoring for detection of atrial fibrillation after TIA: A systematic review and meta-analysis. Int J Stroke. 2017;12(1):33–45.
82. Wang R, Macha K, Haupenthal D, Gaßmann L, Siedler G, Stoll S, et al. Acute care and secondary prevention of stroke with newly detected versus known atrial fibrillation. Eur J Neurol. 2022;29(7):1963–71.

83. Sposato LA, Chaturvedi S, Hsieh CY, Morillo CA, Kamel H. Atrial fibrillation detected after stroke and transient ischemic attack: a novel clinical concept challenging current views. Stroke. 2022;53(3):e94–103.
84. Brambatti M, Connolly SJ, Gold MR, Morillo CA, Capucci A, Muto C, et al. Temporal relationship between subclinical atrial fibrillation and embolic events. Circulation. 2014;129(21):2094–9.
85. Olsen FJ, Christensen LM, Krieger DW, Højberg S, Høst N, Karlsen FM, et al. Relationship between left atrial strain, diastolic dysfunction and subclinical atrial fibrillation in patients with cryptogenic stroke: the SURPRISE echo substudy. Int J Cardiovasc Imaging. 2020;36(1):79–89.
86. Wrigley P, Khoury J, Eckerle B, Alwell K, Moomaw CJ, Woo D, et al. Prevalence of positive troponin and echocardiogram findings and association with mortality in acute ischemic stroke. Stroke. 2017;48(5):1226–32.
87. Boehme AK, Esenwa C, Elkind MSV. Stroke risk factors, genetics, and prevention. Circ Res. 2017;120(3):472–95.
88. Lodder J, Bamford JM, Sandercock PA, Jones LN, Warlow CP. Are hypertension or cardiac embolism likely causes of lacunar infarction? Stroke. 1990;21(3):375–81.
89. Cha MJ, Kim YD, Nam HS, Kim J, Lee DH, Heo JH. Stroke mechanism in patients with non-valvular atrial fibrillation according to the CHADS2 and CHA2 DS2 -VASc scores. Eur J Neurol. 2012;19(3):473–9.
90. Welles CC, Whooley MA, Na B, Ganz P, Schiller NB, Turakhia MP. The CHADS2 score predicts ischemic stroke in the absence of atrial fibrillation among subjects with coronary heart disease: data from the Heart and Soul Study. Am Heart J. 2011;162(3):555–61.
91. Zimetbaum P, Waks JW, Ellis ER, Glotzer TV, Passman RS. Role of atrial fibrillation burden in assessing thromboembolic risk. Circ Arrhythm Electrophysiol. 2014;7(6):1223–9.
92. Chesebro JH, Fuster V, Halperin JL. Atrial fibrillation—risk marker for stroke. N Engl J Med. 1990;323(22):1556–8.
93. Bernstein RA, Kamel H, Granger CB, Piccini JP, Sethi PP, Katz JM, et al. Effect of long-term continuous cardiac monitoring vs usual care on detection of atrial fibrillation in patients with stroke attributed to large- or small-vessel disease: the STROKE-AF randomized clinical trial. JAMA. 2021;325(21):2169–77.
94. Healey JS, Connolly SJ, Gold MR, Israel CW, Van Gelder IC, Capucci A, et al. Subclinical atrial fibrillation and the risk of stroke. N Engl J Med. 2012;366(2):120–9.
95. Yaghi S, Kamel H, Elkind MSV. Atrial cardiopathy: a mechanism of cryptogenic stroke. Expert Rev Cardiovasc Ther. 2017;15(8):591–9.
96. Al-Khatib SM, Allen LaPointe NM, Chatterjee R, Crowley MJ, Dupre ME, Kong DF, et al. Rate and rhythm control therapies in patients with atrial fibrillation: a systematic review. Ann Intern Med. 2014;160(11):760–73.
97. Freedman B, Camm J, Calkins H, Healey JS, Rosenqvist M, Wang J, et al. Screening for atrial fibrillation: a report of the AF-SCREEN international collaboration. Circulation. 2017;135(19):1851–67.
98. Freedman B, Boriani G, Glotzer TV, Healey JS, Kirchhof P, Potpara TS. Management of atrial high-rate episodes detected by cardiac implanted electronic devices. Nat Rev Cardiol. 2017;14(12):701–14.
99. Watson T, Shantsila E, Lip GYH. Mechanisms of thrombogenesis in atrial fibrillation: Virchow's triad revisited. Lancet Lond Engl. 2009;373(9658):155–66.
100. Bukowska A, Hammwöhner M, Corradi D, Mahardhika W, Goette A. Atrial thrombogenesis in atrial fibrillation: Results from atrial fibrillation models and AF-patients. Herzschrittmacherther Elektrophysiol. 2018;29(1):76–83.
101. Di Tullio MR, Sacco RL, Sciacca RR, Homma S. Left atrial size and the risk of ischemic stroke in an ethnically mixed population. Stroke. 1999;30(10):2019–24.

102. Sanfilippo AJ, Abascal VM, Sheehan M, Oertel LB, Harrigan P, Hughes RA, et al. Atrial enlargement as a consequence of atrial fibrillation. A prospective echocardiographic study. Circulation. 1990;82(3):792–7.
103. Keren G, Etzion T, Sherez J, Zelcer AA, Megidish R, Miller HI, et al. Atrial fibrillation and atrial enlargement in patients with mitral stenosis. Am Heart J. 1987;114(5):1146–55.
104. Yaghi S, Song C, Gray WA, Furie KL, Elkind MSV, Kamel H. Left atrial appendage function and stroke risk. Stroke. 2015;46(12):3554–9.
105. Warraich HJ, Gandhavadi M, Manning WJ. Mechanical discordance of the left atrium and appendage. Stroke. 2014;45(5):1481–4.
106. Lee JM, Seo J, Uhm JS, Kim YJ, Lee HJ, Kim JY, et al. Why is left atrial appendage morphology related to strokes? An analysis of the flow velocity and orifice size of the left atrial appendage. J Cardiovasc Electrophysiol. 2015;26(9):922–7.
107. Di BL, Santangeli P, Anselmino M, Mohanty P, Salvetti I, Gili S, et al. Does the left atrial appendage morphology correlate with the risk of stroke in patients with atrial fibrillation? J Am Coll Cardiol. 2012;60(6):531–8.
108. Asinger RW, Koehler J, Pearce LA, Zabalgoitia M, Blackshear JL, Fenster PE, et al. Pathophysiologic correlates of thromboembolism in nonvalvular atrial fibrillation: II. Dense spontaneous echocardiographic contrast (The Stroke Prevention in Atrial Fibrillation [SPAF-III] study). J Am Soc Echocardiogr. 1999;12(12):1088–96.
109. Turgut N, Akdemir O, Turgut B, Demir M, Ekuklu G, Vural O, et al. Hypercoagulopathy in stroke patients with nonvalvular atrial fibrillation: hematologic and cardiologic investigations. Clin Appl Thromb. 2006;12(1):15–20.
110. Mondillo S, Sabatini L, Agricola E, Ammaturo T, Guerrini F, Barbati R, et al. Correlation between left atrial size, prothrombotic state and markers of endothelial dysfunction in patients with lone chronic nonrheumatic atrial fibrillation. Int J Cardiol. 2000;75(2–3):227–32.
111. Li-Saw-Hee FL, Blann AD, Gurney D, Lip GY. Plasma von Willebrand factor, fibrinogen and soluble P-selectin levels in paroxysmal, persistent and permanent atrial fibrillation. Effects of cardioversion and return of left atrial function. Eur Heart J. 2001;22(18):1741–7.
112. Cai H, Li Z, Goette A, Mera F, Honeycutt C, Feterik K, et al. Downregulation of endocardial nitric oxide synthase expression and nitric oxide production in atrial fibrillation. Circulation. 2002;106(22):2854–8.
113. Mihm MJ, Yu F, Carnes CA, Reiser PJ, McCarthy PM, Van Wagoner DR, et al. Impaired myofibrillar energetics and oxidative injury during human atrial fibrillation. Circulation. 2001;104(2):174–80.
114. Lim HS, Willoughby SR, Schultz C, Gan C, Alasady M, Lau DH, et al. Effect of atrial fibrillation on atrial thrombogenesis in humans: impact of rate and rhythm. J Am Coll Cardiol. 2013;61(8):852–60.
115. Hammwöhner M, Ittenson A, Dierkes J, Bukowska A, Klein HU, Lendeckel U, et al. Platelet expression of CD40/CD40 ligand and its relation to inflammatory markers and adhesion molecules in patients with atrial fibrillation. Exp Biol Med Maywood NJ. 2007;232(4):581–9.
116. Van Gelder IC, Healey JS, Crijns HJGM, Wang J, Hohnloser SH, Gold MR, et al. Duration of device-detected subclinical atrial fibrillation and occurrence of stroke in ASSERT. Eur Heart J. 2017;38(17):1339–44.
117. Chew DS, Li Z, Steinberg BA, O'Brien EC, Pritchard J, Bunch TJ, et al. Arrhythmic burden and the risk of cardiovascular outcomes in patients with paroxysmal atrial fibrillation and cardiac implanted electronic devices. Circ Arrhythm Electrophysiol. 2022;15(2):e010304.
118. Aguilar M, Macle L, Deyell MW, Yao R, Hawkins NM, Khairy P, et al. Influence of monitoring strategy on assessment of ablation success and postablation atrial fibrillation burden assessment: implications for practice and clinical trial design. Circulation. 2022;145(1):21–30.
119. Triantafyllou S, Katsanos AH, Dilaveris P, Giannopoulos G, Kossyvakis C, Adreanides E, et al. Implantable cardiac monitoring in the secondary prevention of cryptogenic stroke. Ann Neurol. 2020;88(5):946–55.

120. Boriani G, Vitolo M, Imberti JF, Potpara TS, Lip GYH. What do we do about atrial high rate episodes? Eur Heart J Suppl J Eur Soc Cardiol. 2020;22(Suppl O):O42–52.
121. Sposato LA, Klein FR, Jáuregui A, Ferrúa M, Klin P, Zamora R, et al. Newly diagnosed atrial fibrillation after acute ischemic stroke and transient ischemic attack: importance of immediate and prolonged continuous cardiac monitoring. J Stroke Cerebrovasc Dis. 2012;21(3):210–6.
122. Gladstone DJ, Spring M, Dorian P, Panzov V, Thorpe KE, Hall J, et al. Atrial fibrillation in patients with cryptogenic stroke. N Engl J Med. 2014;370(26):2467–77.
123. Cipriano LE, Sposato LA. Estimating the sensitivity of holter to detect atrial fibrillation after stroke or transient ischemic attack without a gold standard is challenging. Am J Cardiol. 2016;117(2):314–6.
124. Sposato LA, Cipriano LE, Saposnik G, Ruiz Vargas E, Riccio PM, Hachinski V. Diagnosis of atrial fibrillation after stroke and transient ischaemic attack: a systematic review and meta-analysis. Lancet Neurol. 2015;14(4):377–87.
125. Li YG, Bisson A, Bodin A, Herbert J, Grammatico-Guillon L, Joung B, et al. C2 HEST score and prediction of incident atrial fibrillation in poststroke patients: a French Nationwide study. J Am Heart Assoc. 2019;8(13):e012546.
126. Chen LY, Chung MK, Allen LA, Ezekowitz M, Furie KL, McCabe P, et al. Atrial fibrillation burden: moving beyond atrial fibrillation as a binary entity: a scientific statement from the American heart association. Circulation. 2018;137(20):e623–44.
127. Boriani G, Glotzer TV, Santini M, West TM, De Melis M, Sepsi M, et al. Device-detected atrial fibrillation and risk for stroke: an analysis of >10,000 patients from the SOS AF project (stroke prevention strategies based on atrial fibrillation information from implanted devices). Eur Heart J. 2014;35(8):508–16.
128. Ganesan AN, Chew DP, Hartshorne T, Selvanayagam JB, Aylward PE, Sanders P, et al. The impact of atrial fibrillation type on the risk of thromboembolism, mortality, and bleeding: a systematic review and meta-analysis. Eur Heart J. 2016;37(20):1591–602.
129. Chiang CE, Naditch-Brûlé L, Murin J, Goethals M, Inoue H, O'Neill J, et al. Distribution and risk profile of paroxysmal, persistent, and permanent atrial fibrillation in routine clinical practice: insight from the real-life global survey evaluating patients with atrial fibrillation international registry. Circ Arrhythm Electrophysiol. 2012;5(4):632–9.
130. Al-Makhamreh H, Alrabadi N, Haikal L, Krishan M, Al-Badaineh N, Odeh O, et al. Paroxysmal and non-paroxysmal atrial fibrillation in middle eastern patients: clinical features and the use of medications. analysis of the Jordan atrial fibrillation (JoFib) study. Int J Environ Res Public Health. 2022;19(10):6173.
131. Rizos T, Wagner A, Jenetzky E, Ringleb PA, Becker R, Hacke W, et al. Paroxysmal atrial fibrillation is more prevalent than persistent atrial fibrillation in acute stroke and transient ischemic attack patients. Cerebrovasc Dis Basel Switz. 2011;32(3):276–82.
132. Cerasuolo JO, Cipriano LE, Sposato LA. The complexity of atrial fibrillation newly diagnosed after ischemic stroke and transient ischemic attack: advances and uncertainties. Curr Opin Neurol. 2017;30(1):28–37.
133. Gillis AM, Morck M. Atrial fibrillation after DDDR pacemaker implantation. J Cardiovasc Electrophysiol. 2002;13(6):542–7.
134. Mahajan R, Perera T, Elliott AD, Twomey DJ, Kumar S, Munwar DA, et al. Subclinical device-detected atrial fibrillation and stroke risk: a systematic review and meta-analysis. Eur Heart J. 2018;39(16):1407–15.
135. Gorenek B, Bax J, Boriani G, Chen SA, Dagres N, Glotzer TV, et al. Device-detected subclinical atrial tachyarrhythmias: definition, implications and management-an European Heart Rhythm Association (EHRA) consensus document, endorsed by Heart Rhythm Society (HRS), Asia Pacific Heart Rhythm Society (APHRS) and Sociedad Latinoamericana de Estimulación Cardíaca y Electrofisiología (SOLEACE). Europace. 2017;19(9):1556–78.
136. Botto GL, Padeletti L, Santini M, Capucci A, Gulizia M, Zolezzi F, et al. Presence and duration of atrial fibrillation detected by continuous monitoring: crucial implications for the risk of thromboembolic events. J Cardiovasc Electrophysiol. 2009;20(3):241–8.

137. Tran RT, Rankin AJ, Abdul-Rahim AH, Lip GY, Rankin AC, Lees KR. Short runs of atrial arrhythmia and stroke risk: a European-wide online survey among stroke physicians and cardiologists. J R Coll Physicians Edinb. 2016;46(2):87–92.
138. Rankin AJ, Tran RT, Abdul-Rahim AH, Rankin AC, Lees KR. Clinically important atrial arrhythmia and stroke risk: a UK-wide online survey among stroke physicians and cardiologists. QJM Mon J Assoc Physicians. 2014;107(11):895–902.
139. Sposato LA, Cipriano LE, Riccio PM, Hachinski V, Saposnik G. Very short paroxysms account for more than half of the cases of atrial fibrillation detected after stroke and TIA: a systematic review and meta-analysis. Int J Stroke. 2015;10(6):801–7.
140. Swiryn S, Orlov MV, Benditt DG, DiMarco JP, Lloyd-Jones DM, Karst E, et al. Clinical implications of brief device-detected atrial tachyarrhythmias in a cardiac rhythm management device population: results from the registry of atrial tachycardia and atrial fibrillation episodes. Circulation. 2016;134(16):1130–40.
141. Turakhia MP, Ziegler PD, Schmitt SK, Chang Y, Fan J, Than CT, et al. Atrial fibrillation burden and short-term risk of stroke: case-crossover analysis of continuously recorded heart rhythm from cardiac electronic implanted devices. Circ Arrhythm Electrophysiol. 2015;8(5):1040–7.
142. Svendsen JH, Diederichsen SZ, Højberg S, Krieger DW, Graff C, Kronborg C, et al. Implantable loop recorder detection of atrial fibrillation to prevent stroke (The LOOP Study): a randomised controlled trial. Lancet. 2021;398(10310):1507–16.
143. Tsivgoulis G, Triantafyllou S, Palaiodimou L, Grory BM, Deftereos S, Köhrmann M, et al. Prolonged cardiac monitoring and stroke recurrence: a meta-analysis. Neurology. 2022;98(19):e1942–52.
144. Tsivgoulis G, Palaiodimou L, Triantafyllou S, Köhrmann M, Dilaveris P, Tsioufis K, et al. Prolonged cardiac monitoring for stroke prevention: A systematic review and meta-analysis of randomized-controlled clinical trials. Eur Stroke J. 2022;8(1):106–16.
145. Guidoux C, Sibon I, Alamowitch S, Godeneche G, Guillon B, Timsit S, et al. Capacities of atrial fibrillation detection after stroke: a French nationwide survey. Eur Heart J. 2021;42(Sup plement_1):ehab724.2076.
146. Sharobeam A, Churilov L, Parsons M, Donnan GA, Davis SM, Yan B. Patterns of infarction on MRI in patients with acute ischemic stroke and cardio-embolism: a systematic review and meta-analysis. Front Neurol. 2020;11:606521. https://doi.org/10.3389/fneur.2020.606521.
147. Ay H, Oliveira-Filho J, Buonanno FS, Ezzeddine M, Schaefer PW, Rordorf G, et al. Diffusion-weighted imaging identifies a subset of lacunar infarction associated with embolic source. Stroke. 1999;30(12):2644–50.
148. Lip GYH. The ABC pathway: an integrated approach to improve AF management. Nat Rev Cardiol. 2017;14(11):627–8.
149. Proietti M, Romiti GF, Olshansky B, Lane DA, Lip GYH. Improved outcomes by integrated care of anticoagulated patients with atrial fibrillation using the simple ABC (atrial fibrillation better care) pathway. Am J Med. 2018;131(11):1359–1366.e6.
150. Andrade JG, Verma A, Mitchell LB, Parkash R, Leblanc K, Atzema C, et al. 2018 focused update of the canadian cardiovascular society guidelines for the management of atrial fibrillation. Can J Cardiol. 2018;34(11):1371–92.
151. January CT, Wann LS, Calkins H, Chen LY, Cigarroa JE, Cleveland JC, et al. 2019 AHA/ACC/HRS focused update of the 2014 AHA/ACC/HRS guideline for the management of patients with atrial fibrillation: a report of the American College of Cardiology/American Heart Association Task Force on Clinical Practice Guidelines and the Heart Rhythm Society in Collaboration With the Society of Thoracic Surgeons. Circulation. 2019;140(2):e125–51.
152. Boriani G, Glotzer TV, Ziegler PD, De Melis M, Mangoni di S Stefano L, Sepsi M, et al. Detection of new atrial fibrillation in patients with cardiac implanted electronic devices and factors associated with transition to higher device-detected atrial fibrillation burden. Heart Rhythm. 2018;15(3):376–83.
153. Hobbs FR, Taylor CJ, Jan Geersing G, Rutten FH, Brouwer JR. European Primary Care Cardiovascular Society (EPCCS) SPAF working group. European Primary Care

Cardiovascular Society (EPCCS) consensus guidance on stroke prevention in atrial fibrillation (SPAF) in primary care. Eur J Prev Cardiol. 2016;23(5):460–73.

154. Delgado V, Di Biase L, Leung M, Romero J, Tops LF, Casadei B, et al. Structure and function of the left atrium and left atrial appendage: AF and stroke implications. J Am Coll Cardiol. 2017;70(25):3157–72.
155. Casciano JP, Singer DE, Kwong WJ, Fox ES, Martin BC. Anticoagulation therapy for patients with non-valvular atrial fibrillation: comparison of decision analytic model recommendations and real-world warfarin prescription use. Am J Cardiovasc Drugs Drugs Devices Interv. 2012;12(5):313–23.
156. Quinn GR, Severdija ON, Chang Y, Singer DE. Wide variation in reported rates of stroke across cohorts of patients with atrial fibrillation. Circulation. 2017;135(3):208–19.
157. Chao TF, Liu CJ, Chen SJ, Wang KL, Lin YJ, Chang SL, et al. Atrial fibrillation and the risk of ischemic stroke: does it still matter in patients with a CHA2DS2-VASc score of 0 or 1? Stroke. 2012;43(10):2551–5.
158. Krawczyk M, Fridman S, Cheng Y, Fang J, Saposnik G, Sposato LA. Atrial fibrillation diagnosed after stroke and dementia risk: cohort study of first-ever ischaemic stroke patients aged 65 or older. Europace. 2019;21(12):1793–801.
159. Glotzer TV, Hellkamp AS, Zimmerman J, Sweeney MO, Yee R, Marinchak R, et al. Atrial high rate episodes detected by pacemaker diagnostics predict death and stroke: report of the Atrial Diagnostics Ancillary Study of the MOde Selection Trial (MOST). Circulation. 2003;107(12):1614–9.
160. Capucci A, Santini M, Padeletti L, Gulizia M, Botto G, Boriani G, et al. Monitored atrial fibrillation duration predicts arterial embolic events in patients suffering from bradycardia and atrial fibrillation implanted with antitachycardia pacemakers. J Am Coll Cardiol. 2005;46(10):1913–20.
161. Glotzer TV, Daoud EG, Wyse DG, Singer DE, Ezekowitz MD, Hilker C, et al. The relationship between daily atrial tachyarrhythmia burden from implantable device diagnostics and stroke risk: the TRENDS study. Circ Arrhythm Electrophysiol. 2009;2(5):474–80.
162. Perino AC, Fan J, Askari M, Heidenreich PA, Keung E, Raitt MH, et al. Practice variation in anticoagulation prescription and outcomes after device-detected atrial fibrillation. Circulation. 2019;139(22):2502–12.
163. Eckman MH, Singer DE, Rosand J, Greenberg SM. Moving the tipping point: the decision to anticoagulate patients with atrial fibrillation. Circ Cardiovasc Qual Outcomes. 2011;4(1):14–21.
164. Hart RG, Pearce LA, Aguilar MI. Meta-analysis: antithrombotic therapy to prevent stroke in patients who have nonvalvular atrial fibrillation. Ann Intern Med. 2007;146(12):857–67.
165. Hellwig S, Grittner U, Audebert H, Endres M, Haeusler KG. Non vitamin K dependent oral anticoagulants have a positive impact on ischaemic stroke severity in patients with atrial fibrillation. Europace. 2018;20(4):569–74.
166. Macha K, Marsch A, Siedler G, Breuer L, Strasser EF, Engelhorn T, et al. Cerebral ischemia in patients on direct oral anticoagulants. Stroke. 2019;50(4):873–9.
167. Ruff CT, Giugliano RP, Braunwald E, Hoffman EB, Deenadayalu N, Ezekowitz MD, et al. Comparison of the efficacy and safety of new oral anticoagulants with warfarin in patients with atrial fibrillation: a meta-analysis of randomised trials. Lancet Lond Engl. 2014;383(9921):955–62.
168. Wan Y, Heneghan C, Perera R, Roberts N, Hollowell J, Glasziou P, et al. Anticoagulation control and prediction of adverse events in patients with atrial fibrillation: a systematic review. Circ Cardiovasc Qual Outcomes. 2008;1(2):84–91.
169. Connolly SJ, Ezekowitz MD, Yusuf S, Eikelboom J, Oldgren J, Parekh A, et al. Dabigatran versus warfarin in patients with atrial fibrillation. N Engl J Med. 2009;361(12):1139–51.
170. Patel MR, Mahaffey KW, Garg J, Pan G, Singer DE, Hacke W, et al. Rivaroxaban versus warfarin in nonvalvular atrial fibrillation. N Engl J Med. 2011;365(10):883–91.

171. Granger CB, Alexander JH, McMurray JJV, Lopes RD, Hylek EM, Hanna M, et al. Apixaban versus warfarin in patients with atrial fibrillation. N Engl J Med. 2011;365(11):981–92.
172. Wang KL, Lopes RD, Patel MR, Büller HR, Tan DSY, Chiang CE, et al. Efficacy and safety of reduced-dose non-vitamin K antagonist oral anticoagulants in patients with atrial fibrillation: a meta-analysis of randomized controlled trials. Eur Heart J. 2019;40(19):1492–500.
173. Karthikeyan G, Connolly SJ, Yusuf S. Overestimation of stroke risk in rheumatic mitral stenosis and the implications for oral anticoagulation. Circulation. 2020;142(18):1697–9.
174. ACTIVE Writing Group of the ACTIVE Investigators, Connolly S, Pogue J, Hart R, Pfeffer M, Hohnloser S, et al. Clopidogrel plus aspirin versus oral anticoagulation for atrial fibrillation in the atrial fibrillation clopidogrel trial with irbesartan for prevention of vascular events (ACTIVE W): a randomised controlled trial. Lancet Lond Engl. 2006;367(9526):1903–12.
175. Manaktala R, Kluger J. Role of antiplatelet therapy in stroke prevention in patients with atrial fibrillation. J Am Osteopath Assoc. 2017;117(12):761–71.
176. Holmes DR, Reddy VY, Turi ZG, Doshi SK, Sievert H, Buchbinder M, et al. Percutaneous closure of the left atrial appendage versus warfarin therapy for prevention of stroke in patients with atrial fibrillation: a randomised non-inferiority trial. Lancet Lond Engl. 2009;374(9689):534–42.
177. Holmes DR, Doshi SK, Kar S, Price MJ, Sanchez JM, Sievert H, et al. Left atrial appendage closure as an alternative to warfarin for stroke prevention in atrial fibrillation: a patient-level meta-analysis. J Am Coll Cardiol. 2015;65(24):2614–23.
178. Holmes DR, Kar S, Price MJ, Whisenant B, Sievert H, Doshi SK, et al. Prospective randomized evaluation of the watchman left atrial appendage closure device in patients with atrial fibrillation versus long-term warfarin therapy: the PREVAIL trial. J Am Coll Cardiol. 2014;64(1):1–12.
179. Whitlock RP, Vincent J, Blackall MH, Hirsh J, Fremes S, Novick R, et al. Left atrial appendage occlusion study II (LAAOS II). Can J Cardiol. 2013;29(11):1443–7.
180. Tilz RR, Potpara T, Chen J, Dobreanu D, Larsen TB, Haugaa KH, et al. Left atrial appendage occluder implantation in Europe: indications and anticoagulation post-implantation. Results of the European Heart Rhythm Association Survey. Europace. 2017;19(10):1737–42.
181. Borre ED, Goode A, Raitz G, Shah B, Lowenstern A, Chatterjee R, et al. Predicting thromboembolic and bleeding event risk in patients with non-valvular atrial fibrillation: a systematic review. Thromb Haemost. 2018;118(12):2171–87.
182. Eckman MH, Wise RE, Speer B, Sullivan M, Walker N, Lip GYH, et al. Integrating real-time clinical information to provide estimates of net clinical benefit of antithrombotic therapy for patients with atrial fibrillation. Circ Cardiovasc Qual Outcomes. 2014;7(5):680–6.
183. Chao TF, Lip GYH, Lin YJ, Chang SL, Lo LW, Hu YF, et al. Incident risk factors and major bleeding in patients with atrial fibrillation treated with oral anticoagulants: a comparison of baseline, follow-up and delta HAS-BLED scores with an approach focused on modifiable bleeding risk factors. Thromb Haemost. 2018;118(4):768–77.
184. Chao TF, Lip GYH, Liu CJ, Lin YJ, Chang SL, Lo LW, et al. Relationship of aging and incident comorbidities to stroke risk in patients with atrial fibrillation. J Am Coll Cardiol. 2018;71(2):122–32.
185. Chao TF, Liao JN, Tuan TC, Lin YJ, Chang SL, Lo LW, et al. Incident Co-morbidities in patients with atrial fibrillation initially with a CHA2DS2-VASc score of 0 (Males) or 1 (Females): implications for reassessment of stroke risk in initially "low-risk" patients. Thromb Haemost. 2019;119(7):1162–70.
186. Zhang YY, Qiu C, Davis PJ, Jhaveri M, Prystowsky EN, Kowey P, et al. Predictors of progression of recently diagnosed atrial fibrillation in REgistry on Cardiac Rhythm DisORDers Assessing the Control of Atrial Fibrillation (RecordAF)-United States cohort. Am J Cardiol. 2013;112(1):79–84.
187. Jensen M, Suling A, Metzner A, Schnabel RB, Borof K, Goette A, et al. Early rhythm-control therapy for atrial fibrillation in patients with a history of stroke: a subgroup analysis of the EAST-AFNET 4 trial. Lancet Neurol. 2023;22(1):45–54.

188. Schnabel RB, Marinelli EA, Arbelo E, Boriani G, Boveda S, Buckley CM, et al. Early diagnosis and better rhythm management to improve outcomes in patients with atrial fibrillation: the 8th AFNET/EHRA consensus conference. Europace. 2022;25(1):6–27.
189. Pathak RK, Middeldorp ME, Lau DH, Mehta AB, Mahajan R, Twomey D, et al. Aggressive risk factor reduction study for atrial fibrillation and implications for the outcome of ablation: the ARREST-AF cohort study. J Am Coll Cardiol. 2014;64(21):2222–31.
190. Abed HS, Wittert GA, Leong DP, Shirazi MG, Bahrami B, Middeldorp ME, et al. Effect of weight reduction and cardiometabolic risk factor management on symptom burden and severity in patients with atrial fibrillation: a randomized clinical trial. JAMA. 2013;310(19):2050–60.
191. Holmqvist F, Guan N, Zhu Z, Kowey PR, Allen LA, Fonarow GC, et al. Impact of obstructive sleep apnea and continuous positive airway pressure therapy on outcomes in patients with atrial fibrillation-Results from the Outcomes Registry for Better Informed Treatment of Atrial Fibrillation (ORBIT-AF). Am Heart J. 2015;169(5):647–654.e2.
192. Emdin CA, Callender T, Cao J, Rahimi K. Effect of antihypertensive agents on risk of atrial fibrillation: a meta-analysis of large-scale randomized trials. Europace. 2015;17(5):701–10.
193. Chao TF, Liu CJ, Liao JN, Wang KL, Lin YJ, Chang SL, et al. Use of oral anticoagulants for stroke prevention in patients with atrial fibrillation who have a history of intracranial hemorrhage. Circulation. 2016;133(16):1540–7.
194. Nielsen PB, Larsen TB, Skjøth F, Gorst-Rasmussen A, Rasmussen LH, Lip GYH. Restarting anticoagulant treatment after intracranial hemorrhage in patients with atrial fibrillation and the impact on recurrent stroke, mortality, and bleeding: a nationwide cohort study. Circulation. 2015;132(6):517–25.
195. Korompoki E, Filippidis FT, Nielsen PB, Del Giudice A, Lip GYH, Kuramatsu JB, et al. Long-term antithrombotic treatment in intracranial hemorrhage survivors with atrial fibrillation. Neurology. 2017;89(7):687–96.
196. Schreuder FHBM, van Nieuwenhuizen KM, Hofmeijer J, Vermeer SE, Kerkhoff H, Zock E, et al. Apixaban versus no anticoagulation after anticoagulation-associated intracerebral haemorrhage in patients with atrial fibrillation in the Netherlands (APACHE-AF): a randomised, open-label, phase 2 trial. Lancet Neurol. 2021;20(11):907–16.
197. Nielsen PB, Larsen TB, Skjøth F, Lip GYH. Outcomes associated with resuming warfarin treatment after hemorrhagic stroke or traumatic intracranial hemorrhage in patients with atrial fibrillation. JAMA Intern Med. 2017;177(4):563–70.
198. Hemphill JC, Greenberg SM, Anderson CS, Becker K, Bendok BR, Cushman M, et al. Guidelines for the management of spontaneous intracerebral hemorrhage: A Guideline for Healthcare Professionals from the American Heart Association/American Stroke Association. Stroke. 2015;46(7):2032–60.
199. Chiang CE, Chao TF, Choi EK, Lim TW, Krittayaphong R, Li M, et al. Stroke prevention in atrial fibrillation: a scientific statement of JACC: Asia (Part 1). JACC Asia. 2022;2(4):395–411.
200. Kuramatsu JB, Sembill JA, Gerner ST, Sprügel MI, Hagen M, Roeder SS, et al. Management of therapeutic anticoagulation in patients with intracerebral haemorrhage and mechanical heart valves. Eur Heart J. 2018;39(19):1709–23.
201. Kralev S, Schneider K, Lang S, Süselbeck T, Borggrefe M. Incidence and severity of coronary artery disease in patients with atrial fibrillation undergoing first-time coronary angiography. PLoS One. 2011;6(9):e24964.
202. Gargiulo G, Goette A, Tijssen J, Eckardt L, Lewalter T, Vranckx P, et al. Safety and efficacy outcomes of double vs. triple antithrombotic therapy in patients with atrial fibrillation following percutaneous coronary intervention: a systematic review and meta-analysis of non-vitamin K antagonist oral anticoagulant-based randomized clinical trials. Eur Heart J. 2019;40(46):3757–67.
203. Potpara TS, Mujovic N, Proietti M, Dagres N, Hindricks G, Collet JP, et al. Revisiting the effects of omitting aspirin in combined antithrombotic therapies for atrial fibrillation and acute coronary syndromes or percutaneous coronary interventions: meta-analysis of pooled

data from the PIONEER AF-PCI, RE-DUAL PCI, and AUGUSTUS trials. Europace. 2020;22(1):33–46.
204. Sousa-Uva M, Neumann FJ, Ahlsson A, Alfonso F, Banning AP, Benedetto U, et al. 2018 ESC/EACTS Guidelines on myocardial revascularization. Eur J Cardio-Thorac Surg. 2019;55(1):4–90.
205. Yasuda S, Kaikita K, Akao M, Ako J, Matoba T, Nakamura M, et al. Antithrombotic therapy for atrial fibrillation with stable coronary disease. N Engl J Med. 2019;381(12):1103–13.
206. Steffel J, Collins R, Antz M, Cornu P, Desteghe L, Haeusler KG, et al. 2021 European Heart Rhythm Association Practical Guide on the use of non-vitamin K antagonist oral anticoagulants in patients with atrial fibrillation. Europace. 2021;23(10):1612–76.
207. Powers WJ, Rabinstein AA, Ackerson T, Adeoye OM, Bambakidis NC, Becker K, et al. 2018 Guidelines for the early management of patients with acute ischemic stroke: a guideline for healthcare professionals from the American Heart Association/American Stroke Association. Stroke. 2018;49(3):e46–110.
208. Paciaroni M, Agnelli G, Falocci N, Caso V, Becattini C, Marcheselli S, et al. Early recurrence and cerebral bleeding in patients with acute ischemic stroke and atrial fibrillation: effect of anticoagulation and its timing: The RAF study. Stroke. 2015;46(8):2175–82.
209. Kirchhof P, Benussi S, Kotecha D, Ahlsson A, Atar D, Casadei B, et al. 2016 ESC Guidelines for the management of atrial fibrillation developed in collaboration with EACTS. Eur Heart J. 2016;37(38):2893–962.
210. Kimura S, Toyoda K, Yoshimura S, Minematsu K, Yasaka M, Paciaroni M, et al. Practical "1-2-3-4-Day" rule for starting direct oral anticoagulants after ischemic stroke with atrial fibrillation: combined hospital-based cohort study. Stroke. 2022;53(5):1540–9.
211. Oldgren J, Åsberg S, Hijazi Z, Wester P, Bertilsson M, Norrving B, et al. Early versus delayed non-vitamin K antagonist oral anticoagulant therapy after acute ischemic stroke in atrial fibrillation (TIMING): a registry-based randomized controlled noninferiority study. Circulation. 2022;146(14):1056–66.
212. Altavilla R, Caso V, Bandini F, Agnelli G, Tsivgoulis G, Yaghi S, et al. Anticoagulation after stroke in patients with atrial fibrillation. Stroke. 2019;50(8):2093–100.
213. Intercollegiate Stroke Working Party. 2016 National Clinical Guideline for Stroke [Internet]. [cited 2022 Dec 14]. http://guideline.ssnap.org/2016StrokeGuideline/html5/index.html?page=1&noflash
214. Ha JT, Neuen BL, Cheng LP, Jun M, Toyama T, Gallagher MP, et al. Benefits and harms of oral anticoagulant therapy in chronic kidney disease: a systematic review and meta-analysis. Ann Intern Med. 2019;171(3):181–9.
215. Feldberg J, Patel P, Farrell A, Sivarajahkumar S, Cameron K, Ma J, et al. A systematic review of direct oral anticoagulant use in chronic kidney disease and dialysis patients with atrial fibrillation. Nephrol Dial Transplant. 2019;34(2):265–77.
216. Stanifer JW, Pokorney SD, Chertow GM, Hohnloser SH, Wojdyla DM, Garonzik S, et al. Apixaban versus warfarin in patients with atrial fibrillation and advanced chronic kidney disease. Circulation. 2020;141(17):1384–92.
217. Stoica MC, Gáll Z, Gliga ML, Căldăraru CD, Székely O. Oral anticoagulant treatment in patients with atrial fibrillation and chronic kidney disease. Medicina (Mex). 2021;57(5):422.
218. Pokorney SD, Chertow GM, Al-Khalidi HR, Gallup D, Dignacco P, Mussina K, et al. Apixaban for patients with atrial fibrillation on hemodialysis: a multicenter randomized controlled trial. Circulation. 2022;146(23):1735–45.
219. Lee SR, Lee HJ, Choi EK, Han KD, Jung JH, Cha MJ, et al. Direct oral anticoagulants in patients with atrial fibrillation and liver disease. J Am Coll Cardiol. 2019;73(25):3295–308.
220. Violi F, Vestri A, Menichelli D, Di Rocco A, Pastori D, Pignatelli P. Direct oral anticoagulants in patients with atrial fibrillation and advanced liver disease: an exploratory meta-analysis. Hepatol Commun. 2020;4(7):1034–40.

221. Konstantino Y, Zelnik Yovel D, Friger MD, Sahar G, Knyazer B, Amit G. Postoperative atrial fibrillation following coronary artery bypass graft surgery predicts long-term atrial fibrillation and stroke. Isr Med Assoc J IMAJ. 2016;18(12):744–8.
222. Butt JH, Xian Y, Peterson ED, Olsen PS, Rørth R, Gundlund A, et al. Long-term thromboembolic risk in patients with postoperative atrial fibrillation after coronary artery bypass graft surgery and patients with nonvalvular atrial fibrillation. JAMA Cardiol. 2018;3(5):417–24.
223. Biblo LA, Yuan Z, Quan KJ, Mackall JA, Rimm AA. Risk of stroke in patients with atrial flutter. Am J Cardiol. 2001;87(3):346–9. A9
224. Cameli M, Lisi M, Righini FM, Massoni A, Natali BM, Focardi M, et al. Usefulness of atrial deformation analysis to predict left atrial fibrosis and endocardial thickness in patients undergoing mitral valve operations for severe mitral regurgitation secondary to mitral valve prolapse. Am J Cardiol. 2013;111(4):595–601.
225. Schnabel RB, Wild PS, Wilde S, Ojeda FM, Schulz A, Zeller T, et al. Multiple biomarkers and atrial fibrillation in the general population. PLoS One. 2014;9(11):e112486.
226. Han FT, Akoum N, Marrouche N. Value of magnetic resonance imaging in guiding atrial fibrillation management. Can J Cardiol. 2013;29(10):1194–202.
227. Zhang K, Kamtchum-Tatuene J, Li M, Jickling GC. Cardiac natriuretic peptides for diagnosis of covert atrial fibrillation after acute ischaemic stroke: a meta-analysis of diagnostic accuracy studies. Stroke Vasc Neurol. 2021;6(1):128–32.

Chapter 7
Primary Headaches and the Autonomic Nervous System

Pietro Cortelli and Umberto Pensato

7.1 Introduction

Headache is the symptom of head, face, or neck pain and represents the most common neurological symptom, experienced at least once in a lifetime almost universally. Headache disorders are classified as either primary or secondary. Primary headaches are highly prevalent conditions with no underlying cause, yet they can significantly burden a subgroup of patients. Conversely, secondary headaches are less common yet may herald life-threatening conditions and require urgent appropriate diagnostic investigation [1].

Primary headaches are a heterogeneous group, including migraine, tension-type headaches, and trigeminal autonomic cephalalgias (TACs). The exact pathophysiology of primary headaches is not fully understood, yet arguably involves a complex interplay of genetic, environmental, and biochemical factors. Migraine, for example, is thought to be caused by a combination of genetic susceptibility and environmental triggers, leading to changes in the brainstem and the trigeminal nerve that cause pain and other symptoms [2]. Tension-type headache may be related to muscle contractions and changes in neurotransmitter levels [3]. In contrast, cluster headache may involve alterations in the hypothalamus and its regulation of the circadian rhythm [4].

P. Cortelli (✉)
Department of Biomedical and NeuroMotor Sciences (DIBINEM), University of Bologna, Bologna, Italy

IRCCS Istituto delle Scienze Neurologiche di Bologna, Bologna, Italy
e-mail: pietro.cortelli@unibo.it

U. Pensato
IRCCS Humanitas Research Hospital, Milan, Italy

Department of Biomedical Sciences, Humanitas University, Milan, Italy

G. Micieli et al. (eds.), *Autonomic Disorders in Clinical Practice*,
https://doi.org/10.1007/978-3-031-43036-7_7

The autonomic nervous system (ANS) plays a role in the development and progression of primary headaches, particularly in migraine and TACs. Understanding the complex role of the ANS in primary headaches may inform their pathophysiology and treatment [5–7].

In this chapter, we will discuss the role of the ANS from different aspects in migraine and cluster headache (prototype of TACs): (i) pathophysiology, (ii) clinical autonomic manifestations, (iii) interictal autonomic dysfunction, (iv) autonomic modulation as a treatment strategy, and (v) interpretation of primary headaches in a bio-behavioural view.

7.2 Migraine Pathophysiology and the Autonomic Nervous System

Migraine is a complex neurological disorder characterized by recurrent headache attacks that last 4–72 h, typically causing severe pain on one side of the head, with accompanying symptoms such as nausea, vomiting, light and sound sensitivity, and intensifying with physical activity [2]. The migraine attack comprises distinctive consequential phases: prodrome symptoms, aura, headache phase, and postdrome symptoms. The presence of an aura preceding or concomitant to the headache phase distinguishes migraine into two main subtypes: migraine with aura and without aura. Migraine is highly prevalent in the general population, especially young women, and has a significant genetic component [8]. In the past, migraine was believed to be a cerebrovascular disorder; however, current research suggests a much more complex pathophysiology. The exact cause is still not fully understood, but it is thought to involve a primary brain dysfunction leading to activation and sensitization of the trigeminovascular system (TVS) [9]. TVS is composed of trigeminal and upper cervical dorsal root ganglions (first-order neurons), the trigeminocervical complex (second-order neurons), and ascending axonal projections to the midbrain, thalami, and hypothalamus (third-order neurons) [2].

The meninges and the pial cerebral vessels are the main pain-sensitive structures of the head and are innervated by trigeminal terminal ends that contain several neuropeptides, including calcitonin gene-related peptide (CGRP), pituitary adenylate cyclase-activating polypeptide (PACAP) and neuropeptide substance P (SP). Activation of the TVS promotes the blood release of these neuropeptides that are pivotal in migraine pain, as also suggested by the therapeutic efficacy of their inhibitors [10, 11].

Autonomic control of the central autonomic network (CAN) is exerted at every level of the TVS mechanisms [12]. Specifically, connections with the superior salivatory nucleus and the sphenopalatine ganglion are responsible for the cranial autonomic symptoms during migraine attacks, while TVS third-order neurons orchestrate autonomic-behaviour responses. Furthermore, the presence of non-noxious prodromes, such as somnolence, changes in fluid balance, hyperphagia, or food rejection, argues for a primary role of the CAN in the migraine attack generator [2, 8].

7.3 Cluster Headache Pathophysiology and the Autonomic Nervous System

TACs comprise a group of headache disorders characterized by recurrent attacks of strictly unilateral facial pain with predominant accompanying cranial autonomic symptoms [4, 13].

These disorders are distinguished based on clinical features, attack duration and frequency, responsiveness to therapy, and typical triggers (Fig. 7.1) [4, 13]. Cluster headache is the predominant subtype, accounting for more than 90% of the TAC spectrum. The other disorders are hemicrania continua, paroxysmal hemicrania, and short-lasting unilateral neuralgiform headache attack syndromes (SUNHA) [1]. Cluster headache patients experience bouts of headache attacks with circadian and circannual periodicity. The attacks are usually excruciating, accompanied by agitation and restlessness, and last 15–180 min. The underlying pathophysiology of cluster headache, and TACs at large, is complex yet more unveiled than other primary headaches. Interestingly, the autonomic nervous system plays a central role in these disorders. A dysfunctional hypothalamus is the well-known *primum movens* of cluster headache, as suggested by associated neuroendocrine changes, clinical periodicity, functional neuroimaging studies, and response to neuromodulation devices [4, 14–16]. Several hypothalamic nuclei are involved in the pathogenesis, such as the paraventricular nuclei that project to the superior salivatory nucleus (SSN) and the suprachiasmatic nucleus that is responsible for circadian periodicity. The dysfunctional hypothalamus arguably acts as the primary pacemaker and orchestrates the autonomic-behavioural responses of cluster headache attacks by activating the

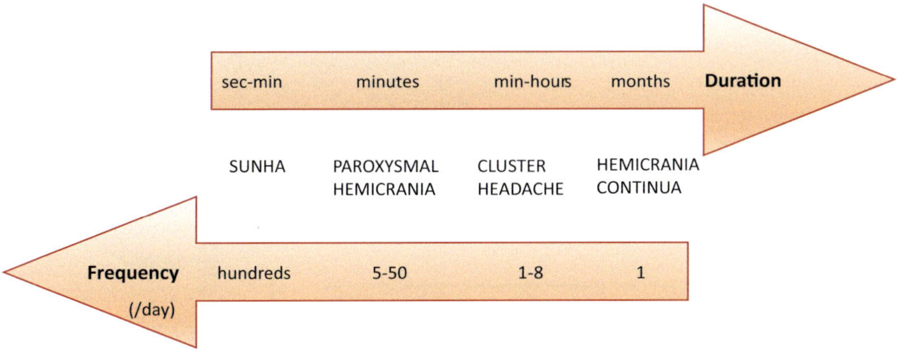

Fig. 7.1 Clinical characteristics of headache attacks frequency and duration in trigeminal autonomic cephalalgias. *SUNHA* short-lasting unilateral neuralgiform headache attack syndromes

trigeminovascular system (TVS) and trigeminal autonomic reflex (TAR) that ultimately influence each other in a vicious circle [4].

7.4 Autonomic Manifestations during Migraine and Cluster Headache Attacks

In primary headaches, trigeminal autonomic symptoms secondary to an enhanced cranial parasympathetic outflow are frequently observed during headache attacks [5, 6]. These autonomic symptoms comprise conjunctival injection, lacrimation, periorbital swelling, ptosis, miosis, nasal congestion, rhinorrhea, and facial sweating. These autonomic manifestations are strictly unilateral and very prominent in all TACs and, consistently, are an essential part of the diagnostic criteria [1]. Nonetheless, these manifestations are frequently observed also in migraine attacks, yet usually milder and bilaterally. Notably, almost half of the migraine patients may display unilateral autonomic symptoms, usually accompanied by more severe pain intensity, potentially representing a distinctive migraine endophenotype with pathophysiological and treatment implications [17].

The trigeminal autonomic reflex (TAR) accounts for these cranial autonomic manifestations observed in primary headaches [5]. The TAR is a physiological reflex with a protective function engendered by any nociceptive stimulation of the trigeminal nerve endings (Fig. 7.2). This reflex protects mainly the eyes and

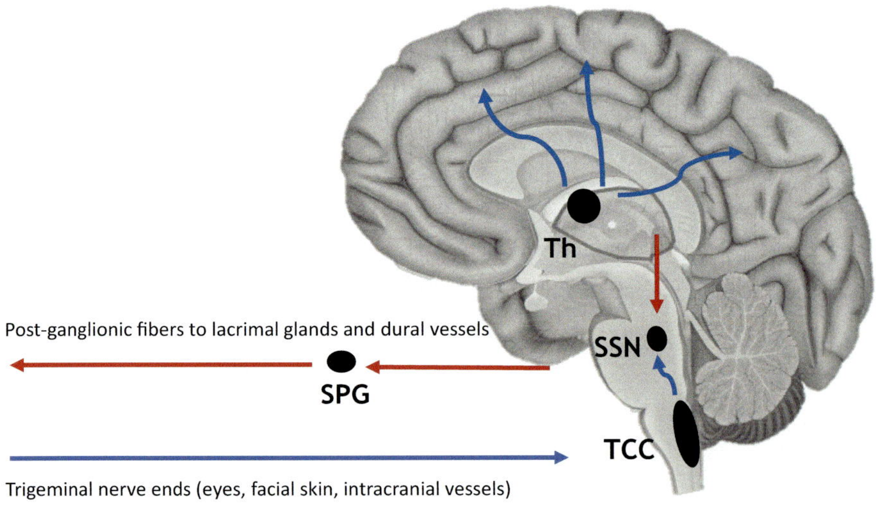

Fig. 7.2 Graphical view of the trigeminal autonomic reflex (TAR). Afferents and efferents components of the reflex are illustrated in blue and red, respectively. *Th* thalamus, *SSN* superior salivatory nucleus, *TCC* trigeminal cervical complex, *SPG* sphenopalatine ganglion

sensitive facial skin areas but is also activated by intracranial structures such as the meninges. The information is transmitted to the trigeminal cervical complex, the thalamic, and cortical areas. Then, the efferents parasympathetic branches arise from the superior salivatory nucleus synapse with the sphenopalatine ganglion (SPG), where post-ganglionic fibres innervate the effector structures, such as lacrimal glands and Dural vessels [5]. The intensity of the autonomic manifestations during headache attacks usually corresponds to the severity of the pain experienced by the patient, further suggesting the protective role of the TAR. While activation of the TAR alone may not cause a primary headache attack, it may contribute to the escalation of headache pain during an attack by triggering centrally-mediated parasympathetic manifestations [18, 19]. Accordingly, several acute and preventive headache treatments target the TAR (see beyond).

7.5 Interictal Autonomic Dysfunction in Migraine and Cluster Headache

Studies on interictal (between headache attacks) autonomic dysfunction in migraine have used various techniques, such as measuring cerebrovascular reactivity, pupil reactivity, cardiovascular reflexes, and biochemical and pharmacological responses. However, these studies have produced inconsistent results with no clear pattern of autonomic dysfunction observed, including hypo- and hyperfunction, as well as normal findings [20]. Therefore, there is currently no apparent autonomic deficit considered intrinsic to migraine headache.

Interictal autonomic dysfunction has also been investigated in cluster headache, mainly during the active cluster phase. A recent review focusing on cardiovascular autonomic changes found no significant or consistent interictal dysfunction except for a moderately increased sympathetic tone in cluster headache patients compared to control subjects [21]. Whereas, a following study demonstrated a prolonged latency of skin response on the affected side of the face, suggesting post ganglionic hypofunction [22].

Collectively, studies investigating ANS dysfunction interictal in both migraine and cluster headache did not reveal significant alterations. Nonetheless, these studies did not consider modulation that headache attacks may involve integrated behavioural responses, where pain perception and modulation are a behavioural motif, and autonomic responses may serve that behaviour [7].

7.6 Primary Headache Treatment and Modulation of the ANS

Modulation of TAR may play a role in treating primary headache disorders such as migraine, cluster headache, and other TACs. Specific therapies, such as indomethacin, oxygen, and neurostimulation of the hypothalamus, sphenopalatine ganglion (SPG), and vagal nerve, have shown promise in impacting TAR and potentially treating these headache disorders [5]. However, more research is still needed to fully understand the relationship between TAR and primary headache disorders and determine the best treatment approach.

Indomethacin is considered an effective treatment for specific primary headaches, such as paroxysmal hemicrania and hemicrania continua [1], due to its ability to inhibit nitrogen oxide-induced Dural vasodilation [23]. This unique property, compared to other non-steroidal anti-inflammatory drugs (NSAIDs) [23], suggests that indomethacin may modulate TAR and its function in primary headache disorders [5]. Further research is needed to fully understand the mechanism behind indomethacin's efficacy in treating these conditions.

Oxygen therapy effectively treats cluster headache attacks [24] and, to a lesser extent, migraine attacks with autonomic symptoms [25]. Preclinical studies have suggested that the brainstem plays a critical role in sensory and autonomic symptoms and that the parasympathetic outflow to the cranial vasculature may be a target for oxygen [26]. The fact that oxygen therapy is effective in both cluster headache and migraine with autonomic symptoms support the idea that it may modulate TAR.

High-frequency stimulation of the SPG is highly effective in treating cluster headache patients who have not responded to other treatments [27]. It works by blocking the parasympathetic discharge. Interestingly, low-frequency stimulation of the SPG, which was thought to trigger cluster headache attacks, was ineffective [18]. This reinforced the concept that the TAR's peripheral activation is insufficient to trigger headache attacks.

Non-invasive vagal nerve stimulation (nVNS) was first attempted on refractory epilepsy [28], yet a concomitant reduction of migraine attacks frequency in epileptic patients was observed. After that, nVNS was tested in migraine and cluster headache and proved consistently effective [29, 30]. The underlying mechanism is not fully unveiled, yet a reduction of autonomic symptoms was observed, thus, modulation of the TAR is possible.

7.7 Primary Headaches as a Reflection of Genetic Darwinian Adaptive Autonomic-Behavioural Responses

Primary headaches are considered painful episodic disorders, yet pain does not represent the full spectrum of clinical manifestations observed during attacks and may even be missing in some rare headaches (e.g., migraine aura without headache) [1].

Therefore, primary headaches can only be fully understood by a comprehensive behavioural view [7]. In this model, the multifaceted phenomena of primary headaches are unified, and the autonomic nervous system's significant role is highlighted not only for the pain but also for the non-headache (prodrome and postdrome) symptoms characteristics of the attacks.

7.7.1 Behaviours Engendered during Primary Headaches

During a migraine attack, patients exhibit a characteristic behaviour where they seek to become as immobile as possible and rest, avoiding physical and mental activity and trying to be in an environment with minimal stimulation [2].

Conversely, during a cluster headache attack, patients exhibit quite the opposite behaviour, characterized by restlessness, psychomotor agitation, aggressiveness, and even self-hurting behaviours [4].

7.7.2 The Behavioural Meaning of Pain

Headache, and pain at large, could be envisaged within the frame of its behavioural significance and utility as a powerful homeostatic emotion. The subjects can perceive pain as either escapable or inescapable and, therefore, is accompanied by opposite autonomic-behaviour responses (Fig. 7.3) [7, 31, 32]. Each type of pain is conveyed by different sensory modalities and pathways. Escapable pain is typically

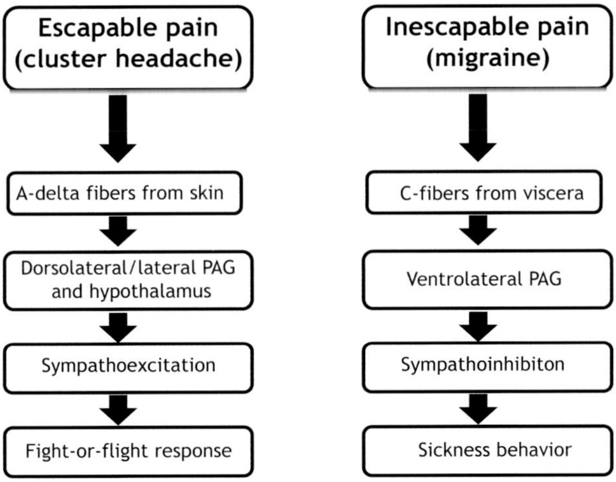

Fig. 7.3 Schematic representation of the different neuronal networks underlying autonomic-behavioural responses of escapable and inescapable pain. *PAG* periaqueductal gray

conveyed by A-delta fibres from the skin, whereas inescapable pain is conveyed by C fibres mainly from deep viscera, serving as visceral homeostatic pain [31, 32]. They also activate different pathways in the central nervous system, specifically in regions such as the periaqueductal Gray (PAG), hypothalamus, amygdala, and forebrain. Escapable pain-activated A-delta fibres project to the dorsolateral/lateral PAG and posterior hypothalamus that coordinate a sympathoexcitation autonomic-behavioural response, namely fight-or-flight defensive response [33]. This manifests with increased production of catecholamines, arterial hypertension, tachycardia, hyperventilation, increased blood flow to the skeletal muscles, aggressiveness, and restlessness. All these features represent an adaptive integrated innate response optimized to fight stressors or flight from potentially threatening situations (escapable pain).

This leads to a fight-or-flight defensive response, with the subjects ready to confront the stressor or run from potentially threatening situations.

Conversely, inescapable pain-activated C fibres project to the ventrolateral PAG that coordinates a sympathoinhibition autonomic-behaviour response, namely sickness behaviour [32]. This leads to hypotension, bradycardia, motor quiescence, lethargy, and disengagement from the environment. These features represent an adaptive integrated innate response optimized to confront stressors in an unavoidable engagement (inescapable pain).

Collectively, these emotional and autonomic responses associated with pain have an evolutionary basis and are part of a defined behavioural programme. Darwin first applied an evolutionary perspective to emotions in animals and humans and identified patterns of emotional behaviours that had evolutionary significance.

7.7.3 The Behavioural Meaning of Migraine and Cluster Headache Attacks

The clinical manifestations observed during primary headache attacks remarkably overlap with the autonomic-behavioural responses shared by all mammalians, suggesting they are evolutionary conserved adaptive strategies [7].

The passive behaviour frequently observed during migraine attacks is likely related to a brain homeostatic imbalance signalled by trigeminal C fibres that help the brain to recover to the homeostasis of the brain itself. This bio-behavioural model of migraine explains the interictal traits distinctive of the migraine brain, such as the deficient brain energy metabolism and deficient habituation in information processing [34]. Therefore, this model views migraine pain as serving as a protective function, as a visceral homeostatic emotion like thirst and hunger that monitors the internal bodily world with an adaptive role. Hints of this fundamental role may come from the persistence of migraine as a frequent genetic trait in the population of reproductive age, potentially underlying an evolutionary advantage of migraineurs [35].

The active behaviour engendered during cluster headache attacks resembles the fight-or-flight defensive response and is arguably related to the activation of trigeminal A-delta fibres.

Therefore, behaviours during migraine and cluster headache attacks should be considered evolutionarily conserved adaptive responses. Nonetheless, even though the behaviours may have evolved for a specific purpose, they may become inappropriate and maladaptive in certain circumstances, such as aggressive or anxiety behaviours [7].

7.8 Conclusions

The ANS plays a pivotal role in primary headaches underlying pathophysiology and its involvement explains several clinical manifestations observed during headache attacks. Additionally, its iatrogenic modulation has important therapeutic implications. The bio-behavioural theory views primary headache attacks as adaptive behavioural responses engendered by a network of pattern generators in the ANS to maintain brain homeostasis. Therefore, to investigate the role of the ANS, it is futile to study autonomic functions during headache attacks separately from the bio-behavioural responses they contribute to.

References

1. Headache classification Committee of the International Headache Society (IHS) the international classification of headache disorders, 3rd edition. Cephalalgia 2018;38:1–211.
2. Ferrari MD, Goadsby PJ, Burstein R, et al. Migraine. Nat Rev Dis Primers. 2022;8:2.
3. Steel SJ, Robertson CE, Whealy MA. Current understanding of the pathophysiology and approach to tension-type headache. Curr Neurol Neurosci Rep. 2021;21:56.
4. Wei DY, Goadsby PJ. Cluster headache pathophysiology insights from current and emerging treatments. Nat Rev Neurol. 2021;17:308–24.
5. Moller M, May A. The unique role of the trigeminal autonomic reflex and its modulation in primary headache disorders. Curr Opin Neurol. 2019;32:438–42.
6. Gevirtz R. The role of the autonomic nervous system in headache: biomarkers and treatment. Curr Pain Headache Rep. 2022;26:767–74.
7. Montagna P, Pierangeli G, Cortelli P. The primary headaches as a reflection of genetic darwinian adaptive behavioral responses. Headache. 2010;50:273–89.
8. Ashina M. Migraine. N Engl J Med. 2020;383:1866–76.
9. Ashina M, Hansen JM, Do TP, Melo-Carrillo A, Burstein R, Moskowitz MA. Migraine and the trigeminovascular system-40 years and counting. Lancet Neurol. 2019;18:795–804.
10. Do TP, Al-Saoudi A, Ashina M. Future prophylactic treatments in migraine: beyond anti-CGRP monoclonal antibodies and gepants. Rev Neurol (Paris). 2021;177:827–33.
11. Christensen CE, Ashina M, Amin FM. Calcitonin gene-related peptide (CGRP) and pituitary adenylate cyclase-activating polypeptide (PACAP) in migraine pathogenesis. Pharmaceuticals (Basel). 2022;15:15.
12. Benarroch EE. Pain-autonomic interactions. Neurol Sci. 2006;27(Suppl 2):S130–3.

13. Nahas SJ. Cluster headache and other trigeminal autonomic Cephalalgias. Continuum (Minneap Minn). 2021;27:633–51.
14. Leone M, Bussone G. A review of hormonal findings in cluster headache. Evidence for hypothalamic involvement. Cephalalgia. 1993;13:309–17.
15. May A, Bahra A, Buchel C, Frackowiak RS, Goadsby PJ. Hypothalamic activation in cluster headache attacks. Lancet. 1998;352:275–8.
16. Leone M, Franzini A, Felisati G, et al. Deep brain stimulation and cluster headache. Neurol Sci. 2005;26(Suppl 2):s138–9.
17. Barbanti P, Aurilia C, Dall'Armi V, Egeo G, Fofi L, Bonassi S. The phenotype of migraine with unilateral cranial autonomic symptoms documents increased peripheral and central trigeminal sensitization. A case series of 757 patients. Cephalalgia. 2016;36:1334–40.
18. Moller M, Haji AA, Hoffmann J, May A. Peripheral provocation of cranial autonomic symptoms is not sufficient to trigger cluster headache attacks. Cephalalgia. 2018;38:1498–502.
19. Guo S, Petersen AS, Schytz HW, et al. Cranial parasympathetic activation induces autonomic symptoms but no cluster headache attacks. Cephalalgia. 2018;38:1418–28.
20. Miglis MG. Migraine and autonomic dysfunction: which is the horse and which is the jockey? Curr Pain Headache Rep. 2018;22:19.
21. Barloese MC. A review of cardiovascular autonomic control in cluster headache. Headache. 2016;56:225–39.
22. Altiokka O, Mutluay B, Koksal A, et al. Evaluation of interictal autonomic function during attack and remission periods in cluster headaches. Cephalalgia. 2016;36:37–43.
23. Summ O, Andreou AP, Akerman S, Goadsby PJ. A potential nitrergic mechanism of action for indomethacin, but not of other COX inhibitors: relevance to indomethacin-sensitive headaches. J Headache Pain. 2010;11:477–83.
24. Cohen AS, Burns B, Goadsby PJ. High-flow oxygen for treatment of cluster headache: a randomized trial. JAMA. 2009;302:2451–7.
25. Jürgens TP, Schulte LH, May A. Oxygen treatment is effective in migraine with autonomic symptoms. Cephalalgia. 2013;33:65–7.
26. Akerman S, Holland PR, Summ O, Lasalandra MP, Goadsby PJ. A translational in vivo model of trigeminal autonomic cephalalgias: therapeutic characterization. Brain. 2012;135:3664–75.
27. Jürgens TP, Barloese M, May A, et al. Long-term effectiveness of sphenopalatine ganglion stimulation for cluster headache. Cephalalgia. 2017;37:423–34.
28. Oliveira T, Francisco AN, Demartini ZJ, Stebel SL. The role of vagus nerve stimulation in refractory epilepsy. Arq Neuropsiquiatr. 2017;75:657–66.
29. Gaul C, Diener HC, Silver N, et al. Non-invasive vagus nerve stimulation for PREVention and acute treatment of chronic cluster headache (PREVA): a randomised controlled study. Cephalalgia. 2016;36:534–46.
30. Tassorelli C, Grazzi L, de Tommaso M, et al. Noninvasive vagus nerve stimulation as acute therapy for migraine: the randomized PRESTO study. Neurology. 2018;91:e364–e73.
31. Keay KA, Bandler R. Distinct central representations of inescapable and escapable pain: observations and speculation. Exp Physiol. 2002;87:275–9.
32. Parry DM, Macmillan FM, Koutsikou S, McMullan S, Lumb BM. Separation of A- versus C-nociceptive inputs into spinal-brainstem circuits. Neuroscience. 2008;152:1076–85.
33. Lumb BM. Hypothalamic and midbrain circuitry that distinguishes between escapable and inescapable pain. News Physiol Sci. 2004;19:22–6.
34. Gross EC, Lisicki M, Fischer D, Sandor PS, Schoenen J. The metabolic face of migraine - from pathophysiology to treatment. Nat Rev Neurol. 2019;15:627–43.
35. Montagna P. Migraine genetics. Expert Rev Neurother. 2008;8:1321–30.

Chapter 8
Gastrointestinal Autonomic Disorders

Andrea Bassi, Michela Bossa, Lucia d'Alba, Carla Greco, Arianna Casini, Clelia Pellicano, Marilia Simonelli, and Stefania Zampatti

8.1 Introduction

The relationship between the nervous system and the digestive system is the subject of increasing scientific interest; after all, the enteric nervous system (ENS) has a number of neurons that is analogous to that of the spinal cord, as well as possessing a degree of independence from the central nervous system (CNS) that is unmatched in organs of other systems.

The ANS is the medium between the CNS and the ENS; the latter is involved in a complex manner in the major functions (i.e., storage/secretion, transit/mixing of

A. Bassi (✉) · M. Bossa · C. Pellicano · S. Zampatti
Department of Clinical Neuroscience and Neurorehabilitation, Foundation Santa Lucia of Rome, Rome, Italy
e-mail: a.bassi@hsantalucia.it; m.bossa@hsantalucia.it; c.pellicano@hsantalucia.it; s.zampatti@hsantalucia.it

L. d'Alba
Unit of Gastroenterology and Digestive Endoscopy, San Camillo-Forlanini Hospital, Rome, Italy

C. Greco
Unit of Endocrinology, Department of Biomedical, Metabolic and Neural Sciences, University of Modena and Reggio Emilia, Modena, Italy
e-mail: carlagreco@unimore.it

A. Casini
Department of Anatomical, Histological, Forensic Medicine and Orthopedic Sciences, Sapienza University of Rome, Rome, Italy
e-mail: arianna.casini@uniroma1.it

M. Simonelli
Phoniatric Service, IRCCS Fondazione Santa Lucia di Rome, Rome, Italy
e-mail: m.simonelli@hsantalucia.it

G. Micieli et al. (eds.), *Autonomic Disorders in Clinical Practice*,
https://doi.org/10.1007/978-3-031-43036-7_8

the food bolus, vase-action of vascular perfusion, and excretion/defecation) of the gastrointestinal (GI) tract. The ENS exhibits a high degree of autonomy from central nervous control; it is the only system in the human body to have evolved to develop its own independent organization, scientific knowledge of which has been given a major boost in the last decade mainly regarding enteric sense-motor functions [1].

The activity of the GI system can be spontaneous or evoked by peripheral stimuli (distension and chemical stimulation) and causes motor responses promoted hierarchically in a primary manner by the ENS (Fig. 8.1). The ENS motor response is conditioned by the ANS, which, in turn, is influenced by the various motor and psychic activities pertaining to the CNS. that the complex regulatory mechanisms (still being studied) are also modulated by extra-neuronal systems such as the immune system, the gut microbiota and the neuroendocrine system. Often, primary neurological diseases (but also secondary neurological diseases determined by non-neurological diseases) result in ANS GI impairment that, in some cases, cannot always be counteracted by vegetative compensatory mechanisms, or modified by therapeutic treatment. The GI dysfunction (Box 8.1) determines clinical disorders that often underlie other diseases that could involve the ANS (Table 8.1) [2].

In the ANS impairment, deficits may involve both classical functional compartments (motor and sensory), but the GI disorders that are most evident, for which more clinical findings are available, are mainly entero-motor dysfunction (rather than entero-secretory deficits and those of the sensory compartment); these disorders include dysphagia, gastroparesis, intestinal pseudo-obstruction, constipation, diarrhea, and fecal incontinence. A separate chapter would deserve the oropharyngeal and the rectal sphincter disorder. The dysphagia and the sialorrhea are often associated with other lesions of head/neck structures, and also rectal sphincter disorder have a co-interaction with similar structures of the urinary system [2].

Neurological and non-neurological diseases affecting the neural axis of entero-motor control (CNS-ANS-ENS structures) are many. Those directly affecting the ANS most frequently are diseases with chronic-neurodegenerative course, diffuse in character, slowly progressive, with involvement of both central and peripheral structures (i.e., Parkinson's disease—[PD], other alpha-synucleinopathies and peripheral diabetic neuropathy). These should also include Multiple Sclerosis (MS), which often has an acute onset due to non-traumatic focal injury [2].

The diagnosis of GI motility disorder in the course of neurological disease involves the identification of the neuro-physio pathological context, as well as the non-modifiable preexisting conditions (i.e., evaluation of the possible presence of

Table 8.1 Clinical presentation of gastrointestinal motor disorder

Esophagus	Stomach	Small intestine	Colon	Anus-rectum
Difficulty swallowing (dysphagia); Retro thoracic retrosternal pain; Regurgitation; Heartburn	Nausea and vomiting; Dyspepsia Epigastralgy	Dyspepsia; Abdominal bloating and distension	Abdominal pain; Constipation; Diarrhea; Abdominal bloating and distension; Flatulence/ bloating	Evacuation effort; Incomplete fractional evacuation; Incontinence or encopresis

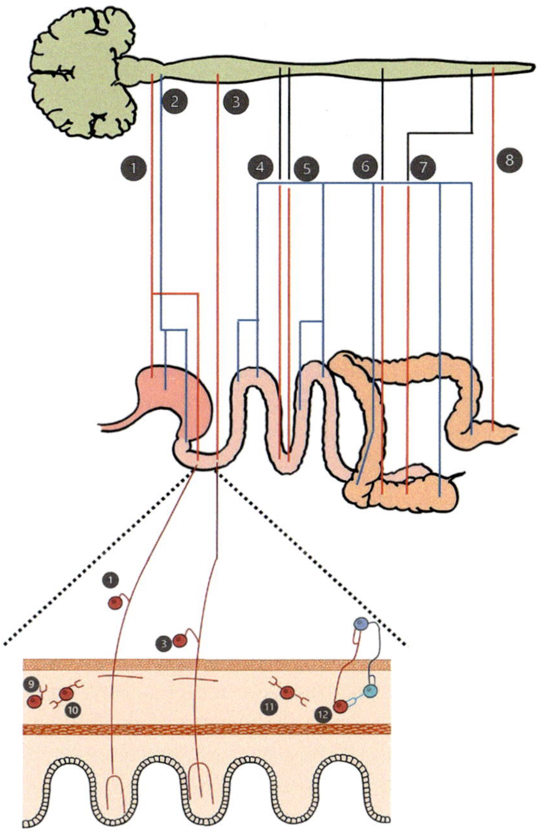

Fig. 8.1 Main extrinsic neural pathways between enteric nervous system and trunk/spinal cord. Main extrinsic motor pathways are shown in blue, afferent pathways in red, and sympathetic preganglionic efferent pathways in black. The motor pathways constitute the parasympathetic and sympathetic nervous systems. In the intestine, sympathetic nerves are inhibitory, parasympathetic nerves are excitatory. In the upper intestinal portions (esophagus and stomach), the main extrinsic sensory nerves are derived from the vagus nerve, while in the lower intestinal portions there is less vagal influence. The main extrinsic sensory nerves in the colon are derived from afferent spinal nerves, whose cell bodies are located in the dorsal root ganglia. (1) vagal afferent; (2) dorsal motor vagal efferent; (3) spinal afferent (*DRG* dorsal root ganglia); (4) coeliac ganglia (sympathetic efferent); (5) superior mesenteric ganglia (sympathetic efferent); (6) inferior mesenteric ganglia (sympathetic efferent); (7) pelvic ganglia (parasympathetic efferent); (8) spinal afferent (DRG). In Microstructures: Intrinsic sensory neurons and extrinsic sensory nerve endings in the enteric nervous system. A wide range of intrinsic sensory neurons and extrinsic sensory nerve endings operate within the enteric nervous system. Dogiel's type I neurons [9] are length-sensitive and tension-insensitive myenteric interneurons. Myenteric interneuron in the myenteric plexus [10]. Extrinsic vagal afferent nerve endings [1] innervate the upper intestine and behave predominantly as slowly adapting voltage receptors. Spinal afferent nerve endings [3] provide very abundant sensory innervation to the lower intestine (distal colon) and are potently activated by stretching and increased muscle tension. Dogiel type II neurons in the myenteric plexus [11] are both chemosensory and mechanosensitive and receive fast and slow synaptic inputs from other enteric neurons. Intestinofugal neurons [12] are generally considered second-order neurons, but they have been shown to be directly mechanosensitive and respond to direct mechanical compression stimuli

congenital or hereditary diseases); as well as potentially modifiable intercurrent conditions determined by non-neurological diseases or other pathologies (i.e., iatrogenic and toxic-food) that secondarily involve the ANS.

Autonomic disorders may occur localized to the GI level, but more often they occur in combination with other autonomic dysfunctions in other body systems (i.e., cardiovascular, thermoregulatory, respiratory, urogenital, pupillomotor, and sudomotor); for example, in parasympathetic dysfunction there may be "sicca" syndrome, light intolerance due to unresponsive dilated pupils, urine retention, erectile dysfunction, resting tachycardia just as sympathetic dysfunction can also be characterized by pupillary miosis, orthostatic intolerance with dizziness or syncope, exercise intolerance, anhidrosis, and heat intolerance.

The examination of the GI system is often strictly the responsibility of the gastroenterology specialist; moreover, clinical investigations for GI motility disorders suffer from the absence of a "gold standard" diagnostic test. Indeed, clinical-instrumental investigations of GI dysfunction often have the limitation of being investigative, invasive, and ultra-specialistic, and the criterion of investigations by refutation is preferred.

Knowledge of the GI autonomic nervous system becomes even more strategic in view of the absence of a specific pharmacological treatment for entero-motor dysfunction. The management of vegetative disorders is aimed at the therapy of the underlying neurological disease, at the search for other modifiable causes, and at the exclusion of non-neurological diseases for which a specific branch specialist is needed. It follows that GI neuro-motor disturbance in the course of neurological disease requires specific expertise, starting with the not obvious restoration of normal hydration, adequate nutrition, and harmonization of pharmacological treatments [3].

In conclusion, GI dysfunction involves a number of disorders that are part of the clinical expression of neurological and not neurological diseases that need, therefore, multidisciplinarity for the purpose of an appropriate diagnostic-therapeutic approach; the aim of the paper is to provide indications for the framing of gastrointestinal autonomic impairment, which can also be pauci- or asymptomatic, how it happens in major neurological diseases.

Box 8.1: Vegetative Gastrointestinal Dysfunction
Inefficient response of the gastrointestinal system to food intake, either at rest (stationarity in metabolic homeostasis with circadian adjustments and adaptations to physiological growth/aging), or during adaptation to psycho-physiological changes (such as during the performance of common life activities in various environmental conditions) or to chronic/acute decline in health status.

8.2 Structures and Gastrointestinal Motility

Neural Structures (Structures and gastrointestinal motility). The ANS, responsible for extrinsic autonomic motor control of the digestive tract, regulates the major functions of the gastrointestinal tract in an integrated and complex manner.

Sympathetic and parasympathetic fibers of the ANS motor neurons innervate the gastrointestinal (GI) smooth muscle, intra-parietal glands, and those attached to the digestive tract (salivary, liver, and pancreas).

The ENS, also called the meta-sympathetic or intrinsic or visceral control, is an intermediary between the ANS and GI effector organs (smooth muscle and glands). The ENS regulates the functioning of GI motility from the medium part of the esophagus to the anal sphincter; it consists of small clusters of cells, the intramural ganglia, which are interconnected and articulate to form two distinct neural plexuses (Auerbach's myenteric plexus and Meissner's submucosal plexus) organized in a complex and finely coordinated neural network. Congenital or acquired abnormalities of the ENS, associated with a lack of intrinsic neurons in the myenteric and submucosal plexuses of the colon, can result in excessive distension and altered motility of the digestive tract, such as congenital megacolon in Hirschsprung's disease [1].

The CNS, mainly through the ANS, modulates and controls GI tract functioning in an uneven manner. The small intestine and large intestine have a greater degree of independence from extrinsic neural afferents than the esophagus and stomach: removal of extrinsic innervation to the stomach results in disorganized and dysregulated gastric activity that often causes symptoms such as nausea and vomiting, discomfort, and abdominal pain with diarrhea; however, after an initial dysfunctional phase, gastric activity regains an adequate level of normalcy [4].

Probably, motor activity also reverberates from the esophagus and stomach into the distal tracts, which are more independent [4], so it is possible to argue that the control systems present a hierarchy of neuronal control: primary regulation determined by the ENS, which in turn is modulated by the structures of the ANS, which in turn is conditioned by various factors (psychic, motor and others pertaining to the CNS) (Diagram 8.1).

Extrinsic Gastrointestinal Neuro-Motor Control (Structures and gastrointestinal motility). The areas of the ANS centrally are in the forebrain, midbrain, hindbrain, and spinal cord; peripherally, the VNS acts through the parasympathetic and sympathetic nervous systems on the ENS. The extrinsic neural control includes parasympathetic and sympathetic nerves of the PNS; a relatively small number of vagal/sacral preganglionic fibers and sympathetic postganglionic fibers are able to interact with the multiple enteric plexus neurons organized in defined circuits pre-established in the wall of the intestine (Fig. 8.1). The extrinsic parasympathetic component is generally excitatory, while the extrinsic sympathetic component has an inhibitory action on the muscles and acts by activating intrinsic inhibitory systems [1]. Intrinsic control of the ENS contains a variety of cellular components (mechanoreceptors and chemoreceptors, interneurons) that process sensory input and control motor units with direct effects on myenteric. In addition, there are brain astroglia-like cells that support neuronal cells and establish a barrier with capillaries in a manner quite similar to the blood-brain barrier [5].

It follows that the hierarchy of neuronal control (Diagram 8.2) relative to intestinal motor activity is as follows: primary regulation is by the Enteric Nervous System (ENS), followed by the ANS and then the Central Nervous System (CNS). Extrinsic control is in turn conditioned by the CNS, which also participates with the somatic

Nervous System (Central, Peripheric,) CNS, PNS				
CNS Brain Brainstem Spinal Cord	Cerebral hemispheres	Telencephalon Diencephalon	Forebrain Central nuclei involved in the regulation of gastrointestinal functions: CeA—Central nucleus of the amygdala BNST—bed nucleus of the stria terminals	
	Brainstem	Mesencephalon	Midbrain The reticular formation.	
	Cerebellum Brainstem	Pons Medulla	Hindbrain Central nuclei involved in the regulation of gastrointestinal functions: PAG—periaqueductal gray; AP—area postrema; dorsal motor nucleus of the vagus; NTS—nucleus of the tractus solitarius; Vestibular N—vestibular nucleus; Trigeminal N—trigeminal nucleus; Raphe N—raphe nuclei	
PNS ANS		Efferent projections from the CNS target skeletal muscle (skeletal motor) or the autonomic nervous system, which is divided into three parts: sympathetic, parasympathetic and enteric. Preganglionic motor neurons (Sympathetic and Parasympathetic) located in the CNS synapse with a postganglionic neuron of Autonomic Nervous System of PNS.		
	Nerves and ganglia	Sympathetic division Parasympathetic division Autonomic responses are mediated by the sympathetic and the parasympathetic systems, which are antagonistic to one another.	Motor efferent compartments, including sympathetic and parasympathetic motor neurons, projecting to the gut wall. Postganglionic sympathetic neurons receive input from the sympathetic neurons in the ILN. Postganglionic parasympathetic neurons from the DMN of the brain stem and from the sacral spinal cord. The postganglionic neurons acts on a target organ.	Sensory afferent compartments: Spinal afferents have their cell bodies in the DRG and project into the dorsal horn of the spinal cord. Vagal afferents have their cell bodies in the nodose and jugular ganglia and project into the nucleus tractus solitarii (NTS) of the brain stem.
Gastrointestinal tract, microstructure				
PNS ANS	Nerves and ganglia	**ENS** **Muscularis propria (externa):** smooth muscle layer; there are usually two layers; the inner layer is circular and the outer layer is longitudinal and is thicker than the inner. The myenteric plexus is located between the two layers of muscle layer.	**Myenteric (Auerbach's) plexus** (Dogiel type I, extrinsic vagal afferent nerve terminals, Dogiel type II) **Sensitive** afferent, STN; **Modulatory** " state " DVM; **Motor** efferent, DVC; tonic *input*, mostly synaptic, inhibitory (GABA) STN vs DVM (tonically active) excitatory *input* (ACh) and (Glu) vs DVM pre-gangliar vagus motor fibers vs ENS ganglia The myenteric plexus primarily regulates gastrointestinal motor activity.	
		Submucosa layer	**Submucosal nerve plexus (Meissner plexus)** The submucosal plexus controls gastrointestinal secretory activity.	
		Mucosa layer		
Gastrointestinal tract, resident neurogenic pathway and activity				

DMN (dorsomedial nucleus); DVC (dorsal vagal complex): dorsal vagal complex formed by the set of area postrema, the STN and the DVM (dorsal vagal motor) nucleus; DRG (dorsal root ganglia); ILN (intermediolateral nucleus); MMC: migrating motor complex; NTS: nucleus tractus solitarii;

Diagram 8.1 Nervous system (central, peripheric) CNS, PNS. *DMN* dorsomedial nucleus, *DVC* dorsal vagal complex: dorsal vagal complex formed by the set of area postrema, the STN and the DVM (dorsal vagal motor) nucleus, *DRG* orsal root ganglia, *ILN* intermediolateral nucleus, *MMC* migrating motor complex, *NTS* nucleus tractus solitarii

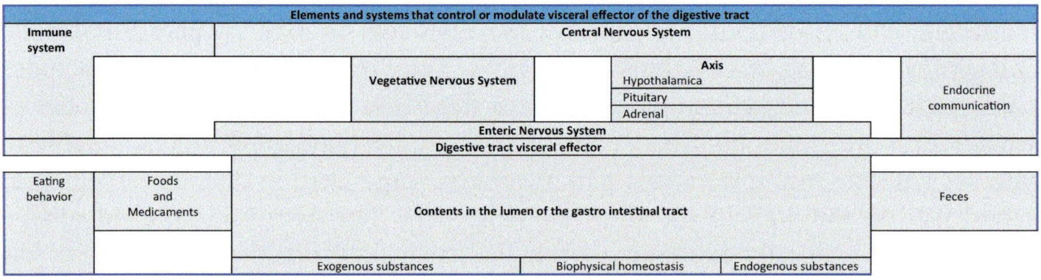

Diagram 8.2 Elements and systems that control or modulate visceral effector of the digestive tract

system in an integrated manner along with the ANS in some activities such as swallowing and defecation. Gut motility is also conditioned by the intrinsic immune system and the endocrine system, including the pituitary-adrenergic axis [5].

The ENS through GI reflexes ensures the proper functioning of the motor activity of the digestive system and coordinates intestinal functions together with the secretory activity.

The GI reflexes (of which the main ones are the peristaltic reflex) promote integrated action (long reflexes, short reflexes and extrinsic reflexes promoted by GI tract peptides), motor function and communication between different parts of the intestine.

Intrinsic Gastrointestinal Activity (Structures and gastrointestinal motility). The digestive tract, just like the heart, contains cells (not neuronal) with spontaneous depolarization (pacemaker-like potential), not induced by vegetative innervation, between the myenteric syncytium: the Interstitial Cells of Cajal (ICC).

These provide different continuous rhythmic activity in the various tracts of the gastrointestinal tract. The electrical rhythmicity they generate is not required for normal gastrointestinal function, at least in the small intestine. These electrical oscillations in smooth muscle are called slow waves of the migratory motor complex (MMC) and result in phasic contractions. The MMC is a cyclic and recurrent motility pattern that is determined in the stomach and progresses in the small intestine, both in wakefulness and sleep, active during fasting, and deactivated in the postprandial digestive phase.

Serotonergic activity contributes to the regulation of slow wave frequency [6] and is reduced in the colonic cells of patients with irritable bowel syndrome. The motor effects of vagotomy on the MMC seem to have an effect delimited to the stomach and not to the small intestine. The affected cells are morphologically similar to star-shaped muscle cells, CCIs, spontaneously generate slow (3/min) electrical waves that propagate into the surrounding musculature, keeping it in a latent state of excitation and regulating its contractile rhythm. CMMs are characterized by three phases illustrated in Fig. 8.2a. About half of the phase III waves originate from the stomach and the other half from the duodenum.

The physiological role of the MMC is not completely known. It is possible that it has a function analogous to muscle tone in the somatic skeletal system; its absence has been associated with gastroparesis, intestinal pseudo-obstruction, and small intestinal bacterial overgrowth. Measurement of gastrointestinal tract motility may be important in the diagnosis of gastrointestinal disorders [7].

In general, afferent information flow from the digestive tract promotes motor actions both during the interdigestive phase and after food intake and related digestive function, up to stool formation and related excretion. Two completely different motor patterns can be identified: an interdigestive motor pattern and a postprandial digestive motor pattern. During the interdigestive phase, there is high muscle tone in the proximal gastric part while recurrent contractions, MMCs, are present in the distal part. This typical contractile pattern appears after gastric emptying from food and originates from a pacemaker area, located on the great curvature between the fundus and the proximal body. The purpose of these phase III contractions is to ensure a pulsatile flow that keeps the stomach and small intestine free of secretions, waste, and microbes during the fasting period, to prepare the stomach to receive the next meal. During the digestive phase, GI smooth muscle can respond to both excitatory and inhibitory motor neurons of different types depending on the motor activity of the digestive system: peristalsis, segmentation movements (or scrambling) and tonic contractions (Fig. 8.2b). Peristalsis occurs according to a coordinated pattern of activity of the smooth muscles of the esophagus and intestine: contraction upstream and relaxation of the distal tract when a bolus distends the intestine, brought about by inhibition of the circular layer and excitation of the longitudinal

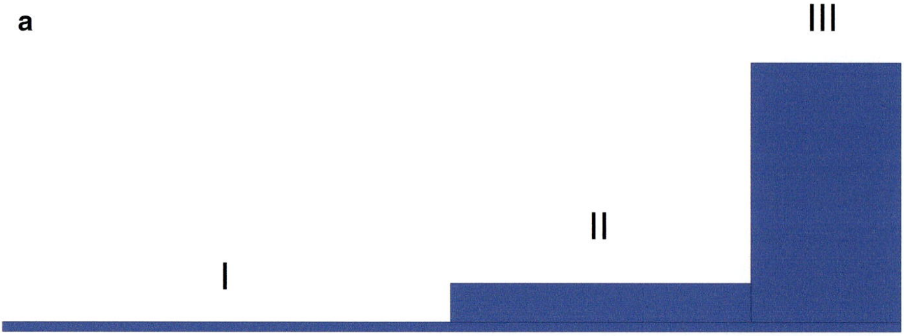

Phase I	60 min, no motor activity
Phase II	20 min, intermittent, and irregular low-amplitude contractions
Phase III	10 min, consists of burst of regular contractions that move down the intestin until the terminal ileum

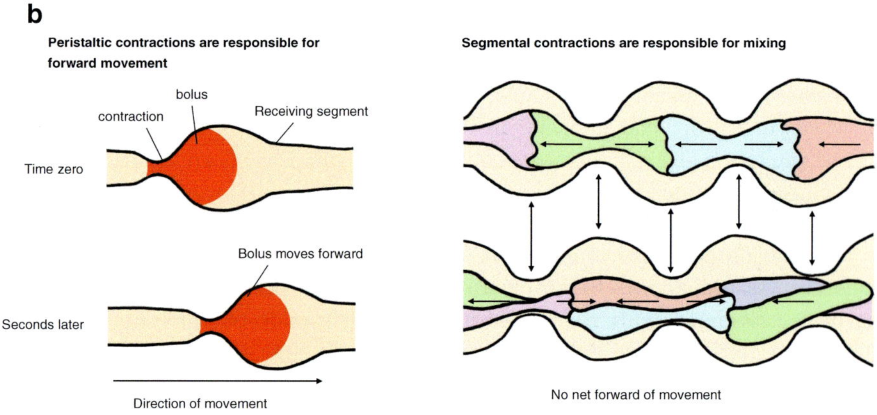

Sustained tonic contractions	Sphinters (passage of material from one segment of the gastrointestinal tract to another)
Peristaltic contractions	GI tract (forward propulsion of material from esophagusto rectum)
Segmental contractions	GI tract (bolus mixing)

Fig. 8.2 (**a**) Motor pattern of the MMC. (**b**) Gastrointestinal motor activity

muscular layer (shortening and widening of the tract); peristalsis normally lets the contents of the digestive tract progress toward the cecum in the aboral direction [8, 9].

Conditioning of intestinal motility (Structures and gastrointestinal motility). Motor function is conditioned by several systems, as well as by psycho-environmental conditions [10].

Numerous endocrine cells are found in the gastrointestinal mucosa that spills into the blood; the endocrine transmission (especially concerning the pituitary-adrenergic axis), intestinal microbiota, immune system,, modulate intestinal motility, through reciprocal interactions with the CNS. They are mostly represented by clear cells (argentaffin or enterochromaffin cells) that produce serotonin through decarboxylation of amine precursors such as 5-hydroxytryptophan; hence, they are referred to by the acronym APUD (Amine Precursor Uptake and Decarboxylation).

Table 8.2 Functions of the intestinal microbiota

Protective action
Pathogen dislocation; competition of nutrients and receptors; production of antimicrobial factors; inhibition of the growth of pathogenic organisms
Metabolic action
Food digestion with SCFA production and energy recovery; regulation of glucose and lipid metabolism (mineral salts); elimination of toxins and drugs; synthesis and absorption of vitamins (folin, biotin, vitamin B12); iron absorption
Immuno-modulatory action
Intestinal barrier fortification; induction of IgA and strengthening of TJ; modulation of inflammation; development of the immune system; modulation in gene expression
Neuro-endocrine action
VNS regulation and development and function; modulation of the endocrine system

SCFA short-chain fatty acids; *Tj* (tight junction) tight junctions

Such cells are located in the lining epithelia of the small and large intestines in the tubules of the gastric, pyloric, duodenal, and pancreatic glands. The numerous diversities of endocrine cells in the gastrointestinal tract allow it to be considered the largest gastro-entero-pancreatic (GEP) endocrine system.

Bacterial colonization of the intestine is critical for the development and maturation of the ENS [13]. Specifically, ENS interacts with the microbiota via serotonin [5-hydroxytryptamine (5-HT)]. 5-HT is produced in both the ENS and Central Nervous System (CNS), is a key neurotransmitter for motor and secretory responses in the ENS, activates local enteric nervous receptors, which determine secretion and propulsive motility, and acts on vagal afferent pathways to modulate contractile activities [14]. Scientific evidence demonstrates the causal link between inflammation of the intestinal mucosa and altered intestinal secretion/motility [15]. Inflammation-related muscle contractile activity decreases by suppressing the inflammatory response with the use of corticosteroids.

In summary, it is well known that the immune system alters intestinal motility, hence the potential beneficial effects of probiotic treatment. Diet, food intake, medication [16] storage and consumption patterns induce physiopathological effects capable of affecting the whole organism, mediated by the gut microbiota (Table 8.2).

8.3 Functional Gastrointestinal Disorders

Functional Gastrointestinal Disorders (FGIDs) are disorders of gut-brain interaction defined by the presence of GI symptoms related to a variable combination of motility disorders, visceral hypersensitivity and altered immune and mucosal function, altered gut microbiota and altered CNS processing in the presence of predisposing psychosocial, genetic and environmental factors [17]. They cause persistent or recurrent symptoms due to abnormalities in gastrointestinal functioning without organic lesions; it is difficult to arrive at a correct classification by common radiographs or endoscopies alone, which are usually normal. Only accurate evaluation of symptoms (Rome IV Criteria) and functional diagnostics studying gastrointestinal movement, microbiota, absorption, and local immunity can give the decisive elements to optimize therapy and personalize it so as to improve the patient's quality of life. Twenty-two FGIDs have been identified by global experts, which can affect any part of the gastrointestinal tract, including the esophagus, stomach, bile duct, and intestine [18]. The most common and most studied FGID is Irritable Bowel Syndrome-abdominal pain associated with altered bowel habits with diarrhea, constipation, or alternation. Other frequent FGIDs include Gastroesophageal Reflux without esophagitis (Non Erosive Reflux Disease NERD) often resistant to therapy, Functional Dyspepsia (Box 8.2), Chronic Abdominal Bloating and Functional Abdominal Pain, Constipation, or Chronic Functional Diarrhea.

Box 8.2: Functional Dyspepsia

Defined by the gastroenterologist, it is an expression of vegetative intestinal dysmotility. According to the Rome IV gastroenterological criteria [19], it is defined by the presence of one or more of the four cardinal symptoms (epigastric pain or burning, postprandial heaviness, and early satiety), not associated with organic, systemic, or metabolic pathology, that has been present for more than 6 months (Fig. 8.3).

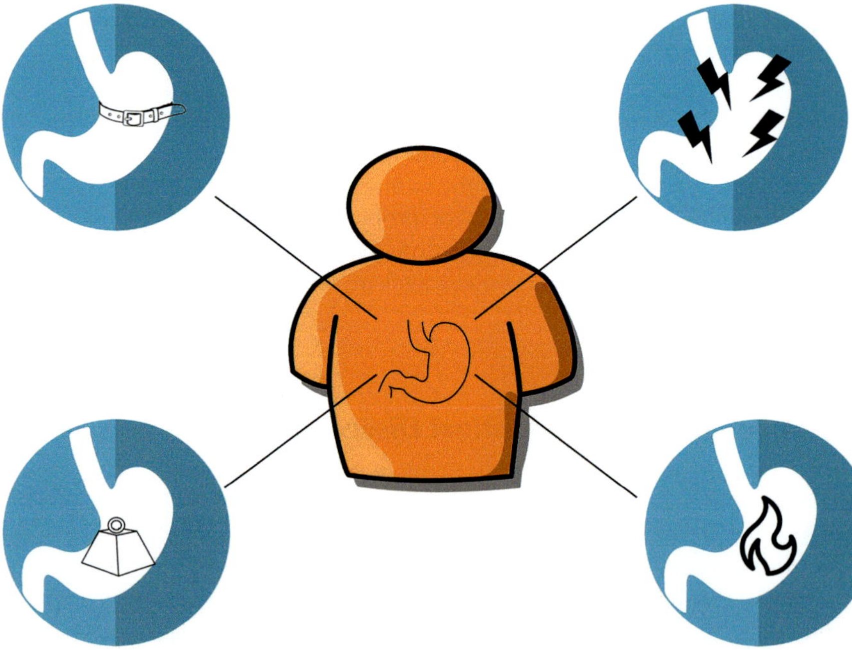

Fig. 8.3 Symptoms of functional dyspepsia according to Rome IV Criteria: epigastric pain, epigastric burning, postprandial fullness, early satiety

8.4 Autonomic Gastrointestinal Dysfunction

GI dysfunction is of strict neurological interest when the GI disorder is among the possible onset manifestations of a neurological disease (i.e., constipation in PD), when it is associated with neurological symptoms/signs not peculiar to the GI district (i.e., functional dyspepsia associated with neurological symptoms), or when it complicates an ongoing neurological disease (i.e., gastroparesis in diabetic neuropathy). GI dysfunction may present in a subclinical form and therefore be difficult to correlate with associated neurological pathology. All segments of the gastrointestinal tract can be affected by GI autonomic dysfunction, contributing to a somewhat variable clinical presentation (Table 8.3) that often, especially for alvus disorders, is not easily reported by the patient [3].

The sympathetic nervous system exerts a predominantly inhibitory effect on GI muscles and is responsible for tonic inhibitory activity on mucosal secretion, as well

Table 8.3 Gastrointestinal motor disorder with vegetative etiopathogenesis

Etiopathogenesis: CNS, VNS, ENS	Main features
Oropharyngeal dysphagia	
Pharyngeal skeletal muscle impairment; disorder of lower motor neuron (e.g., bulbar polio or pseudobulbar palsy), or muscles (e.g., ALS, myasthenia gravis) [2, 20]; oropharyngeal bradykinesia in PD and presence of α-synuclein in motor and sensory nerves [21];	Difficulty swallowing with early aspiration or cough. Often it is accompanied by other symptoms, such as nasopharyngeal regurgitation, voice changes, or the perception of uncoordinated swallowing
Esophageal dysphagia	
Vagal denervation or smooth muscle disease [2, 20] In specific conditions (i.e., MS), dysphagia can be caused by a combination of lesions in several structures: Cerebellum, corticobulbar tract, brainstem and lower cranial nerves, which modulate information to and from the muscles of the respiratory, oropharyngeal and gastrointestinal tracts	Sensation of food or liquid sticking in the esophagus or chest. When it is associated with pain, it takes the name of odynophagia; when it is associated with persistent obstruction and bolus retention, it is classified as food bolus impaction
Gastroparesis	
Gastric motility disorder mainly characterized by uncoordinated antral contractions, pyloric spasm, fundal distention hypersensitivity, and impaired gastric accommodation to a meal, vegetative and vagal neuropathic impairment, and gastric smooth muscle contractility dysfunction The most frequent causes are the idiopathic (60%), and the diabetic (30%) form, successively the post-surgical form. It can be due to vagal myenteric denervation. It may be present in neurological disorders such as stroke, vegetative syndromes, multiple sclerosis, spinal cord injury, neurofibromatosis, peripheral nerve disorders	Continuously or cyclically nausea, vomiting, early satiety, and/or a sense of fullness, it is compatible with gastric retention in the absence of a mechanical obstruction

(continued)

Table 8.3 (continued)

Etiopathogenesis: CNS, VNS, ENS	Main features
Intestinal pseudo-obstruction	
Rare disorder of intestinal motility. It is a severe and disabling disorder characterized by recurrent episodes that mimes the mechanical obstruction, but without organic, systemic, or metabolic disorders, and without physical obstruction detectable by radiographs or surgery The etiology is unknown. The pathogenesis of motor and intestinal transit dysfunctions may involve the impairment of enteric and/or extrinsic nervous system (autonomic neuropathy), of smooth muscle (visceral myopathy), and of interstitial cells of Cajal (intestinal mesenchymal pathy) It may be due by vagal or myenteric denervation, or it may be iatrogenic (narcotics, GLP1 agonists). It may recognize associated to genetic causes: The transmission can be either autosomal dominant (for example mutations of the *ACTG2* gene, for which the patient inherit a single copy of the mutated gene from a parent, or the mutation can be de novo in the affected individual), or linked to the chromosome X (*FLNA*), or autosomal recessive (for example mutations in the *RAD21* and *SGOL1* genes, for which the affected individual inherit two copies of the mutated gene, one from each parent)	Severe chronic 'obstructive' symptoms: Abdominal pain, distention/satiety, nausea/vomiting, intractable diarrhea and/or constipation, malabsorption. These symptoms cause weight loss and/or growth retardation in children. Biological abnormalities usually reflect the level of malabsorption and malnutrition Affected intestinal traits may be confined (only small bowel involvement in most cases) or generalized. Sometimes the disorder also involves other muscles, such as the bladder
Constipation	
Parasympathetic, vagal, sacral, or myenteric denervation injury. It can be classified in constipation with slow or normal transit, and pelvic floor dyssynergia (due to incoordination, altered recto-anal inhibitory reflex, reduced rectal sensitivity, altered rectal compliance in addition to behavioral factors) Other etiological elements of constipation are: Increased bowel transit time (due to drugs and/or loss of supraspinal modulation), anorectal hyposensitivity, a low-fiber diet, weakness of abdominal muscles	Difficult passage of stools and/or infrequent bowel movements (evacuation less than three times a week), hard stools
Fecal incontinence	
Damage of pelvic nerves, sacral roots, cauda equina, or denervation of spinal cord (pelvic floor and anal sphincters). It can result in abnormal rectal sensation or a deficiency of the internal anal sphincter (sympathetic denervation), or the external anal sphincter (sacral parasympathetic neuropathy)	Involuntary loss of stools and intestinal gas, uncontrolled colonic peristalsis, impaired rectal compliance, prolonged recto-anal inhibitory reflex, weakness of the internal and/or external sphincter muscles, and anorectal hyposensitivity

Table 8.3 (continued)

Etiopathogenesis: CNS, VNS, ENS	Main features
Diarrhea	
Autonomic neuropathy, enteric neuropathy, abnormalities of ICCs, oxidative stress, inflammation. It can result in colon hypermotility, dysfunction of the anal sphincters and rectal hyposensitivity	Liquid stools, with blood, mucus, steatorrhea **Symptomatology and signs:** Abdominal cramps, tenesmus, marked borborygmi due to the high peristalsis, pelvic floor dyssynergia, possible alterations of the perineal area

as regulating GI blood flow by vasoconstriction. The parasympathetic, in contrast, can exert both an excitatory and inhibitory effect on muscle tone; this dual and antagonistic characteristic allows for finer and more complex control over GI activity, particularly GI motility related to digestive/secretory/defecatory function. The presence of GI autonomic dysfunction is often underestimated, but in some clinical neurological conditions, it can become crucial, such as in Parkinson's disease (PD), where therapeutic efficacy is linked to good gastric transit efficiency.

The main autonomic GI dysfunctional syndromes are manifested by: thoracic dysphagia with gastroesophageal reflux disease (GERD) is associated, gastroparesis, chronic intestinal pseudo-obstruction, constipation, and anal dysfunction (Table 8.3). Sphincters and valves in the GI tube, in fact, exhibit tonic contraction designed to prevent reflux of gastric contents by compartmentalizing the different tracts of the digestive tract. When such motor mechanisms in the proximal part of the stomach are altered, GERD occurs. In general, however, anorectal dysfunction and oropharyngeal dysphagia are associated with alterations in other apparatuses (i.e., urinary autonomic disorders disturbances in anorectal dysfunction) or secondary to encephalic/spinal lesions, respectively.

Several modifiable factors modulate GI activity, including drugs/food/medications (Table 8.4) taken and endogenously produced toxicants. Therefore, collecting a thorough history is the first fundamental approach for these patients to rule out eating disorders (i.e., incongruous psychiatric ingestion of drugs, foods, or otherwise, as well as prolonged fasting).

Table 8.4 Gastrointestinal motility modifiers (drugs)

Motility inhibitors/constipation-inducing drugs	
Clinical field of use	**Pharmacological Class (some examples)**
Anti-inflammatories/ pain relievers	Opioids (codeine, buprenorphine, fentanyl, hydrocodone, hydromorphone, meperidine, methadone, morphine sulfate, oxycodone, Oxymorphone, tramadol), FANS (indometacine)
Anesthetics	Gas anesthetics
Anorectics	Amphetamine
Neuropsychiatrics	Anxiolitics (benzodiazepine), tricyclic antidepressants (amitriptyline, doxepin, imipramine), MAO inhibitors, antipsychotics (Phenothiazines), antiparkinsonians (levodopa, carbidopa, Pergolide, bromocriptine, amantadine)
Gastroenterologicals	Antiacids (calcium and aluminum salts, e.g., aluminum hydroxide, calcium carbonate), Antidiarrhoics (Loperamide), Antispastic (Diciclοverine, hyoscine as scopolamine); antiulcer (sucralfate, Bismute)
	Anti-arrhythmics (verapamil), Anticonvulsivant/antiepileptic (phenytoin, carbamazepine, gabapentin, oxcarbazepine, Pregabalin), Antihypertensives (clonidine, prazosin, methyldopa, verapamil), calcium antagonists (verapamil, diltiazem, Nifedipine), diuretics (Benzothiazide, potassium-sparing diuretics), lipid-lowering (cholestyramine, colestipol)
Antibiotics	Broad-spectrum antibiotics without probiotic compensation
Chemotherapy	Derivatives of vinca (vinblastine, vincristine), dacarbazine
Orthopedics/ rheumatologists	Calcium salts
Antihistamines	Anti-H1, Difenidramine
Ear/pneumologists	Anticussion (codeine derivatives, e.g., hydrocodone bitartrate, chlorpheniramine polistirex)
Antispasmodics	Anticolinergics (atropine)
Urologicals	Antimuscarinics (Prociclidine, Ossibutinine)
Antihypertensives	Ganglion blockers (Guanethidine)
Others	Hematinics: Iron salts (e.g., ferrous gluconate, ferrous sulfate), barium sulfate, sympathicomimetics (ephedrine, terbutaline)
Drugs with prokinetic action/diarrhea inducers	
Clinical field of use	**Pharmacological class (some examples)**
Gastroenterologics	Prokinetics (metoclopramide, Domperidone, levosulpiride, Bromopride), laxatives (osmotics, lactulose-based, anthraquinones, with lactose or sorbitol, macrogol if inappropriate usage of Prucalopride Linaclotide), proton pump inhibitors, H2-antagonists, magnesium
Antibiotics	Broad-spectrum antibiotics without probiotic compensation
	Diuretics (thiazides)
Anti-inflammatories/ pain relievers	Nonsteroidal (FANS), Opiates, anxiolytics (alprazolam), antidepressants (fluoxetine, lithium), anti-Cholinesterases (donepezil)
Cardiologics	Cardiac antiarrhytmics (propranolol, digoxin, quinidine, procainamide), arterial antihypertensives (ACE inhibitors, hydralazine)
Diabetologics	Oral hypoglycaemics (Clofibrate, metformin)
Anti-cholinergics drugs	Bethanechol, neostigmine
Neurologics	Methyldopa
Others	Prostaglandins, colchicine, thyroxine, uGastrografin

8.5 Neurological Diseases and GI Autonomic Disorders

Extrinsic neurological diseases are defined as those that result in a deficit of extrinsic GI control; Table 8.5 shows the main neurological diseases that result in GI disorders from possible ANS incompetence. The neurological and non-neurological diseases affecting the neural axis of entero-motor control (CNS-VNS structures) are many, but those that directly affect the ANS most frequently are diseases with a chronic-neurodegenerative course, diffuse in character, slowly progressive, with involvement of central and/or peripheral structures (i.e., Parkinson's disease (PD) in alpha-synucleinopathies and peripheral vegetative neuropathy in diabetes). Clinically expressing diseases with chronic progressive course without deficits in neurological extrinsic control, such as immunological endocrine/rheumatological diseases, mainly affect the ENS in addition to the GI structure (Table 8.6). The GI control of ENS exhibits greater autonomy from extrinsic control and within certain limits can compensate for the deficit of ANS; however, when the accommodation capacity of GI autonomic control is impaired, GI disorders result. In cases of acute/subacute GI disorder onset, it is possible that the etiologic agent affecting the nervous system and/or GI system may be lesional. In such cases, it is indicated to evaluate the presence of so-called red flags (Box 8.3), i.e., alarm symptoms, situations in which urgent referral to the gastroenterologist, and first-level examinations should be performed to rule out organic pathology, see later Table 8.12.

Table 8.5 Extrinsic neurological diseases with intestinal dysmotility

Brain diseases	Degenerations of the vegetative system	Spinal cord injury	Peripheral neuropathy	Muscle diseases
Stroke; Head trauma; Neurocognitive syndrome (e.g., Alzheimer's disease; PD); multiple system atrophy; Brainstem injuries;	Pandysautonomy; Familial dysautonomy; Idiopathic orthostatic hypotension and pure autonomic failure; Postural orthostatic tachycardia syndrome;	Spinal cord injury; Multiple sclerosis; Neuromyelitis optica;	Acute peripheral neuropathy; Chronic peripheral neuropathy (i.e., diabetes mellitus; amyloidosis); Paraneoplastic neuropathy; Porphyria; Neurofibromatosis; Nerve lipomatosis; HIV neuropathy; Autoimmune neuropathies ab vs neuronal receptors;	Duchenne/Becker muscular dystrophies; Muscular dystrophies, Polymyositis and dermatomyositis; Mitochondriopathy, Neurogastrointestinal encephalomyopathy, Myotonic dystrophy type 1

Table 8.6 Immunological endocrine/rheumatological diseases with intestinal dysmotility

Autonomic dysfunction	During systemic disease	
		Systemic connectivity
Predominantly sympathetic-stimulatory dysfunction	RAYNAUD'S PHENOMENON GASTROINTESTINAL SYMPTOMS Gastroesophageal reflux symptoms Nasopharyngeal irritation from gas reflux Retrosternal pain (esophagitis/esophageal spasm)	SYSTEMIC SCLEROSIS Rare disease (predominantly female) average age 30/50 years Prevalence 20–40/100000); arterial capillary vasculopathy of the connective tissue of various internal organs and skin including the vasa nervorum with progressive fibrotic evolution
Predominant parasympathetic inbitoria dysfunction	SICK SYNDROME Reduced salivation and reduced tearing GASTROINTESTINAL SYMPTOMS Dysphagia symptoms (especially for dry solid foods)	SJOGREN'S SYNDROME Rare disease with a female predominance, average age 40/50 years. Prevalence 15–25/100000; it predominantly affects the exocrine glands in particular the lacrimal and salivary glands with sclerofibrotic inflammatory progression
Mediators with predominantly sympathetic-stimulatory function	GASTROINTESTINAL SYMPTOMS Gastric hyperacidity, intestinal hypersecretion, pancreatic enzyme secretion and intestinal motility abnormalities	DISEASES OF THE NEUROENDOCRINE SYSTEM Hypothalamic-pituitary-adrenal axis Diffuse endocrine system APUDs that produce serotonin and polypeptides that also function as neurotransmitters

Gastrointestinal autonomic disorders presenting in an acute/subacute mode are often observed in diseases by brain lesion injury (traumatic and nontraumatic) and in the flare-up of chronic-degenerative diseases such as diabetic neuropathy. These disorders will be discussed in other sections.

Box 8.3: "Red Flag"

Age > 50 year;

Familiarity with upper/lower gastrointestinal cancer or chronic inflammatory bowel disease.

High-risk factors for cancer: Previous gastric/colic cancer and/or gastric/colic surgery.

Gastrointestinal bleeding.

Recent onset symptoms (Fever, Progressive and unintentional weight loss, Progressive Dysphagia/Odynephagia, Persistent vomiting, Constipation).

Hematochemical alterations (Ironopenic anemia);

Palpable epigastric/abdominal mass.

8.6 Neurological Diseases and GI Autonomic Disorders: Non-modifiable and Preexisting GI Factors (Aging, Congenital or Inherited GI Diseases)

The impact of aging on the gastrointestinal tract plays a role in worsening GI dysfunction, leading to an age-related selective decline in gut function. In general, nutrient and drug absorption worsens over time, and the defense system against ingested pathogens becomes deficient. Aging is associated with: structural and functional mucosal defense defects, reduced ability to generate protective immunity, and increased incidence of inflammation and oxidative stress. Changes in gut function associated with aging have particular implications for esophageal, gastric, and colonic motility, leading to changes in taste and reduced esophageal sphincter motility and gastric emptying. Older individuals, therefore, are particularly susceptible to malnutrition, postprandial hypotension, dysphagia, constipation, and fecal incontinence. Decreased numbers of myenteric plexus nerve cells, which affect the absorption and plication (surface area) of the small intestine, due to villous degeneration, can lead to reduced nutrient absorption.

Knowledge and evaluation of genetically determined conditions are essential for the appropriate characterization of the disease. Certain factors may alert the clinician, suggesting the search for genetic conditions. These include the age of onset of the autonomic disorder, location, and the possible presence of associated neurological disorders. Tables 8.7 and 8.8 show some of the main recognizable enteric phenotypes and the corresponding clinical-instrumental evaluations useful for correct diagnostic framing or the genes (and thus transmission patterns) to be evaluated.

Table 8.7 Enteric neuronal phenotypes associated with pediatric neuro-intestinal disease

Disease	Epidemiology onset	Autonomic dysfunction (main symptoms)	Clinical-instrumental indications
Congenital achalasia	Incidence 1–3:100000 Insidious onset, mean age at diagnosis 7y	Dysphagia, reflux and regurgitation, chest pain (due to lack of relaxation of the lower esophageal sphincter)	Endoscopy, Esophageal manometry Esophagus x-ray
Hirschsprung disease	1:5000 born alive Infancy onset	Neonatal onset: Abdominal pain, constipation, progressive abdominal distension, vomiting and diarrhea Childhood-onset: Severe constipation and failure to thrive	Anorectal manometry, showing the absence of the anal inhibitory reflex; Rectal biopsy (rectal mucosa and submucosa) showing aganglionosis, thickening of extrinsic nerve fibers, and overexpression of acetylcholinesterase.

(continued)

Table 8.7 (continued)

Disease	Epidemiology onset	Autonomic dysfunction (main symptoms)	Clinical-instrumental indications
Spina bifida	1: 2000 newborns Onset at birth	Two main forms: Open or cystic spina bifida and occult spina bifida (asymptomatic or paucisymptomatic). Open spina bifida involves the spine and spinal cord, it may be present a pocket in the skin that contains only the meninges (meningocele) or also the spinal cord (myelomeningocele). Usually located in the lumbar or sacral portion of the spine, the clinical picture varies according to the region involved. In general, there is paraplegia (paralysis of the lower limbs), hydrocephalus, the Arnold-Chiari malformation, urinary and anorectal incontinence	Prenatal ultrasound and/or MRI
Neuronal intestinal dysplasia, type B	Unknown prevalence Childhood-onset (rarely adult)	Severe constipation or bowel obstruction	Rectal biopsy (rectal mucosa and submucosa) showing colonic submucosal hyperganglionosis
Pediatric gastroparesis	Unknown prevalence Childhood-onset (mean age 8 years)	Nausea, vomiting, abdominal pain, early satiety and/or feeling of fullness	4-h gastric scintigraphy to evaluate gastric emptying rate
CIPO (chronic intestinal pseudo-obstruction)	1:100.000	Abdominal pain, distension/ satiety, nausea/vomiting, diarrhea and/or intractable constipation, malabsorption	Clinical diagnosis, supported by radiography showing intestinal dilatation and air-fluid levels (endoscopy, manometry, laboratory tests, biopsy)

CIPO chronic intestinal pseudo-obstruction [2, 22]

Table 8.8 Genetic diseases with vegetative impairment and gastrointestinal disfunction

Disease	Gene (inheritance)	Locus	OMIM
Neuropathy hereditary sensory and autonomic (HSAN)	HSAN5 – *NGF* (AR)	1p13.2	162030
	CIPA – *NTRK1* (AR)	1q23.1	191315
	HSN2C – *KIF1A* (AR)	2q37.3	601255
	HSN1B (gene unknown) (AD)	3p24-p22	608088
	HSAN7 – *SCN11A* (AD)	3p22.2	604385
	HSAN2B – *RETREG1* (AR)	5p15.1	613114
	HSAN6 – *DST* (AR)	6p12.1	113810
	HSAN1A – *SPTLC1* (AD)	9q22.31	605712
	HSAN3 – *ELP1* (AR)	9q31.3	603722
	HSAN8 – *PRDM12* (AR)	9q34.12	616458
	HSN1F – *ATL3* (AD)	11q13.1	609369
	HSAN2A – *WNK1* (AR)	12p13.33	605232
	HSN1D – *ATL1* (AD)	14q22.1	606439
	HSAN1C – *SPTLC2* (AD)	14q24.3	605713
	HSAN9 – *TECPR2* (AR)	14q32.31	615000
	HSN1E – *DNMT1* (AD)	19p13.2	126375
Hereditary sensory and vegetative neuropathies are a group of disorders of different prevalence. The age at onset is generally related to the model of transmission. In particular, early onset/infantile forms generally recognize an autosomal recessive (AR) etiology, adult-onset forms are generally autosomal dominant (AD) (i.e., HSAN1A – OMIM#162400). Adult-onset forms show a phenotype with minimal vegetative dysfunctions. Clinical phenotype of HSAN1A can include abdominal pain, diarrhea, and weight loss. The neonatal/infantile-onset forms have a phenotype with several signs of gastric vegetative impairment. Gastrointestinal dysfunction and vomiting crises are one of the diagnostic criteria in HSAN3 (OMIM#223900) (present in 40% of patients), the gastroesophageal reflux is typical in HSAN2A (OMIM#201300) and HSAN9 (OMIM#615031)			
Familial amyloid polyneuropathy (FAP)	*TTR* (AD)	18q12.1	176300
Familial amyloid polyneuropathy (FAP) is also known as amyloid or transthyretin polyneuropathy (*TTR*). FAP is an adult-onset progressive sensorimotor and vegetative neuropathy. Worldwide there are different prevalences of FAP: It is a very frequent disorder (about 5%) in East Africa, and among African Americans, instead in European and Caucasian populations, it has a frequency of about 1:100,000, with some geographical variations. It is characterized by incomplete penetrance with geographical variations. Age at onset and symptoms at onset varies greatly. Patients with adulthood (third to fifth decades) onset often show sensory neuropathy. Patients with earlier onset frequently show symptoms with gastrointestinal involvement (attacks of nausea and vomiting, delayed gastric emptying). About 3% of patients with amyloidosis have gastrointestinal amyloid neuropathy, which can cause dysphagia, constipation, diarrhea, and steatorrhea			
Familial autonomic neuropathy	ERBB3 (AR)	12q13.2	190151
Familial visceral neuropathy (OMIM # 243180) is a rare disorder with neonatal onset. Generally, it is transmitted with an autosomal recessive pattern. The phenotype involves a vegetative intestinal disfunction, with secondary gastric involvement. Vomiting is secondary to aganglionosis or hypoganglionosis of the colon			

(continued)

Table 8.8 (continued)

Disease	Gene (inheritance)	Locus	OMIM
Mitochondrial neurogastrointestinal encephalopathy (MNGIE)	TYMP (AR)	22q13.33	131222
	RRM2B (AR)	8q22.3	604712
	POLG (AR)	15q26.1	174763
Mitochondrial neurogastrointestinal encephalopathy (MNGIE) syndrome is characterized by the association of impaired gastrointestinal motility, peripheral neuropathy, chronic progressive external ophthalmoplegia, and leukoencephalopathy. Onset typically occurs in early adulthood (within the fourth decade); gastric symptoms are often present at onset and include cramps, vomiting, diarrhea, intestinal pseudo-obstruction, dysphagia, and gastroparesis			
Ehlers-Danlos syndrome (EDS) type 3 hypermobile	Nessun gene conosciuto		%130020
Ehlers-Danlos syndrome is a heterogeneous group of disorders characterized by fragility of connective tissues, that results in cutaneous, ligament, joint, vascular and/or organic manifestations. Hypermobile Ehlers-Danlos syndrome shows features of a vegetative disorder with impaired gastrointestinal function. Mainly manifestation (33%–67%) includes a functional disorder of the intestine, with frequent gastroesophageal reflux and gastritis. Some patients may show delayed gastric emptying, that can be exacerbated by opioids			
17q12 microdeletion syndrome		17q12	# 614527
17q12 microdeletion syndrome is a rare chromosomal abnormality syndrome resulting from partial deletion of the long arm of chromosome 17. Clinically, it is characterized by cystic kidney disease, juvenile diabetes, and neurodevelopmental disorders (cognitive impairment, developmental delay, and autism spectrum disorder). Less frequently, there are Müllerian aplasia in females, macrocephaly, mild facial dysmorphism (high forehead, deep-set eyes, and plump cheeks), and transient hypercalcemia. Onset is typically in neonatal/infantile age. Patients may have gastroesophageal reflux and dysphagia, in some cases associated with esophageal abnormalities or duodenal atresia			
Episodic ataxia (EA)	EA1 – *KCNA1* (AD)	12p13.32	176260
	EA2 – *CACNA1A* (AD)	19p13.13	601011
	EA3 (gene unknown) (AD)		%606554
	EA4 (gene unknown) (AD)		%606552
	EA5 – *CACNB4* (AD)	2q23.3	601949
	EA6 – *SLC1A3* (AD)	5p13.2	600111
	EA7 (gene unknown) (AD)		%611907
	EA8 (gene unknown) (AD)		%616055
	EA9 – *SCN2A* (AD)	2q24.3	182390
Hereditary episodic ataxia (EA) is a group of neurological disorders characterized by recurrent episodes of ataxia and dizziness that may be progressive. Weakness, dystonia, and ataxia may be present in the interictal period. Nine types of AE have been described so far (AE type 1 to AE type 9), with types 1 and 2 being the most frequent (estimated prevalence 1:500,000). The age of onset is highly variable between the different forms, from typical childhood in EA1 and EA2, to adulthood (third-sixth decade) for EA4. GI symptoms include nausea and vomiting and are typically present in the forms EA3, EA4, EA6, and EA9			
Neurofibromatosis type 1 (NF1)	*NF1* (AD)	17q11.2	613113
The phenotype of neurofibromatosis type 1 include constipation, generally secondary to gastrointestinal malignancies (neurogenic malignancies, disorder of interstitial cells of Cajal, neuroendocrine tumors, adenocarcinomas). It is one of the most frequent genetic pathologies, with a worldwide prevalence of about 1:3000. The age of onset is generally infantile, and dermatological signs (cafè-au-lait spots, cutaneous neurofibromas) are typically the onset manifestations			

Table 8.8 (continued)

Disease	Gene (inheritance)	Locus	OMIM
Duchenne and Becker muscular dystrophies (DMD/BMD)	*DMD* (XL)	Xp21.2-p21.1	300377
Dystrophinopathies are a group of X-linked muscular diseases with great phenotypic variability. Distrophinopathies include severe phenotypes such as Duchenne muscular dystrophy (DMD), milder phenotypes such as Becker muscular dystrophy (BMD), and dilated cardiomyopathy (DCM) and paucisymptomatic or asymptomatic phenotypes such as isolated hyperkalemia. The prevalence is variable according to the different phenotypes but generally varies between 1:5000 and 1:20000. In some cases, dystrophinopathies may be associated with gastroparesis with impaired pharyngoesophageal swallowing			
Myotonic dystrophy type 1 (DM1)	*DMPK* (AD)	19q13.32	605377
Myotonic dystrophy type 1 is a multisystemic genetic disorder characterized by a wide range of muscular (muscle weakness, myotonia) and systemic (cerebral, endocrine, cardiac, gastrointestinal, uterine, cutaneous and immunological districts) manifestations. The disease is characterized by anticipation: The phenotype is more severe in patients with an early onset than in patients with onset in adulthood. GI manifestations include dysphagia, GI reflux, and megacolon. In childhood-onset forms, gastrointestinal disorders are very frequent (malnutrition and fecal incontinence), furthermore it can be present some intestinal disorders can be associated with inflammation of the myenteric plexus and alteration of smooth muscle (chronic intestinal pseudo-obstructions and megacolon)			
Fabry disease (FD)	*GLA* (XL)	Xq22.1	300644
Fabry disease (FD) is a progressive, hereditary, multisystemic lysosomal storage disease characterized by neurologic, cutaneous, renal, cardiovascular, cochleovestibular, and cerebrovascular manifestations. The age of onset is highly variable, the classic form has an onset in childhood/adolescence, and the atypical forms (renal and cardiac variant) have an onset in adulthood (after 25 years). The frequency varies worldwide, with higher frequencies in Italian and Chinese populations. In particular, in Italy, the incidence is 1:3100, with a ratio of 11:1 between the atypical form and the classic form. The gastrointestinal symptoms are typical of the classic form and are due to the deposition of glycosphingolipids in small intestine vessels and in intestinal vegetative ganglia. Clinical manifestations of GI impairment include episodic diarrhea, nausea, vomiting, bloating and abdominal cramps, and intestinal malabsorption			
Achalasia-Addisonianism-Alacrima syndrome (triple A syndrome)	*AAAS* (AR) *GMPPA* (AR)	12q13 2q35	605378 615495
Triple A syndrome is a very rare multisystemic disorder characterized by adrenal insufficiency with isolated glucocorticoid deficiency, achalasia, alacrimia, vegetative dysfunction, and neurodegeneration. The prevalence is not known. Onset occurs between the neonatal period and adulthood. In the neonatal period, phenotype is characterized by alacrimia and achalasia of the cardia; in childhood and adolescence patients show achalasia and adrenal insufficiency (which can cause hypoglycemia and seizures); in adulthood there is a diffuse neurological involvement, with alterations of the vegetative nervous system and polyneuropathy Alachrymia, achalasia, and adrenal insufficiency are the three cardinal features of the triple A syndrome, but they may not be present altogether, or they may be associated with vegetative dysfunction and other neurological signs ("double A" or "quad A," respectively). The neurological signs are very heterogeneous: Vegetative disorders (dyshidrosis, and digestive, sexual, circulatory and urinary disorders), pyramidal syndrome and peripheral neuropathy (gait disturbance, sensory deficits), bulbar and facial deficits (insufficient velum, atrophy or paresis of the tongue, orbicularis oculi muscle dysfunction, and oropharyngeal dysphagia)			

OMIM online mendelian inheritance in man, *AR* autosomal recessive, *AD* autosomal dominant, *XL* X-linked

8.7 Neurological Diseases and GI Autonomic Disorders: Clinical Expression of Gastrointestinal Autonomic Dysfunction

The mode of onset of GI vegetative disorders can be variable. Neurological diseases with chronic-neurodegenerative courses with diffuse character have slowly progressive GI disorder expression (i.e., alpha-synucleinopathies and peripheral autonomic neuropathy). In contrast, neurological diseases with acute/subacute onset of GI disorder frequently recognize a traumatic or nontraumatic lesional etiology (see "Acute/subacute onset" section); except for flare-ups of alpha-synucleinopathies, peripheral neuropathy or the like. However, the latter diseases may be neurodegenerative in nature (e.g., MS).

Acute/subacute onset (Clinical expression of gastrointestinal vegetative dysfunction). Acute/subacute GI autonomic disorders may occur as a complication of an ongoing neurological disease but also as an expression of an acute condition, e.g., in patients with Chagas disease (a tropical parasitosis characterized by extensive injury of the myenteric plexus), in drug intoxications (e.g., metformin in diabetics), in ganglionitis, or after vagotomy. Acute/subacute onset GI vegetative disorders may have a lesional etiology, which may be traumatic or nontraumatic.

Acute/subacute onset, injury with traumatic VNS injury may involve the encephalon (head injury), spinal cord injury (SCI), and/or spinal and cranial nerve injury, along with related complications (Box 8.4) [23–26].

Box 8.4: Chronic GI Complications from Trauma

Chronic GI dysfunction occurs in 27–62% of patients with spinal cord injury. GI dysfunction is a multifactorial consequence of neurogenic circuits and loss of central (supraspinal) control. Specifically, while post-SCI loss of descending control to lumbosacral reflex circuits is generally considered to play an important role in colonic and anorectal dysfunction, gastric dysmotility is seen as an indirect pathology and secondary to the vagal afferent signaling defect after SCI. Specifically, emerging data indicate a reduced sensitivity of vagal afferents to gastrointestinal neuroactive peptides, neurotransmitters, and possibly macronutrients, while the loss of descending pathways to lumbosacral segmental circuits overlaps with pathophysiological remodeling of the colonic intrinsic neurocircuitry. GI disorders after SCI are mainly related to motility disturbance. Upper GI motility disturbances are rare in the chronic phase after injury, while colonic and anorectal dysfunction are common and result from disruption of supraspinal control, sacral parasympathetic activation at the colon with reduced postprandial motor responses, pelvic floor dysfunction, and anal sphincters, leading to defecation disturbances or fecal incontinence. The most common symptoms are constipation, distention, abdominal pain, rectal bleeding, hemorrhoids, fecal incontinence, and vegetative hyperreflexia. A biliary stone is observed in 17%–31% of cases [26].

Complications often present in individuals with SCI at the bowel level result in the condition of "neurogenic bowel." In turn, vegetative dysreflexia, evoked by enteric tube distention, as in severe constipation conditions, triggers increased sympathetic discharge below the level of injury that can be life-threatening, particularly in individuals with SCI at or above the T5-T6 spinal cord. These lesions result in major dysfunction of the colorectum, bladder, and sexual function. The most commonly associated symptoms are slow colonic transit, constipation, and/or bowel obstruction, sometimes associated with episodes of overflow incontinence [26].

In SCI occurring above the mid-thoracic spinal segments, pathophysiologic reductions in emptying and motility of the upper gastrointestinal tract are observed. Studies on gastric motor function have demonstrated a reduction in basal contractions after high spinal cord injury, above T3 but not less than T9 from thoracic contusion in animal guinea pigs, persisting up to 6 weeks after T3-SCI. CCK, released from lipid- and protein-sensitive enteroendocrine cells in the duodenum, has been implicated in the regulation of motility. It is capable of activating the terminals of C-type vagal afferent fibers that project to nucleus cells of the solitary tract in addition to acting on nodose ganglion cells and centrally within the dorsal vagal complex. Activation at each of these levels results in gastro inhibition [28, 29].

Acute/subacute onset, injury with non-traumatic etiology (i.e., MS) recognizes multiple causes: tumors, vascular disease, toxic-parenchymal conditions, and inflammatory conditions; in addition, in the spine, degeneration of the fibrocartilaginous disc and/or osteo-articular arthritic component may result in spinal canal stenosis and/or spinal radiculopathy. Among non-traumatic injuries, acute CNS ischemia due to blood vessel occlusion and/or hemorrhagic bleeding has an important role epidemiologically and by extent of sequelae (Box 8.5).

Compared with traumatic lesional etiologies, nontraumatic ones tend to be age-dependent; some of them affect the structures of the CNS by autoimmune mechanisms (such as autoimmune autonomic ganglionopathy), but also by toxic/iatrogenic mechanisms (as in those from antidiabetic drugs or in carbon monoxide intoxications).

Autonomic dysfunction is a common and significant cause of disability in MS patients, as it produces not only gastrointestinal dysfunction but also cardiovascular, bladder, sexual, thermoregulatory, and pupillary dysfunction, probably also contributing to one of the pivotal symptoms of MS: fatigue [30, 31]. Multiple sclerosis (MS) is an inflammatory-neurodegenerative disease that can have a progressive chronic course. Autonomic dysfunction in MS is attributed to several factors: demyelination in areas of the CNS involved in control or modulation of the ANS, altered interactions between the autonomic and immune systems, and Epstein-Barr virus (EBV) infection.

It has been shown that in the prodromal stages (up to 10 years before the onset of signs and/or symptoms), MS patients experience four main symptoms: pain, cognitive symptoms/fatigue, psychiatric symptoms, and autonomic dysfunction affecting the upper gastrointestinal, urinary, and anorectal tracts [32]. In MS, an increase in catecholamine production takes place in response to hyperactivation of the immune system [33]. It has also been found that autonomic dysfunction in MS follows a dual pattern: while disease activity (demonstrable as clinical relapses/presence of demyelinating lesions on radiological examinations) is associated with sympathetic system dysfunction, disease progression (demonstrable as increased neurological disability) is associated with parasympathetic system dysfunction [34].

The main gastrointestinal autonomic symptoms in MS involve both the upper and lower gastrointestinal tracts and are dysphagia, fecal incontinence, constipation, and diarrhea (Table 8.9).

Box 8.5: Main Causes of Injuries of the Brain and Spinal Cord

Acute cerebral ischemia. Dysphagia in stroke is the most common occurrence; it can be brought on by involvement of motor neurons of the related cranial nerves of swallowing (trigeminal V, facial VII, glossopharyngeal IX, vagus X, accessory XI, and hypoglossal XII). Over time, it can complicate with malnutrition or ab ingestis pneumonia, normally of the oropharyngeal type, thus not caused by a VNS disorder. Conversely, pseudo-obstruction of the colon could have a vegetative basis, although this represents a rare occurrence. The second most incident gastrointestinal symptom is constipation, which affects about 45% of subjects in the acute phase and persists at least in the subsequent rehabilitation phases. This disorder is prevalent in brain, rather than brainstem, localizations; it is associated with decreased rectal sensitivity and overall delay of colonic transit in at least ¼ of cases [26, 27].

Brainstem lesions. Brainstem lesions can present in the acute phase, even in the absence of intracranial hypertension, with various gastrointestinal complaints: isolated gastrointestinal motor dysfunction or vomiting from the involvement of the vomiting center on the floor of the fourth ventricle. Compression of the brainstem and lower cranial nerves can cause neurogenic dysphagia in patients with Arnold-Chiari malformations. The presence of more widespread vegetative dysfunction, in particular if adrenergic pathways are involved, is always an indication to look for a CNS lesion [26].

Table 8.9 Symptoms and signs of gastrointestinal vegetative dysfunction in Multiple Sclerosis and complications

Disease	Epidemiology	Clinical presentation	Evaluation
Oropharyngeal dysphagia	**Frequency:** 30–40% [35, 36] More common in adults moderately and severely impaired (expanded disability status scale, EDSS score: 8–9) [37]	**Symptomatology**: Coughing during or after eating and/or drinking, food sticking in their mouth and/or throat, throat clearing, gagging, drooling, slowness and fatigue while eating, dyspnea, weight loss and any episodes of either unexplained fever or pneumonia **Complications**: Reduced eating desire; social withdrawal; mealtime anxiety/distress; critical impact in quality of life (QoL) of the patients [38] Dehydration, malnutrition, and food aspiration [39], increased risk of ab ingestis pneumonia, morbidity, and death; reduced ability to perform activities of daily living (ADL)	See Table 8.14 for clinical exam and instrumental tests
Faecal incontinence	**Frequency:** About 50% of the patients [40, 41] **Type** – Passive: If the patient has not awareness of the incontinence – Urge incontinence: If fecal incontinence is accompanied by a degree of urgency	**Symptomatology**: Fecal incontinence, associated or not with urinary incontinence **Complications**: Perianal dermatitis (anal eczema, perianal eczema), pruritus ani, pressure sores, higher risk of urinary and vaginal infections	See Table 8.14 for clinical exam and instrumental tests
Constipation	**Frequency:** 18–43% [40, 41] More common in the early stages of the disease and with a low level of disability (lower EDSS scores: 0–3,5): Severe constipation is often the first symptom of MS	**Symptomatology**: Absence of evacuation stimulus, presence of hard stools, difficulty in expelling stools **Complications**: Intestinal occlusion, hemorrhoids, thrombosis hemorrhoidal, rectal prolapse	See Table 8.14 for clinical exam and instrumental tests

(continued)

Table 8.9 (continued)

Disease	Epidemiology	Clinical presentation	Evaluation
Diarrhea	Higher prevalence of diarrhea in patients with MS which present: – Comorbidity: IBD (Crohn's disease, ulcerative colitis), probably due to genetic predisposition, damage to the intestinal microbial flora and the role of the immune system present at the gastrointestinal level [42, 43, 44] – Therapy with dimethyl fumarate used in relapsing-remitting forms [45]	**Symptomatology**: Abdominal cramps, tenesmus **Complications:** Dehydration and hydroelectrolytic imbalance	See Table 8.14 for clinical exam and instrumental tests

8.8 Chronic Progressive Course and Exacerbation (Clinical Expression of Gastrointestinal Autonomic Dysfunction)

Neurological disorder presentation can occur acute/subacutely, as is observed in pathologies with lesional etiology; one of the distinguishing features in chronic-degenerative pathologies could be the intra-individual fluctuation of the disorders over time, as it is observed frequently in diabetic neuropathy.

In some pathological conditions, gastrointestinal disorders can progress slowly with progressive chronic features, as it has been observed in degenerative neurological diseases, such as PD and SM. Other systemic pathologies can cause peripheral neuropathy determined by the involvement of small-fibers, as it occurs in DM, and they have a chronic progressive course. The related autonomic disorders can progress over time to become frankly disabling, while gastrointestinal autonomic disorders must often be subclinical or clinically irrelevant and therefore it has to be actively investigated.

Neurodegenerative diseases, such as α-synucleinopathies, alter gastrointestinal function with a chronic progressive course. In PD, GI symptoms are observed in the very early stages of the disease, in the "premotor" phase of the disease. GI symptoms involve the entire digestive tract and are evident throughout the course of the disease. Indeed, constipation, in particular, may precede the onset of motor symptoms, even more than 10 years. The GI tract seems to play a crucial role in the neurodegenerative process leading to PD, being an entrance door from the external environment to the ENS. Indeed, α-synuclein would spread with a rostro caudal gradient, from the GI, at the ENS, and through the sympathetic and parasympathetic nervous system to the CNS, causing the typical neuropathological changes of PD [46] (Table 8.10).

Table 8.10 Symptoms and signs of gastrointestinal autonomic dysfunction in Parkinson's disease and complications

Disease	Epidemiology	Clinical presentation	Evaluation
Drooling	**Frequency:** 10–81% of patients From impaired swallowing of saliva rather than from increased production;	**Symptomatology:** Anamnestic evidence of hypersalivation, loss of saliva, sialorrhea; **Complications:** Psychosocial discomfort; wounds, skin lesions, angular cheilitis, skin infections;	See Table 8.14 for clinical exam and instrumental tests
Dysphagia	**Frequency:** More than 80% of patients during the course of their disease; all phases are affected (oral, pharyngeal and esophageal); the onset of severe dysphagia in the first year of the disease is a red flag for atypical Parkinsonism (Multy systemic atrophy-MSA; progressive Supranuclear palsy-PSP);	**Symptomatology**: Coughing during or after eating and/or drinking; weight loss, drooling, recurrent respiratory infections; chronic inflammatory state not otherwise justified; inefficacy of drug dose that can be stuck in valleculae; **Complications**: Aspiration pneumonia;	*Questionnaires: The swallowing disturbance questionnaire* (SDQ) and the Munich dysphagia test-Parkinson's disease (MDT-PD) [47, 48]; See Table 8.14 for clinical exam and instrumental tests
Reduced gastric emptying/ gastroparesis	**Frequency:** Up to 100% of patients	**Symptomatology:** Nausea, bloating, reduced effectiveness of dopaminergic drugs**;** **Complications:** Lack of efficacy of dopaminergic therapy; nutritional and weight changes;	See Table 8.14 for clinical exam and instrumental tests
Faecal incontinence	**Frequency:** 10–24% of patients	**Symptomatology**: Loss of stools; **Complications**: Recurrent urinary and vaginal infections; psychosocial discomfort;	See Table 8.14 for clinical exam and instrumental tests
Constipation/ reduced intestinal transit	**Frequency:** 20–89% of patients; it can be a premotor symptom of PD	**Symptomatology**: Abdominal bloating; **Complications**: Fecal impaction; bowel obstruction;	See Table 8.14 for clinical exam and instrumental tests
Difficulty in defecation	**Frequency:** 60% of patients; it can be due to the impaired release (dystonic phenomenon) of the anal sphincter;	**Symptomatology**: Excessive effort, pain and incomplete evacuation; **Complications:** Pain and failure to evacuate;	See Table 8.14 for clinical exam and instrumental tests

Peripheral sensory and autonomic neuropathy of large and small fibers may be present in metabolic disorders (DM, hypothyroidism, uremia), cobalamin deficiency, infections, immune-mediated conditions (gammopathies, vasculitis, and celiac disease), neurotoxic exposure (alcoholism and drug treatment), and in inherited conditions (inherited sensory and autonomic neuropathy, Fabry disease, and transthyretin-mediated hereditary amyloidosis).

Gastrointestinal autonomic symptoms occur frequently in DM and result in a major impact on quality of life. In particular, DM represents the most common cause of chronic gastroparesis, a condition of altered gastric motility resulting in delayed gastric emptying in the absence of mechanical obstruction [46, 49] (Table 8.11). The pathogenesis is complex and heterogeneous, being determined by

Table 8.11 Symptoms and signs of gastrointestinal autonomic dysfunction in Diabetes Mellitus and complications

Disease	Epidemiology	Clinical presentation	Evaluation
Functional dyspepsia	Prevalence up to 50% in DM1 and DM2	**Symptoms:** Epigastric fullness, early satiety, nausea, vomiting, pyrosis, abdominal pain **Signs and complications:** Hypo-hyper-nutrition, effect on glycemic control, weight modifications	See Table 8.14 for instrumental tests
Gastroparesis	Prevalence 9.6% in men and 37.8% in women (defined by scintigraphy; Olmsted County) Incidence 5.2% in DM1 and 1% in DM2 over 10 years (Olmsted County)	**Symptoms:** Dysphagia, nausea, vomiting, abdominal bloating, post-meal fullness, early satiety, abdominal pain, weight loss **Signs and complications:** Impaired balance between intestinal absorption of glucose and the action of exogenously administered insulin, or other antidiabetics; poor glycemic control (episodes of ketoacidosis); dehydration and nutritional deficiencies; weight modifications	**Questionnaire** Gastroparesis cardinal symptom index (GCSI) Gastrointestinal domain of the composite vegetative symptom score 31 (COMPASS 31) See Table 8.14 for instrumental tests
Diarrhea	Prevalence 15.6%	**Signs and complications**: Fecal incontinence, abdominal pain, dehydration and nutritional deficiencies, bowel malabsorption, weight modifications	Intestinal diary recording: Frequency and characteristics (liquid stools, with blood, with mucus, steatorrhea) See Table 8.14 for instrumental tests
Faecal incontinence	Prevalence 1–8.6%	**Signs and complications**: Possible association with diarrhea	Intestinal diary recording Perineum evaluation and RE See Table 8.14 for instrumental tests

Table 8.11 (continued)

Disease	Epidemiology	Clinical presentation	Evaluation
Costipation	Prevalence 30%	**Symptoms and complications:** Feeling of incomplete evacuation, need for manual maneuvers during defecation, possible association with diarrhea	Intestinal diary recording Perineum evaluation and RE See Table 8.14 for instrumental tests

Abbreviations in table: *DM1* type 1 diabetes mellitus, *DM2* type 2 diabetes mellitus; RE, rectal exploration

vegetative neuropathy and enteric neuropathy, abnormalities of *interstitial cells of Cajal*, and acute fluctuations in blood glucose. These mechanisms result in reduced *fundus* release, antral hypomotility with subsequent dilatation, and pylorospasm, all of which are responsible for dyspeptic symptoms. Moreover, unpredictable gastric emptying can impair the balance between intestinal absorption of glucose from food and the action of exogenously administered insulin, as well as other antidiabetics, resulting in postprandial glycemic fluctuations and poor glycemic control.

Chronic diarrhea and fecal incontinence, in addition to symptoms of gastroparesis, are common in diabetic patient [50, 51]. Hypo- and hyper-colonic motility have been demonstrated in DM and together with internal anal sphincter dysfunction, contribute to fecal incontinence [50, 51]. The management of diabetic patient with gastrointestinal autonomic symptoms, due to the above, is often suboptimal: therapy aims to control gastric symptoms, improve glycemic control, and promote maintenance of optimal hydration and nutritional status. Treatment is essentially based on dietary and behavioral measures and use of prokinetic drugs, although these are not effective in all patients. Surgery and gastric electrostimulation represent alternative forms of therapy to be reserved for cases refractory to drug therapy.

8.9 Laboratory and Instrumental Tests for the Diagnosis of Dysmotility of the Gastrointestinal System

Currently, we do not have a commercially available in vivo diagnostic test for the diagnosis of enteric dysmotility, and GI symptoms are generally not predictive of objective motility dysfunction. This condition would always recommend a specialized objective evaluation by verifying the type and extent of GI motor disturbance; available clinical-instrumental diagnostic findings that can provide useful information to support the diagnosis of enteric dysmotility are helpful in guiding its treatment. However, although the finding of GI motor impairment in a patient with GI dysmotility significantly increases the likelihood of enteric neuropathy, some patients may have enteric dysmotility despite normal motility measurements. The pathophysiology underlying GI system dysmotility varies among patient groups, but the methods of assessing dysfunction are overall identical.

Table 8.12 Instrumental tests for diagnosis of vegetative dysmotility of the GI system

First-line testing
Esophagogastroduodenoscopy; Anoscopy/colonoscopy; colon-CT; X-ray barium enema
Further insights
(a) Radiological tests (X-ray video-Fluoroscopy; Scintigraphic gastric emptying; intestinal transit time study; Defecography or defeco-MRI)
(b) Functional/metabolic tests (high-resolution esophageal, gastroduodenal, anorectal manometry; balloon expulsion test; wireless motility capsule; Fibrolaryngoscopy)
(c) Hydrogen and methane breath test

Diagnosis involves exclusion of primarily gastro-enterological disease; then, identification of neurologic disease and its distribution; and documentation of segmental bowel dysfunction, usually using noninvasive imaging, transit measurements, or intraluminal measurements of pressor activity and motility coordination.

In patients with moderate symptoms without any warning symptoms, noninvasive motility testing should be considered in the first instance. Otherwise, however, digestive endoscopy is one of the most widely used methods to which the patient should be referred immediately. This technique is both diagnostic and therapeutic, useful for the study of many gastroenterological pathologies, as it allows not only a direct view, from the inside, of certain organs but also allows histologic typing or/and removal of lesions by biopsy or endoscopic operative techniques (e.g., polypectomy) (Table 8.12).

8.10 Laboratory and Instrumental Tests for the Diagnosis of Dysmotility of the Gastrointestinal System: First-Line Testing

This group of tests is indicated to rule out organic pathologies. The symptoms of GI motor disorders are nonspecific, and dysmotility cannot be differentiated from organic pathology on the basis of the patient's history alone. For example, epigastric pain, early satiety, and abdominal fullness are typical symptoms of gastroparesis but may also be due to gastroduodenal ulcers or gastric cancer. Therefore, it is important to first rule out other etiologies, especially mucosal and obstructive lesions, by appropriate investigations such as upper and lower gastrointestinal endoscopy, imaging techniques, and laboratory investigations. Such tests are mandatory in patients with warning symptoms (i.e., age, low hemoglobin levels, weight or blood loss, consistent episodes of vomiting, recent onset constipation).

First-line testing***:*** ***Virtual colonoscopy*** is a simple low-dose x-ray CT scan. The anatomical data acquired in a few seconds with the CT scan are then processed by specific software, which reconstructs the bowel virtually and three-dimensionally on the screen, allowing "navigation" within it, but also visualizing the thickness of the colon wall and other organs.

Table 8.13 First-line test to disprove GI organic pathologies

	Esophagogastroduodenoscopy EGDS	Colonoscopy/ anoscopy	COLON-CT	Double-contrast opaque enema
Evaluated bodies	Esophagus stomach duodenum	Anus-rectum, colon, terminal ileum	Colon	Colon
Biopsies	Yes	Yes	NO	NO
Operating procedures	Yes	Yes	NO	NO
RX	NO	NO	Yes	Yes
Preparation	Yes	Yes	Yes	Yes

First-line testing*: Double-contrast opaque schism* is a technique that is now rarely performed because it has been replaced by colonoscopy and virtual colonoscopy. It is an x-ray of the colon and rectum performed by using first a suspension of water and barium introduced rectally and then air, which allows the structure of the organ in which it is placed, i.e., the colon in toto, to be visible on x-rays. It is indicated in suspicion of an abnormality in the rectum or colon, or in cases of irregular bowel function (sudden onset of constipation even alternating with diarrhea). It may show neoplasms and diverticula (small extroversions of the intestinal wall) and mucosal changes (Table 8.13).

8.11 Laboratory and Instrumental Tests for the Diagnosis of Dysmotility of the Gastrointestinal System: Further Investigation

Radiological tests are indicated to assess swallowing dynamics, morphology of the esophagus and esophago-gastric junction, to measure gastric and gastrointestinal emptying time, to morpho-functionally evaluate all pelvic floor structures and study their dysfunction underlying symptoms. Functional/metabolic tests are useful to assess the motor activity and sensitivity of the GI system. Finally, a niche examination, Breath tests are tests that through exhaled breath provide reliable indications of various diseases, such as lactose intolerance, bacterial contamination, malabsorption.

Radiological tests. X-ray videofluoroscopy (or radiologic study of swallowing or morphodynamic Rx of swallowing) is a radiologic investigation, indicated in cases of dysphagia, which is minimally invasive, well-tolerated, easily performed, lasting only a few minutes and with minimal radiologic exposure. It allows, by video recording, to accurately study the entire dynamics of the complex mechanism of swallowing, esophageal motility, the presence of endoluminal pathology, and the position of the gastroesophageal junction. It is also of great help in identifying the most useful rehabilitation techniques for the purpose of improving swallowing efficiency and reducing the risk of aspiration. The test allows precise correlation between pressure events (esophageal contractions) and the actual propagation of the radio-opaque bolus from the oral cavity to the pharynx, esophagus and, through the cardia, to the stomach. It can be performed with boluses of various sizes and nature (liquid or solid). The technique in recent years has evolved a great deal thanks in part to the recent introduction of digital elements that make it possible to acquire, using minimal doses of radiation the entire investigation, from the introduction of the meal into the oral cavity to the passage of the bolus into the stomach and the first loops of the mesenterial tenuous, with dynamic reconstructions of up to 15 images per second.

Scintigraphic gastric emptying; it is indicated in patients with early satiety, nausea, vomiting, regurgitation, bloating, postprandial fullness, visible upper abdominal distension, abdominal pain and weight loss, in whom a risk factor such as long-standing diabetes mellitus has been identified, in suspected gastroparesis and in all cases in which objective evidence of delayed gastric emptying is required. Scintigraphy is the gold standard for measuring gastric emptying: it involves the use of harmless radioactive materials administered with a meal or beverage or intravenously. Radiation emitted by the radiopharmaceutical (99mTc-Nanocolloid) is detected by the gamma chamber and transformed into images. Alternatively, 13C gastric emptying breath tests can be used [52].

Several substrates including octanoic acid (medium chain fatty acid) and Spirulina platensis (edible seaweed) are labeled with a stable carbon (nonradioactive-13C) Unclear and subsequently incorporated into the solid component of low-calorie meals. After transiting the stomach, these are digested and absorbed in the proximal small intestine and metabolized by the liver so that 13C is excreted from the lungs and its increase from baseline in breath samples can be measured by mass spectrometry. Thus, alterations in the 13C:12C ratio in breath samples collected at multiple postprandial time points reflect gastric emptying. Given the strong correlation with scintigraphy obtained simultaneously, the 13C spirulina technique has been approved by the U.S. Food and Drug Administration (FDA). It is a noninvasive, repeatable, simple and relatively inexpensive technique and can be centralized. The main limitations are artifacts in patients with intestinal malabsorption and liver or lung disease.

8.12 Laboratory and Instrumental Tests for the Diagnosis of Dysmotility of the Gastrointestinal System: Other Diagnostic Options in Highly Specialized Centers

8.12.1 Two/Three-Dimensional Transabdominal Ultrasound

Intestinal Transit Time Study, measures the rate at which fecal waste moves in the colon by monitoring intestinal progression of radiopaque markers administered p.o. (20 markers × 3 days every 24 h) with direct Rx of the abdomen [53]. The patient, after having had a spontaneous or provoked evacuation (in this case preferably by enema) 24–36 h before the start of the investigation and maintaining usual eating habits, should take during breakfast 20 radiopaque markers (1 sachet), at 9 a.m. for 3 consecutive days. Each day, the indicators will have a different form. On day 4 and, if necessary, on days 7 and 10, the patient will undergo a direct examination of the abdomen, in postero-anterior projection, on large-format film (35 × 43), taking care to include in the radiograms the entire pelvic excavation (including the pubic symphysis) and the two colic flexures. A radiogram in lateral projection (on 24x39 film) will be performed, including sacrum and coccyx, where the indicators reach the pelvic excavation. The day and time of any evacuations should be reported on a sheet throughout the investigation. Once the radiograms have been taken, a line passing through the vertebral spinous apophysis on the P-A radiogram and one perpendicular to the sacrum, passing through the S1-S2 intervertebral space on the lateral radiogram, should be drawn so as to roughly distinguish right colon (CD: cecum, ascending and mid-transverse) from left colon (CS: left mid-transverse, descending and sigma) and rectum (Re). Then it will be necessary to count and report the number of radiopaque indicators of each type present in the CD, CS and Re, respectively. Data analysis: (i) the parameters considered are total oro-anal transit time, which is equal to the evacuation time of 80% of the indicators administered (of at least one type); (ii) normal values in adults <96 h, children <33 h; (iii) segmental transit of the CD, CS and Re is assessed by the transit index, which is the average percentage of indicators cleared daily from each segment considered; normal values are in adults CD < 82, CS < 62, Re < 64, children < 60 for all segments.

Defecography and Defeco-RMN, are indicated for the diagnosis of organic and functional pelvic floor pathology. Defecography is the radiologic study that simulates defecation, allowing its pathophysiology to be studied and related disorders to be highlighted by video recording of evacuation after rectal filling with barium. It allows visualization of the pelvic floor and wall of the rectum in both basal and dynamic conditions and the detection of functional and anatomical changes that are only evident during evacuation effort. Rx of the pelvis in lateral projection: at rest, in contraction, in ponzation, and during evacuation. Defeco RMN: Allows morphological evaluation with simultaneous study of various segments of the pelvis and soft tissues in both static and dynamic.

8.13 Laboratory and Instrumental Tests for the Diagnosis of Dysmotility of the Gastrointestinal System: Subsequent Insights Functional/Metabolic Testing

High-resolution esophageal manometry, allows the motility of the esophagus and upper and lower esophageal sphincter to be studied by introducing a catheter into the viscera that can measure pressure changes occurring in the lumen of the organ. It is indicated in the presence of nonorganic dysphagia, non-cardiac chest pain, GERD, systemic diseases (collagenopathies, amyloidosis, diabetes, etc.).

High-resolution esophageal manometry represents an advancement of the classic technique to study the muscular function of the esophagus: the probe incorporates up to 36 sensors, which allow the entire esophagus to be scanned from the pharynx to the stomach and allow precise measurement of pressure, esophageal peristalsis, and upper and lower esophageal sphincter activity. The examination is performed by introducing, through the nostril a flexible nasogastric tube about 5 mm in diameter. The patient will be lying down and will have to swallow water or solids when required. The investigation takes 20 min. This procedure is considered safe.

High-resolution gastroduodenal manometry is an invasive and expensive technique, but it provides important information about the frequency and strength of antral and proximal bowel contractions, antra-duodenal coordination, and the presence or absence of stage III MMC. It is performed only in specialized centers dedicated to research.

High-resolution anorectal manometry is a method that can provide important data on the physiology and pathology of the defecatory act. It studies the prevailing pressures in the rectum and anal canal at rest, during stimulation and dynamic testing, gives information on anorectal function expendable in clinical practice, for diagnostic, evaluative and therapeutic-rehabilitative purposes. It also assesses rectal sensitivity. It is commonly used in cases of fecal incontinence, difficulty evacuating, anal fissure, rectal prolapse, hemorrhoids, or rectal pain. Currently, high-resolution manometry allows measurement and analysis of the pressure activity of the rectum and anal sphincter with a single placement of a catheter and allows reconstruction of the anal canal through the 36-point recorder readings that ensure optimal diagnostic accuracy. Technique of execution: a tube of about 5 mm in diameter is introduced into the rectum for about 10 cm after evacuation enemas. The patient will be lying on the left side, with thighs overlapping and flexed on the trunk at 90°. The investigation takes 20–30 min. It has virtually no complications or contraindications.

The balloon expulsion test is to assess expulsive capacity in suspected abdominopelvic dyssynergy. This test is not a standardized method, but it is part of the tests indicated by the guidelines to be performed in cases of defecatory difficulty. The method is simple and inexpensive; it is performed by filling a rectal balloon with 50 ml of warm water, sitting the patient on the sanitary vessel, or a comfortable one, and recording the time of expulsion, which must be less than 2 min.

The Wireless Motility Capsule (WMC) is a noninvasive technique to indirectly measure gastric emptying and intestinal transit times. Once ingested, the capsule records pH, pressure, and temperature signals that are analyzed by an external receiver. This smart pill has the limitation that, being a large indigestible solid, even when ingested with a test meal, it does not reflect the emptying of its calorically digestible components as it is eliminated separately during the fasting state. However, it does allow the assessment of global transit abnormalities that may be useful in the evaluation and management of comorbidities, such as constipation, that are associated with gastroparesis [54]. In studies conducted, WMC has enabled correct diagnosis in more than 50% of patients with suspected gastroparesis (or slow intestinal transit). In a recent study WMC detected delayed gastric emptying in 10% more individuals and in almost twice as many diabetics as scintigraphy [55].

Fiberoptic Endoscopic Evaluation of Swallowing (FEES), is an additional instrumental examination for the study of vegetative gastrointestinal dysfunction dysphagia, also called functional dyspepsia [56]. It has the advantage of being a well-tolerated, modestly invasive outpatient procedure that can be performed even in uncooperative patients.

The main goals of FEES are to identify the oropharyngeal swallowing deficits underlying neurogenic dysphagia, to evaluate the efficacy and safety of oral feed ing, to identify rehabilitative and adaptive therapeutic maneuvers, along with the most appropriate food consistencies and postural strategies for the individual patient. FEES also makes it possible to detect indirect signs of esophageal dysphagia such as post-deglutition reflux that can occur because of GI autonomic dysfunction; by allowing to examine of the entire intake of a meal in real time, it also enables the detection of swallowing muscle fatigue with late esophageal regurgitation [57].

The method therefore allows for a complete evaluative picture of the larynx and pharynx morphology, motility, and functions [58]. It follows that the evaluation of pharyngeal stagnations, in relation to their location, extent, management, degree of penetration and aspiration into the larynx, is particularly indicated in pathologies such as PD and Parkinsonism, where the differential diagnosis between oropharyngeal dysphagia and indirect pharyngeal phase impairment due to gastropharyngeal-laryngeal reflux from related esophageal autonomic dysfunction, both of which are present but not always simultaneously, is necessary because of the different therapeutic approach that ensues (Box 8.6).

Box 8.6: FEES in the Evaluation of the Patient with Vegetative Dysphagia

FEES in the evaluation of the patient with v dysphagia allows for an evaluation of GERD, an extremely common pathology characterized by typical symptoms (heartburn and regurgitation) and influenced by diet, stress, and lifestyle, and which, due to the alterations induced on the pharyngolaryngeal mucosa, simulates pharyngeal deglutition alterations that are actually absent.

This type of reflux always originates from the stomach and, due to incompetence of the upper esophageal sphincter (SES), is able to reach the mucosa of the larynx and pharynx [59]. These structures are extremely sensitive to gastric juice, so inflammation sets in very rapidly for even minute amounts of refluxed material, resulting in the symptoms described earlier.

The atypical symptomatology of GERD is represented by dry, hacking cough; pharyngeal foreign body sensation (throat knot); difficulty swallowing saliva; mucous stagnation sensation; hoarseness or voice disturbance; need to have to clear the voice frequently; dry mouth and throat; and sore and burning throat. The above symptoms always require consultation by an Otolaryngologist or Phoniatrician, whose history and clinical evaluation should be complemented by fibroendoscopy with swallowing tests.

At FEES signs suggestive of gastroesophageal reflux are hyperemia of the mucosa of the arytenoid cartilages, inter-aritenoid mucosa, true vocal cords, tracheal mucosa; inter-aritenoid pachydermia; ulcers of the mucosa of the arytenoid cartilages, inter-aritenoid mucosa; laryngeal granulomas; of the mucosa of the arytenoid cartilages, inter-aritenoid mucosa. However, the swallowing act both spontaneous and on demand of saliva and food, appears normal.

However, the significance of endoscopic exploration in subjects with vegetative dysfunction is also to avert the presence of swallowing deficits that could give rise to the same symptoms (i.e., aspiration cough in the dysphagic oropharyngeal subject) of different prognostic impact as well as a therapeutic approach.

In the GI dysfunction of patients with Parkinsonism, FEES can detect characteristic dysphagia signs such as predeglutory dropping, bolus fragmentation, stagnation in the glossoepiglottic vallecula and piriform sinus, delayed pharyngeal phase initiation, and deficits in laryngeal movement, bolus penetration (when it reaches the vocal cords), and aspiration (when the bolus passes the true vocal cords). The extent, location, and management of stagnation influence the risk of penetration and aspiration [60].

Being able to assess numerous swallowing acts and detect altered swallowing parameters even in patients at an unadvanced stage of disease, FEES is a highly sensitive method that also allows early diagnosis of asymptomatic dysphagia [61]. In addition to the standard FEES protocol, specific testing protocols have been developed and validated for various neurogenic disorders; the FEES-L-Dopa-Test is for the evaluation of L-Dopa-sensitive dysphagia in patients with Parkinson's syndrome [62].

Several useful scales are also available for quantifying salient endoscopic findings such as the Aspiration and Penetration Scale (PAS), according to Rosenbek [63], the Yale Residual Scale [64], and the Secretion Severity Scale [60].

8.14 Laboratory and Instrumental Tests for the Diagnosis of Dysmotility of the Gastrointestinal System: Ultra-Specialty Evaluation

Hydrogen breath test (H2-breath test) and respiratory methane test are used for the study of bacterial contamination of the small intestine and for the diagnosis of malabsorption of certain sugars (lactose, sorbitol, glucose). In case of bloating, distension, alterations in alvus. They also provide important data on intestinal transit times. They are noninvasive, easy to perform, and excellently tolerated by patients. They are based on the failure of the intestinal mucosa to absorb certain sugars, resulting in the production of hydrogen (H2) and methane (CH4), which are found in the exhaled air [65].

8.15 Suggestions for the Management of Gastro-Enteric Failure

Functional dyspepsia, as an expression of intestinal dysmotility, is a clinical problem that is not easy to treat because the available drugs are often ineffective; moreover, to the little benefit adduced, one can add the side effects inherent in any therapy.

Some relevant GI autonomic dysfunctions benefit from treatment with resolution of the problem or, at least, management of the disorders determined by the underlying disease. Thus, in addition to treatment of the underlying neurological disease, management focuses mainly on restoration of normal hydration and nutrition and pharmacological treatment of GI neuromuscular deficit. The main autonomic dysfunction syndromes with recalls of pathogenesis and diagnostic-therapeutic suggestions are presented in Table 8.14 [2].

Table 8.14 Visceral dysfunctional syndromes: reminders of pathogenesis and diagnostic-therapeutic suggestions

Clinical presentation	Neurological mechanism	Diagnosis/assessment	Management
Oropharyngeal dysphagia	Pharyngeal skeletal muscles; lower motor neuron (i.e., bulbar polio or pseudobulbar palsy) or muscle (e.g., ALS, myasthenia gravis)	**Physical exam:** Dentition, movement of the uvula (IX and X cranial nerves) Jaw snap **Instrumental examination:** Video fluoroscopy; HR esophageal manometry; FEES	Nutritional support Prevention of pulmonary aspiration
Thoracic dysphagia, GERD	Vagal denervation Or smooth muscle disease	**Instrumental examination:** Video fluoroscopy; FEES; HR esophageal manometry; PH impedancemetry of the 24 h	PPI Prokinetics Antacids

(continued)

Table 8.14 (continued)

Clinical presentation	Neurological mechanism	Diagnosis/assessment	Management
Dyspepsia nausea-vomiting (gastroparesis)	Vagal, myenteric denervation; Drug iatrogenic (narcotics, GLP-1 agonists)	**Instrumental examination:** Gastric emptying test (scintigraphy/GEBT) GD manometry Self-tests	Hydration and nutrition support Prokinetic therapy and antiemetics in refractory patients pyloromyotomy feeding PEG nasogastric tube
Abdominal pain, distension/satiety, nausea/vomiting, diarrhea and/or intractable constipation, malabsorption (chronic intestinal pseudo-obstruction)	I wander Myenteric denervation Drug iatrogens (narcotics, GLP-1 agonists)	**Physical exam:** EO abdomen; E.R EMG (myopathy/neuropathy) **Instrumental examination:** Gastric emptying test (scintigraphy/GEBT) GD manometry EMG (myopathy/neuropathy)	Prokinetics for gastroparesis + enteral or parenteral nutrition Treating small intestinal bacterial overgrowth related to myopathic disease small intestine transplant
Constipation	Vagal or sacral parasympathetic Myenteric denervation	**Physical exam:** EO abdomen; E.R Associated neuropathy or spinal disease **Instrumental examination:** HR anorectal manometry with balloon expulsion Colon transit times Vedi note del testo	Diet Osmotic laxatives Secretory or prokinetic Pelvic floor rehabilitation TAI (transanal irrigation) Rarely colectomy or colostomy
Fecal incontinence	Pelvic nerves Sacred roots Cauda equina and spinal cord injury, pelvic floor and anal sphincters	**Physical exam:** Rectal exploration **Instrumental examination:** HR anorectal manometry EMG (myopathy/neuropathy)	Medicines Diet Pelvic floor rehabilitation Hygiene and skin care TAI Sphincter reconstruction and rarely colostomy or ileostomy

Table 8.14 (continued)

Clinical presentation	Neurological mechanism	Diagnosis/assessment	Management
Passive diarrhea/ incontinence	Loss of sympathetic inhibitory control (may manifest with bowel motor activity, including diarrhea)	**Physical exam:** Abdomen exam Rectal exploration **Instrumental examination:** Chemical/physical and cultural and parasitological examination of feces Laboratory tests (i.e., celiac disease, pancreatic enzymes, dysthyroidism) Colonoscopy with ileoscopy + esophagoduodenoscopy with biopsy Anorectal manometry	Medicines Diet Pelvic floor rehabilitation Hygiene and skin care TAI Sphincter reconstruction and rarely colostomy or ileostomy

ALS amyotrophic lateral sclerosis, *EO* objective examination, *ER* digital rectal exploration, *GD* gastroduodenal, *GEBT* gastric emptying with breath test, *GERD* gastroesophageal reflux disease, *HR MAR* high-resolution anorectal manometry, *PEG* percutaneous endoscopic gastrostomy

In the absence of protocols validated through randomized, controlled trials, research has turned toward the study and evaluation of para pharmaceuticals capable of modifying GI activity; today a wide range of dietary supplements based on nutrients or other substances with a "physiological" effect (e.g., plant extracts and preparations) are also available; as well as other "natural" products (Table 8.15). These are to date widely consumed in the population and aimed at seeking health and wellness benefits [66].

Although in the body, the main responsible for the contractility of gastrointestinal muscles, as already mentioned, is acetylcholine, most prokinetic drugs act at higher levels than it itself is released, resulting in important systemic side effects that limit the use of cholinergic agonists. For the treatment of all propulsive-type motor disturbances of the gastrointestinal tract, to stimulate motility of both stomach and intestines, in cases of GERD, dyspepsia, nausea, vomiting, and constipation from slowed transit, prokinetics capable of more selectively coordinating contractile activity and transit of intestinal contents are currently used. Those mainly involved are dopaminergic (D2) subtype, serotonergic (5-HT3 and 5-HT4), muscarinic-type cholinergic and motilin receptors.

Prokinetic drugs that act on dopaminergic receptors block the effects of dopamine, which normally reduce motility in the gastrointestinal tract. Their activity results in increased motility and reduced nausea and vomiting, the latter mechanism mediated by activity on dopaminergic receptors centrally. The activity on serotonergic receptors is agonist, which causes stimulation of peristalsis and gastric emptying.

Table 8.15 Parapharmaceutical drugs capable of modifying GI activity

Symptom	Active ingredient	Action
Gerd-dyspepsia	Iberis Amara, Matricaria chamomilla Carum carvi, Mentha piperita Glycyrrhiza glabra Melissa officinalis Chelidonium majus Silybum marianum Angelica archangelica, Perilla, ginger, melatonin, alginate, pectin carbenoxolone	Mucoprotective effects Prokinetic effects Anti-inflammatory effects Enzymatic effects
Nausea-vomiting	Ginger Vitamina B6 Perilla	– Prokinetic effect at the gastroduodenal level – Essential for the synthesis of serotonin – Prokinetic and anti-inflammatory effects
Diarrhea	Probiotics Diosmectide Psillium/guar gum Berberine	– They colonize the intestine and compete with pathogens (bacteria, viruses and protozoa) responsible for acute and/or chronic diarrhea (secretory/inflammatory) – Clay that covers the mucous membrane and protects it by increasing the resistance of the mucus and binding to pathogens, bacteria, viruses and toxins. – Mass forming – Antimicrobial, eubiotic and intestinal antisecretive actions; reduces intestinal motility
Constipation	Senna cascara aloe Lactulose Psyllium	– Anthraquinone laxatives – Osmotic laxative – Mass forming
Bloating	Probiotics Charcoal	They compete with the methanogenic microbiota The porosity is exploited to trap substances and gases in order to avoid their absorption or accumulation in the digestive system

GERD gastroesophageal reflux disease

Serotonin is important for both motor and secretory functions of the gastrointestinal tract, so it is found in high concentrations. Activity on muscarinic receptors stimulates smooth muscle contraction, so there is increased motility. Finally, motilin is a hormone that promotes the flow of intestinal contents, as it acts by stimulating the release of acetylcholine. Metoclopramide reduces nausea and vomiting, often in cases from chemotherapy therapies, by facilitating gastric emptying; it can be administered either orally or parenterally. Domperidone has a more specific action on D2 receptors at the gastric level unlike Metoclopramide, increasing gastric emptying.

It can also be used in the treatment of acid reflux in children. Second-generation prokinetics include those that act on serotonergic receptors (Cisapride, Renzapride, and Zacopride). Finally, third-generation ones include Prucalopride and the antibiotic Erythromycin. The latter owes its effect to its agonist action on motilin receptors. Third-generation drugs do not act on dopaminergic receptors and therefore lack the antiemetic effect and related adverse reactions.

Regardless of the mechanism of action, among the most widely used prokinetics are Betanechol; Neostigmine; Levosulpiride; Linaclotide; Domperidone; Bromopride; Metoclopramide.

8.16 Conclusion

The relationship between the nervous system and the digestive system is also ensured by the ANS. Extrinsic GI autonomic dysfunction can complicate the course of various vegetative nervous system disorders; recognizing and treating autonomic disorder is important. Autonomic dysfunction of other body districts (e.g., cardio autonomic disorders with reduced heart rate variability, arrhythmias, increased blood pressure variability, and neurogenic orthostatic hypotension), moreover, is associated with increased morbidity and mortality.

The activity of the GI system is promoted from the periphery and has a complex and peculiar peripheral control system through the ENS; this has a high degree of independence from the CNS. In GI disorders in the course of neurological disease, multidisciplinary management with the gastroenterologist is advisable. GI motility dysfunction is a varied and frequent disorder in both gastroenterology and neurology, although often underdiagnosed by neurologists. GI autonomic dysfunction may be driven by an ANS deficiency. Excluding other non-ANS pathologies, the mode of onset of GI autonomic disorders, its expression, and clinical progression can be helpful in the diagnosis and management of GI disorder; it can sometimes present in slowly progressive subtle ways, as when autonomic dysfunction may be the first sign of an underlying paraneoplastic condition.

The tempestive recognition of GI dysfunction is important to provide early administration of treatments which, however, are currently limited, as well as to allow prevention of GI complications in the course of neurological disease. Finally, autonomic tests support monitoring the course of autonomic disorders and the treatment response, even if specific GI tests should be performed in a multidisciplinary program with the support of gastroenterological experts.

References

1. Spencer NJ, Hu H. Enteric nervous system: sensory transduction, neural circuits and gastrointestinal motility. Nat Rev Gastroenterol Hepatol. 2020;17(6):338–51.
2. Camilleri M. Gastrointestinal motility disorders in neurologic disease. Clin Invest. 2021;131(4):e143771.
3. Kornum S, Terkelsen AJ, Bertoli D, Klinge MW, Høyer KL, Kufaishi HHA, Borghammer P, Drewes AM, Brock C, Krogh K. Assessment of gastrointestinal autonomic dysfunction: present and future perspectives Ditte. J Clin Med. 2021;10:1392.
4. Browning KN, Travagli RA. Central nervous system control of gastrointestinal motility and secretion and modulation of gastrointestinal functions. Compr Physiol. 2014;4(4):1339–68.
5. Silverthorn DU. Human physiology. San Francisco, CA: Pearson Education, Inc.; 2007. p. 94111.
6. Lychkova AE. Serotonin regulation of motor function of the small intestine. Eksp Klin Gastroenterol. 2011;3:130–5.
7. Deloose E, Janssen P, Depoortere I, Tack J. The migrating motor complex: control mechanisms and its role in health and disease. Nat Rev Gastroenterol Hepatol. 2012;9(5):271–85.
8. Chu S, Schubert ML. Gastric secretion. Curr Opin Gastroenterol. 2013;29:636–41.
9. Di Mario F, Goni E. Gastric acid secretion: changes during a century. Best Pract Res Clin Gastroenterol. 2014;28:953–65.
10. Huizinga JD, Chen JH. The myogenic and neurogenic components of the rhythmic segmentation motor patterns of the intestine. Front Neurosci. 2014;8(78):1–3.
11. Track NS. The gastrointestinal endocrine system. Can Med Assoc J. 1980;122(3):287–92.
12. Andersson-Rolf A, Clevers H, Dayton TL. Diffuse hormonal systems. 2021. In: Feingold KR, Anawalt B, Boyce A, Chrousos G, de Herder WW, Dhatariya K, Dungan K, Hershman JM, Hofland J, Kalra S, Kaltsas G, Koch C, Kopp P, Korbonits M, Kovacs CS, Kuohung W, Laferrère B, Levy M, McGee EA, McLachlan R, Morley JE, New M, Purnell J, Sahay R, Singer F, Sperling MA, Stratakis CA, Trence DL, Wilson DP, editors. Endotext [Internet]. South Dartmouth, MA: MDText.com, Inc.; 2000.
13. Heiss Christina N, Olofsson LE. The role of the gut microbiota in development, function and disorders of the central nervous system and the enteric nervous system. J Neuroendocrinol. 2019;31(5):e12684.
14. Rouphael C, Arora Z, Thota PN, Lopez R, Santisi J, Funk C, Cline M. Role of wireless motility capsule in the assessment and management of gastrointestinal dysmotility in patients with diabetes mellitus. Neurogastroenterol Motil. 2017;29(9)
15. Collins SM. The immunomodulation of enteric neuromuscular function: implications for motility and inflammatory disorders. Gastroenterology. 1996;111(6):1683–99.
16. Redondo-Useros EN, González-Zancada N, Díaz LE, Gómez-Martínez S, Marcos A. Microbiota and lifestyle: A special focus on diet. Nutrients. 2020;12(6):1776.
17. Schmulson MJ, Drossman DA. What is new in Rome IV. J Neurogastroenterol Motil. 2017;23(2):151–63.
18. Drossman DA, Hasler WL. Rome IV-functional GI disorders: disorders of gut-brain interaction. Gastroenterology. 2016;150(6):1257–61.
19. Stanghellini V, Chan FKL, Hasler WL. Gastroduodenal disorders. Gastroenterology. 2016;150:1380–92.
20. Triggs J, Pandolfino J. Recent advances in dysphagia management. F1000Res. 2019;29(8):Faculty Rev-1527.
21. Pfeiffer RF. Gastrointestinal dysfunction in Parkinson's disease. Curr Treat Options Neurol. 2018;20(12):54.
22. Westfal ML, Goldstein AM. Pediatric enteric neuropathies: diagnosis and current management. Curr Opin Pediatr. 2017;29(3):347–53.

23. Jaglal SB, Munce SEP, Guilcher SJ, Couris CM, Fung K, Craven BC, Verrier M. Health system factors associated with rehospitalizations after traumatic spinal cord injury: a population-based study. Spinal Cord. 2009;47:604–9.
24. Coggrave M, Norton C, Cody JD. Management of incontinence and constipation in adults with central neurological diseases. Cochrane Database Syst Rev. 2014;(1):CD002115.
25. Kuric J, Lucas CE, Ledgerwood AM, Kiraly A, Salciccioli GG, Sugawa C. Nutritional support: a prophylaxis against stress bleeding after spinal cord injury. Paraplegia. 1989;27(2):140–5.
26. Posillico SE, Golob JF, Rinker AD, Kreiner LA, West RS, Conrad-Schnetz KJ, Kelly ML, Claridge JA. Bedside dysphagia screens in patients with traumatic cervical injuries: an ideal tool for an under-recognized problem. J Trauma Acute Care Surg. 2018;85(4):697–703.
27. Wheeler TL, de Groat W, Eisner K, Emmanuel A, French J, Grill W, Kennelly MJ, Krassioukov A, Gallo Santacruz B, Biering-Sørensen F, Kleitman N, Bowel and Bladder Workshop Participants. Translating promising strategies for bowel and bladder management in spinal cord injury. Exp Neurol. 2018;306:169–76.
28. Holmes GM, Blanke EN. Gastrointestinal dysfunction after spinal cord injury. Exp Neurol. 2019;320:113009.
29. Johnston JR, Freeman KG, Edwards GL. Activity in nodose ganglia neurons after treatment with CP 55,940 and cholecystokinin. Physiol Rep. 2018;6(23):e13927.
30. Racosta JM. Autonomic nervous system dysfunction and fatigue in multiple sclerosis: common pathophysiology or spurious association? Clin Auton Res. 2019;29(3):261–2.
31. Flachenecker P, Rufer A, Bihler I, Hippel C, Reiners K, Toyka KV, Kesselring J. Fatigue in MS is related to sympathetic vasomotor dysfunction. Neurology. 2003;61(6):851–3.
32. Habek M, Krbot SM. Autonomic nervous system: a key player in prodromal multiple sclerosis? Clin Auton Res. 2020;30(2):97–9.
33. Cosentino M, Marino F. Adrenergic and dopaminergic modulation of immunity in multiple sclerosis: teaching old drugs new tricks? J Neuroimmune Pharmacol. 2013;8(1):163–79.
34. Habek M. Immune and autonomic nervous system interactions in multiple sclerosis: clinical implications. Clin Auton Res. 2019;29(3):267–75.
35. Bergamaschi R, Crivelli P, Rezzani C, Patti F, Solaro C, Rossi P, Restivo D, Maimone D, Romani A, Bastianello S, Tavazzi E, D'Amico E, Montomoli C, Cosi V. The DYMUS questionnaire for the assessment of dysphagia in multiple sclerosis. J Neurol Sci. 2008;269(1–2):49–53.
36. Marchese-Ragona R, Restivo DA, Marioni G, Ottaviano G, Masiero S, Staffieri A. Evaluation of swallowing disorders in multiple sclerosis. Neurol Sci. 2006;27:S335–7.
37. Calcagno P, Ruoppolo G, Grasso MG, De Vincentiis M, Paolucci S. Dysphagia in multiple sclerosis prevalence and prognostic factors. Acta Neurol Scand. 2002;105(1):40–3.
38. Ekberg O, Hamdy S, Woisard V, Wuttge-Hannig A, Ortega P. Social and psychological burden of dysphagia: its impact on diagnosis and treatment. Dysphagia. 2002;17(2):139–46.
39. Poorjavad M, Derakhshandeh F, Etemadifar M, Soleymani B, Minagar A, Maghzi AH. Oropharyngeal dysphagia in multiple sclerosis. Mult Scler. 2010;16(3):362–5.
40. Johns JS, Krogh K, Ethans K, Chi J, Querée M, Eng JJ. Spinal cord injury research evidence team. Pharmacological management of neurogenic bowel dysfunction after spinal cord injury and multiple sclerosis: A systematic review and clinical implications. J Clin Med. 2021;10(4):882.
41. Preziosi G, Gordon-Dixon A, Emmanuel A. Neurogenic bowel dysfunction in patients with multiple sclerosis: prevalence, impact, and management strategies. Degener Neurol Neuromuscul Dis. 2018;6(8):79–90.
42. Dziadkowiec KN, Stawinski P, Radadiya D, Al Abbasi B, Shaun I. Is multiple sclerosis an extra-intestinal manifestation of inflammatory bowel disease? Food for Thought Cureus. 2020;12(7):e9485.
43. Alkhawajah MM, Caminero AB, Freeman HJ, Oger JJF. Multiple sclerosis and inflammatory bowel diseases: what we know and what we would need to know! Multiple Scler J. 2013;19:259–65.

44. Singh S, Kumar N, Loftus EV Jr, Kane SV. Neurologic complications in patients with inflammatory bowel disease: increasing relevance in the era of biologics. Inflamm Bowel Dis. 2013;19:864–72.
45. Naismith RT, Wundes A, Ziemssen T, Jasinska E, Freedman MS, Lembo AJ, Selmaj K, Bidollari I, Chen H, Hanna J, Leigh-Pemberton R, Lopez-Bresnahan M, Lyons J, Miller C, Rezendes D, Wolinsky JS, EVOLVE-MS-2 Study Group. Diroximel fumarate demonstrates an improved gastrointestinal tolerability profile compared with dimethyl fumarate in patients with relapsing–remitting multiple sclerosis: results from the randomized, double-blind, phase III EVOLVE-MS-2 study. CNS Drugs. 2020;34(2):185–96.
46. Parkman HP, Hasler WL, Fisher RS, American Gastroenterological Association. American Gastroenterological Association medical position statement: diagnosis and treatment of gastroparesis. Gastroenterology. 2004;127(5):1589–91.
47. Simons JA, Fietzek UM, Waldmann A, Warnecke T, Schuster T, Ceballos-Baumann AO. Development and validation of a new screening questionnaire for dysphagia in early stages of Parkinson's disease. Parkinsonism Relat Disord. 2014;20(9):992–8.
48. Manor Y, Giladi N, Cohen A, Fliss D, Cohen T. Validation of a swallowing disturbance questionnaire for detecting dysphagia in patients with Parkinson's disease. Mov Disord. 2007;22(13):1917–21.
49. Camilleri M, Parkman HP, Shafi MA, Abell TL, Gerson L, American College of Gastroenterology. Clinical guideline: management of gastroparesis. Am J Gastroenterol. 2013;108(1):18–37.
50. Bytzer P, Talley NJ, Hammer J, Young LJ, Jones MP, Horowitz M. GI symptoms in diabetes mellitus are associated with both poor glycemic control and diabetic complications. Am J Gastroenterol. 2002;97(3):604–11.
51. Bytzer P, Talley NJ, Leemon M, Young LJ, Jones MP, Horowitz M. Prevalence of gastrointestinal symptoms associated with diabetes mellitus: a population-based survey of 15,000 adults. Arch Intern Med. 2001;161(16):1989–96.
52. Fox Mark R, Kahrilas Peter J, Sabine R, Gyawali CP, Mark SS, Rao Satish S, Jutta K, Camilleri M. Clinical measurement of gastrointestinal motility and function: who, when and which test? Nat Rev Gastroenterol Hepatol. 2018;15(9):568–79.
53. Metcalf AM, Phillips SF, Zinsmeister AR, Maccarty RL, Beart RW, Wolff BG. Simplified assessment of segmental colonic transit. Gastroenterology. 1987;92:40–7.
54. Grover M, Farrugia G, Stanghellini V. Gastroparesis: a turning point in understanding and treatment. Gut. 2019;8(12):2238–50.
55. Keller J, Bassotti G, Clarke J, Dinning P, Fox M, Grover M, Hellström PM, Ke M, Layer P, Malagelada C, Parkman HP, Scott SM, Tack J, Simren M, Törnblom H, Camilleri M. International working group for disorders of gastrointestinal motility and function. advances in the diagnosis and classification of gastric and intestinal motility disorders. Nat Rev Gastroenterol Hepatol. 2018;15(5):291–308.
56. Dziewas R, Allescher HD, Aroyo I, Bartolome G, Beilenhoff U, Bohlender J, Breitbach-Snowdon H, Fheodoroff K, Glahn J, Heppner HJ, Hörmann K, Ledl C, Lücking C, Pokieser P, Schefold JC, Schröter-Morasch H, Schweikert K, Sparing R, Trapl-Grundschober M, Wallesch C, Warnecke T, Werner CJ, Weßling J, Wirth R, Pflug C. Diagnosis and treatment of neurogenic dysphagia - S1 guideline of the German Society of Neurology. Neurol Res Pract. 2021;3(1):23.
57. Farneti D, Genovese E. Correlations between bedside and instrumental endoscopic parameters in determining severity of dysphagia: an integrated clinical evaluation of safety and efficiency. Acta Otorhinolaryngol Ital. 2020;40(4):277–81.
58. Schindler A, Baijens LWJ, Geneid A, Pizzorni N. Phoniatricians and otorhinolaryngologists approaching oropharyngeal dysphagia: an update on FEES. Eur Arch Otorhinolaryngol. 2021;15:1–16.
59. Poelmans J, Feenstra L, Demedts I, Rutgeerts P, Tack J. The yield of upper gastrointestinal endoscopy in patients with suspected reflux-related chronic ear, nose, and throat symptoms. Am J Gastroenterol. 2004;99:1419–26.

60. Murray J, Langmore SE, Ginsberg S, Dostie A. The significance of accumulated oropharyngeal secretions and swallowing frequency in predicting aspiration. Dysphagia. 1996;11:99–103.
61. Buhmann C. Pill swallowing in Parkinson's disease: a prospective study based on flexible endoscopic evaluation of swallowing. Parkinsonism Relat Disord. 2019;62:51–6.
62. Warneckeet T, Suttrup I, Schroder JB, Osada N, Oelenberg S, Hamacher C, Suntrup S, Dziewas R. Levodopa responsiveness of dysphagia in advanced Parkinson's disease and reliability testing of the FEES-levodopa-test. Parkinsonism Relat Disord. 2016;28:100–6.
63. Rosenbek JC, Robbins J, Roecker EB, Coyle JL, Wood JL. A penetration-aspiration scale. Dysphagia. 1996;11:93–8.
64. Neubauer PD, Rademaker AW, Leder SB. The yale pharyngeal residue severity rating scale: an anatomically defined and image-based tool. Dysphagia. 2015;30(5):521–8.
65. Paolo U-S, Oppia F, Lai M, Cabras F. Hydrogen breath tests: are they really useful in the nutritional management of digestive disease? Nutrients. 2021;13(3):974.
66. Dossett ML, Cohen EM, Cohen J. Integrative medicine for gastrointestinal disease. Prim Care. 2017;44(2):265–80.

Chapter 9
Autonomic Dysfunction in Sleep Disorders

Marco Bozzali, Raffaele Manni, Alberto Romagnolo, and Michele Terzaghi

9.1 Sleep and Autonomic Nervous System: Anatomo-Functional Correlates

The autonomic nervous system (ANS) is involved in the control of a wide range of bodily functions. Main ANS interactions include those with the cardiovascular system (i.e., heart rate, blood pressure), the gastroenteric tract (e.g., smooth muscle contraction, gland secretion), the neuroendocrine system, the nociceptive pathways, large neuronal networks subserving awareness and behavioural responses. Anatomically, the ANS consists of a number of structures that are connected to each other and distributed along the neural axis. These structures include several cortical areas whose main role is to regulate the whole ANS. Taken altogether, they are defined as the "Central Autonomic Network" (CAN), which consists of a set of hierarchically organised structures. Within the neural axis, the ANS is composed by the following structures: nuclei located in the medulla and in the inferior portion of the pons, whose main role is to mediate cardiovascular, breathing, gastrointestinal, and micturition reflexes; nuclei located in the superior part of the pons and

M. Bozzali (✉) · A. Romagnolo
'Rita Levi Montalcini' Department of Neuroscience, University of Torino, Turin, Italy

SC Neurologia 2U, AOU City of Health and Science, Turin, Italy
e-mail: marco.bozzali@unito.it; alberto.romagnolo@unito.it

R. Manni
Department of Brain and Behavioral Sciences, University of Pavia, Pavia, Italy
e-mail: raffaele.manni@mondino.it

M. Terzaghi
Department of Brain and Behavioral Sciences, University of Pavia, Pavia, Italy

Unit of Sleep Medicine and Epilepsy, IRCCS Istituto Mondino Foundation, Pavia, Italy
e-mail: michele.terzaghi@mondino.it

G. Micieli et al. (eds.), *Autonomic Disorders in Clinical Practice*,
https://doi.org/10.1007/978-3-031-43036-7_9

midbrain, which modulate nociceptive inputs, awareness and behavioural responses; the hypothalamus, which integrates autonomic, endocrine as well behavioural responses to environmental stimuli. The CAN includes the insular and anterior cingulate cortices, which regulate the autonomic function in response to emotional stimuli. This means that the ANS as a whole regulates a wide range of functions that operate in waking as well as in sleep state, with the final goal of maintaining homeostasis in conditions of reduced metabolic needs, and promoting adaptation mechanisms against environmental perturbations [1, 2].

Wakefulness and sleep represent two opposite conditions in terms of motor activity and environmental interaction. In sleeping state, the ANS activity exhibits profound changes of both types, tonic and phasic, in the framework of a dynamic interaction with the mechanisms of sleep regulation. Such a strict interaction is based on structural and functional mechanisms. Hierarchically, the hypothalamus is the most important ANS node for the control of sleeping cycles. Its nuclei regulate neuroendocrine responses, the control of internal body temperature, the sense of hunger and fulfilment, and the sleep-wake cycles. Autonomic neurons within the hypothalamus (i.e., lateral and periventricular nuclei) together with those from the cranial part of the brainstem are anatomically located near the ventrolateral preoptic nucleus of the thalamus, which is implicated in sleep regulation [3]. The autonomic neurons from the hypothalamus project to the spinal cord, thus contributing to vasoconstriction. They are also believed to play a cardinal role during sleep-related postural modifications by controlling changes of blood pressure and heart rate. Moreover, the suprachiasmatic nucleus of the hypothalamus projects to a set of hypothalamic nuclei that are implicated in autonomic functions (i.e., paraventricular nuclei) as well as in sleep regulation (ventrolateral preoptic area) [4, 5]. Interestingly, the suprachiasmatic nucleus is defined as "internal clock" for its prominent role in controlling circadian rhythms. It subserves the circadian control of the CAN [6] that, in turn, has dynamic interactions with the so-called sleep-generator neurons, which are located in the brainstem, diencephalon, and in cerebral cortex [7]. In the lateral part of the hypothalamus, there are neurons producing hypocretin, which are believed to play a stabilisation role in the wake-sleep switching by promoting the waking state. These neurons project specific structures of the ANS, including the periaqueductal grey formation, the nucleus of the solitary tract, the ambiguus nucleus, and the dorsal nucleus of the vagus nerve. In their capacity, they modulate various autonomic functions, such as blood pressure and heart rate regulation [8]. Acetylcholine and noradrenaline, which are the two principal neurotransmitters involved in autonomic functions, also play a regulation role in the wake-sleep cycles. Cholinergic projections from the pedunculopontine and the lateroposterior tegmental nuclei of the pons project to the thalamus and are implicated in promoting REM sleep. Conversely, noradrenergic neurons from the locus coeruleus are inhibited during both the non-REM phases of sleep and the tonic phases of REM sleep. Their activity increases during the phasic intervals of REM sleep. During physiological sleep, several autonomic modifications occur with sudden changes from a predominant parasympathetic to a predominant sympathetic tone. Parasympathetic tone is increased during the non-REM phases of sleep and, even more, during the REM phases. Conversely, the sympathetic tone is generally reduced in all these phases, and presents with peaks of activity during the phasic phases of REM sleep only [9, 10]. The autonomic tone that characterises the non-REM phases of sleep is associated with a homeostatic trend towards reduction of muscular activity and metabolism. These adjustments are mediated by baro- and chemo-reflexes, and by hypothalamic driven changes in internal body temperature. Due to parasympathetic effect, the heart rate and blood pressure get reduced in non-REM sleep, the muscular tone of vessels reduces (vasodilatation), the vagal tone and baroreflex sensitivity increase, and breathing frequency becomes more regular. These features indicate that non-REM sleep is a state of homeostatic stability and general recovery. In the transition between the different phases of sleep, sudden episodes of increased parasympathetic activity may occur and result in the so-called respiratory sinus arrhythmia with heart rate pauses [11]. In REM sleep phases, there is a predominant sympathetic activity that results in hypertension peaks, irregular heart and breathing rates, and dysregulation of body temperature. Heart rate and blood pressure become variable with an average increase compared to that observed in non-REM sleep [5, 12]. All autonomic manifestations that have been described so far occur not only in night sleep but also during daytime naps [13–15]. Sleep architecture is due to fluctuations of awareness [16], whose temporal organisation characterises the so-called sleep cycles. Awareness is associated with a predominant sympathetic activity with increased muscular tone, heart rate and blood pressure [17]. The circadian organisation of the waking state in temporal periods allows sleep continuation to be preserved. However, the strict association between sleep and autonomic variability plays the double role in allowing prompt awakening from sleep and to directly control the cardiovascular reflexes. The autonomic activity mediated by baroreceptors may indeed induce awakening from sleep [18, 19], and awakening may in turn modulate baroreceptor activity. This reciprocal interaction facilitates well-defined transitions between sleeping and awaking states [20]. Nonetheless, age-related modifications of ANS activity occur over the lifespan. These changes are mainly due to a progressive loss of neurons devoted to promoting awakening in the elderly [21]. For anatomical and functional reasons, the ANS is strictly associated with mechanisms underlying the wake-sleep rhythms. The presence of sleep disorders may disentangle the autonomic activity from the mechanisms of sleep regulation, with an increase in sympathetic tone. When the sleep is fragmented by frequent episodes of awakening, which are associated with increased sympathetic activity and sudden hypertension peaks, a state of hyper-awareness may occur, which is associated with an increased risk for morbidity and mortality. In the case these episodes are particularly frequent, higher heart rate and blood pressure values may also be transferred into the awaking state, with an average increase of sympathetic tone and blood pressure in day time. This is the pathophysiological mechanism by which sleep disorders may increase the risk of pathologically relevant events, by inducing failure of cardiovascular regulation at nighttime [22, 23]. On the other hand, a reduced activity of neurons devoted to induce the awakening state may account for drowsiness and for the need of daytime naps, which are typical of elderly individuals [21]. Similarly, a failure of the physiological process of blood pressure reduction overnight may represent a negative prognostic factor for cardiovascular disease [24]. Finally, the clinical relevance of an impaired control of the circadian rhythms of ANS activity is suggested by a higher incidence of cardiovascular events in the morning time [25].

9.2 Principal Sleep Disorders

Sleep disorder taxonomy is currently based on the third edition of the International Classification of Sleep Disorders (ICSD-3) [26], which includes the following nosological categories:

Insomnia. This category includes both, transient and chronic types of insomnia according to their duration, which may last shorter (i.e., transient) or longer (i.e., chronic) than 3 months. Even though the ICSD-3 does not clarify this point, the total sleep duration is an important phenotypic feature to be considered. Insomnia may either coexist with a reduced total duration of sleep (i.e., shorter than 6 h) or be itself longer than 6 h. Such a distinction is believed to have direct implications for individual long-term health conditions, with the former phenotype being associated with a less favourable prognosis.

Sleep-related breathing disorders. These include a wide range of pathological conditions that may be divided into obstructive apnoea (most frequent syndromes), central apnoea, hypoventilation and hypoxic disorders.

Central Hypersomnia. This category includes the following clinical conditions: (1) narcolepsy type 1, associated with cataplexy and reduced CSF concentrations of hypocretin (orexin); (2) narcolepsy type 2, which does not associate with cataplexy; (3) Idiopathic hypersomnia; (4) the Kleine-Levin syndrome (extremely rare); (5) hypersomnia associated to medical, genetic, psychiatric or iatrogenic conditions.

Circadian rhythm disorders. This category includes a heterogeneous range of conditions, including: i) those disorders characterised by an anticipated (i.e., falling asleep at night or waking up at the morning earlier than normal) or a delayed sleep phase (i.e., falling asleep late, in the early hours of the morning); ii) those disorders associated with irregular sleep phases or due to professional or touristic needs/circumstances (e.g., night-work; jet lag).

Parasomnias. This category includes i) those conditions that are not REM related (arousal disorders; confusional arousal; sleepwalking; pavor nocturnus; nocturnal sleep-related eating disorders); ii) those conditions that are REM sleep-related (REM behavioural disorder; hypnotic paralysis; nightmare disorder); iii) other conditions (e.g., nocturnal enuresis; somniloquy).

Sleep-related movement disorders. This category includes some frequent conditions, such as restless legs syndrome (RLS), periodic limb movement disorder, and bruxism.

Other sleep disorders. This category includes all disorders that are not part of the categories listed above.

Almost all sleep disorders are characterised by ANS involvement to some extent. As explained above, this is due to the strict anatomical and physiological link between sleep, its phases, and the ANS.

The next paragraph aims to review those sleep disorders which are most frequently seen in clinical practice and for which ANS involvement is most remarkable or supported by scientific evidence. Moreover, particular attention is paid to a possible association between autonomic dysregulation and cardiovascular risk (Table 9.1).

9.3 ANS Impairment in Sleep Disorders

9.3.1 Insomnia

Insomnia consists of difficulty in either falling or staying asleep and is associated with daytime symptoms such as fatigability, drowsiness, irritability, concentration and memory problems. In its transient and chronic form, insomnia afflicts up to 35% and 10% respectively of the world population. The strongest risk factors for insomnia include ageing and female gender. ANS involvement in the pathophysiology of insomnia seems to be strictly associated with an excessive activation of arousal mechanisms in the so-called "hyperarousal condition." This association has been demonstrated by electrophysiological (i.e., increased beta and gamma activity on EEG recordings), functional neuroimaging (PET imaging), and neuroendocrine studies [27]. Experimental and epidemiological studies indicate the presence of sympathetic hyperactivity as linked to the hyperarousal condition. This relationship is supported by evidence of increased endothelial damage [28], and might (at least partially) account for the increased risk of developing hypertension and other cardiovascular diseases in patients suffering from sympathetic hyperactivity [29]. This means that an early characterisation and treatment of insomnia and cardiovascular comorbidities might reduce patient mortality [30]. However, the precise mechanism underlying the link between hyperarousal and increased sympathetic tone still needs to be fully clarified [31]. Some studies suggest a concomitant contribution of reduced parasympathetic tone, especially in patients suffering from insomnia with reduced total duration of sleep (less than 6 h) [32]. Generally, patients with insomnia show increased heart rate in waking state as well during sleep alongside an increased systolic blood pressure overnight, with a consequent non-dipper pattern of sleep [33, 34]. An increased risk for cardiovascular accidents seems to be more remarkable in patients with reduced total duration of sleep [35].

Table 9.1 Principal characteristics of the most frequently observed sleep disorders associated to ANS involvement. For each of them, there are summarized here predominant sympthetic or parasympathetic involvement, principal autonomic alterations, pathophysiological mechanisms, clinical symptoms and signs, association with cardiovascular risk factors, and available therapies

Sleep disorder	Sympathetic/ parasympathetic involvement	Main autonomic alterations	Supposed pathogenetic mechanisms	Daytime autonomic symptoms/signs	Association with cardiovascular risk	Treatment of autonomic dysfunction
Insomnia	Increased sympathetic activity Reduced parasympathetic activity (possible)	• Nighttime systolic BP increase and blunted day-to-night BP dipping (non-dipper pattern) • HR increase, blunted nigh-time HR reduction	• Sympathetic overactivity associated with hyperarousal • Reduced parasympathetic activity only in patients with short sleep duration phenotype (sleep <6 h)	• HR increase	• Increased cardiovascular risk (in particular in patients with short sleep duration phenotype)	/
Obstructive sleep apnoea	Increased sympathetic activity	• Nighttime HR fluctuation (HR reduction during apnoea, tachycardia on resumption of breathing) • Blunted day-to-night BP dipping (non-dipper pattern)	• Hypoxia-induced chemoreflex overstimulation • Reduced baroreflex sensitivity • Attenuated NST inhibitory effect on the sympathetic efferent neurons • Possible bottom-up influence on vigilance central control areas (→ excessive daytime sleepiness)	• HR and BP increase • Increased levels of plasma and urine catecholamines	• Increased cardiovascular and stroke risk	CPAP: • Reduces sympathetic overactivity • Reduces BP values

Sleep disorder	Sympathetic/parasympathetic involvement	Main autonomic alterations	Supposed pathogenetic mechanisms	Daytime autonomic symptoms/signs	Association with cardiovascular risk	Treatment of autonomic dysfunction
Narcolepsy	Alteration of both sympathetic and parasympathetic activity (possible)	• Blunted day-to-night BP dipping (non-dipper pattern), with increased systolic BP during REM sleep • Increased HR	• Controversial data on sympathetic-vagal imbalance (sympathetic hyperactivity or inhibition, parasympathetic inhibition) • Possible influence of orexin on autonomic regulation	• HR increase (controversial data)	• Unknown, but possible increase of cardiovascular risk in patients with non-dipper pattern	/
Idiopathic hypersomnia	Increased parasympathetic activity	• HR reduction during sleep • HR increase associated with arousal	• Possible role of hypothalamus, basal forebrain, and medial frontal cortex • Possible role of histaminergic system	• HR reduction • Orthostatic hypotension	• Unknown	/

(continued)

Table 9.1 (continued)

Sleep disorder	Sympathetic/ parasympathetic involvement	Main autonomic alterations	Supposed pathogenetic mechanisms	Daytime autonomic symptoms/signs	Association with cardiovascular risk	Treatment of autonomic dysfunction
REM sleep behaviour disorder	Mixed alteration, mainly reduced sympathetic activity	• Blunted HR increase during movement and arousal • Nighttime BP increase and blunted day-to-night BP dipping (non-dipper pattern)	• Reduced sympathetic activation and reduced parasympathetic inhibition during the NREM-REM sleep transition • Reduced cardiac sympathetic innervation • Possible anatomic correlation between the REM sleep and autonomic control nuclei in the brainstem	• Orthostatic hypotension • Both sympathetic and vagal alterations at the cardiovascular reflex tests	• Unknown, but possible increase of cardiovascular risk in patients with non-dipper pattern	/
Restless legs syndrome	Increased sympathetic activity (possible)	• HR and BP increase associated with PLMS	• PLMS-induced enhancement of sympathetic activity • Possible reduction of dopaminergic inhibitory activity on the sympathetic system	• Mild HR and BP increase • Increased levels of plasma and urine catecholamines	• Increased cardiovascular and stroke risk, with unclear association with arterial hypertension • Possible sharing, between RLS and cardiovascular diseases, of common risk factors (smoking, metabolic syndrome)	• Possible role of dopamine agonists?

BP blood pressure, *CPAP* continuous positive airway pressure, *HR* heart rate, *NST* nucleus of solitary tract, *PLMS* periodic limb movements during sleep, *RLS* restless legs syndrome

9.3.2 Obstructive Sleep Apnoea

The obstructive sleep apnoea (OSA) syndrome is characterised by recurrent episodes of breathing stops (i.e., apnoea) and/or remarkable reduction of oronasal airflow (hypopnoea). These events are determined by mechanic occlusion of the higher airflow pathways, which causes periodic oxyhemoglobin desaturations and sleep fragmentation. This condition is most commonly observed in adult age with a prevalence of 18% in individuals older than 60 years. Nonetheless, OSA syndrome is increasingly observed also in teenagers and children suffering from tonsil hypertrophy and early obesity. The ANS involvement in OSA is strictly associated with the presence and severity of apnoea. Heart rate fluctuates with a pattern of reduction during apnoea, and increases immediately after its termination. Nocturnal blood pressure is increased with frequent detections of a non-dipper pattern (i.e., less than 10% decrease from daytime blood pressure values) [36, 37]. From a pathophysiological viewpoint, it has been observed an increased sensitivity of the chemoreflex [38] and a reduced sensitivity of the baroreflex in the presence of recurrent apnoea [39]. Together, these effects are associated with an increased sympathetic tone on autonomic tests, and increased plasma levels of norepinephrine [40]. These observations account for the increased prevalence of hypertension, cardiovascular disease and cerebrovascular accidents in patients with OSA [41]. As a chronic effect of OSA, a reduced sensitivity of the baroreflex might induce abnormalities in the bottom-up mechanisms of regulation that brainstem structures operate through their connection with cortical areas devoted to the maintenance of awareness. This would explain the excessive daytime sleepiness of patients with OSA [42]. Clinically, the presence of daytime sleepiness in patients with OSA is regarded as a reliable marker for the presence of hypertension and a higher risk for cardiovascular disease [43]. Continuous Positive Airway Pressure (CPAP) is an efficacious treatment for patients with OSA. The continuous use of CPAP reduces patients' sympathetic tone, although clear-cut evidence of its impact on reducing the risk for cardiovascular and cerebrovascular disease still needs to be demonstrated [41, 44].

9.3.3 Narcolepsy Type 1

Narcolepsy type 1 is a form of primary hypersomnia that is clinically characterised by excessive daytime sleepiness and the occurrence of sudden episodes of falling asleep (described by patients as incoercible), with a 15–20 min duration, and facilitated by low environmental stimulation. Narcolepsy type 1 (differently from narcolepsy type 2) also presents with episodes of catalepsy, which are characterised by sudden muscular tone reductions and possible falls. These symptoms are due to the intrusion of REM sleep features into the waking state. In patients suffering from narcolepsy type 1, there is a remarkable reduction of CSF levels of hypocretin (orexin) (i.e., a hypothalamic peptide implicated in wake-sleep rhythm regulation).

Narcolepsy's type 1 prevalence is about 0.1% in the general population. The mechanisms for ANS involvement in patients with narcolepsy type 1 are mainly related to reduced production of orexin. This reflects abnormal regulation (physiologically mediated by orexin) of several ANS structures, such as the insula, amigdala, and the anterior cingulate cortex [45]. In narcolepsy's type 1 brains, there is an unbalance between sympathetic and vagal activity in nighttime as well as in daytime, whose predominance in either direction remains to be clarified. This unbalance might be due to sympathetic hyper- [46] or hypoactivity [47], or parasympathetic hypoactivity [48]. The nocturnal blood pressure profile of patients with narcolepsy type 1 presents with a non-dipping pattern, which is likely due to an increase of systolic pressure (particularly in non-REM phases of sleep). Patient heart rate is generally higher than that observed in healthy individuals [49–51]. It still remains to be clarified whether patients with narcolepsy type 1 present with a higher risk for cardiovascular disease, as their abnormal pattern of nocturnal blood pressure levels would suggest.

9.3.4 Idiopathic Hypersomnia

Idiopathic hypersomnia is a disorder of juvenile-onset (it typically affects individuals younger than 25 years) whose aetiology remains obscure. It is characterised by the presence of increased daytime sleepiness with the need of frequent and prolonged naps (lasting for a few hours), which are reported to be scarcely laughter. An additional feature is the protracted nocturnal sleep with difficulty in waking up. In contrast to what is observed in narcolepsy type 1, patients with hypersomnia show CSF levels of orexin within the normal range, and do not suffer from an early onset of REM sleep. Idiopathic hypersomnia is an extremely rare condition with a prevalence of 1–5/10000 individuals. Nonetheless, this disorder is frequently associated with autonomic symptoms, such as orthostatic hypotension. This is the reason why hypersomnia is included in the present book chapter. The autonomic involvement in idiopathic hypersomnia is likely related to a parasympathetic hyperactivity, which is persistently present in waking as well as in sleep state. This is supported by evidence of heart rate variability (HRV) evaluations [52]. Moreover, it has been observed an increased heart rate during arousal [52], which probably reflects a temporary increase in sympathetic activity. In the waking state, episodes of orthostatic hypotension are frequently observed. A recent case-control study reports a higher frequency of autonomic symptoms in patients with idiopathic hypersomnia with significant correlations with the severity of their daytime sleepiness and quality of life [53]. A possible cause for the autonomic dysregulation observed in patients with idiopathic hypersomnia might be found in abnormal central control of their hypothalamic nuclei and medial prefrontal cortex. In more detail, the histaminergic system from the hypothalamus that regulates the release of orexin seems to be involved in the autonomic dysregulation observed in these patients. It remains unclear an association between these autonomic abnormalities and an increased risk for cardio- and cerebrovascular disease.

9.3.5 REM Behaviour Disorder

REM behaviour disorder (RBD) is a parasomnia characterised by movements and vocalisation during sleep, which may be of great intensity and accompanied by kicks, punches, leaps, and falls off the bed. These manifestations occur during the REM phase of sleep due to dissociation with the physiological muscular atonia. Patients make their dreams come true for a duration that ranges from 1 to 20 min. Although such a disorder may present in isolation as an idiopathic form of RBD (iRBD), it is more often regarded as the clinical onset of a neurodegenerative disease involving the brainstem, with alpha-synucleinopathies as the most common form. The rate of phenoconversion from RBD to alpha-synucleinopathy approaches 90% of cases in 10–15 years from clinical onset. Patients suffering from RBD in either form, iRBD or RBD associated with alpha-synucleinopathies present with some autonomic dysfunctions [54]. However, it remains controversial whether the autonomic impairment in patients with iRBD is due to a common pathophysiological process of neurodegeneration [55], or whether iRBD should only be regarded as a marker of potential phenoconversion from iRBD to alpha-synucleinopathies [56]. The vast majority of studies report a sympathetic-vagal imbalance in waking state as well as during sleep, in patients with RBD [57]. This imbalance seems to be dominated by reduction of sympathetic activity [58], even though parasympathetic abnormalities have also been described [54]. The dysfunction of both autonomic sections (sympathetic and parasympathetic) is due to the involvement of their central as well as peripheral branches [59, 60]. Such abnormalities impact the physiological increase of heart rate in response to movements during sleep as well as in an awake state. Additionally, they induce an increase of nocturnal blood pressure with a poor reduction of nictemeral changes, with a non-dipper pattern [55]. In waking phases, patients present with a higher prevalence of orthostatic hypotension [61].

The importance of an association between dysautonomia and RBD in relation to its prognostic value of phenoconversion to alpha-synucleinopathies and development of cardio- and cerebrovascular disease is still under discussion and needs further evidence based on future prospective studies [55].

9.3.6 Restless Leg Syndrome

Restless leg syndrome (RLS) is characterised by "annoying sensations" and "restlessness feeling" in the lower limbs, which are exacerbated by rest and mitigated by voluntary movement. Symptoms are more frequently experienced in the evening, especially before falling asleep. In 90% of cases RLS associates with periodic limb movements of sleep (PMLS). RLS affects 5–10% of the general population in all age groups. This condition is most frequently idiopathic, but it may also be associated with other neurological and non-neurological conditions, and drugs' administration. The autonomic involvement in RLS appears to be associated with an altered sympathetic-vagal balance, which is predominantly due to increased sympathetic activity in waking condition as well as during sleep [41, 62]. Sympathetic hyperactivity seems to be associated with increased frequency of PLMS episodes, and increases of heart rate and blood pressure values [63, 64]. However, there is some evidence suggesting that sympathetic activation is promoted or caused by PLMS [63]. Additionally, a specific role may be played by a reduction of inhibitory dopaminergic tone from the hypothalamus to spinal cord motor neurons and autonomic neurons from the intermediolateral nuclei (i.e., sympathetic preganglionic pathway) [65]. Such a hypothesis suggests a common pathophysiological mechanism for PMLS and autonomic dysfunction, thus supporting some evidence that treatment with dopamine agonists improves both types of symptoms [66]. Similarly to other sleep disorders, RLS is also associated with an increased risk for cardiovascular disease, even though the underlying pathophysiology still remains to be clarified [67]. A clear-cut link with an increased parasympathetic tone is indeed uncertain [67]. Alternatively, it is possible that such an association may be due to sharing of risk factors between RLS and cardiovascular disease [68].

9.4 Clinical Approach to Dysautonomia in Patients with Sleep Disorder

Autonomic dysfunctions are frequently observed in patients suffering from sleep disorder. As illustrated above, ANS involvement encompasses the whole range of sleep disorders, thus indicating the existence of common anatomical pathways subserving the autonomic and sleep regulation, as well as common pathophysiological mechanisms. In clinical practice, cardiovascular dysautonomia invariably presents with abnormalities and dysregulation of heart rate and blood pressure, although a prominent or causative role of sympathetic or parasympathetic dysfunction remains uncertain. On the other hand, dysautonomia, whenever present, may strongly contribute to increasing the clinical risk of patients carriers of other risk factors for cardio- and cerebrovascular disease, such as ageing, smoking, obesity, metabolic syndrome. Additionally, in the case of dysautonomia causing orthostatic hypotension, there is an increased risk of patient falls and traumatic injuries. These considerations indicate that a timely diagnosis of dysautonomia, which frequently associated with sleep disorders, is of cardinal importance for the identification of patients at higher risk for cardio- and cerebrovascular disease and for optimising their therapies, with the final goal of reducing patient morbidity and mortality.

In this view, an early evaluation of dysautonomia in patients complaining of sleep disorders is strongly recommended. In the absence of validated guidelines, we propose here a practical approach to investigate dysautonomia in patients complaining of sleep disorders.

9.4.1 Clinical History Collection

This part should explicitly investigate the following aspects:

- The presence of vascular risk factors and comorbidities.
- Symptoms and/or signs suggestive for cardiovascular autonomic dysregulation.
- Previous detection of increased or reduced blood pressure values. In the latter case (hypotension), it is relevant to understand whether low blood pressure values are present in specific conditions, such as after lunch/dinner (i.e., postprandial hypotension) or when standing up (i.e., orthostatic hypotension).
- The presence of headache over night or when waking up.
- Increased nocturnal diuresis.
- Episodes of dizziness, vertigo, feeling of neck or shoulder muscle fatigue.
- Episodes of visual loss, fainting, or syncope when standing up (orthostatism).

Particular attention should be paid when examining patients suffering from insomnia, OSA, or RLS. These conditions are indeed more frequently associated with dysautonomia.

9.4.2 First Level Assessments

In the case of a clinical history suggestive for cardiovascular dysautonomia, or in the presence of remarkable risk factors for vascular disease, a screening assessment should be performed by Ambulatory Blood Pressure Monitoring (24 h recording). This simple assessment, which is available in most clinical settings, provides a comprehensive picture of the circadian fluctuations of blood pressure and heart rate. This allows the presence of diurnal and nocturnal hypertension to be documented, alongside supine hypertension, increased blood pressure variability, hypotension events (e.g., postprandial hypotension), changes in nocturnal dipping.

Overall, this simple screening may suggest:

- The presence of cardiovascular dysautonomia (particularly relevant is the absence or inversion of nocturnal dipping);
- Possible needs for starting hypertension medication or adjusting ongoing therapies.

In the case hypertension is demonstrated, additional investigations are needed to identify/exclude impairment of specific organs/systems. Principal post-screening assessments include:

- Doppler Ultrasound of the cerebral arteries;
- Kidney function tests;
- Neuroimaging (CT or MRI brain scanning).

9.4.3 Patient Referral to Specialised Centres for Cardiovascular Dysautonomia

Should the Ambulatory Blood Pressure Monitoring assessment demonstrate abnormalities suggestive for cardiovascular dysautonomia, patient referral to a Specialised Centre for cardiovascular dysautonomia is strongly recommended for a comprehensive autonomic investigation.

References

1. Silvani A, Dampney RA. Central control of cardiovascular function during sleep. Am J Physiol Heart Circ Physiol. 2013;305(12):H1683–92.
2. Benarroch EE. Control of the cardiovascular and respiratory systems during sleep. Auton Neurosci. 2019;218:54–63.
3. Saper CB. The central autonomic nervous system: conscious visceral perception and autonomic pattern generation. Annu Rev Neurosci. 2002;25:433–69.
4. Burgess H, Trinder J, Kim Y, Luke D. Sleep and circadian influences on cardiac autonomic nervous system activity. Am J Phys. 1997;273(4):H1761–8.
5. Trinder J, Waloszek J, Woods M, Jordan A. Sleep and cardiovascular regulation. Pflugers Arch. 2012;463(1):161–8.
6. Albrecht U. Timing to perfection: the biology of central and peripheral circadian clocks. Neuron. 2012;74(2):246–60.
7. Lowey AD. Anatomy of the autonomic nervous system: an overview. In: Lowey AD, Spyer KM, editors. Central regulation of autonomic functions. New York: Oxford University Press; 1990. p. 3–16.
8. Shirasaka T, Nakazato M, Matsukura S, Takasaki M, Kannan H. Sympathe- tic and cardiovascular actions of orexins in conscious rats. Am J Phys. 1999;277(6):R1780–5.
9. Parmeggiani PL, Morrison AR. Alterations of autonomic functions during sleep. In: Lowey AD, Spyer KM, editors. Central regulation of autonomic functions. New York: Oxford University Press; 1990.
10. Chokroverty BS. Physiological changes in sleep. In: Chokroverty S, Ferini-Strambi L, editors. Oxford textbook of sleep disorders. Oxford: Oxford University Press; 2017. p. 43–52.
11. Guilleminault C, Quera-Salva MA, Goldberg MP. Pseudohypersomnia and pre-sleep behaviour with bilateral paramedian thalamic lesions. Brain. 1993;116:1549–63.
12. Trinder J. Cardiac activity and sympathovagal balance during sleep. Sleep Med Clin. 2007;2(2):199–208.
13. Cellini N, Whitehurst LN, McDevitt EA, Mednick SC. Heart rate variability during daytime naps in healthy adults: autonomic profile and short-term reliability. Psychophysiology. 2016;53(4):473–81.
14. Cellini N, Torre J, Stegagno L, Sarlo M. Cardiac autonomic activity during daytime nap in young adults. J Sleep Res. 2018;27(2):159–64.

15. Whitehurst LN, Naji M, Mednick SC. Comparing the cardiac autonomic activity profile of daytime naps and nighttime sleep. Neurobiol Sleep Circadian Rhythms. 2018;5:52–7.
16. Smerieri A, Parrino L, Agosti M, Ferri R, Terzano MG. Cyclic alternating pattern sequences and non-cyclic alternating pattern periods in human sleep. Clin Neurophysiol. 2007;118(10):2305–13.
17. Sforza E, Jouny C, Ibanez V. Cardiac activation during arousal in humans: further evidence for hierarchy in the arousal response. Clin Neurophysiol. 2000;111(9):1611–9.
18. Cole RJ. Postural baroreflex stimuli may affect eeG arousal and sleep in humans. J Appl Physiol. 1989;67:2369–75.
19. Silvani A, Calandra-Buonaura G, Benarroch EE, et al. Bidirectional interactions between the baroreceptor reflex and arousal: an update. Sleep Med. 2015;16:210–6.
20. Bangash MF, Xie A, Skatrud JB, Reichmuth KJ, Barczi SR, Morgan BJ. Cerebrovascular response to arousal from NReM and ReM sleep. Sleep. 2008;31(3):321–7.
21. Katzman R, Terry R. Normal aging of the nervous system. In: Katzman R, editor. The neurology of aging. Philadelphia, PA: Davis; 1983.
22. Wolk R, Gami AS, Garcia-Touchard A, Somers VK. Sleep and cardiovascular disease. Curr Probl Cardiol. 2005;30(12):625–62.
23. Yano Y, Kario K. Nocturnal blood pressure and cardiovascular disease: a review of recent advances. Hypertens Res. 2012;35(7):695.
24. Staessen JA, Wang JG, Thijs L. Cardiovascular protection and blood pressure reduction: a meta-analysis. Lancet. 2001;358(9290):1305–15.
25. Thosar SS, Butler MP, Shea SA. Role of the circadian system in cardiovascular disease. J Clin Invest. 2018;128(6):2157–67.
26. American Academy of Sleep Medicine. The international classification of sleep disorders 3rd ed (ICSD-3). Derien, IL: AASM; 2014.
27. Riemann D, Spiegelhalder K, Feige B, et al. The hyperarousal model of insomnia: a review of the concept and its evidence. Sleep Med Rev. 2010;14(1):19–31.
28. Tobaldini E, Fiorelli EM, Solbiati M, Costantino G, Nobili L, Montano N. Short sleep duration and cardiometabolic risk: from pathophysiology to clinical evidence. Nat Rev Cardiol. 2019;16(4):213–24.
29. Carter JR, Grimaldi D, Fonkoue IT, Medalie L, Mokhlesi B, Van Cauter E. Assessment of sympathetic neural activity in chronic insomnia: evidence for elevated cardiovascular risk. Sleep. 2018;41(9):zsy126.
30. Grimaldi D, Goldsteinb MR, Carterc JR. Insomnia and cardio-vascular autonomic control. Auton Neurosci 2019; 220: 102551. Review.
31. Ferini Strambi L, Marelli S, Salsone M. Primary insomnia and dysautonomia. In: Chokroverty S, Cortelli P, eds. Autonom Nervous Syst Sleep. 2021;14:165–71.
32. Spiegelhalder K, Fuchs L, Ladwig J, et al. Heart rate and heart rate variability in subjectively reported insomnia. J Sleep Res. 2011;20(1Pt 2):137–45.
33. Irwin M, Clark C, Kennedy B, Christian Gillin J, ziegler M. Nocturnal catecholamines and immune function in insomniacs, depressed patients, and control subjects. Brain Behav Immun. 2003;17(5):365–72.
34. Maiolino G, Bisogni V, Soranna D, et al. Sleep Disorders Working Group of the Italian Society of Hypertension. Effects of insomnia and restless legs syndrome on sleep arterial blood pressure: a systematic review and meta-analysis. Sleep Med Rev. 2021;59:101497.
35. Vgontas AN, Fernandez-Mendoza J, Liao D, Bixler EO. Insomnia with objective short sleep duration: the most biologically severe phenotype of the disorder. Sleep Med Rev. 2013;17(4):241–54.
36. Somers VK, Me D, Clary MP, Abboud FM. Sympathetic neural mechanisms in obstructive sleep apnea. J Clin Invest. 1995;96:1897–904.
37. Portaluppi F, Provini F, Cortelli P, et al. Undiagnosed sleep-disordered breathing among male nondippers with essential hypertension. J Hypertens. 1997;15(11):1227–33.

38. Somers VK, Mark AL, Zavala DC, Abboud FM. Influence of ventilation and hypocapnia on sympathetic nerve responses to hypoxia in normal humans. J Appl Physiol. 1989;67:2095–100.
39. Parati G, Di Rienzo M, Bonsignore MR, et al. Autonomic cardiac regulation in obstructive sleep apnea syndrome: evidence from spontaneous baroreflex analysis during sleep. J Hypertens. 1997;15(12 Pt 2):1621–6.
40. Cortelli P, Parchi P, Sforza E, et al. Cardiovascular autonomic dysfunction in normotensive awake subjects with obstructive sleep apnea syndrome. Clin Auton Res. 1994;4:57–62.
41. Calandra-Buonaura G, Provini F, Guaraldi P, Plazzi G, Cortelli P. Cardiovascular autonomic dysfunctions and sleep disorders. Sleep Med Rev. 2016;26:43–56.
42. Lombardi C, Parati G, Cortelli P, et al. Daytime sleepiness and neural cardiac modulation in sleep-related breathing disorders. J Sleep Res. 2008;17(3):263–70.
43. Kapur VK, Resnick HE, Gottlieb DJ, Sleep Heart Health Study Group. Sleep disordered breathing and hypertension: does self-reported sleepiness modify the association? Sleep. 2008;31:1127–32.
44. Cepeda-Valery B, Acharjee S, Romero-Corral A, Pressman GS, Gami AS. Obstructive sleep apnea and acute coronary syndromes: aetiology, risk, and management. Curr Cardiol Rep. 2014;16:535.
45. Grimaldi D, Silvani A, Benarroch EE, Cortelli P. Orexin/hypocretin system and autonomic control: new insights and clinical correlations. Neurology. 2014;82:271–8.
46. Grimaldi D, Pierangeli G, Barletta G, et al. Spectral analysis of heart rate variability reveals an enhanced sympathetic activity in narcolepsy with cataplexy. Clin Neurophysiol. 2010;121:1142–7.
47. Fronczek R, Overeem S, Reijntjes R, Lammers GJ, van Dijk JG, Pijl H. Increased heart rate variability but normal resting metabolic rate in hypocretin/orexin-deficient human narcolepsy. J Clin Sleep Med. 2008;4:248–54.
48. Silvani A, Grimaldi D, Barletta G, et al. Cardiovascular variability as a function of sleep-wake behaviour in narcolepsy with cataplexy. J Sleep Res. 2013;22(2):178–84.
49. Grimaldi D, Calandra-Buonaura G, Provini F, et al. Abnormal sleep- cardiovascular system interaction in narcolepsy with cataplexy: effects of hypocretin deficiency in humans. Sleep. 2012;35(4):519–28.
50. Dauvilliers Y, Jaussent I, Krams B, et al. Non-dipping blood pressure profile in narcolepsy with cataplexy. PLoS One. 2012;7(6):e38977.
51. van der Meijden WP, Fronczek R, Reijntjes RH, et al. Time- and state- dependent analysis of autonomic control in narcolepsy: higher heart rate with normal heart rate variability independent of sleep fragmentation. J Sleep Res. 2015;24(2):206–14.
52. Sforza E, Roche F, Barthelemy JC, Pichot V. Diurnal and nocturnal cardiovascular variability and heart rate arousal response in idiopathic hypersomnia. Sleep Med. 2016;24:131–6.
53. Miglis MG, Schneider L, Kim P, Cheung J, Trotti LM. Frequency and severity of autonomic symptoms in idiopathic hypersomnia. J Clin Sleep Med. 2020;16(5):749–56.
54. Lee H, Cho YW, Kim HA. The severity and pattern of autonomic dysfunction in idiopathic rapid eye movement sleep behaviour disorder. Mov Disord. 30(13):1843–8.
55. Terzaghi M, Pilati L, Ghiotto N, et al. Twenty-four-hour blood pressure profile in idiopathic ReM sleep behaviour disorder. Sleep. 2022;45(2):zb239.
56. Pilotto A, Romagnolo A, Tuazon JA, et al. Orthostatic hypotension and ReM sleep behaviour disorder: impact on clinical outcomes in α-synucleinopathies. J Neurol Neurosurg Psychiatry. 2019;90(11):1257–63.
57. Barone DA, Ebben MR, Samie A, Mortara D, Krieger AC. Autonomic dysfunction in isolated rapid eye movement sleep without atonia. Clin Neurophysiol. 2015;126(4):731–5.
58. Postuma RB, Lanfranchi PA, Blais H, Gagnon JF, Montplaisir JY. Cardiac autonomic dysfunction in idiopathic ReM sleep behaviour disorder. Mov Disord. 2010;25(14):2304–10.
59. Palma JA, Urrestarazu E, Alegre M, et al. Cardiac autonomic impairment during sleep is linked with disease severity in Parkinson's disease. Clin Neurophysiol. 2013;124(6):1163–8.

60. Kashihara K, Imamura T, Shinya T. Cardiac 123I-MIBG uptake is reduced more markedly in patients with ReM sleep behaviour disorder than in those with early stage Parkinson's disease. Parkinsonism Relat Disord. 2010;16(4):252–5.
61. Frauscher B, Nomura T, Duerr S, et al. Investigation of autonomic function in idiopathic ReM sleep behaviour disorder. J Neurol. 2012;259(6):1056–61.
62. Izzi F, Placidi F, Romigi A, et al. Is the autonomic nervous system involved in restless legs syndrome during wakefulness? Sleep Med. 2014;15(11):1392–7.
63. Guggisberg AG, Hess CW, Mathis J. The significance of the sympathetic nervous system in the pathophysiology of periodic leg movements in sleep. Sleep. 2007;30:755–66.
64. Pennestri MH, Montplaisir J, Colombo R, Lavigne G, Lanfranchi PA. Nocturnal blood pressure changes in patients with restless legs syndrome. Neurology. 2007;68:1213–8.
65. Clemens S, Rye D, Hochman S. Restless legs syndrome: revisiting the dopamine hypothesis from the spinal cord perspective. Neurology. 2006;67:125–30.
66. Manconi M, Ferri R, Zucconi M, et al. Effects of acute dopamine-agonist treatment in restless legs syndrome on heart rate variability during sleep. Sleep Med. 2011;12(1):47–55.
67. Kato M, Phillips BG, Sigurdsson G, Narkiewicz K, Pesek CA, Somers VK. Effects of sleep deprivation on neural circulatory control. Hypertension. 2000;35:1173–5.
68. Schlesinger I, Erikh I, Avizohar O, Sprecher E, Yarnitsky D. Cardiovascular risk factors in restless legs syndrome. Mov Disord. 2009;24:1587–92.

Chapter 10
Autonomic Dysfunctions in Temporal Lobe Epilepsy

Michele Terzaghi, Elena Capriglia, Annalisa Rubino, and Raffaele Manni

10.1 Introduction

Approximately 60% of all epileptic patients suffer from focal epilepsy, and in about one-third of these patients, the epileptogenic focus resides in the temporal lobe [1].

Autonomic symptoms and signs are frequently seen in epilepsy [2–9] and can accompany various types of focal, generalized, motor, and nonmotor seizures [10]. This symptomatology may be prevalent at the onset of a focal seizure, which has allowed recognition by the International League Against Epilepsy (ILAE) as a distinct type of seizure (focal onset autonomic seizure) [10]: "focal autonomic seizures may present with gastrointestinal sensations, feeling hot or cold, hot flashes, piloerection (goose bumps), palpitations, sexual arousal, respiratory changes, or other autonomic effects" [10].

Autonomic dysfunctions during epileptic seizures result from an alteration of the Central Autonomic Network (CAN) [7]. The CAN be divided into two subsystems: one is the brainstem/medulla system, which responds typically to nonconscious stimuli, and one is the cortical/subcortical autonomic system, responding to conscious stimulation. The brainstem/medulla system is connected to internal sensors, such as baro- and chemoreceptors, and includes the nuclei of the solitary tract,

M. Terzaghi (✉)
Department of Brain and Behavioral Sciences, University of Pavia, Pavia, Italy

Unit of Sleep Medicine and Epilepsy, Mondino Foundation IRCCS, Pavia, Italy
e-mail: michele.terzaghi@mondino.it

E. Capriglia
Department of Brain and Behavioral Sciences, University of Pavia, Pavia, Italy
e-mail: elena.capriglia01@universitadipavia.it

A. Rubino · R. Manni
Unit of Sleep Medicine and Epilepsy, Mondino Foundation IRCCS, Pavia, Italy
e-mail: annalisa.rubino@mondino.it; raffaele.manni@mondino.it

G. Micieli et al. (eds.), *Autonomic Disorders in Clinical Practice*,
https://doi.org/10.1007/978-3-031-43036-7_10

ambiguous, dorsal vagal, pre-Bötzinger/Bötzinger complex, parabrachial, and Kölliker-Fuse nuclei, the rostral and caudal ventral respiratory group, the serotonergic raphe, and mesencephalic periaqueductal gray/reticular formation. The cortical/subcortical autonomic system is activated by external stimulation by initiating the appropriate response via the brainstem/medulla system and its leading components are hypothalamus, thalamus (in particular, ventral posterior medial and lateral nuclei), the mesial prefrontal cortex and the insular cortex [11]. Animal and human clinical studies suggested an important role of posterior insula in cortical and cortical/brainstem autonomic integration [12].

Temporal lobe epilepsy (TLE), particularly when associated with mesial temporal sclerosis, may be related to structural brain abnormalities beyond the epileptogenic focus in cortical and subcortical regions belonging to CAN [13–16]. It can be speculated that the loss of neurons in the epileptogenic focus in TLE may cause damage to white matter tracts that connect the focus to extra-focal brain areas, thus causing atrophy of distant but anatomically connected brain regions such as the mesial prefrontal cortex and insula [15].

The anterior cingulate, insular, posterior orbito-frontal and the prefrontal cortices are fundamental in influencing the autonomic nervous system at the cortical level along with the amygdala and the hypothalamus [17, 18]. In epileptic patients, ictal discharges occurring in or propagating to these structures can lead to increased sympathetic outflows, thus resulting in autonomic dysfunction [19].

TLE can be associated with a wide range of autonomic alterations, which can occur before, during or after the epileptic seizure (Table 10.1). The climax of these alterations could be represented by sudden unexpected death in epilepsy (SUDEP) [11]; SUDEP is the main cause of premature death (10–50%) in epileptic patients

Table 10.1 Autonomic dysfunctions in temporal lobe epilepsy

Cardiovascular	Respiratory	Gastrointestinal	Cutaneous	Sexual	Urinary
Ictal sinus tachycardia	Ictal hyperventilation	Epigastric auras	Ictal flushing	Sexual auras	Ictal urinary urge and urination
Ictal bradyarrhythmias and ictal asystole	Ictal oxygen desaturation, ictal hypoventilation, bradypnea, ictal central apnea	Ictal vomiting and retching in adults	Ictal pallor	Genital automatisms	Peri-ictal drinking
	Postictal nosewiping	Ictal vomiting in children	Ictal sweating		
	Peri-ictal coughing	Peri-ictal spitting	Ictal piloerection		
		Ictal hypersalivation			
		Ictal flatulence			
		Ictal urge to defecate			

[20–22]. The observations in patients dying from SUDEP suggested a postictal breakdown of autonomic control, consisting in a severe alteration of the respiratory and cardiac function, leading to a generalized EEG suppression and eventually to terminal cardio-respiratory arrest [23, 24].

A study made by Mueller et al. investigated TLE patients with and without MTS; in two patients who died from SUDEP, the brainstem was studied with deformation-based morphometry and graph analysis. The authors found volume loss in the dorsal mesencephalon, suggesting more extensive brainstem damage and network disruption in these subjects [11]. Volume loss was more represented at the level of the periaqueductal gray, colliculi, raphe, and reticular formation, extending into the diencephalon, particularly in the medial posterior thalamus [11]. In patients with TLE and mesial temporal sclerosis, this volume loss was even more severe and widespread, extending into the dorsal section of the pons and in the upper medulla oblongata. These changes were also associated with an impaired interconnection between the altered areas [11].

Two subtypes of TLE are currently recognized, according to the structures initially involved during seizures: the first and most common is medial TLE (MTLE), the second one, less frequent, is lateral (or neocortical) TLE (LTLE or NTLE) [25]. In MTLE, seizures originate in the temporal medial structures such as the hippocampus, entorhinal cortex, amygdala and parahippocampal gyrus [26]. In LTLE the epileptic discharge arises in the temporal neocortex, which includes the superior, medial, inferior circumvolutions, the temporo-occipital and temporo-parietal junctions [25, 27, 28].

10.2 Cardiovascular Manifestations

10.2.1 Ictal Sinus Tachycardia

Sinus tachycardia is the exceeding of the heart rate compared to the normal range for a resting heart. The upper threshold in adults is generally considered 100 beats per minute (bpm) [29]. Ictal sinus tachycardia can be defined as the occurrence of sinus tachycardia before, during or shortly after the onset of ictal discharges [18].

The temporal lobe is the brain region that most frequently gives rise to ictal sinus tachycardia [19]. Heart rate changes associated with seizures were reported in 78% [30] and 62% [31] of temporal lobe onset seizures versus 22% and 11%, respectively, of extratemporal seizures.

No significant difference in the degree of heart rate increase has been reported between seizures originating from the mesial or lateral temporal lobe structures, although heart rate changes precede EEG discharges more frequently in lateral temporal lobe seizures than mesial seizures [32]. Similarly, Di Gennaro et al. [33] and Mayer et al. [34] reported that the onset of ictal heart rate increase occurred earlier in mesial than in lateral temporal seizures in adult and pediatric populations, respectively.

When evaluating lateralization as a potential influencing factor on the occurrence and/or degree of ictal heart rate changes, while a different effect has been shown by stimulating the right or left insula (i.e., stimulation of the left insula causes bradycardia while stimulation of the right insula results in tachycardia) [35], there is no evidence for such an effect for the temporal lobe [19]. A study with subdural electrodes showed no difference in ictal heart rate in seizures originating in the right or left temporal lobe, while preictal tachycardia was observed more often in right temporal seizures compared to left temporal seizures [36]. Moreover, it has been shown that ictal tachycardia occurs earlier if the seizure originates in the right temporal lobe compared to contralateral and if seizures arise from the hippocampal formation [37].

10.2.2 Ictal Bradyarrhythmias and Ictal Asystole

Bradyarrhythmias range from mild asymptomatic sinus bradycardia (<60 bpm) to more severe forms (pronounced sinus bradycardia, sinus arrest, atrioventricular block) and prolonged asystole [2, 3, 7].

Bradyarrhythmias are much less frequent during epileptic seizure than tachyarrhythmias [2, 3, 7, 9, 38] and cardiac asystole occurs even more rarely [39].

In a study with surface EEG, most patients with ictal bradyarrhythmias presented seizure focus on the temporal lobe [40]. Most cases of ictal asystole were related to seizure onset from the temporal lobe, up to 80–82% of the cases reviewed by Tényi et al. [41, 42] and up to 90% of those reviewed by van der Lende et al. [38]. Van der Lende et al. did not find a consistent lateralization [38]. Ictal asystole could be the direct consequence of epileptic activity stimulating CAN or an indirect effect evoking a vasovagal reflex. This phenomenon could be self-limited because the cerebral anoxia caused by asystole could be a potential mechanism of seizure termination; indeed, seizures characterized by ictal asystole usually have a shorter duration than those without [38, 43].

Moreover, one study indicates that interictal cardiovascular autonomic function is also altered, manifested by impaired heart rate responses to stimuli such as deep breathing, Valsalva maneuver, and tilting, in refractory and well-controlled TLE, even if interictal autonomic dysfunction is more evident in refractory TLE [44].

10.3 Respiratory Manifestations

10.3.1 Ictal Hyperventilation

It is a symptom that may occasionally occur in TLE. It is more frequent if the origin of the seizure is in the mesial temporal lobe compared to seizures originating in the temporal neocortex; this could be explained by considering the important connectivity between mesial temporal lobe structures and the hippocampus and autonomic nuclei of the brainstem [45].

10.3.2 Ictal Oxygen Desaturation, Ictal Hypoventilation, Bradypnea, Ictal Central Apnea

Ictal hypoxemia has been reported in some epileptic patients and may contribute to SUDEP. Electrical stimulation of CAN-related brain regions (the hippocampal gyrus, the ventral and medial temporal pole, the anterior portion of the insula, and the anterior limbic gyrus) results in inhibition of respiratory movements [46]. Some studies have shown that electrical stimulation of mesial temporal structures causes central apnea [47, 48].

Desaturation is correlated with the onset of temporal lobe seizure [49, 50]. The occurrence of low blood oxygen levels is more frequent if the epileptic discharge spreads to the contralateral hemisphere. The descending pathways from the limbic areas to the brainstem respiratory center are primarily ipsilateral [51], so seizure-related bilateral impairment of these descending pathways may be a requirement for respiratory inhibition [50].

Bradypnea in epileptic patients is defined as a 10% decrease in respiratory rate from the interictal baseline [52]. Ictal bradypnea has been demonstrated in temporal lobe seizures in adults and children [52, 53]. Bradypnea was not preceded or followed by changes in respiratory rate, and no differences were found between right- and left-sided seizures [53]. No changes in respiratory control during the interictal period are described in literature [53].

Ictal central apnea consists of cessation of respiratory movements for more than 10 s in absence of generalized tonic/clonic movements. It is more frequent in TLE than in extratemporal epilepsies; moreover, ictal central apneas have a longer duration and hypoxemia is more severe when correlated to TLE [54].

10.3.3 Postictal Nose Wiping

It is a postictal symptom of reliable lateralizing significance in focal epilepsy originating in the temporal lobe. It occurs in 40–50% of patients with TLE, less frequent in extratemporal epilepsies, and the hand used to perform nose wiping is ipsilateral to seizure onset side [55–59]. More frequently associated with seizures that originate in the nondominant temporal lobe, it has been proposed as a purposeful reaction to increased upper airway secretion during seizures, with the use of the ipsilateral hand because the contralateral hand exhibits postictal weakness or neglect [55]. Wennberg with intracerebral electrodes has demonstrated the crucial role of the amygdala in the induction of postictal nose wiping and that seizures restricted to hippocampus did not result in nose wiping [56].

10.3.4 Peri-Ictal Coughing

Ictal coughing is rare (0.16% of patients) [60], while postictal coughing is a frequent sign in TLE, in up to 40% of patients, and it is associated with mesial temporal seizure onset [61–65]. No lateralizing significance has been demonstrated [60–65].

It is often associated with other vegetative phenomena, including salivation and retching, and it is therefore considered a reactive phenomenon to excessive autonomic stimulation caused by respiratory secretions. If, on the other hand, it occurs without other accompanying autonomic symptoms, it is thought to be directly generated by CAN activation during seizures [60–66].

10.4 Gastrointestinal Manifestations

10.4.1 Epigastric Auras

Epigastric aura is associated in 73.6% of cases with TLE and tends to correlate with MTLE [28, 45, 67]. If it is followed by ictal oral and manual automatisms, it is highly indicative of TLE (98.3% of probability) [67]. Initially, some studies have reported that the presence of epigastric aura was more frequent with nondominant temporal lobe involvement [68, 69], but it is currently agreed that epigastric auras have no localizing significance [62, 67, 70–72].

10.4.2 Ictal Vomiting and Retching in Adults

This is a rare seizure manifestation of TLE in adults, indicating seizure onset in the nondominant hemisphere [7, 73–79], even if several cases of ictal vomiting derived from the dominant temporal lobe were reported [80–82]. Some studies have failed to find a lateralizing significance of ictal vomiting [9, 83].

TLE was suspected in a case report of a 64-year-old man reporting intractable intermittent nausea and vomiting since the age of 59. The patient was screened for gastrointestinal, psychiatric, infectivological, and rheumatological dysfunction, all without pathological findings. Brain MRI was normal and routine scalp EEG demonstrated stereotyped, monomorphous intermittent paroxysmal theta and delta sequences on the left temporal derivations. Treatment with carbamazepine resulted in complete regression of the described episodes [84].

It has been proposed that ictal vomiting may be due to the activation of a complex cortical network that includes medial and lateral portions of the temporal lobe (especially the lateral superior temporal cortex), the insula, and the occipital lobe [7, 75, 77, 79]. These findings are consistent with those obtained from cortical stimulation studies, during which abdominal sensations were elicited through the stimulation of various brain areas, although vomiting could not be elicited through the stimulation of a single brain area [85, 86]. In a study based on the use of subdural grid electrodes, Kramer et al. showed that ictal vomiting is associated with the spread of seizure activity to the lateral and superior parts of the temporal lobe [75]. In the case of a 26-year-old male undergoing presurgical evaluation for refractory focal epilepsy, investigated with bilateral intracranial electrodes that included insular leads, it was shown that the occurrence of ictal vomiting correlated with exclusive involvement of the anterior part of both insular lobes [87]. Furthermore, ictal SPECT in patients presenting with ictal vomiting revealed hypoperfusion of the medial and lateral regions of the temporal lobe, with involvement of the lateral superior temporal cortex, again suggesting insular cortex involvement [79]. However, a more recent study did not confirm insular involvement in the development of this symptomatology: during stereo-EEG recording in a 4-year-and-7-month-old female, vomiting was related to a seizure originating in the mesial temporal structures without insular propagation [88].

10.4.3 Ictal Vomiting in Children

Unlike adults, who rarely experience ictal vomiting during seizures, ictal vomiting is a more frequent occurrence in children and may accompany a large number of different epilepsies [89]. The mechanism that causes vomiting in idiopathic focal epilepsies of childhood has been attributed by Guerrini et al. to an infrasylvian spread of seizure to nondominant temporal lobe [76]. In this study, three children with brain lesions between 10 and 13 years of age during photic stimulation manifested a seizure in the right occipital lobe that spread to the ipsilateral mesial temporal limbic structures and associated vomiting in the final stages of the seizure.

10.4.4 Peri-Ictal Spitting

It is a rare symptom occurring in 0.3–2% of temporal lobe seizures [8, 64, 90–92]. Most authors reported ictal spitting in seizures arising from the nondominant temporal lobe [90, 92, 93], but it has also been found in seizures arising from the dominant temporal lobe [8, 91, 94]. In a case report, a 28-year-old patient was studied with bilateral intracerebral and strip electrodes, and the epileptogenic focus was found in the left mesial temporal lobe [95]. However, the symptomatogenic area for ictal spitting has been shown to be the right hemisphere, based on the observation that the spitting occurred only after the epileptic discharge had spread to the right temporal lobe [95].

Awareness may or may not be retained during an ictal spitting. It is considered a pure motor automatism and not a symptom in response to gustatory aura; in fact, patients do not report ictal gustatory hallucination during the episode [7]. It is not associated with other symptoms such as ictal vomiting or coughing, suggesting that different brain areas are activated to mediate these symptoms [90].

10.4.5 Ictal Hypersalivation

Ictal hypersalivation in TLE appeared to be a prominent manifestation of complex focal seizures in 10 of the 590 patients (1.7%) in the cohort of patients studied by Shah et al. [96]. These patients had MTLE with hippocampal atrophy (7 with nondominant TLE and with 3 dominant TLE), and the authors found that ictal hypersalivation indicated seizure onset in the nondominant temporal lobe [96]. However, other authors have failed to replicate this result. In a study by Janszky et al., hypersalivation occurred in 12% of the patients, with equal frequency in seizure originating in the dominant or nondominant temporal lobe [8]. Hoffmann et al. observed ictal hypersalivation in 9.4% of seizures originating in the mesial and none in those originating in the lateral part of the temporal lobe; the comparison between left (11.4%) and right (6.9%) mesial temporal origin was statistically not significant [65].

10.4.6 Ictal Flatulence

A rare symptom, occurring in 0.6% of patients (2/327) of the series studied by Strzelczyk et al. [97]. Ictal flatulence indicates a temporal or/and insular involvement during seizure, without lateralizing value, and may be associated with other autonomic signs and symptoms [97–99].

10.4.7 Ictal Urge to Defecate

Reported in a few case reports, it seems to indicate seizure onset in the nondominant temporal lobe [100, 101].

10.5 Cutaneous Manifestations

10.5.1 Ictal Flushing

Metz et al. studied a 59-year-old man with TLE who presented with transient paroxysms of flushing, hypertension, tachycardia and increased plasma catecholamine levels during seizures, anticipated by an epigastric aura [102].

10.5.2 Ictal Pallor

It is a symptom observed in TLE, in patients with atrophy of the amygdala. It may be associated with ictal fear and anticipated by epigastric aura, palpitations and mydriasis [103].

10.5.3 Ictal Sweating

Ictal sweating is reported in the case of a 42-year-old man with seizures since the age of 33 years. The etiology of his epilepsy was anti-Ma2 positive autoimmune encephalitis associated with a testicular teratoma. MRI of this patient showed left insular hyperintense swelling and MTS. Clinically, seizures were characterized by an aura of a tingling sensation in the right face, followed by difficulty in left-right discrimination and aphasia and the appearance of profuse sweating of the left face; this was the first description of unilateral sweating during temporal seizures [104]. In 2019, another case report of a 60-year-old man with an episode of cyclical sweating was published. The EEG study showed left temporal lobe interictal discharges and rhythmic activity in the 6-Hz range during the episodes [105].

10.5.4 Ictal Piloerection

It occurs in 0.4–1.2% of patients with refractory seizures, especially in patients with TLE [106, 107]. Unilateral piloerection is most frequently associated with an ipsilateral seizure onset zone, whereas bilateral ictal piloerection has no lateralizing significance [108]. The insula or amygdala appears to have a pivotal role in the development of this symptomatology [108].

10.6 Sexual Manifestations

10.6.1 Sexual Auras

They are more frequent in women, suggesting a gender-specific organization of sexual function within the limbic system [109–113]. Orgasmic auras, although occurring more frequently in seizures arising from the nondominant temporal lobe, have no lateralizing significance [114, 115]. Chaton et al. documented an association between a spontaneous orgasmic aura and ictal discharges restricted to the right amygdala without involvement of the orbitofrontal, temporal basal and insular cortices, thus confirming the central role of the amygdala in human sexuality [116].

10.6.2 Genital Automatisms

More prevalent in men than women, they are related to temporal lobe seizures [117]. The manifestations, due to temporal lobe involvement, are more subtle than sexual automatisms (i.e., hypermotor movements) of frontal lobe seizures [118]. Genital automatisms have a high lateralizing value to the ipsilateral hemisphere and are mostly concordant with other unilateral hand automatisms [117].

10.7 Urinary Symptoms

10.7.1 Ictal Urinary Urge and Urination

Ictal urinary urgency and urination is a rare symptom, occurring in 0.4–3% of patients with TLE [8, 119–123]. In most patients, including two patients studied with intracranial electrodes [121, 123], seizure onset could be lateralized to the nondominant temporal lobe [119, 120, 122]; only one study failed to localize the ictal urinary stimulus [8]. The lateralization to the nondominant hemisphere may be explained by a hemispheric-specific representation of central bladder control. An Ictal SPECT study performed during ictal urinary urge demonstrated hypoperfusion of the superior temporal gyrus and insular cortex [119]. This hypothesis is further supported by PET studies in normal subjects in which urination was associated with activation of the right dorsal pontine tegmentum and right inferior frontal gyrus, whereas during the filled bladder condition the right frontal operculum and/or right anterior insula were activated [124]. Therefore, epileptic activity within the insular cortex could be responsible for a full bladder sensation and the resulting ictal urinary urge. Alternatively, ictal urinary urgency could be mediated by the propagation of epileptic activity to frontal lobe structures, i.e., the right inferior frontal gyrus, which are responsible for suprapontine bladder control [7].

10.7.2 Peri-Ictal Drinking

Defined as the action of drinking during or within 2 min after an electroclinical seizure, it is reported in 7–15% of patients with focal epilepsy [8, 9, 64, 125–130]. In the study made by Pietrafusa et al., all patients suffered from TLE and 75% of them had right hemisphere involvement. The discharge propagation went from the mesial temporal structures to the hypothalamus, possibly causing thirst activation and water-seeking [130]. The lateralization to the nondominant hemisphere could be explained by asymmetric representation of the CAN responsible for fluid control, thirst and water-seeking behavior [126]. Alternatively, patients with nondominant TLE are more often able to react to external stimuli and could therefore respond to the unpleasant sensation of thirst by water-seeking [64].

References

1. Manford M, Hart YM, Sander JW, Shorvon SD. National General Practice Study of epilepsy (NGPSE): partial seizure patterns in a general population. Neurology. 1992;42(10):1911–7. https://doi.org/10.1212/WNL.42.10.1911.
2. Freeman R, Schachter SC. Autonomic epilepsy. Semin Neurol. 1995;15(2):158–66. https://doi.org/10.1055/s-2008-1041019.

3. Freeman R. Cardiovascular manifestations of autonomic epilepsy. Clin Auton Res. 2006;16(1):12–7. https://doi.org/10.1007/s10286-006-0278-y.
4. Liporace JD, Sperling MR. Simple autonomic seizures. In: Engel Jr J, Pedley TA, editors. Epilepsy: a comprehensive textbook. Philadelphia, PA: Lippincott-Raven Publishers; 1997. p. 549–55.
5. Reeves AL. Autonomic activity in epilepsy: diagnostic considerations and implications. J Epilepsy. 1997;10:111–6.
6. Lesser RP, Lüders H, Dinner DS, Morris HHI. Simple partial seizures. In: Lüders H, Lesser RP, editors. Epilepsy: electroclinical syndromes. London: Springer; 1987. p. 223–78.
7. Baumgartner C, Lurger S, Leutmezer F. Autonomic symptoms during epileptic seizures. Epileptic Disord. 2001;3(3):103–16.
8. Janszky J, Fogarasi A, Toth V, Magalova V, Gyimesi C, Kovacs N, Schulz R, Ebner A. Peri-ictal vegetative symptoms in temporal lobe epilepsy. Epilepsy Behav. 2007;11(1):125–9. https://doi.org/10.1016/j.yebeh.2007.04.015.
9. Baysal-Kirac L, Baykan B. Current view of autonomic findings during epileptic seizures. Turk J Neurol. 2015;21:147–53.
10. Fisher RS, Cross JH, French JA, Higurashi N, Hirsch E, Jansen FE, Lagae L, Moshé SL, Peltola J, Roulet Perez E, Scheffer IE, Zuberi SM. Operational classification of seizure types by the international league against epilepsy: position paper of the ILAE Commission for Classification and Terminology. Epilepsia. 2017;58(4):522–30. https://doi.org/10.1111/epi.13670.
11. Mueller SG, Bateman LM, Laxer KD. Evidence for brainstem network disruption in temporal lobe epilepsy and sudden unexplained death in epilepsy. NeuroImage Clin. 2014;5:208–16. https://doi.org/10.1016/j.nicl.2014.06.010.
12. Nagai M, Hoshide S, Kario K. The insular cortex and cardiovascular system: a new insight into the brain-heart axis. J Am Soc Hypertens. 2010;4(4):174–82.
13. Scanlon C, Mueller SG, Cheong I, Hartig M, Weiner MW, Laxer KD. Grey and white matter abnormalities in temporal lobe epilepsy with and without mesial temporal sclerosis. J Neurol. 2013;260(9):2320–9.
14. Mueller SG, Laxer KD, Barakos J, Cheong I, Garcia P, Weiner MW. Widespread neocortical abnormalities in temporal lobe epilepsy with and without mesial sclerosis. NeuroImage. 2009;46(2):353–9.
15. Mueller SG, Laxer KD, Barakos J, Cheong I, Garcia P, Weiner MW. Subfield atrophy pattern in temporal lobe epilepsy with and without mesial sclerosis detected by high-resolution MRI at 4 tesla: preliminary results. Epilepsia. 2009;50(6):1474–83.
16. Bernhardt BC, Worsley KJ, Besson P, Concha L, Lerch JP, Evans AC, Bernasconi N. Mapping limbic network organization in temporal lobe epilepsy using morphometric correlations: insights on the relation between mesiotemporal connectivity and cortical atrophy. NeuroImage. 2008;42(2):515–24.
17. Devinsky O. Diagnosis and treatment of temporal lobe epilepsy. Rev Neurol Dis. 2004;1(1):2–9.
18. Jansen K, Lagae L. Cardiac changes in epilepsy. Seizure. 2010;19(8):455–60.
19. Eggleston KS, Olin BD, Fisher RS. Ictal tachycardia: the head-heart connection. Seizure. 2014;23(7):496–505. https://doi.org/10.1016/j.seizure.2014.02.012.
20. Shorvon S, Tomson T. Sudden unexpected death in epilepsy. Lancet. 2011;378(9808):2028–38.
21. Tomson T, Nashef L, Ryvlin P. Sudden unexpected death in epilepsy: current knowledge and future directions. Lancet Neurol. 2008;7(11):1021–31.
22. Ryvlin P, Nashef L, Lhatoo SD, Bateman LM, Bird J, Bleasel A, et al. Incidence and mechanisms of cardiorespiratory arrests in epilepsy monitoring units (MORTEMUS): a retrospective study. Lancet Neurol. 2013;12(10):966–77.
23. Bateman LM, Spitz M, Seyal M. Ictal hypoventilation contributes to cardiac arrhythmia and SUDEP: report on two deaths in video-EEG–monitored patients. Epilepsia. 2010;51(5):916–20.

24. Seyal M, Hardin KA, Bateman LM. Postictal generalized EEG suppression is linked to seizure-associated respiratory dysfunction but not postictal apnea. Epilepsia. 2012;53(5):825–31.
25. Bartolomei F, Wendling F, Vignal JP, Kochen S, Bellanger JJ, Badier JM, Le Bouquin-Jeannes R, Chauvel P. Seizures of temporal lobe epilepsy: identification of subtypes by coherence analysis using stereo-electro-encephalography. Clin Neurophysiol. 1999;110(10):1741–54. https://doi.org/10.1016/s1388-2457(99)00107-8.
26. Kanner AM, Campos M. Epilepsia del lóbulo temporal. Epilepsias Diagnóstico Tratamiento. 2004;16:263–7.
27. Williamson PD. Anatomic classification of localization-related epilepsies. Epilepsy. 1998:2405–16.
28. Maillard L, Vignal JP, Gavaret M, Guye M, Biraben A, McGonigal A, Chauvel P, Bartolomei F. Semiologic and electrophysiologic correlations in temporal lobe seizure subtypes. Epilepsia. 2004;45(12):1590–9. https://doi.org/10.1111/j.0013-9580.2004.09704.x.
29. Custer JW, Rau RE. Johns Hopkins: the harriet lane handbook. Philadelphia, PA: Elsevier Inc; 2008.
30. Garcia M, D'Giano C, Estelles S, Leiguarda R, Rabinowicz A. Ictal tachycardia: its discriminating potential between temporal and extratemporal seizure foci. Seizure. 2001;10(6):415–9.
31. Weil S, Arnold S, Eisensehr I, Noachtar S. Heart rate increase in otherwise subclinical seizures is different in temporal versus extratemporal seizure onset: support for temporal lobe autonomic influence. Epileptic Disord. 2005;7(3):199–204.
32. Schernthaner C, Lindinger G, Pötzelberger K, Zeiler K, Baumgartner C. Autonomic epilepsy—the influence of epileptic discharges on heart rate and rhythm. Wien Klin Wochenschr. 1999;111(10):392–401.
33. Di Gennaro G, Quarato PP, Sebastiano F, Esposito V, Onorati P, Grammaldo LG, et al. Ictal heart rate increase precedes EEG discharge in drug-resistant mesial temporal lobe seizures. Clin Neurophysiol. 2004;115(5):1169–77.
34. Mayer H, Benninger F, Urak L, Plattner B, Geldner J, Feucht M. EKG abnormalities in children and adolescents with symptomatic temporal lobe epilepsy. Neurology. 2004;63(2):324–8.
35. Oppenheimer SM, Gelb A, Girvin JP, Hachinski VC. Cardiovascular effects of human insular cortex stimulation. Neurology. 1992;42(9):1727.
36. Saleh Y, Kirchner A, Pauli E, Hilz MJ, Neundörfer B, Stefan H. Temporallappenepilepsien. Einfluss der Fokusseite auf die autonome regulation der Herzfrequenz? [Temporal lobe epilepsy: effect of focus side on the autonomic regulation of heart rate?]. Nervenarzt. 2000;71(6):477–80. https://doi.org/10.1007/s001150050610.
37. Hirsch M, Altenmüller DM, Schulze-Bonhage A. Latencies from intracranial seizure onset to ictal tachycardia: a comparison to surface EEG patterns and other clinical signs. Epilepsia. 2015;56(10):1639–47. https://doi.org/10.1111/epi.13117
38. van der Lende M, Surges R, Sander JW, Thijs RD. Cardiac arrhythmias during or after epileptic seizures. J Neurol Neurosurg Psychiatry. 2016;87(1):69–74. https://doi.org/10.1136/jnnp-2015-310559.
39. Rocamora R, Kurthen M, Lickfett L, Von Oertzen J, Elger CE. Cardiac asystole in epilepsy: clinical and neurophysiologic features. Epilepsia. 2003;44(2):179–85. https://doi.org/10.1046/j.1528-1157.2003.15101.x.
40. Tinuper P, Bisulli F, Cerullo A, Carcangiu R, Marini C, Pierangeli G, Cortelli P. Ictal bradycardia in partial epileptic seizures: autonomic investigation in three cases and literature review. Brain. 2001;124(Pt 12):2361–71. https://doi.org/10.1093/brain/124.12.2361.
41. Tényi D, Gyimesi C, Kupó P, Horváth R, Bóné B, Barsi P, Kovács N, Simor T, Siegler Z, Környei L, Fogarasi A, Janszky J. Ictal asystole: a systematic review. Epilepsia. 2017;58(3):356–62. https://doi.org/10.1111/epi.13644.
42. Baumgartner C, Koren J, Britto-Arias M, Schmidt S, Pirker S. Epidemiology and pathophysiology of autonomic seizures: a systematic review. Clin Auton Res. 2019;29(2):137–50. https://doi.org/10.1007/s10286-019-00596-x.

43. Schuele SU, Bermeo AC, Alexopoulos AV, Burgess RC. Anoxia-ischemia: a mechanism of seizure termination in ictal asystole. Epilepsia. 2010;51(1):170–3. https://doi.org/10.1111/j.1528-1167.2009.02168.x.
44. Ansakorpi H, Korpelainen JT, Suominen K, Tolonen U, Myllylä VV, Isojärvi JI. Interictal cardiovascular autonomic responses in patients with temporal lobe epilepsy. Epilepsia. 2000;41(1):42–7. https://doi.org/10.1111/j.1528-1157.2000.tb01503.x.
45. Foldvary N, Lee N, Thwaites G, Mascha E, Hammel J, Kim H, Friedman AH, Radtke RA. Clinical and electrographic manifestations of lesional neocortical temporal lobe epilepsy. Neurology. 1997;49(3):757–63. https://doi.org/10.1212/wnl.49.3.757.
46. Kaada BR, Jasper H. Respiratory responses to stimulation of temporal pole, insula, and hippocampal and limbic gyri in man. AMA Arch Neurol Psychiatry. 1952;68(5):609–19.
47. Lacuey N, Zonjy B, Londono L, Lhatoo SD. Amygdala and hippocampus are symptomatogenic zones for central apneic seizures. Neurology. 2017;88(7):701–5. https://doi.org/10.1212/WNL.0000000000003613.
48. Dlouhy BJ, Gehlbach BK, Kreple CJ, Kawasaki H, Oya H, Buzza C, Granner MA, Welsh MJ, Howard MA, Wemmie JA, Richerson GB. Breathing inhibited when seizures spread to the amygdala and upon amygdala stimulation. J Neurosci. 2015;35(28):10281–9. https://doi.org/10.1523/JNEUROSCI.0888-15.2015.
49. Blum AS, Ives JR, Goldberger AL, Al-Aweel IC, Krishnamurthy KB, Drislane FW, Schomer DL. Oxygen desaturations triggered by partial seizures: implications for cardiopulmonary instability in epilepsy. Epilepsia. 2000;41(5):536–41. https://doi.org/10.1111/j.1528-1157.2000.tb00206.x.
50. Bateman LM, Li CS, Seyal M. Ictal hypoxemia in localization-related epilepsy: analysis of incidence, severity and risk factors. Brain J Neurol. 2008;131(Pt 12):3239–45. https://doi.org/10.1093/brain/awn277.
51. Hopkins DA, Holstege G. Amygdaloid projections to the mesencephalon, pons and medulla oblongata in the cat. Exp Brain Res. 1978;32(4):529–47.
52. O'Regan ME, Brown JK. Abnormalities in cardiac and respiratory function observed during seizures in childhood. Dev Med Child Neurol. 2005;47(1):4–9.
53. Jansen K, Varon C, Van Huffel S, Lagae L. Ictal and interictal respiratory changes in temporal lobe and absence epilepsy in childhood. Epilepsy Res. 2013;106(3):410–6. https://doi.org/10.1016/j.eplepsyres.2013.07.008.
54. Lacuey N, Zonjy B, Hampson JP, Rani MRS, Zaremba A, Sainju RK, Gehlbach BK, Schuele S, Friedman D, Devinsky O, Nei M, Harper RM, Allen L, Diehl B, Millichap JJ, Bateman L, Granner MA, Dragon DN, Richerson GB, Lhatoo SD. The incidence and significance of periictal apnea in epileptic seizures. Epilepsia. 2018;59(3):573–82. https://doi.org/10.1111/epi.14006.
55. Leutmezer F, Serles W, Lehrner J, Pataraia E, Zeiler K, Baumgartner C. Postictal nose wiping: a lateralizing sign in temporal lobe complex partial seizures. Neurology. 1998;51(4):1175–7. https://doi.org/10.1212/wnl.51.4.1175.
56. Wennberg R. Electroclinical analysis of postictal noserubbing. Can J Neurol Sci. 2000;27(2):131–6.
57. Hirsch LJ, Lain AH, Walczak TS. Postictal nosewiping lateralizes and localizes to the ipsilateral temporal lobe. Epilepsia. 1998;39(9):991–7. https://doi.org/10.1111/j.1528-1157.1998.tb01449.x.
58. Geyer JD, Payne TA, Faught E, Drury I. Postictal nose-rubbing in the diagnosis, lateralization, and localization of seizures. Neurology. 1999;52(4):743–5. https://doi.org/10.1212/wnl.52.4.743.
59. Dupont S, Samson Y, Nguyen-Michel VH, Zavanone C, Navarro V, Baulac M, Adam C. Lateralizing value of semiology in medial temporal lobe epilepsy. Acta Neurol Scand. 2015;132(6):401–9. https://doi.org/10.1111/ane.12409.
60. Asadi-Pooya AA, Shabo L, Wyeth D, Nei M. Ictal coughing: clinical features and differential diagnoses. Epilepsy Behav. 2017;73:51–3. https://doi.org/10.1016/j.yebeh.2017.04.044.

61. Van Ness P, Marotta J, Kucera A, Klem G, Chee M. Postictal cough is a sign of temporal-lobe epilepsy. Neurology. 1993;43(4):A273–4. Philadelphia, PA: Lippincott-Raven Publ
62. Gil-Nagel A, Risinger MW. Ictal semiology in hippocampal versus extrahippocampal temporal lobe epilepsy. Brain J Neurol. 1997;120(Pt 1):183–92. https://doi.org/10.1093/brain/120.1.183.
63. Fauser S, Wuwer Y, Gierschner C, Schulze-Bonhage A. The localizing and lateralizing value of ictal/postictal coughing in patients with focal epilepsies. Seizure. 2004;13(6):403–10. https://doi.org/10.1016/j.seizure.2003.09.007.
64. Musilová K, Kuba R, Brázdil M, Tyrlíková I, Rektor I. Occurrence and lateralizing value of "rare" peri-ictal vegetative symptoms in temporal lobe epilepsy. Epilepsy Behav. 2010;19(3):372–5. https://doi.org/10.1016/j.yebeh.2010.07.010.
65. Hoffmann JM, Elger CE, Kleefuss-Lie AA. The localizing value of hypersalivation and postictal coughing in temporal lobe epilepsy. Epilepsy Res. 2009;87(2–3):144–7. https://doi.org/10.1016/j.eplepsyres.2009.08.005.
66. Wennberg R. Postictal coughing and noserubbing coexist in temporal lobe epilepsy. Neurology. 2001;56(1):133–4. https://doi.org/10.1212/wnl.56.1.133-a.
67. Henkel A, Noachtar S, Pfänder M, Lüders HO. The localizing value of the abdominal aura and its evolution: a study in focal epilepsies. Neurology. 2002;58(2):271–6. https://doi.org/10.1212/wnl.58.2.271.
68. Gupta AK, Jeavons PM, Hughes RC, Covanis A. Aura in temporal lobe epilepsy: clinical and electroencephalographic correlation. J Neurol Neurosurg Psychiatry. 1983;46(12):1079–83. https://doi.org/10.1136/jnnp.46.12.1079.
69. Taylor DC, Lochery M. Temporal lobe epilepsy: origin and significance of simple and complex auras. J Neurol Neurosurg Psychiatry. 1987;50(6):673–81. https://doi.org/10.1136/jnnp.50.6.673.
70. Palmini A, Gloor P. The localizing value of auras in partial seizures: a prospective and retrospective study. Neurology. 1992;42(4):801–8. https://doi.org/10.1212/wnl.42.4.801.
71. Fried I, Spencer DD, Spencer SS. The anatomy of epileptic auras: focal pathology and surgical outcome. J Neurosurg. 1995;83(1):60–6. https://doi.org/10.3171/jns.1995.83.1.0060.
72. Marks WJ Jr, Laxer KD. Semiology of temporal lobe seizures: value in lateralizing the seizure focus. Epilepsia. 1998;39(7):721–6. https://doi.org/10.1111/j.1528-1157.1998.tb01157.x.
73. Mitchell WG, Greenwood RS, Messenheimer JA. Abdominal epilepsy. Cyclic vomiting as the major symptom of simple partial seizures. Arch Neurol. 1983;40(4):251–2. https://doi.org/10.1001/archneur.1983.04050040081017.
74. Fiol ME, Leppik IE, Mireles R, Maxwell R. Ictus emeticus and the insular cortex. Epilepsy Res. 1988;2(2):127–31. https://doi.org/10.1016/0920-1211(88)90030-7.
75. Kramer RE, Lüders H, Goldstick LP, Dinner DS, Morris HH, Lesser RP, Wyllie E. Ictus emeticus: an electroclinical analysis. Neurology. 1988;38(7):1048–52. https://doi.org/10.1212/wnl.38.7.1048.
76. Guerrini R, Ferrari AR, Battaglia A, Salvadori P, Bonanni P. Occipitotemporal seizures with ictus emeticus induced by intermittent photic stimulation. Neurology. 1994;44(2):253–9. https://doi.org/10.1212/wnl.44.2.253.
77. Devinsky O, Frasca J, Pacia SV, Luciano DJ, Paraiso J, Doyle W. Ictus emeticus: further evidence of nondominant temporal involvement. Neurology. 1995;45(6):1158–60. https://doi.org/10.1212/wnl.45.6.1158.
78. Kotagal P, Lüders HO, Williams G, Nichols TR, McPherson J. Psychomotor seizures of temporal lobe onset: analysis of symptom clusters and sequences. Epilepsy Res. 1995;20(1):49–67. https://doi.org/10.1016/0920-1211(94)00055-2.
79. Baumgartner C, Olbrich A, Lindinger G, Pataraia E, Gröppel G, Bacher J, Aull S, Serles W, Hoffmann M, Leutmezer F, Czech T, Prayer D, Pietrzyk U, Asenbaum S, Podreka I. Regional cerebral blood flow during temporal lobe seizures associated with ictal vomiting: an ictal SPECT study in two patients. Epilepsia. 1999;40(8):1085–91. https://doi.org/10.1111/j.1528-1157.1999.tb00823.x.

80. Chen C, Yen DJ, Yiu CH, Shih YH, Yu HY, Su MS. Ictal vomiting in partial seizures of temporal lobe origin. Eur Neurol. 1999;42(4):235–9. https://doi.org/10.1159/000008114.
81. Schäuble B, Britton JW, Mullan BP, Watson J, Sharbrough FW, Marsh WR. Ictal vomiting in association with left temporal lobe seizures in a left hemisphere language-dominant patient. Epilepsia. 2002;43(11):1432–5. https://doi.org/10.1046/j.1528-1157.2002.40701.x.
82. Schindler K, Wieser HG. Ictal vomiting in a left hemisphere language-dominant patient with left-sided temporal lobe epilepsy. Epilepsy Behav. 2006;8(1):323–7. https://doi.org/10.1016/j.yebeh.2005.10.014.
83. Tarnutzer AA, Mothersill I, Imbach LL. Ictal nausea and vomiting - is it left or right? Seizure. 2018;61:83–8. https://doi.org/10.1016/j.seizure.2018.08.011.
84. Terzaghi M, Sartori I, Rustioni V, Manni R. Cyclic vomiting syndrome in adults: disregarding a possible epileptic component? Neurogastroenterol Motil. 2009;21(1):95–6. https://doi.org/10.1111/j.1365-2982.2008.01211.x.
85. Penfield W, Jasper H. Epilepsy and the functional anatomy of the human brain, vol. 47. Boston, MA: Little, Brown & Co.; 1954. p. 704.
86. Van Buren JM. The abdominal aura. A study of abdominal sensations occurring in epilepsy and produced by depth stimulation. Electroencephalogr Clin Neurophysiol. 1963;15:1–19. https://doi.org/10.1016/0013-4694(63)90035-x.
87. Catenoix H, Isnard J, Guénot M, Petit J, Remy C, Mauguière F. The role of the anterior insular cortex in ictal vomiting: a stereotactic electroencephalography study. Epilepsy Behav. 2008;13(3):560–3. https://doi.org/10.1016/j.yebeh.2008.06.019.
88. Pietrafusa N, de Palma L, De Benedictis A, Trivisano M, Marras CE, Vigevano F, Specchio N. Ictal vomiting as a sign of temporal lobe epilepsy confirmed by stereo-EEG and surgical outcome. Epilepsy Behav. 2015;53:112–6. https://doi.org/10.1016/j.yebeh.2015.10.009.
89. Pal DK, Ferrie C, Addis L, Akiyama T, Capovilla G, Caraballo R, de Saint-Martin A, Fejerman N, Guerrini R, Hamandi K, Helbig I, Ioannides AA, Kobayashi K, Lal D, Lesca G, Muhle H, Neubauer BA, Pisano T, Rudolf G, Seegmuller C, et al. Idiopathic focal epilepsies: the "lost tribe". Epileptic Disord. 2016;18(3):252–88. https://doi.org/10.1684/epd.2016.0839.
90. Voss NF, Davies KG, Boop FA, Montouris GD, Hermann BP. Spitting automatism in complex partial seizures: a nondominant temporal localizing sign? Epilepsia. 1999;40(1):114–6. https://doi.org/10.1111/j.1528-1157.1999.tb01998.x.
91. Vojvodic N, Ristic AJ, Bascarevic V, Popovic L, Parojcic A, Koprivsek K, Sveljo O, Sokic D. Ictal spitting in left temporal lobe epilepsy and fMRI speech lateralization. Clin Neurol Neurosurg. 2013;115(4):495–7. https://doi.org/10.1016/j.clineuro.2012.06.009.
92. Kellinghaus C, Loddenkemper T, Kotagal P. Ictal spitting: clinical and electroencephalographic features. Epilepsia. 2003;44(8):1064–9. https://doi.org/10.1046/j.1528-1157.2003.67302.x.
93. Ozkara C, Hanoglu L, Eşkazan E, Kulaksizogvlu IB, Ozyurt E. Ictal spitting during a left emporal lobe-originated complex partial seizure: a case report. Epileptic Disord. 2000;2(3):169–72.
94. Quevedo-Diaz M, Campo AT, Vila-Vidal M, Principe A, Ley M, Rocamora R. Ictal spitting in non-dominant temporal lobe epilepsy: an anatomo-electrophysiological correlation. Epileptic Disord. 2018;20(2):139–45. https://doi.org/10.1684/epd.2018.0963.
95. Park SM, Lee SA, Kim JH, Kang JK. Ictal spitting in a patient with dominant temporal lobe epilepsy: supporting evidence of ictal spitting from the nondominant hemisphere. Eur Neurol. 2007;57(1):47–9. https://doi.org/10.1159/000097010.
96. Shah J, Zhai H, Fuerst D, Watson C. Hypersalivation in temporal lobe epilepsy. Epilepsia. 2006;47(3):644–51. https://doi.org/10.1111/j.1528-1167.2006.00480.x.
97. Strzelczyk A, Nowak M, Bauer S, Reif PS, Oertel WH, Knake S, Hamer HM, Rosenow F. Localizing and lateralizing value of ictal flatulence. Epilepsy Behav. 2010;17(2):278–82. https://doi.org/10.1016/j.yebeh.2009.12.010.
98. Penfield W, Faulk ME Jr. The insula; further observations on its function. Brain. 1955;78(4):445–70. https://doi.org/10.1093/brain/78.4.445.

99. Vittal NB, Singh P, Azar NJ. Ictal flatulence: seizure onset in the nondominant hemisphere. Epilepsy Behav. 2009;16(4):663–5. https://doi.org/10.1016/j.yebeh.2009.09.019.
100. Koubeissi MZ, Crone NE, Lesser RP. Seizures manifesting as an urge to defecate, with an ictal discharge in the right hemisphere. Epilepsia. 2005;46(8):1330–2. https://doi.org/10.1111/j.1528-1167.2005.17505.x.
101. Taieb G, Renard D, Labauge P, Janicot F, Briere C. Ictal urge to defecate associated with a right-sided mesial temporal cavernoma. Epilepsy Behav. 2012;24(2):272–3. https://doi.org/10.1016/j.yebeh.2012.04.112.
102. Metz SA, Halter JB, Porte D Jr, Robertson RP. Autonomic epilepsy: clonidine blockade of paroxysmal catecholamine release and flushing. Ann Intern Med. 1978;88(2):189–93. https://doi.org/10.7326/0003-4819-88-2-189.
103. Cendes F, Andermann F, Gloor P, Gambardella A, Lopes-Cendes I, Watson C, Evans A, Carpenter S, Olivier A. Relationship between atrophy of the amygdala and ictal fear in temporal lobe epilepsy. Brain. 1994;117(Pt 4):739–46. https://doi.org/10.1093/brain/117.4.739.
104. Franco AC, Noachtar S, Rémi J. Ictal ipsilateral sweating in focal epilepsy. Seizure. 2017;50:4–5. https://doi.org/10.1016/j.seizure.2017.05.009.
105. Chelmowski MK, Morris GL 3rd. Cyclical sweating caused by temporal lobe seizures. Ann Intern Med. 2019;170(11):813–4. https://doi.org/10.7326/L18-0425.
106. Stefan H, Pauli E, Kerling F, Schwarz A, Koebnick C. Autonomic auras: left hemispheric predominance of epileptic generators of cold shivers and goose bumps? Epilepsia. 2002;43(1):41–5. https://doi.org/10.1046/j.1528-1157.2002.21001.x.
107. Rocamora R, Becerra JL, Fossas P, Gomez M, Vivanco-Hidalgo RM, Mauri JA, Molins A. Pilomotor seizures: an autonomic semiology of limbic encephalitis? Seizure. 2014;23(8):670–3. https://doi.org/10.1016/j.seizure.2014.04.013.
108. Loddenkemper T, Kellinghaus C, Gandjour J, Nair DR, Najm IM, Bingaman W, Lüders HO. Localising and lateralising value of ictal piloerection. J Neurol Neurosurg Psychiatry. 2004;75(6):879–83. https://doi.org/10.1136/jnnp.2003.023333.
109. Aull-Watschinger S, Pataraia E, Baumgartner C. Sexual auras: predominance of epileptic activity within the mesial temporal lobe. Epilepsy Behav. 2008;12(1):124–7. https://doi.org/10.1016/j.yebeh.2007.07.007.
110. Bente D, Kluge E. Sexuelle Reizzustände im Rahmen des Uncinatus-Syndroms; ein klinischer Beitrag zur Pathophysiologie und Pathobiologie des Archicortex [Sexual irritation conditions in the scope of uncinatus syndrome; a clinical contribution to pathophysiology and pathobiology of archicortex]. Archiv Psychiatrie Nervenkrankheiten. 1953;190(4):357–76. https://doi.org/10.1007/BF01225303.
111. Currier RD, Little SC, Suess JF, Andy OJ. Sexual seizures. Arch Neurol. 1971;25(3):260–4. https://doi.org/10.1001/archneur.1971.00490030086010
112. Freemon FR, Nevis AH. Temporal lobe sexual seizures. Neurology. 1969;19(1):87–90. https://doi.org/10.1212/wnl.19.1.87.
113. Rémillard GM, Andermann F, Testa GF, Gloor P, Aubé M, Martin JB, Feindel W, Guberman A, Simpson C. Sexual ictal manifestations predominate in women with temporal lobe epilepsy: a finding suggesting sexual dimorphism in the human brain. Neurology. 1983;33(3):323–30. https://doi.org/10.1212/wnl.33.3.323.
114. Janszky J, Szücs A, Halász P, Borbély C, Holló A, Barsi P, Mirnics Z. Orgasmic aura originates from the right hemisphere. Neurology. 2002;58(2):302–4. https://doi.org/10.1212/wnl.58.2.302.
115. Janszky J, Ebner A, Szupera Z, Schulz R, Hollo A, Szücs A, Clemens B. Orgasmic aura—A report of seven cases. Seizure. 2004;13(6):441–4. https://doi.org/10.1016/j.seizure.2003.09.005.
116. Chaton L, Chochoi M, Reyns N, Lopes R, Derambure P, Szurhaj W. Localization of an epileptic orgasmic feeling to the right amygdala, using intracranial electrodes. Cortex. 2018;109:347–51. https://doi.org/10.1016/j.cortex.2018.07.013.

117. Dede HÖ, Bebek N, Gürses C, Baysal-Kıraç L, Baykan B, Gökyiğit A. Genital automatisms: reappraisal of a remarkable but ignored symptom of focal seizures. Epilepsy Behav. 2018;80:84–9. https://doi.org/10.1016/j.yebeh.2017.12.023.
118. Mascia A, Di Gennaro G, Esposito V, Grammaldo LG, Meldolesi GN, Giampà T, Sebastiano F, Falco C, Onorati P, Manfredi M, Cantore G, Quarato PP. Genital and sexual manifestations in drug-resistant partial epilepsy. Seizure. 2005;14(2):133–8. https://doi.org/10.1016/j.seizure.2004.12.002.
119. Baumgartner C, Gröppel G, Leutmezer F, Aull-Watschinger S, Pataraia E, Feucht M, Trinka E, Unterberger I, Bauer G. Ictal urinary urge indicates seizure onset in the nondominant temporal lobe. Neurology. 2000;55(3):432–4. https://doi.org/10.1212/wnl.55.3.432.
120. Loddenkemper T, Foldvary N, Raja S, Neme S, Lüders HO. Ictal urinary urge: further evidence for lateralization to the nondominant hemisphere. Epilepsia. 2003;44(1):124–6. https://doi.org/10.1046/j.1528-1157.2003.26202.x.
121. Gurgenashvili K, Massey SL, Grant M, Piatt J Jr, Legido A, Valencia I. Intracranial localisation of ictal urinary urge epileptogenic zone to the non-dominant temporal lobe. Epileptic Disord. 2011;13(4):430–4. https://doi.org/10.1684/epd.2011.0476.
122. Yilmaz S, Gokben S, Turhan T, Serdaroglu G, Tekgul H. Ictal urinary urge: localization and lateralization value in a pediatric case. Child's Nerv Syst. 2015;31(12):2383–5. https://doi.org/10.1007/s00381-015-2816-1.
123. Rengarajan R, Shamim S. Urinary urge seizure semiology localization by intracranial monitoring. Proc (Bayl Univ Med Cent). 2018;31(1):109–11. https://doi.org/10.1080/08998280.2017.1400880.
124. Blok BF, Sturms LM, Holstege G. Brain activation during micturition in women. Brain. 1998;121(Pt 11):2033–42. https://doi.org/10.1093/brain/121.11.2033.
125. Szucs A, Fogarasi A, Rásonyi G, Kelemen A, Narula L, Tóth V, Janszky J, Halász P. Peri-ictal water drinking in temporal lobe epilepsy: is it a reliable lateralizing sign? Epilepsy Behav. 2007;11(4):578–81. https://doi.org/10.1016/j.yebeh.2007.07.012.
126. Trinka E, Walser G, Unterberger I, Luef G, Benke T, Bartha L, Ortler M, Bauer G. Peri-ictal water drinking lateralizes seizure onset to the nondominant temporal lobe. Neurology. 2003;60(5):873–6. https://doi.org/10.1212/01.wnl.0000049459.83589.6c.
127. Rémillard GM, Andermann F, Gloor P, Olivier A, Martin JB. Water-drinking as ictal behavior in complex partial seizures. Neurology. 1981;31(2):117–24. https://doi.org/10.1212/wnl.31.2.117.
128. Errguig L, Lahjouji F, Belaidi H, Jiddane M, Elkhamlichi A, Dakka T, Ouazzani R. Peri-ictal water drinking and other ictal vegetative symptoms: localizing and lateralizing the epileptogenic zone in temporal lobe epilepsy? Two case reports and review of the literature. Rev Neurol. 2013;169(11):903–10. https://doi.org/10.1016/j.neurol.2013.06.005.
129. Sheikh Z, Olango W, Raval B, Marks D. Ictal water-seeking in nondominant temporal lobe seizures. Neurology. 2016;86(19):1847–8. https://doi.org/10.1212/WNL.0000000000002662.
130. Pietrafusa N, Trivisano M, de Palma L, Serino D, Moavero R, Benvenga A, Cappelletti S, Boero G, Vigevano F, La Neve A, Specchio N. Peri-ictal water drinking: a rare automatic behaviour in temporal lobe epilepsy. Epileptic Disord. 2015;17(4):384–96. https://doi.org/10.1684/epd.2015.0776.

Chapter 11
Autonomic Involvement in Childhood Epilepsy

Pasquale Parisi, Vittorio Sciruicchio, Daniela D'Agnano, Vincenzo Raieli, Giovanni Di Nardo, and Alessandro Ferretti

Abbreviations

ASMs	Anti-seizure medications
CAN	Central autonomic network
DEE	Developmental and epileptic encephalopathies
EDA	Electrodermal activity
EEG	Electroencephalogram
EE-SWAS	Epileptic encephalopathy with spike-and-wave activation in sleep
HRV	Heart rate variability
IA	Ictal apnoea
ILAE	International League Against Epilepsy
PGES	Postictal generalized EEG suppression
SeLEAS	Self-limited epilepsy with autonomic seizures

P. Parisi (✉) · G. Di Nardo · A. Ferretti
Pediatrics,Unit, Department of Neuroscience, Mental Health and Sense Organs (NESMOS), Faculty of Medicine and Psychology, Sapienza University, Sant'Andrea Hospital, Rome, Italy
e-mail: pasquale.parisi@uniroma1.it; giovanni.dinardo@uniroma1.it; alessandro.ferretti@uniroma1.it

V. Sciruicchio · D. D'Agnano
Children Epilepsy and EEG Center, PO, San Paolo ASL (Azienda Sanitaria Locale), Bari, Italy
e-mail: vittorio.sciruicchio@asl.bari.it

V. Raieli
Child Neurology and Psychiatry Unit—ISMEP, ARNAS Civico, Palermo, Italy

G. Micieli et al. (eds.), *Autonomic Disorders in Clinical Practice*,
https://doi.org/10.1007/978-3-031-43036-7_11

SeLECTS	Self-limited epilepsy with centrotemporal spikes
SeLFE	Self-limited focal epilepsies of childhood
SUDEP	Sudden unexpected death in epilepsy
TCSs	Tonic-clonic seizures
TLE	Temporal lobe epilepsy
VNS	Vagus nerve stimulation

11.1 Introduction

Epileptic seizures are characterized by recurrent, paroxysmal, and unprovoked episodes of cerebral cortical dysfunction, due to abnormal excessive or synchronous neuronal activity in the brain [1]. During seizures involuntary movements, sensory phenomena, altered levels of consciousness, behavior abnormalities, impairments in cognitive function, and abnormal autonomic phenomena may occur. Many different autonomic symptoms appear during epileptic seizures, some of which are rarely considered life-threatening. In 2007, an international working group of expert researchers defined autonomic seizure as "an epileptic seizure characterized by altered autonomic function of any type at seizure onset or in which manifestations consistent with altered autonomic function are prominent (qualitatively dominant or clinically important) even if not present at seizure onset". The same researchers suggested the following terminology to define autonomic status epilepticus: "an autonomic seizure which lasts more than 30 min, or a series of such seizures over a 30-min period without full recovery between seizures" [2]. The latter condition is typically observed in epilepsy previously named Panayiotopoulos syndrome (PS). Other focal seizures, especially in childhood, may manifest only as autonomic symptoms or signs [3]. The International League Against Epilepsy (ILAE) recently contributed to the classification of autonomic symptoms present in both focal and generalized seizures. The most recent edition of the ILAE's classification (2017) presents a three-level model, beginning with seizure type and progressing to epilepsy diagnosis (focal epilepsy, generalized epilepsy, combined generalized and focal epilepsy, and unknown epilepsy group). The last level is that of epileptic syndrome: a specific syndrome diagnosis can be made based on clinical seizure types, neurologic manifestations, and electroencephalographic (EEG) patterns, often supported by specific etiological findings (structural, genetic, metabolic, immunological, and infectious) [4]. The syndromes often have age-dependent presentations and a range of specific comorbidities (Fig. 11.1). In clinical practice, epileptic syndrome identification is important for appropriate antiepileptic drug selection, prognosis, and parent counseling.

The expanded ILAE 2017 operational classification encourages the identification of seizure type. Focal seizures with retained or impaired awareness may optionally be characterized by one of the motor-onset or non-motor-onset symptoms listed in Fig. 11.2. In this operational classification, non-motor focal seizures may manifest as autonomic dysfunction, behavior arrest, cognitive, emotional, or sensory

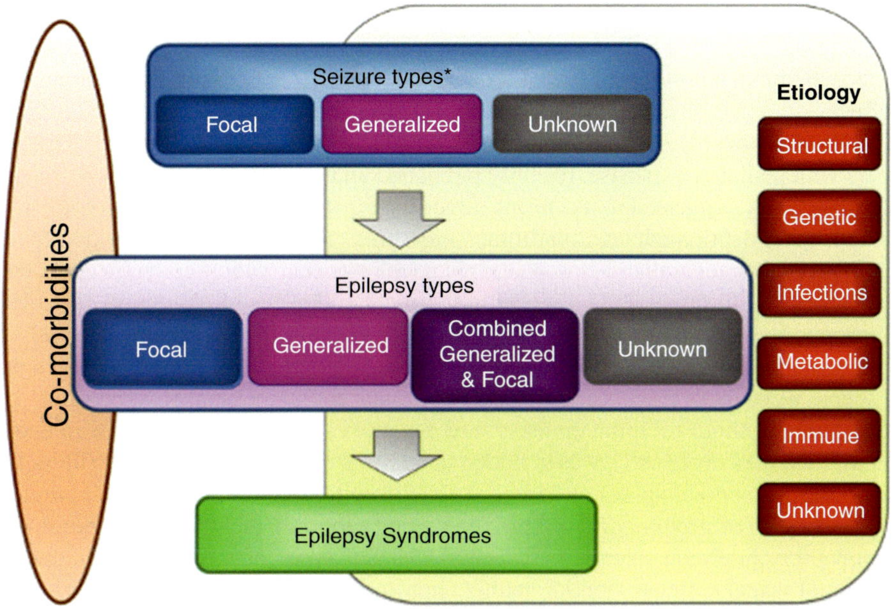

Fig. 11.1 Framework for classification of the epilepsies according to the ILAE 2017. (From Scheffer et al. 2017 [5] with permission)

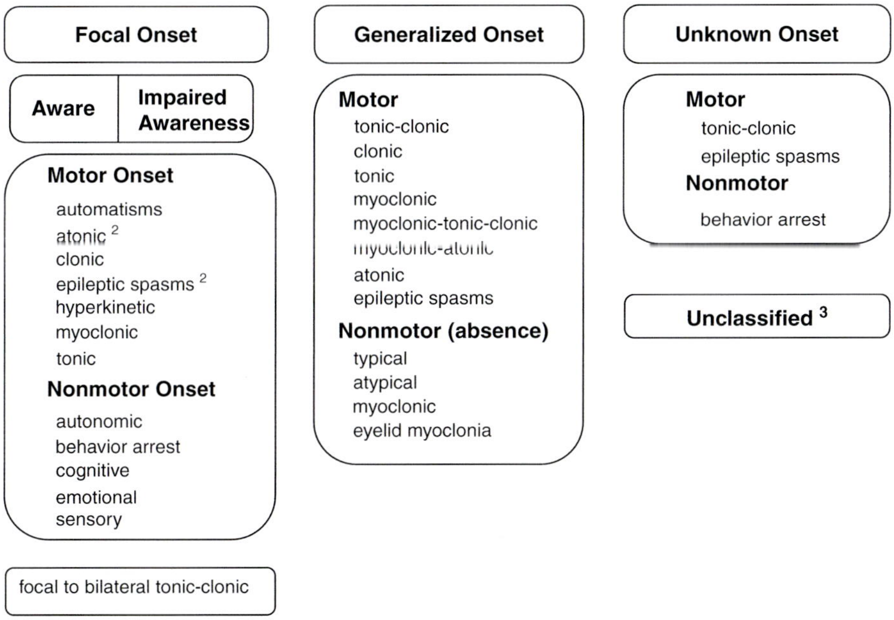

Fig. 11.2 Scheme of the new operational classification of seizure types promoted by ILAE 2017 (from Fisher et al. 2017 [4] with permission).[2] The degree of impaired awareness is often not specified.[3] Unclassifiable due to lack of information or inability to classify the episode into a category

dysfunction. According to this classification, "focal autonomic seizures can present with gastrointestinal sensations, a sense of heat or cold, flushing, piloerection (goosebumps), palpitations, sexual arousal, respiratory changes, or other autonomic effects" [5].

Based on the 2017 seizure classification, an ILAE Task Force composed of members with pediatric expertise, recently published an update on the taxonomy of syndromes. They suggested to use terms directly describing the seizure semiology and classified epileptic pediatric syndromes into three categories: (1) self-limited focal epilepsies; (2) generalized epilepsies; (3) developmental and/or epileptic encephalopathies [6]. In the context of self-limited focal epilepsies of childhood (SeLFE), the authors described syndromes with specific clinical, seizure semiology, and electroencephalographic (EEG) features. Based on their long-term prognosis two subgroups were identified. In the first subgroup, Panayiotopoulos syndrome, or early-onset benign occipital epilepsy now renamed self-limited epilepsy with autonomic seizures (SeLEAS), was included in addition to benign epilepsy of childhood with centrotemporal spikes or benign Rolandic epilepsy, now renamed self-limited epilepsy with centrotemporal spikes. The second subgroup included two syndromes: idiopathic childhood occipital epilepsy—Gastaut type, now renamed childhood occipital visual epilepsy, and idiopathic photosensitive occipital lobe epilepsy, now renamed photosensitive occipital lobe epilepsy. Clinically significant autonomic symptoms and signs can also accompany seizures of focal, generalized, and/or unknown onset. SeLEAS, known as Panayiotopoulos syndrome, is a model of autonomic epilepsy specific to childhood (see below). Furthermore, ictal autonomic manifestations are frequently underreported either because they are unrecognized, given their predominantly nocturnal onset, or forgiven. In a recent prospective survey, only 11% of documented autonomic features were recalled by the patient [7]. The clinical range and significance of autonomic dysfunction during seizures are not fully understood and, in many cases, seizures are classified by the earliest prominent motor or nonmotor onset feature [8]. As reported elsewhere in this book, the central autonomic network (CAN) is often involved during the propagation of both focal and generalized seizures. A wide variety of clinical events are thought to be mediated by cortical discharges recruiting CAN pathways [9]. In addition, as already mentioned and reported in several studies, autonomic symptoms and signs are frequently childhood-related because of a susceptibility to autonomic seizures due to a lower seizure threshold of subcortical components, related to a supposed immaturity of CAN [2, 10]. Assessment of autonomic functions involved in seizures results in two outcomes: first, a better localization and management of epilepsies; second, the correct framing of some autonomic disorders co-occurring in sudden unexpected death in epilepsy (SUDEP) could facilitate the use of measures that would help to reduce mortality of people with epilepsy. This chapter will focus on autonomic signs and symptoms in epileptic seizures and the most common forms of epilepsy associated with autonomic phenomena will be considered (SeLEAS or Panayiotopoulos syndrome and Temporal lobe epilepsy). In addition, the clinical aspects underlying SUDEP will be described.

11.2 Autonomic Seizures: The Role of Central Autonomic Network

Clinical features of seizures in epilepsy result from the recruitment or dysfunction of specific areas of the brain. These areas may have a functional relationship to anatomically close areas, but seizures can also propagate to distant areas of the brain. In other words, a network dysfunction, due to poor integration of neurons, facilitates the aberrant generation and propagation of neuronal discharges. Autonomic changes are frequent manifestations of epileptic seizures [11, 12]. During seizures, autonomic symptoms may be the only ones or predominant clinical features, as in simple autonomic seizures, or accompany both focal and generalized seizures. In all these cases, autonomic seizures are characterized by recurrent stereotypical symptoms affecting the cardiovascular, neuroendocrine, respiratory, genitourinary, sexual, gastrointestinal systems, and/or cutaneous and pupillary symptoms. Direct activation of the CAN by epileptic discharges, rather than the motor or behavioral effects of the seizures themselves may cause autonomic symptoms and signs [11]. The role of the CAN and possible dysfunction of this area is assessed by functional neuroimaging, particularly functional magnetic resonance imaging [13]. The CAN is an integral component of an internal regulation system that includes the insular cortex, orbitofrontal cortex, anterior cingulate cortex, amygdala, hypothalamus, periaqueductal grey matter, parabrachial complex nucleus, the nucleus of the solitary tract, ventrolateral reticular formation of the medulla, and medullary raphe. The CAN is characterized by reciprocal interconnections and receives converging visceral and somatosensory information, through which the brain controls visceromotor, neuroendocrine, pain, and behavioral responses essential for survival [14]. From a functional and methodological point of view, this network is a structure divided into three main components in relation to distinctive regions of the central nervous system:

(a) The spinal cord contains neuronal bodies and Projections causing the elementary segmental reflex control of the autonomic nervous system functions (Fig. 11.3).
(b) At the brainstem level, the nucleus of the solitary tract, the ventrolateral medulla, and the parabrachial nucleus of the dorsolateral pons are involved in cardiovascular, respiratory, gastrointestinal, and genitourinary autonomic systems regulation. The periaqueductal grey in the midbrain region integrates autonomic control with pain Modulation and behavioral responses to stress and sleep (Fig. 11.3).
(c) Finally, at the forebrain level, the hypothalamus integrates autonomic, endocrine, and sleep functions, while the anterior limbic circuit (anterior cingulate cortex, amygdala, and insular cortices) integrates bodily sensation and pain with the emotional autonomic response [14] (Fig. 11.3).

These regions control the peripheral autonomic function through both direct and indirect connections with centers in the lower brainstem [13, 15].

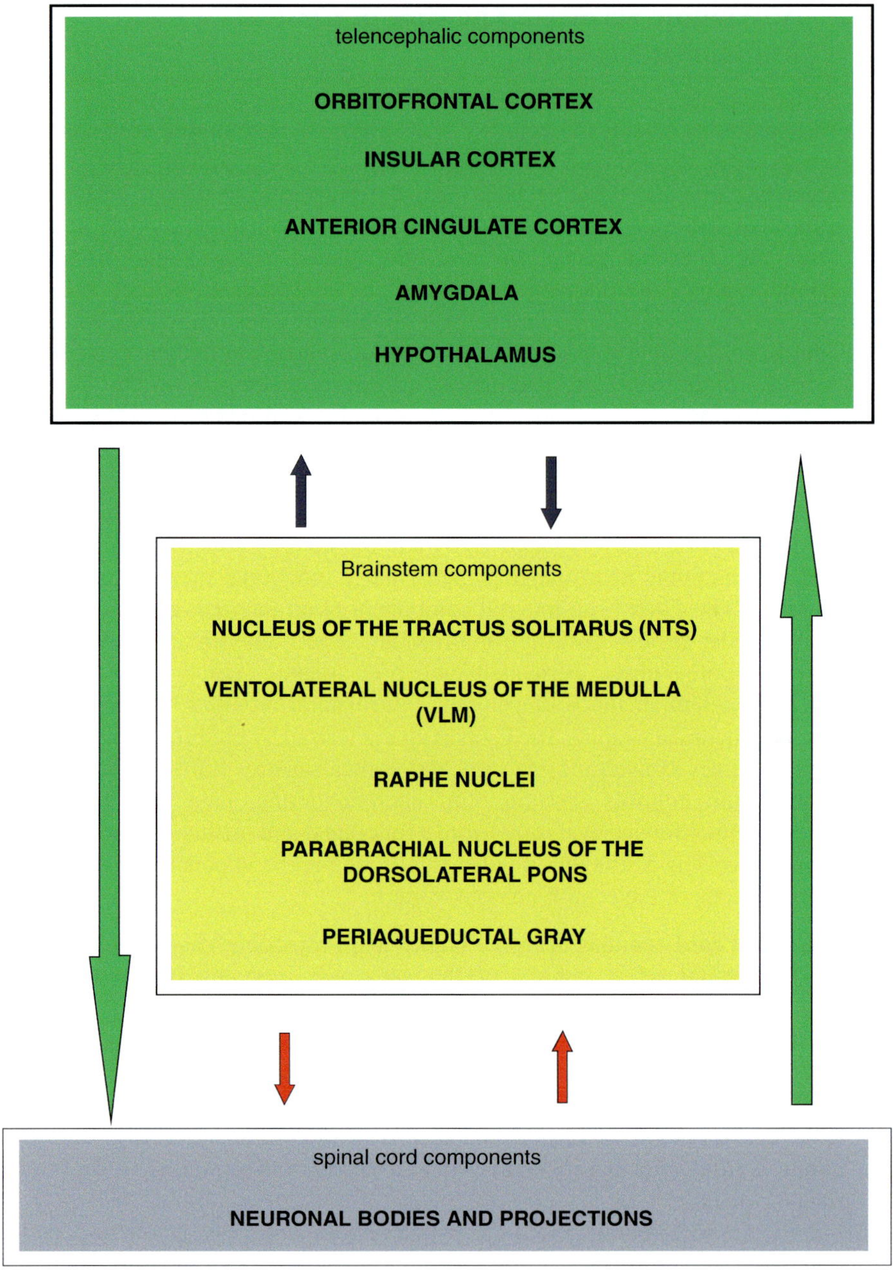

Fig. 11.3 Principal components of the Central Autonomic Network (CAN) from the cerebral neocortex to the spinal cord. The lower segments of the CAN are regulated by the higher centers. There exist reciprocal connections between the structures. The CAN which exerts a modulating influence on the peripheral autonomic system is directly influenced by the limbic system and the epileptic foci. The real organization of CAN is much more complex than presented here

Structures responsible for the sympathetic response include the noradrenergic neurons of the locus coeruleus and the ventrolateral medulla oblongata. The parabrachial region, nucleus ambiguous, the nucleus of the vagus nerve, corpus amygdaloideum, and periaqueductal grey matter influence parasympathetic mechanisms. Other areas play a role in both modalities [16].

The area postrema, also known as the chemoreceptor trigger zone, is one of the regions linked to vomiting. The motor elements of vomiting are controlled by the dorsal vagal nucleus, the nucleus of the solitary tract, the parvocellular reticular formation, and the ventral respiratory groups [14]. Extensive functional neuroimaging studies show that the autonomic symptoms, especially in self-limiting forms of epilepsy are related to the lower seizure threshold caused by the hyperexcitability of specific autonomic circuits connected with motor or sensory responses. Otherwise, primary epileptogenic activity may spread to higher-order brain areas when reaching the symptomatogenic threshold resulting in focal seizures that could evolve into generalized seizures [17]. In general, the autonomic disturbances present in different epileptic seizures can be classified according to their presentation during a seizure so that ictal and post-ictal forms can be distinguished. The autonomic signs have an early ictal onset when the cortex early involved in the central autonomic network. Conversely, the autonomic symptoms occur in the post-event or later in the ictal period [18].

11.3 Autonomic Changes in the Ictal Phase

11.3.1 Cardiovascular Symptoms

Since the first description of the relationship between the brain and heart in people with epilepsy more than a century ago, several studies have shown that seizures, both generalized and focal, induce autonomic dysfunction of the cardiovascular system [19, 20]. Cardiovascular alterations, specifically seizure-related cardiac arrhythmias, play an important role in determining the excess of mortality in patients with epilepsy and they have been implicated as potential pathomechanisms of SUDEP. Ictal sinus tachycardia can be observed in 82% of patients with epilepsy, as reported in a previous review. The authors reported that the average percentage of seizures associated with significant heart rate changes is similar for generalized (64%), including generalized tonic–clonic seizures, and focal onset seizures (71%) [21]. Focal seizures evolving to bilateral tonic–clonic seizures show a higher ictal heart rate as compared to focal seizures with impaired awareness [22]. Since the earliest observations in the rat, some authors demonstrated that cardiac regulation involved the right insula for sympathetic control and the left insula for parasympathetic control [23, 24]. These findings are still debated [25]. In a study using intracranial electrodes, the EEG signal precedes other seizure manifestations, but ictal tachycardia was reported to be an early sign, especially in right mesial temporal onset seizures [26]. In childhood epilepsy, available studies on ictal tachycardia are limited but no significant differences seem to be in the frequencies of ictal tachycardia in adults versus children [10]. Some authors reported ictal tachycardia in TLE seizures in 98% and confirmed right hemispheric lateralization of sympathetic cardiac control [27]. A recent study suggested that epilepsy duration is an independent risk factor for ECG changes and that cardiac alterations may be a time-dependent phenomenon [28]. Ictal Bradycardia occurs less commonly during seizures than tachycardia and is observed in <5% of seizures [29]. In a cohort of 49 children, similar results were reported (3.7% of seizures had ictal bradycardia) [30]. Occasionally the bradycardia may be severe enough to cause sinus arrest and asystole. Cardiac asystole is infrequent. In a previous study, in a large cohort, cardiac asystole occurred in 7 out of 2003 patients (0.34%), undergoing long-term video EEG/ECG monitoring [31]. This is in line with the reported 0.27–0.4% of patients suffering ictal asystole during prolonged video EEG telemetry [32]. In two different systematic reviews, it was reported that all patients examined, 103 cases in the first and 157 in the second, who presented with ictal asystole suffered from focal epilepsy [33, 34]. Prolonged cerebral hypoperfusion induced by asystole may result in the onset of syncope. Ictal asystole with subsequent syncope predominantly happens in people with temporal lobe epilepsy [33, 35]. In a cortical stimulation study, Oppenheimer et al. confirmed that bradycardia appears during stimulation of the left insular cortex. This result suggested that seizures occurring in the left hemisphere are more frequently associated with ictal bradycardia [23]. In the 20 s after the end of the electroencephalographic discharge, such as the postictal period, ictal asystole can occur. In the aforementioned review, 13 patients presented with postictal asystole, among them 85% presented focal seizures evolving into bilateral tonic-clonic seizures (TCSs) [33]. During the ictal and peri-ictal periods, other cardiac arrhythmias, including atrial flutter/atrial fibrillation and postictal ventricular fibrillation, were identified [2, 33, 36, 37]. Postictal ventricular fibrillation is preceded mainly by focal to bilateral seizures. In these conditions, increasing sympathetic activity, peri-ictal QTc prolongation and other predisposing cardiac conditions may be contributing factors anti-seizure medications (ASMs), such as sodium channel blockers, including carbamazepine, lacosamide, lamotrigine, and phenytoin, may play an important role in determining variation in heart rate frequency, firstly bradycardia, particularly at high dosages [22, 38]. However, Lamberts et al., suggested that concomitant heart disease more than epileptic features may lead to cardiovascular symptoms [39].

11.3.2 Respiratory Manifestations

Automatic mechanisms of respiration are controlled by the central respiratory oscillators located in the lower brain stem, under the control of forebrain cortical areas (hippocampal formation; anterior cingulate gyrus; insula; basal forebrain; and the motor area). Focal seizures localized in these cortical areas could affect respiration and early experimental stimulation studies, show that the activation of these areas results in irregular breathing patterns, end-expiratory apnoea, and hyperpnoea [40]. Due to anatomical location, temporal lobe epilepsy is commonly associated with apnoea and oxygen desaturations [41, 42]. Hyperventilation is a common underdiagnosed sign of seizures because monitoring of respiratory activity is not always performed during electroencephalographic recording. In a polygraphic video-EEG recordings study, on 57 pre-surgery patients, authors reported that central apnoea with oxygen desaturation and increased CO2 levels occur in around one-third of seizures [43]. The authors also observed that ictal oxygen desaturations of <90%, <80%, and <70% were shown in 33.2%, 10.2%, and 3.6% of all seizures. In this study, the degree of desaturation was significantly correlated with temporal lobe seizure onset, right hemispheric seizure lateralization, duration, and contralateral spread [43]. In a study based on cardiorespiratory monitoring and video EEG monitoring, ictal central apnoea preceded EEG seizure onset in 54.3% of cases and it was the only clinical manifestation in 16.5% of seizures [41]. The onset of central ictal apnoea (IA) depends on the quickness of the seizure spreading from one temporal lobe to the contralateral. Patients with TLE with contralateral diffusion are at the highest risk of seizure-related respiratory dysfunctions [44]. Other respiratory-related autonomic phenomena during seizures include stridor, postictal nose wiping, peri-ictal coughing, and other respiratory manifestations (i.e., laryngospasm, nocturnal choking, and laryngeal constriction) [3]. Unilateral postictal nose-wiping was reported as a symptom of localizing and lateralizing in focal epilepsy. Indeed, it occurs in 40–50% of patients with temporal lobe epilepsy and it is highly predictive (92%) of seizure onset ipsilateral to the used hand [45, 46]. Nose wiping happens during seizures originating in the non-dominant temporal lobe and can be interpreted as a purposeful reaction to rhinorrhoea. The use of the hand ipsilateral to the hemisphere of seizure onset is due to a contralateral postictal weakness or neglect [45]. Furthermore, a depth electrode study has demonstrated that the involvement of the amygdala is crucial for the induction of postictal nose wiping [47]. Ictal coughing is a rare autonomic symptom, reported only in 0.16% of a large cohort of patients, without clear localization or lateralization [48]; conversely, post ictal coughing has been reported in 25% of patients [49]. The simultaneous presence of hypersalivation and retching could be a response to excessive autonomic stimulation and subsequent increased respiratory secretions and, in the absence of additional autonomic symptoms, suggest direct activation of CAN. Usually, the origin of these phenomena is in the mesial portion of the temporal lobe, unclear is the lateralization [47, 50]. Most anecdotal observations deal with symptoms such as laryngospasm, referred to seizures originating from the frontal operculum [51] and choking sensation due to frontal lobe seizures, which are often misdiagnosed with OSAS [52].

11.3.3 Gastrointestinal Symptoms

In adulthood, gastrointestinal auras are the most common symptoms of focal epilepsy [11, 53]. In the most recent systematic review, the authors suggest that, in 83% of cases, the gastrointestinal aura originates from the temporal lobe, specifically the mesial temporal lobe. In previous studies, authors reported that abdominal feelings are associated with focal seizures originating from the non-dominant temporal lobe, but this data has not been confirmed [54, 55].

11.3.3.1 Ictal Vomiting in Adults

Ictal vomiting and ictal retching are rarely reported during focal seizures in adulthood (approximately 2% in temporal lobe epilepsies) [56]. While many studies suggest that ictal nausea, and vomiting, are linked to seizure onset in the non-dominant hemisphere, indicating a functional hemispheric asymmetry for gastrointestinal motility control [57, 58], this assumption is still debated and several authors described an involvement of left (dominant) temporal lobe [59–61]. According to the study by Tarnutzer [62], the evaluation of ictal video EEG, shows no significant differences between left and right temporal lobe localization and suggests that ictal vomiting has no lateralization value. In conclusion, ictal vomiting has been obtained by stimulating the left temporal mesial structures (amygdala, hippocampus, and insula cortex), particularly the insular cortex. However, studies conducted with intracranial electrical stimulation of the insular cortex have not been able to elicit vomiting [63, 64].

11.3.3.2 Ictal Vomiting in Childhood

Autonomic symptoms, mostly vomiting, are the hallmark of SeLEAS. Unlike adults, in whom ictal vomiting is rare and appears later, in childhood, it occurs as the only symptom mimicking other clinical disorders, such as sleep disorders, episodic syndromes that may be associated with migraine, gastroesophageal reflux disease, encephalitis, syncope, or metabolic disease. In these clinical disorders emesis is the predominant clinical feature at the onset of the seizure [65].

11.3.4 Cutaneous Manifestations

During focal seizures, flushing, pallor, sweating, and pilomotor erection, often associated with sensations of warmth and cold may arise. Among them, although skin flushing is part of the symptoms of seizures in Panayiotopoulos Syndrome, it is less frequently reported than pallor. In a retrospective review of medical charts seizures and videotaping, authors detected skin flushing in 19 children out of 100 who underwent surgical treatment and showed it has no lateralizing or localized value [66]. In the same study by Fogarasi et al., ictal pallor was reported in about 10% of children with focal seizures both temporal and extratemporal epilepsy mainly in TLE. Ictal pallor has a high predictive value in localizing seizure onset from the left temporal lobe, especially in younger patients [66]. It is due to vasoconstriction in the skin circulation and usually, it is underdiagnosed because of the difficulty in recognizing this symptom in video monitoring. Ictal piloerection is a rare manifestation that occurs in 0.4 1.2% of patients, mainly in people with temporal lobe epilepsy. Ictal piloerection may be distributed unilaterally or bilaterally. Unilateral piloerection is most frequently associated with the ipsilateral seizure onset zone, while bilateral ictal piloerection has no hemispheric predominance [67]. The location of the symptomatogenic zone remains unclear, but probably the insula and amygdala play an important role. The etiology of ictal piloerection includes malignant brain tumors, autoimmune encephalitis, especially limbic encephalitis, and hippocampal sclerosis [68, 69]. Finally, another cutaneous manifestation described is sweating. In a young man, ipsilateral facial sweating secondary to anti-Ma2 autoimmune encephalitis is associated with testicular neoplasia [70].

11.3.5 Sexual and Genital Manifestations

Sexual and genital manifestations can occur mainly during or after focal seizures. According to Leutmezer [71] can be subdivided into (a) sexual auras, (b) sexual automatisms, (c) genital auras, and (d) genital automatisms. The authors use the term "sexual" to refer to symptoms/signs with erotic content, while "genital" refers to symptoms/signs interesting the genitals without erotic components.

According to the last seizure classification, sexual auras can be classified: focal emotional seizures and sexual automatisms as focal emotional or focal hyperkinetic seizures; genital auras as focal sensory seizures; and genital automatisms as focal seizures with automatisms [4]. Sexual auras consist of erotic and pleasurable thoughts, orgasms, and penile erection that may occur before a seizure with temporal onset (more frequently non-dominant lobe temporal) without absolute lateralizing location. Sexual auras happen especially in female subjects. The area involved is the right amygdala which confirms its key role in human sexuality [72]. Genital auras are reported in a few cases in the literature and consist of disagreeable feelings or genital pain, sometimes associated with ictal orgasm. The cortical areas involved are the postcentral gyrus, interhemispheric fissure, and perisylvian region [73]. Sexual automatisms consist of hypermotor movements of the pelvis and truncal, combined with masturbatory activity. These manifestations typically occur in frontal lobe seizures [74]. Genital automatisms, such as repetitive manipulation of the genitals, occur most frequently in temporal lobe epilepsy, usually ipsilateral to the side of the hand used in manipulation [75, 76]. Unlike sexual auras, prevalent in women, genital automatisms usually occur in males [77]. This finding confirms the different organization of sexual functions between the two sexes within the limbic network [78].

The ictal urinary urge is a rare symptom, and his pathophysiological mechanism is not entirely clear. In previous studies, evaluating scalp video-EEG monitoring or functional imaging, demonstrated a localization in the non-dominant hemisphere, specifically, the temporal lobe [11, 79, 80]. It is not clear why ictal urinary urgency is commoner in right hemisphere epilepsy, but it confirms the presumed asymmetry of central autonomic influences on the bladder.

11.3.6 Miscellaneous

Other vegetative symptoms reported in temporal lobe epilepsies include spitting, ictal hypersalivation, and peri-ictal water drinking. Spitting is a rare symptom (appearing in up to 2%) present both in seizures arising in the nondominant temporal lobe and the dominant one [53, 81–83]. The symptomatogenic zone was recognized in areas controlling emotional behavior but this area could not be considered a lateralizing sign of a nondominant temporal lobe [83]. Ictal hypersalivation is a common feature in self-limited focal epilepsies of childhood particularly in self-limited epilepsy with centrotemporal spikes and in early-onset benign occipital epilepsy [84, 85]. As demonstrated in a previous study, increased salivation is a rare manifestation in patients with intractable epilepsy. In a small series of 10 adults, the authors show that this uncommon sign is a localizing feature for mesial temporal seizures, mainly those that originate in the non-dominant hemisphere [86]. Peri-ictal water drinking is a rare and under-recognized sign because it is a usual habitual action. In patients with temporal lobe epilepsy, it seems to be due to the involvement of the non-dominant hemisphere. This data reflects the asymmetrical control of neural networks concerned with fluid balance, thirst, and water-seeking. The peri-ictal water drinking could be due to the propagation of epileptiform discharges from mesial temporal structures to the hypothalamus that cause thirst and consequently water-seeking [87, 88].

11.4 Lobe Temporal Epilepsy

Temporal lobe epilepsy (TLE) is one of the most common forms of focal epilepsy in adolescence and adulthood [89], representing about 40% of all epilepsies in adult people (usually with a positive family history) [90] and the 60–75% of all patients with drug-resistant epilepsy [91] among which approximately two-thirds require surgical management [92]. TLE includes a heterogeneous group of disorders that share the localization of the epileptogenic zone in the temporal lobe, either in the lateral or in the mesial portion. Mesial TLE is probably the best-known electro-clinical pattern of all epilepsies [93] since TLE commonly arises from the mesial temporal lobe (hippocampus, amygdala, and parahippocampal gyrus) and is observed in about 80% of people with TLE [93, 94]. A wide variety of clinical events is associated with the involvement of medial temporal lobe networks. Focal seizure symptomatology is usually preceded by an epileptic aura that appears before the loss of awareness and may also represent the only clinical feature. Aura is usually composed of subjective symptoms without objective signs, which reflects the initial seizure discharge in the brain. Often it is misunderstood so that the diagnosis of epilepsy is made long after the onset of these symptoms.

Several old stimulation and observational studies demonstrated the correlation between specific cortical areas and autonomic function [95, 96] even if there is no clear topographic pattern of the autonomic effects. It is well known that the insular cortex, anterior cingulum, supplementary sensorimotor area, posterior orbitofrontal cortex, or amygdala are involved in alterations in heart and respiratory rate, mydriasis, piloerection, genitourinary symptoms [97, 98]. In addition, in drug-resistant TLE, the occurrence of recurrent and uncontrolled seizures that repeatedly activate CAN structures can result in epilepsy-related autonomic dysfunction. So that the autonomic dysfunction observed in TLE becomes more prominent with the progression of the disease as well as the increased seizure frequency [99]. In the focal aware seizures may be recognized alterations in heart and respiratory rate, abdominal discomfort, and/or rising epigastric sensation and ictus emeticus. The latter identifies the triad symptomatology consisting of nausea, retching, and vomiting, which, rather rare in temporal epilepsy, is instead typical of Panayiotopoulos syndrome. Other autonomic symptoms such as pallor, flushing, mydriasis, piloerection, sweating, and genitourinary symptoms may be present but they are ignored because less frequently reported by patients or by witnesses.

The symptomatogenic zone involved in the abdominal aura (the most reported type of autonomic aura) is the anterior insular cortex, frontal operculum, mesial temporal structures, and supplementary motor area [100]. Regarding focal aware seizures, in addition to the autonomic symptoms described, cognitive (e.g., deja vu, jamais vu), emotional state (e.g., fear) or sensory (e.g., olfactory, gustatory, visual, auditory) symptoms may also be present. Sensory auras, primarily olfactory, referred to as "uncinate fits" are typically described as unpleasant odors often associated with gustatory phenomena [101]. Although olfactory aura is historically reported as a typical TLE aura, it is a rare phenomenon occurring in only 5% of patients [102] and it is related to involvement in cortical areas such as the amygdala, olfactory bulb, insular cortex, and orbitofrontal cortex [98, 100]. The visual auras are usually caused by a dysregulation affecting the posterior regions of the temporal lobe. Visual auras include both simple and complex manifestations: the first one is due to the activation of the contralateral primary visual cortex and contiguous visual association areas; the second one involves the temporo-occipital junction or the basal temporal cortex [103]. Another feature of temporal lobe epilepsy is the presence of auditory phenomena. These auditory hallucinations, described as sounds or in the complex forms of hearing voices or songs, in the former case, can be attributed to activation of Heschel's gyrus, while in the latter, they are attributed to activation of the temporal associative cortex. In mesial temporal lobe epilepsy, fear is one of the most common affective symptoms. Several pieces of evidence suggest the amygdala is the symptomaticogenic area of fear, but some studies reported other regions (mesial frontal regions, occipital, and parietal lobes) as the origin of this affective symptom [104–107]. Although autonomic symptoms are typical features in temporal lobe seizures, some of them may be also reported in frontal lobe epilepsy. Epigastric sensations are one of the reported symptoms of basal frontal epilepsy as gustatory, cardiac, and respiratory manifestations that are described in patients with frontal, insular, and opercular lobe epilepsy. Cold shivering and piloerection, infrequent symptoms of focal seizures, although most often associated with a left temporal lobe focus can also occur with a right temporal, as well as a frontal or parietal lobe focus [9]. Frontal lobe localization may also be suggested by urinary incontinence during focal epilepsy with secondary generalization [108]. Differential diagnosis between frontal or temporal lobe epilepsy could be challenging when ictal tachycardia is present. A recent study investigated the differences between TLE and FLE patients with ultra-short-term heart rate variability (HRV) analysis and found different HRV profiles in the pre-ictal, ictal, and postictal intervals in the two groups: the temporal lobe epilepsy patients exhibited elevated sympathetic or vagal activity during the pre-ictal and postictal condition, while the FLE patients showed a marked increment and decrement in sympathetic tone during the ictal period [109].

11.5 Autonomic Seizures and Autonomic Status Epilepticus in Self-Limited Epilepsy with Autonomic Seizure

The primary cause of autonomic seizures and autonomic status epilepticus in children is SeLEAS, formerly known as Panayiotopoulos syndrome or early onset benign occipital epilepsy [6, 110, 111]. SeLEAS is characterized by the onset in early childhood of focal autonomic seizures followed by a stereotypical onset and progression that are often prolonged. The epilepsy is self-limited, with remission typically within a few years from onset [2]. The mean duration of the disease is approximately 3 years [112]. The usual age at onset is between 3 and 6 years (70% of cases), and ranges from 1 to 14 years [113], with a peak at 5 years [113, 114]. The likelihood of having seizures after the age of 12 years is exceptional [114]. Antecedent and birth history are normal. Neurological examination, development, and cognition are normal [115, 116]. Both sexes are affected equally. SeLEAS accounts for 5% of childhood epilepsies between 1 and 14 years and 13% of childhood epilepsies between 3 and 6 years [117]. A history of febrile seizures is seen in 5–17% of patients. Seizure frequency is typically low, with approximately 25% of children having a single seizure only [118], the median total number of fits is two to three, and the prognosis is invariably excellent, with remission usually occurring within 1 year from onset [114, 118]. Focal autonomic seizures, with or without impaired awareness, are mandatory for diagnosis. Awareness is usually preserved at seizure onset and may fluctuate in degree of impairment as the seizure progresses. In a typical presentation, the child, able to speak and understand, complains "I feel sick," looks pale, and shows autonomic symptoms and signs [110]. Autonomic features at onset may vary, but most frequently include retching, pallor, flushing, nausea, malaise, or abdominal pain. Vomiting, the most common autonomic manifestation, occurs in approximately 75% of children [6]. In others, only nausea or retching occurs, and in a few, emesis may not be apparent. Other autonomic manifestations may occur concurrently or appear later during the seizure such as pupillary (mydriasis, and, less often, miosis), temperature, and cardiorespiratory (breathing, pallor, cyanosis, and heart rate) changes. Incontinence of urine and/or feces, hypersalivation, and modifications of intestinal motility were also reported. Syncope may rarely occur. Seizures frequently evolve with eye and/or head deviation, generalized hypotonia, and focal clonic (hemiclonic) or focal to bilateral tonic–clonic seizure activity. More than 70% of seizures occur from sleep; the child may wake up with similar complaints while still aware or else may be found vomiting, conscious, confused, or unresponsive [110]. Seizures are often prolonged and can last longer than 30 min [113, 119, 120]. Electroencephalography is the most useful test in autonomic seizures. Multifocal spikes with high amplitude sharp-slow wave complexes (>200 μV) at various locations and predominant in the occipital regions can be present at disease onset [121] (Fig. 11.4). In some cases, the background activity could be normal [6]. During follow-up, abnormalities might move to either centrotemporal or frontopolar regions. Generalized abnormalities may also be seen [110, 122]. If persistent focal slowing is present, a structural brain abnormality should be sought as an alternative etiology. Diffuse slowing is not seen except in the postictal period [113, 120, 123, 124]. EEG abnormalities are activated both by sleep deprivation and by sleep when abnormalities often have a wider field and may be bilaterally synchronous. If seizures are recorded, ictal onset varies, but most have posterior onset [121]. The ictal pattern shows rhythmic slow activity intermixed with small spikes and/or fast activity [125]. Neuroimaging, if performed, shows no causal lesion. Brain MRI should be considered in cases with recurrent seizures or atypical presentations. Symptomatic autonomic epilepsy caused by heterogeneous brain lesions has been observed [113, 117, 126]. Nonspecific MRI findings should not exclude a diagnosis of SeLEAS [6]. Approximately 20% of patients may evolve to other self-limited focal epilepsies (SeLFEs), most commonly self-limited epilepsy with centrotemporal spikes (SeLECTS) [118]. Rarely, SeLEAS may evolve into epileptic encephalopathy with spike-and-wave activation in sleep (EE-SWAS). SeLEAS is probably genetically determined; however, no causative gene variants have been detected so far. There is a higher prevalence of febrile seizures in first-degree relatives and case reports of siblings with other SeLFEs [127]. SeLEAS does not usually require treatment, as the course of the disease is, in most cases, mild, and the prognosis is good [16]. It is crucial to differentiate the disease from other forms of epilepsy, especially occipital and structural epilepsy, and non-epileptic disorders [121]. Autonomic seizures and autonomic status epilepticus are easy to diagnose because of the characteristic clustering of clinical seizure semiology, which is often supported by interictal EEG findings. The main problem is to

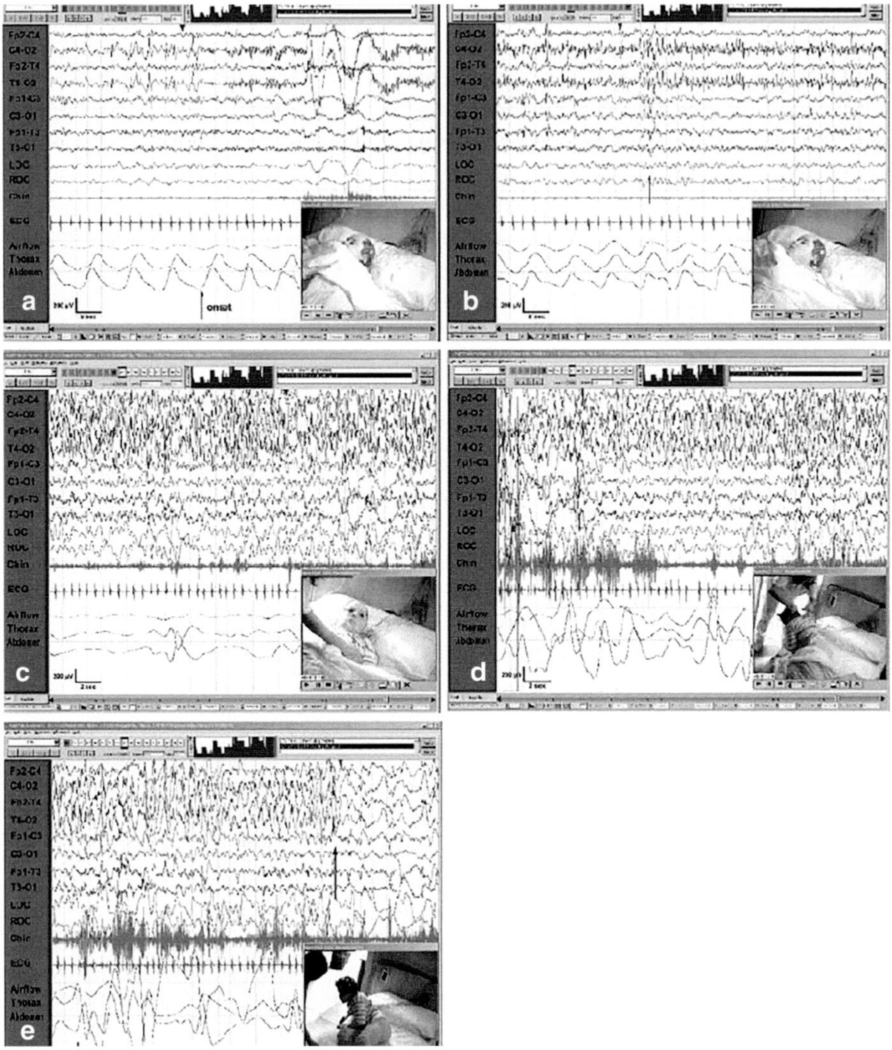

Fig. 11.4 Ictal registration of a child with self-limited epilepsy with autonomic seizures (SeLEAS) (from Parisi P, et al. 2007 [121]): polygraphic recording included scalp EEG (8 channels), electro-oculogram (LOC and ROC), chin electromyogram, ECG, nasal and oral airflow, thorax and abdominal movements. During sleep stage two, the seizure started (see arrow) with a run of fast spikes at 7 Hz involving principally the right occipital region (**a**), associated with tachycardia as the sole manifestation (minimal clinical manifestation: movement of the left arm). (**b**) Soon after the start and for approximately 10 min, with no clinical manifestations associated, the EEG showed the persistence of spike-and-wave at 3–4 Hz localized almost exclusively over the right occipital region, with rare spreading (see arrow) to the other EEG derivations. (**c**) A tonic conjugate deviation of the eyes to the left accompanied at the EEG by a rich content in high-amplitude slow waves in the theta and delta ranges predominate in the right hemisphere. (**d**) Ictal vomiting occurs 11 min after the onset of the seizure. (**e**) As repetitive vomiting stopped, the low-amplitude high frequency suddenly disappeared (see arrow) with the presence of post-ictal low-frequency components. (From Parisi P et al. Neurol Sci 2007; 28 [2]:72–9 with permission)

recognize emetic symptoms, ictal syncope, and other autonomic manifestations as seizure events and not to dismiss them or erroneously consider them as unrelated to the seizure and a feature of encephalitis, migraine, syncope, or gastroenteritis [128]. Autonomic seizures and autonomic status epilepticus are important to differentiate between SeLEAS and symptomatic causes. In SeLEAS, neurological state and mental state are normal and brain imaging is unremarkable. Conversely, in symptomatic cases, there are often abnormal neurological or mental symptomatology, abnormal brain imaging, and EEG background abnormalities [113].

11.6 Autonomic Dysfunctions in Developmental and Epileptic Encephalopathies

Autonomic symptoms could be encountered in several developmental and epileptic encephalopathies (DEE) and may represent either an epileptic manifestation or, more frequently, may develop apart from the epileptic disorder strongly correlated with the burden of functional impairments [129]. Rett syndrome is a neurodevelopmental disorder that primarily affects females, characterized by consistently reported seizures and paroxysmal autonomic symptoms mostly in patients carrying the methyl-CpG-binding-protein 2 (MeCP2) or CDKL5 mutation [130, 131]. Autonomic features encompass peripheral vasomotor disturbances, breathing dysfunction during wakefulness, apnoea, and cardiac dysautonomia with susceptibility to arrhythmias [132]. Epilepsy is a core symptom of Rett syndrome, with prevalence as high as 60–90% [133]; however, the analysis of video-EEG demonstrated that the majority of clinically reported seizures did not have an autonomic correlate [134]. Dravet syndrome is an epileptic encephalopathy that develops in the first year of life presenting multiple seizure types [135]. The diagnosis is clinical, but most cases carry a mutation in the SCN1A gene encoding for neuronal sodium channels [10]. Half of the patients had temperature regulation problems; other features of autonomic dysfunction such as sweating, pupillary dilation, flushing, gastroparesis, and heart rate changes are also more commonly described in children with Dravet syndrome than controls [135, 136]. As compared to age- and sex-matched control groups of other epileptic syndromes and healthy controls, patients with Dravet syndrome displayed a relative predominance of sympathetic over parasympathetic activity when investigating the electrical characteristics of cardiac function [137]. Autonomic signs are also reported in most patients with the SCN8A mutation, mainly as the first manifestation of focal or focal to bilateral tonic/tonic-clonic seizure [138]. A stereotyped sequence of appearance has been frequently described with some signs occurring within the first seconds (flushing of the face, sometimes associated with sialorrhea, bradycardia, and hypopnea) and others such as tachycardia, polypnea, perioral cyanosis, and pallor that followed later during the seizure [138]. Tonic seizures with long-lasting apnea requiring ventilation are believed to be one of the characteristic features of patients with this mutation [139]. Likewise, a case of SCN8A-related encephalopathy with ictal asystole requiring cardiac pacemaker implantation has been described [140]. Manifestations such as breathing dysfunction, apnoea, and cardiac dysautonomia with susceptibility to arrhythmias may underlie a brainstem dysfunction and/or a channelopathy linking neural and cardiac dysfunction and may account for the higher risk of SUDEP described in patients with some DEE as compared to the general population [141]. Aspects of dysautonomic function may provide biomarkers of DEE disease severity [129] or may predict the onset of a DEE. A recent study characterizes the temporal changes in heart rate variability, a surrogate of a marker of autonomic functional state, in infants at risk of Infantile epileptic spasm syndrome (an age-dependent epileptic syndrome characterized by clusters of clinical spasms and typical electroencephalogram features) finding that certain early HRV metrics may be predictive of the clinical onset of the disease [142].

11.7 Involvement of the Autonomic Nervous System in SUDEP

People with epilepsy have a 24-fold increased risk of dying suddenly compared with the general population [143] and among the causes of premature deaths in patients with epilepsy, SUDEP represents a major cause [143, 144]. SUDEP is defined as the "sudden, unexpected, witnessed or unwitnessed, nontraumatic and non-drowning death, occurring in benign circumstances, in an individual with epilepsy, with or without evidence for a seizure and excluding documented status epilepticus, in which postmortem examination does not reveal a cause of death" [145]. SUDEP is an important risk in patients with intractable epilepsy, with a variable reported incidence across the studies [146, 147]. The reported incidence does not vary between the pediatric (1.11–1.45 per 1000 person-years in children and adolescents with epilepsy) [148, 149] and adult (1.20 per 1000 person-years with epilepsy) [146] populations. However, the studies that have identified the incidence of SUDEP have not considered the different and multiple causes and types of epilepsy. The pathophysiology of SUDEP remains unknown, most cases of sudden death are unwitnessed and post-mortem examinations are often lacking [39, 150]. The potential mechanisms proposed involve prominent primary or secondary involvement of the autonomic nervous system in the form of central or obstructive apnea or both, cardiac arrhythmia, autonomic dysregulation, and hypoxia. Available data from witnessed and monitored SUDEP cases suggest that, in most cases, a convulsive seizure triggers catastrophic cardio-respiratory dysfunction that results in death [151, 152]. The autonomic system collapse, beginning with a respiratory dysfunction followed by heart failure, supports the notion that the brainstem structures that control autonomic function are involved in the mechanism of SUDEP [153]. The MORTEMUS study, which is the largest study to date describing cardiorespiratory function at the time of death in epilepsy, reported all SUDEP deaths occurring after a convulsive seizure [151]. In those cases, a seizure appeared to trigger progressive bradycardia and apnea beginning during the immediate postictal period; terminal apnea occurred before terminal asystole in all cases. It is arguable that more severe and drug-resistant disease has a greater risk of SUDEP [154, 155]. Nevertheless, SUDEP can occur early in the disease course or in individuals with a condition that is usually considered benign [156, 157] and, there are cases of non-seizure–related SUDEP, which reveal that a seizure is not necessary to trigger severe terminal cardiorespiratory dysfunction resulting in death [158]. In a cohort of three patients with refractory epilepsy, all patients died in the epilepsy monitoring unit during continuous video-EEG monitoring [158] and there was no clinical seizure and no ictal change on EEG preceding death. In all cases, there was progressive cardiorespiratory dysfunction associated with suppression of the EEG. In two cases there was tachycardia and tachypnea preceding bradypnea and bradycardia followed by terminal apnea, which was then followed by terminal asystole, a pattern that is similar to the progression of cardiorespiratory dysfunction noted in the MORTEMUS study [151]. These data suggest that catastrophic autonomic network dysfunction may occur due to initial severe brainstem dysfunction, which may be responsible for the highly abnormal cardiorespiratory patterns [159]. Interestingly, in focal and generalized epilepsies, autonomic functional changes were observed not only during the ictal period, but also during interictal and postictal periods where all aspects of the autonomic function, including parasympathetic, sympathetic, and adrenal medullary systems may be affected [9]. The magnitude of the sympathetic activation and parasympathetic suppression in each type of seizure or epilepsies may also be an important factor to be considered, as they may influence the probability risk of SUDEP [160]. HRV, which reflects the balance between sympathetic and parasympathetic activity in the autonomic nervous system, provides a physiological perspective for the examination of cardiac pathologies [161]. Patients with epilepsy often have interictal autonomic dysfunction, as is observable from the HRV abnormalities reported in both focal (particularly in temporal lobe epilepsy) and generalized epilepsy [162–165]. Children with drug-resistant epilepsy showed lower HRV values compared to children with controlled epilepsy or healthy children [166]. However, the chronically reduced parasympathetic effect may predispose drug-resistant epileptic children to a more severe stress response during seizures [166]. Patients with Dravet syndrome, which is highly associated with drug-resistant epilepsy and SUDEP, also have reduced HRV [137, 167]. In support, concurrent seizure activity in the temporal lobes significantly increased the heart rate and decreased the HRV in patients with refractory epilepsy, suggesting that there was an autonomic imbalance that tended to sympathetic dominance due to seizures [168]. There is also one case report of a man with refractory epilepsy and SUDEP in whom serial studies showed a sudden increase in parasympathetic activity, as measured by high-frequency power and the ratio between cardiac vagal index and cardiac sympathetic index during the 1 day to 30 min preceding death [169]. However, thus far, there are no clear specific HRV biomarkers for SUDEP. Surges et al. (2009) compared HRV in seven patients with SUDEP with HRV in seven control patients and found no significant differences in interictal HRV measures between the groups [170]. Although the MORTEMUS and other available SUDEP data suggest that primary cardiogenic causes of SUDEP are rare, it is still possible that abnormal HRV might contribute to SUDEP in a minority of cases. Each autonomic sign should be evaluated in the context of preceding autonomic manifestations. For example, asystole could be the first ictal expression, but could also follow IA or ictal hypotension. IA was thought to be a possible mechanism of SUDEP [171, 172]. However, several observations indicate that IA is not invariably linked to SUDEP [31, 173, 174]. Another important aspect to consider is the seizure type and the timing of the event. For instance, ictal asystole is predominantly seen in focal seizures of temporal lobe onset, whereas postictal asystole is strongly associated with TCSs, including both primary generalized TCSs and focal-to-bilateral TCSs [33]. The same holds for apnoea: ictal central apnoea is strongly linked to focal temporal lobe seizures, whereas postictal central apnoea is seen only in the context of TCSs (41 42). Eyewitness reports suggest that around 10% of witnessed SUDEP events occur in the absence of apparent seizure activity [39, 152, 175, 176], indicating that seizures are not required as proximate triggers for SUDEP. It is reasonable to assume that in some or even most of these cases, sudden death was caused by cardiac arrhythmias. Retrospective analysis of multi-day ECG data obtained during video-EEG monitoring from patients who subsequently died due to SUDEP found that SUDEP patients had greater increases in heart rate during seizures than in other refractory control epilepsy patients [177]. Heart rate alterations are the most studied and probably the most frequent ictal autonomic signs, with a prevalence of 38–100% [21]. The degree of autonomic change varies according to the seizure type. Ictal tachycardia seems to be more prominent in seizures originating from the temporal and orbitofrontal cortex and in TCSs [22, 168, 178–183]. Depth EEG recordings in people with temporal lobe epilepsy (TLE) indicate that ictal tachycardia coincides with seizure activity in the anterior hippocampus and amygdala [181]. The spread of seizure activity to subregions of the ipsilateral and contralateral hemispheres correlates with heart rate increase [168, 182, 184]. Heart rate alterations could be the earliest clinical sign of seizure onset and it might be a significant tool for seizure detection [183]. In multi-day recordings in patients admitted to epilepsy monitoring units, almost 40% of patients had ictal cardiac arrhythmias or repolarization abnormalities, including bundle branch block, atrial fibrillation, supraventricular tachycardia, asystole, and other abnormalities [36, 185]. In a prospective cohort study, patients with chronic epilepsy showed significantly higher T-wave alternation and lower HRV values compared to patients with newly diagnosed epilepsy [186]. Furthermore, cardiac repolarization abnormalities are found in epilepsy patients also in association with seizures [38, 187, 188]. Convulsive and longer seizures may increase the risk for ictal Electrocardiogram abnormalities [36]. Ventricular tachyarrhythmias may occur more frequently in patients with epilepsy (possibly related to increased risk of cardiovascular disease in this population) and could be an underestimated cause of SUDEP [39, 189, 190]. In a monitored patient without cardiac pathologies, who experienced sudden onset of ventricular tachycardia (VT) and ventricular fibrillation (VF) following a focal-to-bilateral TCS [38] a SUPED was documented. However, most of the VT/VF events occurred in patients with pre-existing or acute heart conditions [39]. However, most forms of cardiac arrhythmias can be observed in people with epilepsy, particularly in association with seizures [191]. Ictal bradycardia has been reported to occur in up to 6.4% of focal seizures and up to 13.6% of people with epilepsy undergoing video-EEG monitoring [191]. Long-term EKG recording (between 4 and 22 months) via implantable loop recorders in patients with refractory epilepsy suggest that ictal and interictal bradycardia may occur relatively commonly in this population, with 8/39 patients in both studies combined having bradycardia or asystole [155, 192]. Other ictal cardiovascular manifestations, such as blood pressure, lack precise prevalence because they are not routinely assessed during EEG recordings. The resting awake interictal heart rate (HR) and blood pressure (BP) in SUDEP cases and control epilepsy groups (refractory and controlled) are similar but there is a trend toward a higher diastolic BP and more stable (less variable) HR over time in individuals who subsequently died due to SUDEP [193]. However, increases in blood pressure can be seen across all focal seizure types and in focal-to-bilateral TCSs [194]. While these findings need to be confirmed in larger populations, they again support the possibility that patients at risk for SUDEP may have underlying autonomic dysfunction, which may increase their risk for death in the setting of a seizure. Blood pressure is regulated by the baroreflex, whereby significant deterioration in its sensitivity has been observed in the early postictal period following bilateral/generalized convulsive seizures [195]. This may be due to increased muscle contractions, a large amount of catecholamine released, and impaired brainstem function [195]. While most cases of SUDEP were probably caused by a cardiorespiratory failure during the early postictal period following generalized convulsive seizures, recent studies have reported that impaired baroreflex sensitivity may also cause life-threatening systemic blood pressure to decrease after generalized convulsive seizures [196]. In addition to the cardiological autonomic involvement, the respiratory one has also been underlined by scientific evidence. The MORTEMUS study provides clear evidence of respiratory dysfunction in SUDEP. In patients with SUDEP in the MORTEMUS series, convulsive seizures were followed by terminal apnea and then asystole [151]. In total, 75% of people who succumb to SUDEP are found in the prone position, (which is likely to further aggravate postictal breathing disturbances) [151, 197] and are unwitnessed, though there is often evidence of a recent seizure (e.g., tongue bite, urinary incontinence, or body positioning to suggest a recent seizure) at the time of death [197–199]. Ictal central apnea strongly correlates with focal epilepsy, particularly temporal lobe epilepsy. In 56 patients with focal epilepsy, approximately one-third of focal seizures with or without generalization were accompanied by desaturations below 90% [43]. In another cohort, ictal central apnea occurred in 47% of 109 patients (36.5% of 312 seizures), most notably in temporal lobe epilepsy [41]. Dlouhy et al. (2015) found that electrical stimulation of the amygdala in patients undergoing intracranial EEG monitoring resulted in central apnea [200]. It has also been observed that seizures spreading to the amygdala may cause central apnea and oxygen desaturation in patients with persistent epilepsy [200]. In pediatric patients with refractory epilepsy who underwent intracranial electroencephalography, apnea formation was found to occur simultaneously with the spread of the seizure to the amygdala area responsible for respiratory suppression [201]. This suggests that there may be a functional link between the amygdala and respiration in the brainstem which may cause respiratory loss as a result of epileptiform activity. In a study by Park et al., focal to the bilateral tonic–clonic seizures or generalized tonic–clonic seizures which caused ictal/postictal hypoxemia more than 125 s had a statistically significant association with high-risk cardiac arrhythmias (nonsustained ventricular tachycardia, bradyarrhythmia, and sinus pauses). The odds ratio for the occurrence of arrhythmia was 7.86 for desaturation durations ≥125 s versus desaturations <125 s ($p = 0.005$). The odds ratio increased to 13.09 for desaturation durations ≥150 s ($p < 0.001$) [202]. These studies show that the peri-ictal respiratory decline may be the critical initial node in the series of terminal events resulting in sudden death. Animal models have been studied to identify the basic neurobiological mechanisms of respiratory arrest with seizures. It has been well-studied that 5-hydroxytryptamine (5-HT) neurons play a critical role in maintaining respiratory drive. Provoked audiogenic seizures in DBA/2 mice which lack several 5 HT receptor proteins in the brainstem lead to death due to respiratory arrest, which can be prevented with oxygenation [203]. Notably, seizure-related death is reduced using selective serotonin reuptake inhibitors (SSRI) [204, 205]. Additionally, adenosine antagonists may also significantly reduce ictal apnea [206]. Reduced 5-HT levels and immature 5-HT neurons in the medulla have also been noted in infants who died of sudden infant death syndrome (SIDS), which suggests a possible role of 5-HT axis dysfunction as a cause of sudden unexplained death [207]. Further investigation is needed to evaluate whether SSRIs and adenosine antagonists might have a role in reducing ictal apnea in humans. Another characteristic feature of the early postictal phase was the generalized flattening of the EEG trace (postictal generalized EEG suppression, PGES). The origin and clinical importance of PGES are not yet fully understood [208], but it might be a condition for the neurovegetative breakdown in TCS-related SUDEP. Clinical and electrophysiological data obtained from children with epilepsy revealed that PGES was associated with peri-ictal tachycardia and hypoxemia [209]. However, in a clinical study examining generalized convulsive seizures retrospectively, the percentage of postictal unresponsiveness, including oropharyngeal immobility, was found to be higher in patients with PGES after seizures [210]. This suggests that postictal immobility and PGES are associated with peri-ictal respiratory disorders [211]. Electrodermal activity (EDA) measures changes in the electrical conductance of the skin due to sympathetic neuronal activity [212]. One study evaluating primarily children found that there is a surge of EDA (correlating with increased sympathetic activation) and suppression of high-frequency power of HRV (correlating with parasympathetic suppression) after tonic–clonic seizures [160]. This post-ictal autonomic dysregulation correlated to increased duration of PGES in this study. These data suggest that PGES, which may be a biomarker for SUDEP, could be associated with significant autonomic dysfunction during the critical post-ictal period when SUDEP most often occurs. Additional investigation showed that age may affect the degree of sympathetic and parasympathetic activity following seizures [213]. Adults tend to have longer durations of PGES Sarkis et al. also found that adults had longer durations of PGES and that the duration of PGES correlated with the degree of sympathetic activation as measured by EDA [213]. However, after controlling for PGES duration, pediatric patients were found to have stronger sympathetic activation as well as greater parasympathetic suppression than adults. These age-dependent findings may correlate with the variable incidence of SUDEP seen in different age groups. From the brain structural view, a volume loss of brainstem regions, a structure with a crucial role in autonomic control, has been also observed in SUDEP cases compared to controls [214] suggesting a possible link between structural and functional autonomic pathology. SUDEP victims show significant tissue loss in areas essential for cardiorespiratory recovery and enhanced volumes in areas that trigger hypotension or impede respiratory patterning [215]. In detail, substantial bilateral gray matter loss appeared in SUDEP cases in the medial and lateral cerebellum. The periaqueductal gray, left posterior and medial thalamus, left hippocampus, and bilateral posterior cingulate also showed volume loss in SUDEP [215]. In a retrospective study, posterior thalamic grey matter volume, an area mediating oxygen regulation, was reduced in cases of SUDEP and subjects at high risk, when compared to controls [216]. The T1 images of individuals with temporal lobe epilepsy (TLE) revealed a volume loss in the dorsal mesencephalon region, which plays a role in autonomic control [214]. While the 3T magnetic resonance imaging (MRI) findings of patients with focal epilepsy showed large atrophy in the autonomic nuclei of the medulla oblongata's periaqueductal gray area instead [153]. Also, some neurotransmitters may play a role in the etiopathogenesis of SUDEP. Acetylcholine (ACh), the main stimulant of the autonomic nervous system, mediates signal transmission through cholinergic and nicotinic receptors. Accumulating evidence indicates that dysfunction of nicotinic ACh receptors, which are widely expressed in hippocampal and cortical neurons, may be significantly implicated in the pathogenesis of epilepsy [217]. It has also been reported that M1 muscarinic receptors in the medial septum region of the hippocampus integrate the inputs of vagal afferents from the brainstem into the hippocampus [218]. In this context, it is important to investigate the possible effects of M1 receptors on epilepsy and SUDEP [219]. On the other hand, deficits in serotonergic signaling might also be involved in seizure-related breathing disturbances. Animal data suggest that postictal deficits in serotonergic neurotransmission can impair the arousal reaction to postictally elevated CO2 levels and cause hypoventilation or respiratory arrest [207], which can be prevented by the administration of serotonin reuptake inhibitors [220]. Moreover, in a post-mortem study, the depletion of brainstem neurons involved in serotonin and galanin signaling was greater in SUDEP cases than in controls [221].

11.7.1 Genetic Epilepsy and SUDEP

A growing body of evidence points to a genetic susceptibility to cardiorespiratory and autonomic dysfunction in epilepsy. Animal data suggest that an ion channelopathy may cause both epilepsy and alter the autonomic control of the heart [222].

Epilepsy-related alterations in the cardiac expression of sodium (Nav1.1/1.5), potassium (Kv4.2/4.3), calcium (NCX1), and cationic (HCN2/4) channels have thus been reported in animal models [223]. It remains to be determined whether or not this mechanism is associated with impaired vegetative regulation in patients with epilepsy and especially, with the risk of SUDEP. In an analysis of the entire exome sequencing of 61 SUDEP cases, mutations known to cause long QT syndrome were found in 7% of cases and an additional 15% had candidate variants in potentially predisposing genes to malignant cardiac arrhythmias [224]. Similarly, the effect of the SCN1A mutation on heart function may partly explain the increased risk of mortality in Dravet syndrome [225–227]. Other genetic defects might contribute to both epilepsy and cardiac arrhythmias in some individuals, for example, SCN5A, KCNQ1, and KCNH2 [172, 228, 229]. For individuals with pathogenic variants in genes including SCN1A, SCN1B, SCN8A, SCN2A, GNB5, KCNA1, and DEPDC5, there are varying degrees of evidence to suggest an increased risk for sudden death. Why the risk for sudden death is higher is not completely clear; however, in many cases, pathogenic variants in these genes are also associated with autonomic dysfunction, which is hypothesized as a contributing factor to SUDEP [230]. Several ion channel genes whose mutations are involved in cardiac arrhythmias are also expressed in the brain (Fig. 11.5) [231]. For example, the SCN5A gene, whose mutation is associated with long QT syndrome, is also expressed in the brain and is associated with epilepsy [232].

Gene	Protein	Effect on brain	Effect on heart
KCNQ1	Potassium channel Kv7.1	Epilepsy	Long QT syndrome
KCNQ2	Potassium channel Kv7.2	Benign neonatal epilepsy; epileptic encephalopathy	Long QT syndrome
KCNH2	Potassium channel Kv11.1	Epilepsy	Long QT syndrome, Short QT syndrome
KCNJ2	Potassium channel Kir2.1	Epilepsy, autism spectrum disorder	Short QT syndrome, Long QT syndrome
KCNA1	Potassium channel Kv1.1	Epilepsy, ataxia	Atrial fibrillation, AV blocks
SCN1A	Sodium channel Nav1.1	Dravet syndrome	Likely increased risk of peri-ictal arrhythmia
SCN2A	Sodium channel Nav1.2	Benign neonatal epilepsy; epileptic encephalopathy	Likely increased risk of arrhythmia
SCN5A	Sodium channel Nav1.5	Epilepsy	Long QT syndrome, Brugada syndrome
SCN8A	Sodium channel Nav1.6	Epileptic encephalopathy, movement disorders	Ventricular arrhythmias
SCN10A	Sodium channel Nav1.8	Epileptic encephalopathy	Long QT syndrome, Brugada syndrome
HCN1	Hyperpolarization-activated cationic channel HCN1	Epileptic encephalopathy	Sick sinus syndrome
HCN4	Hyperpolarization-activated cationic channel HCN4	Benign myoclonic epilepsy in infancy, generalized epilepsy	Sick sinus syndrome
CACNA1C	L-type calcium channel Cav1.2 alpha 1	Epileptic encephalopathy, Timothy syndrome	Long QT syndrome, Short QT syndrome, Brugada syndrome, idiopathic VF
CACNA2D1	L-type calcium channel Cav1.2 alpha 2-delta 1	Epilepsy	Brugada syndrome, Short QT syndrome
RYR2	Ryanodine receptor 2 (intracellular calcium channel)	Epilepsy	CPVT

Fig. 11.5 Main channelopathies associated with epilepsy and arrhythmias. *AV* atrioventricular, *CPVT* catecholaminergic polymorphic ventricular tachycardia, *VF* ventricular fibrillation. (From Costagliola G, et al. 2021 [231] with permission)

11.7.2 Detection and Prevention of SUDEP

Seizure control is the most important potentially modifiable risk factor of SUDEP. To best participate in their care, patients should be knowledgeable about the potential risks of seizures, including SUDEP. The American Academy of Neurology and American Epilepsy Society recommend that clinicians counsel epilepsy patients regarding SUDEP. Survey studies of epilepsy patients and family members of SUDEP patients have shown that they prefer to know about the risk factors of SUDEP during the early phase of management [233, 234]. Unfortunately, some data suggest that only a small minority of neurologists counsel all of their patients about SUDEP [235]. Ictal autonomic changes and interictal autonomic dysfunction might serve as diagnostic clues, providing targets for seizure detection. Retrospective studies suggest that heart rate alterations can be prevented by improving seizure control using ASMs [236–238]. ASMs often serve as a double-edged sword for epileptic patients. Although ASMs are mainly designed to help epileptic patients control their seizures, some might worsen their condition leading to other health complications [239], including cardiorespiratory dysfunctions such as myocardial infarction [20, 240], arrhythmias [20], respiratory depression [239], and even cardiovascular death or SUDEP [240]. This has been particularly reported with sodium channel blockers [20], including the risk of an atrioventricular block with carbamazepine [241], sinus pause and hypotension with rapid administration of phenytoin [20, 242] or atrioventricular block or atrial fibrillation with lacosamide [243–245]. However, no formal relationship has been established between these drug-related adverse events and ictal arrhythmias [20]. A meta-analysis by Ryvlin reported that adjunctive ASMs might reduce the SUDEP risk by seven times when given to patients with intractable epilepsy [246]. The impact of epilepsy surgery on the risk of SUDEP is more controversial [146], however, lower mortality rates were observed in successful versus failed TLE surgery [155, 247–249]. In patient with drug-resistant epilepsy, pacemaker implantation is advisable to reduce the risk of falls and life-treating injuries, although some individuals might not benefit from these devices' injuries [188, 236, 250–252]. Of course, ASM adherence and surgical interventions, when appropriate, may improve seizure control and reduce the risk of SUDEP. The effect of vagus nerve stimulation (VNS) on autonomic function remains uncertain. Heart changes associated with VNS are rare. Few cases of VNS-induced bradycardia have been reported. In addition, data on the alterations in the parasympathetic tone of the cardiovascular system induced by VNS are contradictory [253]. VNS was associated with a reduced SUDEP risk [254, 255]. VNS seems to reduce abnormally elevated levels of T-wave alternans, thereby stabilizing the electrical properties of the heart [256]. However, whether this intervention could help to reduce the risk of sudden cardiac death due to ventricular tachycardia and ventricular fibrillation (VT/VF) is currently unknown. Prone position and post-ictal immobility are often cited in SUDEP cases, and some data suggest that nocturnal supervision might reduce the risk of SUDEP [257]. A Cochrane Review and the American Academy of Neurology–American Epilepsy Society SUDEP guidelines concluded that only very-low-certainty (Grading of Recommendations Assessment, Development, and Evaluation) and level C (modified Grading Recommendations Assessment) evidence was available to support the preventive impact of nocturnal supervision on SUDEP risk [146, 258]. This evidence was derived from retrospective case–control studies [254, 257, 259] and is supported by the observation that the majority of SUDEP events occur at night, during sleep in non-supervised individuals [151, 175, 199]. Epilepsy monitoring unit data from the MORTEMUS study also suggests that an immediate nonspecific postictal intervention from a caregiver is likely to prevent SUDEP [151]. Nursing interventions such as stimulating and turning the patient to the lateral position and suction with or without supplemental oxygenation have been reported to shorten the duration of peri-ictal hypoxemia and seizure duration [260, 261]. However, currently, no guidelines exist on the use of supplemental oxygen with seizures, and the potential benefits must be weighed against the significant cost and risks of home oxygen. Currently, there have been efforts to utilize the autonomic response to treat/reduce seizures and eventually SUDEP risk, in drug-resistant epilepsy patients. For example, autonomic biofeedback therapy has shown some promising results in reducing seizure frequency in drug-resistant temporal lobe epileptic patients by using their galvanic skin response (a measure of sympathetic activation) [262]. This suggests that changes in autonomic network control such as blood pressure and heart rate may be monitored to not only predict and measure seizures but also be harnessed for treatment strategies against epilepsy. These autonomic responses may also be used to record and monitor nocturnal seizures which may help to deter SUDEP [263]. Over the past 10 years, there has been a growing interest in the potential applications of mobile health technologies for seizure detection, with the objective of faster caregivers' intervention and decreased risk of seizure-related injuries [161, 179, 264]. While detection of generalized TCSs has shown promising results with utilization either alone or in combination with accelerometers, automatic video detection, surface EMG, and bed alarms [265, 266], these approaches are much less sensitive for focal seizures. While it is clear that pacemaker implantation can be very helpful in preventing ictal syncope (i.e., syncope due to ictal asystole with subsequent hypotension and cerebral hypoperfusion) and falls, it is not clear that pacemaker implantation can prevent SUDEP. Schuele et al. found that when pacemakers were implanted in patients with ictal asystole and followed for 5 years, the risk of recurrent asystole appears to be low and that asystole may be a benign event [267, 268]. In this panorama, an interesting perspective remains the development of technologies capable of early detection of autonomic alterations and providing warnings of different types of seizures, thus reducing the risk of SUDEP.

References

1. Fisher RS, van Emde BW, Blume W, Elger C, Genton P, Lee P, Engel J Jr. Epileptic seizures and epilepsy: definitions proposed by the International League Against Epilepsy (ILAE) and the International Bureau for Epilepsy (IBE). Epilepsia. 2005;46(4):470–2. https://doi.org/10.1111/j.0013-9580.2005.66104.x.
2. Ferrie CD, Caraballo R, Covanis A, Demirbilek V, Dervent A, Fejerman N, Fusco L, Grünewald RA, Kanazawa O, Koutroumanidis M, Lada C, Livingston JH, Nicotra A, Oguni H, Martinovic Z, Nordli DR Jr, Parisi P, Scott RC, Specchio N, Verrotti A, Vigevano F, Walker MC, Watanabe K, Yoshinaga H, Panayiotopoulos CP. Autonomic status epilepticus in Panayiotopoulos syndrome and other childhood and adult epilepsies: a consensus view. Epilepsia. 2007;48(6):1165–72. https://doi.org/10.1111/j.1528-1167.2007.01087.x. Epub 2007 Apr 18.
3. Baumgartner C, Koren J, Britto-Arias M, Schmidt S, Pirker S. Epidemiology and pathophysiology of autonomic seizures: a systematic review. Clin Auton Res. 2019;29(2):137–50. https://doi.org/10.1007/s10286-019-00596-x. Epub 2019 Feb 25.
4. Fisher RS, Cross JH, French JA, Higurashi N, Hirsch E, Jansen FE, Lagae L, Moshé SL, Peltola J, Roulet Perez E, Scheffer IE, Zuberi SM. Operational classification of seizure types by the International League Against Epilepsy: position paper of the ILAE Commission for Classification and Terminology. Epilepsia. 2017;58(4):522–30. https://doi.org/10.1111/epi.13670. Epub 2017 Mar 8.
5. Scheffer IE, Berkovic S, Capovilla G, Connolly MB, French J, Guilhoto L, Hirsch E, Jain S, Mathern GW, Moshé SL, Nordli DR, Perucca E, Tomson T, Wiebe S, Zhang YH, Zuberi SM. ILAE classification of the epilepsies: position paper of the ILAE Commission for Classification and Terminology. Epilepsia. 2017;58(4):512–21. https://doi.org/10.1111/epi.13709. Epub 2017 Mar 8.
6. Specchio N, Wirrell EC, Scheffer IE, Nabbout R, Riney K, Samia P, Guerreiro M, Gwer S, Zuberi SM, Wilmshurst JM, Yozawitz E, Pressler R, Hirsch E, Wiebe S, Cross HJ, Perucca E, Moshé SL, Tinuper P, Auvin S. International League Against Epilepsy classification and definition of epilepsy syndromes with onset in childhood: position paper by the ILAE Task Force on Nosology and Definitions. Epilepsia. 2022;63(6):1398–442. https://doi.org/10.1111/epi.17241. Epub 2022 May 3.
7. Mielke H, Meissner S, Wagner K, Joos A, Schulze-Bonhage A. Which seizure elements do patients memorize? A comparison of history and seizure documentation. Epilepsia. 2020;61(7):1365–75. https://doi.org/10.1111/epi.16550. Epub 2020 Jun 9.
8. Panayiotopoulos CP. Epileptic seizures and their classification. In: A clinical guide to epileptic syndrome and their treatment. 2nd ed. London: Springer-Verlag; 2007. p. 17–56.
9. Devinsky O. Effects of seizures on autonomic and cardiovascular function. Epilepsy Curr. 2004;4(2):43–6. https://doi.org/10.1111/j.1535-7597.2004.42001.x.
10. Moseley BD. Seizure-related autonomic changes in children. J Clin Neurophysiol. 2015;32(1):5–9. https://doi.org/10.1097/WNP.0000000000000138.
11. Baumgartner C, Lurger S, Leutmezer F. Autonomic symptoms during epileptic seizures. Epileptic Disord. 2001;3(3):103–16.
12. Freeman R, Schachter SC. Autonomic epilepsy. Semin Neurol. 1995;15(2):158–66. https://doi.org/10.1055/s-2008-1041019.
13. Sklerov M, Dayan E, Browner N. Functional neuroimaging of the central autonomic network: recent developments and clinical implications. Clin Auton Res. 2019;29(6):555–66. https://doi.org/10.1007/s10286-018-0577-0. Epub 2018 Nov 23.
14. Benarroch EE. The central autonomic network: functional organization, dysfunction, and perspective. Mayo Clin Proc. 1993;68(10):988–1001. https://doi.org/10.1016/s0025-6196(12)62272-1.

15. Bennaroch EE. The autonomic nervous system: basic anatomy and physiology. Contin Lifelong Learn Neurol. 2007;13(6 (Autonomic Disorders)):13–32.
16. Zontek A, Paprocka J. Gastrointestinal and autonomic symptoms—how to improve the diagnostic process in Panayiotopoulos syndrome? Children (Basel). 2022;9(6):814. https://doi.org/10.3390/children9060814.
17. Graziosi A, Pellegrino N, Di Stefano V, Raucci U, Luchetti A, Parisi P. Misdiagnosis and pitfalls in Panayiotopoulos syndrome. Epilepsy Behav. 2019;98(Pt A):124–8. https://doi.org/10.1016/j.yebeh.2019.07.016. Epub 2019 Jul 29.
18. Goodman JH, Stewart M, Drislane FW. Autonomic disturbances. In: Engel J, Pedley TA, editors. Epilepsy, a comprehensive textbook, vol. 3. 2nd ed. Lippincott William & Wilkins; 2008. p. 1999–2005.
19. Russell AE. Cessation of the pulse during the onset of epileptic fits, with remarks on the mechanism of fits. Lancet. 1906;168:152–4. https://doi.org/10.1016/S0140-6736(01)30477-4.
20. Shmuely S, van der Lende M, Lamberts RJ, Sander JW, Thijs RD. The heart of epilepsy: current views and future concepts. Seizure. 2017;44:176–83. https://doi.org/10.1016/j.seizure.2016.10.001. Epub 2016 Oct 26.
21. Eggleston KS, Olin BD, Fisher RS. Ictal tachycardia: the head-heart connection. Seizure. 2014;23(7):496–505. https://doi.org/10.1016/j.seizure.2014.02.012. Epub 2014 Mar 6.
22. Surges R, Cho CA, Walker MC. Enhanced QT shortening and persistent tachycardia after generalized seizures. Neurology. 2010;74(5):421–6. https://doi.org/10.1212/WNL.0b013e3181ccc706.
23. Oppenheimer SM, Gelb A, Girvin JP, Hachinski VC. Cardiovascular effects of human insular cortex stimulation. Neurology. 1992;42(9):1727–32. https://doi.org/10.1212/wnl.42.9.1727.
24. Oppenheimer S, Cechetto D. The insular cortex and the regulation of cardiac function. Compr Physiol. 2016;6(2):1081–133. https://doi.org/10.1002/cphy.c140076.
25. Chouchou F, Mauguière F, Vallayer O, Catenoix H, Isnard J, Montavont A, Jung J, Pichot V, Rheims S, Mazzola L. How the insula speaks to the heart: cardiac responses to insular stimulation in humans. Hum Brain Mapp. 2019;40(9):2611–22. https://doi.org/10.1002/hbm.24548. Epub 2019 Feb 28.
26. Hirsch M, Altenmüller DM, Schulze-Bonhage A. Latencies from intracranial seizure onset to ictal tachycardia: a comparison to surface EEG patterns and other clinical signs. Epilepsia. 2015;56(10):1639–47. https://doi.org/10.1111/epi.13117. Epub 2015 Aug 18.
27. Mayer H, Benninger F, Urak L, Plattner B, Geldner J, Feucht M. EKG abnormalities in children and adolescents with symptomatic temporal lobe epilepsy. Neurology. 2004;63(2):324–8. https://doi.org/10.1212/01.wnl.0000129830.72973.56.
28. Chan SW, Dervan LA, Watson RS, Anderson AE, Lai YC. Epilepsy duration is an independent factor for electrocardiographic changes in pediatric epilepsy. Epilepsia Open. 2021;6(3):588–96. https://doi.org/10.1002/epi4.12519. Epub 2021 Jul 19.
29. Leutmezer F, Schernthaner C, Lurger S, Potzelberger K, Baumgartner C. Electrocardiographic changes at the onset of epileptic seizures. Epilepsia. 2003;44:348–54.
30. Moseley B, Bateman L, Millichap JJ, Wirrell E, Panayiotopoulos CP. Autonomic epileptic seizures, autonomic effects of seizures, and SUDEP. Epilepsy Behav. 2013;26(3):375–85. https://doi.org/10.1016/j.yebeh.2012.08.020. Epub 2012 Oct 23.
31. Lanz M, Oehl B, Brandt A, Schulze-Bonhage A. Seizure induced cardiac asystole in epilepsy patients undergoing long term video-EEG monitoring. Seizure. 2011;20(2):167–72. https://doi.org/10.1016/j.seizure.2010.11.017. Epub 2010 Dec 22.
32. Rocamora R, Kurthen M, Lickfett L, Von Oertzen J, Elger CE. Cardiac asystole in epilepsy: clinical and neurophysiologic features. Epilepsia. 2003;44(2):179–85. https://doi.org/10.1046/j.1528-1157.2003.15101.x.
33. van der Lende M, Surges R, Sander JW, Thijs RD. Cardiac arrhythmias during or after epileptic seizures. J Neurol Neurosurg Psychiatry. 2016;87(1):69–74. https://doi.org/10.1136/jnnp-2015-310559. Epub 2015 Jun 2.

34. Tényi D, Gyimesi C, Kupó P, Horváth R, Bóné B, Barsi P, Kovács N, Simor T, Siegler Z, Környei L, Fogarasi A, Janszky J. Ictal asystole: a systematic review. Epilepsia. 2017;58(3):356–62. https://doi.org/10.1111/epi.13644. Epub 2016 Dec 18.
35. Schuele SU, Bermeo AC, Alexopoulos AV, Locatelli ER, Burgess RC, Dinner DS, Foldvary-Schaefer N. Video-electrographic and clinical features in patients with ictal asystole. Neurology. 2007;69(5):434–41. https://doi.org/10.1212/01.wnl.0000266595.77885.7f.
36. Nei M, Ho RT, Sperling MR. EKG abnormalities during partial seizures in refractory epilepsy. Epilepsia. 2000;41:542–8.
37. Zijlmans M, Flanagan D, Gotman J. Heart rate changes and ECG abnormalities during epileptic seizures: prevalence and definition of an objective clinical sign. Epilepsia. 2002;43(8):847–54. https://doi.org/10.1046/j.1528-1157.2002.37801.x.
38. Surges R, Shmuely S, Dietze C, Ryvlin P, Thijs RD. Identifying patients with epilepsy at high risk of cardiac death: signs, risk factors and initial management of high risk of cardiac death. Epileptic Disord. 2021;23(1):17–39. https://doi.org/10.1684/epd.2021.1254.
39. Lamberts RJ, Blom MT, Wassenaar M, Bardai A, Leijten FS, de Haan GJ, Sander JW, Thijs RD, Tan HL. Sudden cardiac arrest in people with epilepsy in the community: circumstances and risk factors. Neurology. 2015;85(3):212–8. https://doi.org/10.1212/WNL.0000000000001755. Epub 2015 Jun 19.
40. Van Buren JM. Some autonomic concomitants of ictal automatism; a study of temporal lobe attacks. Brain. 1958;81(4):505–28. https://doi.org/10.1093/brain/81.4.505.
41. Lacuey N, Zonjy B, Hampson JP, Rani MRS, Zaremba A, Sainju RK, Gehlbach BK, Schuele S, Friedman D, Devinsky O, Nei M, Harper RM, Allen L, Diehl B, Millichap JJ, Bateman L, Granner MA, Dragon DN, Richerson GB, Lhatoo SD. The incidence and significance of periictal apnea in epileptic seizures. Epilepsia. 2018;59(3):573–82. https://doi.org/10.1111/epi.14006. Epub 2018 Jan 16.
42. Vilella L, Lacuey N, Hampson JP, Rani MRS, Loparo K, Sainju RK, Friedman D, Nei M, Strohl K, Allen L, Scott C, Gehlbach BK, Zonjy B, Hupp NJ, Zaremba A, Shafiabadi N, Zhao X, Reick-Mitrisin V, Schuele S, Ogren J, Harper RM, Diehl B, Bateman LM, Devinsky O, Richerson GB, Tanner A, Tatsuoka C, Lhatoo SD. Incidence, recurrence, and risk factors for peri-ictal central apnea and sudden unexpected death in epilepsy. Front Neurol. 2019;10:166. https://doi.org/10.3389/fneur.2019.00166.
43. Bateman LM, Li CS, Seyal M. Ictal hypoxemia in localization-related epilepsy: analysis of incidence, severity and risk factors. Brain. 2008;131(Pt 12):3239–45. https://doi.org/10.1093/brain/awn277. Epub 2008 Oct 24.
44. Seyal M, Bateman LM. Ictal apnea linked to contralateral spread of temporal lobe seizures: intracranial EEG recordings in refractory temporal lobe epilepsy. Epilepsia. 2009;50:2557–62.
45. Leutmezer F, Serles W, Lehrner J, Pataraia E, Zeiler K, Baumgartner C. Postictal nose wiping: a lateralizing sign in temporal lobe complex partial seizures. Neurology. 1998;51(4):1175–7. https://doi.org/10.1212/wnl.51.4.1175.
46. Hirsch LJ, Lain AH, Walczak TS. Postictal nosewiping lateralizes and localizes to the ipsilateral temporal lobe. Epilepsia. 1998;39(9):991–7. https://doi.org/10.1111/j.1528-1157.1998.tb01449.x.
47. Wennberg R. Electroclinical analysis of postictal noserubbing. Can J Neurol Sci. 2000;27(2):131–6.
48. Asadi-Pooya AA, Shabo L, Wyeth D, Nei M. Ictal coughing: clinical features and differential diagnoses. Epilepsy Behav. 2017;73:51–3. https://doi.org/10.1016/j.yebeh.2017.04.044. Epub 2017 Jun 12.
49. Musilová K, Kuba R, Brázdil M, Tyrlíková I, Rektor I. Occurrence and lateralizing value of "rare" peri-ictal vegetative symptoms in temporal lobe epilepsy. Epilepsy Behav. 2010;19(3):372–5. https://doi.org/10.1016/j.yebeh.2010.07.010. Epub 2010 Aug 25.
50. Hoffmann JM, Elger CE, Kleefuss-Lie AA. The localizing value of hypersalivation and postictal coughing in temporal lobe epilepsy. Epilepsy Res. 2009;87(2–3):144–7. https://doi.org/10.1016/j.eplepsyres.2009.08.005. Epub 2009 Sep 11.

51. Cannistraro RJ, Middlebrooks EH, Brinkmann BH, Feyissa AM. Paroxysmal epileptic laryngospasms: frequent nightly awakenings. Neurol Clin Pract. 2018;8(6):e46–8. https://doi.org/10.1212/CPJ.0000000000000554.
52. Terzaghi M, Sartori I, Cremascoli R, Rustioni V, Manni R. Choking in the night due to NFLE seizures in a patient with comorbid OSA. J Clin Sleep Med. 2014;10(10):1149–52. https://doi.org/10.5664/jcsm.4122.
53. Janszky J, Fogarasi A, Toth V, Magalova V, Gyimesi C, Kovacs N, Schulz R, Ebner A. Peri-ictal vegetative symptoms in temporal lobe epilepsy. Epilepsy Behav. 2007;11(1):125–9. https://doi.org/10.1016/j.yebeh.2007.04.015. Epub 2007 Jun 20.
54. Ye BS, Cho YJ, Jang SH, Lee MK, Lee BI, Heo K. The localizing and lateralizing value of auras in lesional partial epilepsy patients. Yonsei Med J. 2012;53(3):477–85. https://doi.org/10.3349/ymj.2012.53.3.477.
55. Marks WJ Jr, Laxer KD. Semiology of temporal lobe seizures: value in lateralizing the seizure focus. Epilepsia. 1998;39(7):721–6. https://doi.org/10.1111/j.1528-1157.1998.tb01157.x.
56. Kramer RE, Lüders H, Goldstick LP, Dinner DS, Morris HH, Lesser RP, Wyllie E. Ictus emeticus: an electroclinical analysis. Neurology. 1988;38(7):1048–52. https://doi.org/10.1212/wnl.38.7.1048.
57. Devinsky O, Frasca J, Pacia SV, Luciano DJ, Paraiso J, Doyle W. Ictus emeticus: further evidence of nondominant temporal involvement. Neurology. 1995;45(6):1158–60. https://doi.org/10.1212/wnl.45.6.1158.
58. Schindler K, Wieser HG. Ictal vomiting in a left hemisphere language-dominant patient with left-sided temporal lobe epilepsy. Epilepsy Behav. 2006;8(1):323–7. https://doi.org/10.1016/j.yebeh.2005.10.014. Epub 2005 Dec 6.
59. Kotagal P, Lüders HO, Williams G, Nichols TR, McPherson J. Psychomotor seizures of temporal lobe onset: analysis of symptom clusters and sequences. Epilepsy Res. 1995;20(1):49–67. https://doi.org/10.1016/0920-1211(94)00055-2.
60. Chen C, Yen DJ, Yiu CH, Shih YH, Yu HY, Su MS. Ictal vomiting in partial seizures of temporal lobe origin. Eur Neurol. 1999;42(4):235–9. https://doi.org/10.1159/000008114.
61. Schäuble B, Britton JW, Mullan BP, Watson J, Sharbrough FW, Marsh WR. Ictal vomiting in association with left temporal lobe seizures in a left hemisphere language-dominant patient. Epilepsia. 2002;43(11):1432–5. https://doi.org/10.1046/j.1528-1157.2002.40701.x.
62. Tarnutzer AA, Mothersill I, Imbach LL. Ictal nausea and vomiting—is it left or right? Seizure. 2018;61:83–8. https://doi.org/10.1016/j.seizure.2018.08.011. Epub 2018 Aug 12.
63. Isnard J, Guénot M, Sindou M, Mauguière F. Clinical manifestations of insular lobe seizures: a stereo-electroencephalographic study. Epilepsia. 2004;45(9):1079–90. https://doi.org/10.1111/j.0013-9580.2004.68903.x.
64. Pugnaghi M, Meletti S, Castana L, Francione S, Nobili L, Mai R, Tassi L. Features of somatosensory manifestations induced by intracranial electrical stimulations of the human insula. Clin Neurophysiol. 2011;122(10):2049–58. https://doi.org/10.1016/j.clinph.2011.03.013. Epub 2011 Apr 14.
65. Carbonari G, Tonti G, Di Pisa V, Franzoni E, Cordelli DM. Pediatric epilepsies misdiagnosed as gastrointestinal disorders. Epilepsy Behav. 2018;83:137–9. https://doi.org/10.1016/j.yebeh.2018.03.034. Epub 2018 Apr 26.
66. Fogarasi A, Janszky J, Tuxhorn I. Ictal pallor is associated with left temporal seizure onset zone in children. Epilepsy Res. 2005;67(3):117–21. https://doi.org/10.1016/j.eplepsyres.2005.09.001. Epub 2005 Oct 17.
67. Loddenkemper T, Kellinghaus C, Gandjour J, Nair DR, Najm IM, Bingaman W, Lüders HO. Localising and lateralising value of ictal piloerection. J Neurol Neurosurg Psychiatry. 2004;75(6):879–83. https://doi.org/10.1136/jnnp.2003.023333.
68. Rocamora R, Becerra JL, Fossas P, Gomez M, Vivanco-Hidalgo RM, Mauri JA, Molins A. Pilomotor seizures: an autonomic semiology of limbic encephalitis? Seizure. 2014;23(8):670–3. https://doi.org/10.1016/j.seizure.2014.04.013. Epub 2014 May 2.

69. Fisch L, Mégevand P, Badoud S, Seeck M, Burkhard PR. Pilomotor seizure: when paroxysmal gooseflesh heralds brain tumor. Neurology. 2012;78(15):1189. https://doi.org/10.1212/WNL.0b013e31824f80f5. Erratum in: Neurology. 2012 Jul 10;79(2):199. Badoud, A [corrected to Badoud, S].
70. Franco AC, Noachtar S, Rémi J. Ictal ipsilateral sweating in focal epilepsy. Seizure. 2017;50:4–5. https://doi.org/10.1016/j.seizure.2017.05.009. Epub 2017 May 12.
71. Leutmezer F, Serles W, Bacher J, Gröppel G, Pataraia E, Aull S, Olbrich A, Czech T, Baumgartner C. Genital automatisms in complex partial seizures. Neurology. 1999;52(6):1188–91. https://doi.org/10.1212/wnl.52.6.1188.
72. Janszky J, Szücs A, Halász P, Borbély C, Holló A, Barsi P, Mirnics Z. Orgasmic aura originates from the right hemisphere. Neurology. 2002;58(2):302–4. https://doi.org/10.1212/wnl.58.2.302.
73. York GK, Gabor AJ, Dreyfus PM. Paroxysmal genital pain: an unusual manifestation of epilepsy. Neurology. 1979;29(4):516–9. https://doi.org/10.1212/wnl.29.4.516.
74. Spencer SS, Spencer DD, Williamson PD, Mattson RH. Sexual automatisms in complex partial seizures. Neurology. 1983;33(5):527–33. https://doi.org/10.1212/wnl.33.5.527.
75. Dobesberger J, Walser G, Unterberger I, Embacher N, Luef G, Bauer G, Benke T, Bartha L, Ulmer H, Ortler M, Trinka E. Genital automatisms: a video-EEG study in patients with medically refractory seizures. Epilepsia. 2004;45(7):777–80. https://doi.org/10.1111/j.0013-9580.2004.44003.x.
76. Mascia A, Di Gennaro G, Esposito V, Grammaldo LG, Meldolesi GN, Giampà T, Sebastiano F, Falco C, Onorati P, Manfredi M, Cantore G, Quarato PP. Genital and sexual manifestations in drug-resistant partial epilepsy. Seizure. 2005;14(2):133–8. https://doi.org/10.1016/j.seizure.2004.12.002.
77. Dede HÖ, Bebek N, Gürses C, Baysal-Kıraç L, Baykan B, Gökyiğit A. Genital automatisms: reappraisal of a remarkable but ignored symptom of focal seizures. Epilepsy Behav. 2018;80:84–9. https://doi.org/10.1016/j.yebeh.2017.12.023. Epub 2018 Feb 2.
78. Rémillard GM, Andermann F, Testa GF, Gloor P, Aubé M, Martin JB, Feindel W, Guberman A, Simpson C. Sexual ictal manifestations predominate in women with temporal lobe epilepsy: a finding suggesting sexual dimorphism in the human brain. Neurology. 1983;33(3):323–30. https://doi.org/10.1212/wnl.33.3.323.
79. Gurgenashvili K, Massey SL, Grant M, Piatt J Jr, Legido A, Valencia I. Intracranial localisation of ictal urinary urge epileptogenic zone to the non-dominant temporal lobe. Epileptic Disord. 2011;13(4):430–4. https://doi.org/10.1684/epd.2011.0476.
80. Loddenkemper T, Foldvary N, Raja S, Neme S, Lüders HO. Ictal urinary urge: further evidence for lateralization to the nondominant hemisphere. Epilepsia. 2003;44(1):124–6. https://doi.org/10.1046/j.1528-1157.2003.26202.x.
81. Vojvodic N, Ristic AJ, Bascarevic V, Popovic L, Parojcic A, Koprivsek K, Sveljo O, Sokic D. Ictal spitting in left temporal lobe epilepsy and fMRI speech lateralization. Clin Neurol Neurosurg. 2013;115(4):495–7. https://doi.org/10.1016/j.clineuro.2012.06.009. Epub 2012 Jul 3.
82. Quevedo-Diaz M, Campo AT, Vila-Vidal M, Principe A, Ley M, Rocamora R. Ictal spitting in non-dominant temporal lobe epilepsy: an anatomo-electrophysiological correlation. Epileptic Disord. 2018;20(2):139–45. https://doi.org/10.1684/epd.2018.0963.
83. Kellinghaus C, Loddenkemper T, Kotagal P. Ictal spitting: clinical and electroencephalographic features. Epilepsia. 2003;44(8):1064–9. https://doi.org/10.1046/j.1528-1157.2003.67302.x.
84. Fejerman N, Caraballo RH, Dalla BB. Benign childhood epilepsy with centrotemporal spikes. In: Benign focal epilepsies in infancy, childhood and adolescence. Surrey: John Libbey Eurotext Limited; 2007. p. 113.
85. Fejerman N, Caraballo RH. Early-onset benign childhood occipital epilepsy (Panayiotopoulos type). In: Benign focal epilepsies in infancy, childhood and adolescence. Surrey: John Libbey Eurotext Limited; 2007. p. 220.

86. Shah J, Zhai H, Fuerst D, Watson C. Hypersalivation in temporal lobe epilepsy. Epilepsia. 2006;47(3):644–51. https://doi.org/10.1111/j.1528-1167.2006.00480.x.
87. Denton D, Shade R, Zamarippa F, Egan G, Blair-West J, McKinley M, Fox P. Correlation of regional cerebral blood flow and change of plasma sodium concentration during genesis and satiation of thirst. Proc Natl Acad Sci U S A. 1999;96(5):2532–7. https://doi.org/10.1073/pnas.96.5.2532.
88. Trinka E, Walser G, Unterberger I, Luef G, Benke T, Bartha L, Ortler M, Bauer G. Peri-ictal water drinking lateralizes seizure onset to the nondominant temporal lobe. Neurology. 2003;60(5):873–6. https://doi.org/10.1212/01.wnl.0000049459.83589.6c.
89. Hauser WA, Annegers JF, Rocca WA. Descriptive epidemiology of epilepsy: contributions of population-based studies from Rochester, Minnesota. Mayo Clin Proc. 1996;71(6):576–86. https://doi.org/10.4065/71.6.576.
90. Cendes F. Progressive hippocampal and extrahippocampal atrophy in drug resistant epilepsy. Curr Opin Neurol. 2005;18(2):173–7. https://doi.org/10.1097/01.wco.0000162860.49842.90.
91. Blümcke I, Thom M, Wiestler OD. Ammon's horn sclerosis: a maldevelopmental disorder associated with temporal lobe epilepsy. Brain Pathol. 2002;12(2):199–211. https://doi.org/10.1111/j.1750-3639.2002.tb00436.x.
92. Blair RD. Temporal lobe epilepsy semiology. Epilepsy Res Treat. 2012;2012:751510. https://doi.org/10.1155/2012/751510. Epub 2012 Mar 7.
93. Tatum WO 4th. Mesial temporal lobe epilepsy. J Clin Neurophysiol. 2012;29(5):356–65. https://doi.org/10.1097/WNP.0b013e31826b3ab7.
94. Bercovici E, Kumar BS, Mirsattari SM. Neocortical temporal lobe epilepsy. Epilepsy Res Treat. 2012;2012:103160. https://doi.org/10.1155/2012/103160. Epub 2012 Jul 16.
95. Van Buren JM. Sensory, motor and autonomic effects of mesial temporal stimulation in man. J Neurosurg. 1961;18:273–88. https://doi.org/10.3171/jns.1961.18.3.0273.
96. Lathers CM, Schraeder PL. Review of autonomic dysfunction, cardiac arrhythmias, and epileptogenic activity. J Clin Pharmacol. 1987;27(5):346–56. https://doi.org/10.1002/j.1552-4604.1987.tb03030.x.
97. Loddenkemper T, Kotagal P. Lateralizing signs during seizures in focal epilepsy. Epilepsy Behav. 2005;7(1):1–17. https://doi.org/10.1016/j.yebeh.2005.04.004.
98. Foldvary-Schaefer N, Unnwongse K. Localizing and lateralizing features of auras and seizures. Epilepsy Behav. 2011;20(2):160–6. https://doi.org/10.1016/j.yebeh.2010.08.034.
99. Athira SB, Pal P, Nair PP, Nanda N, Aghoram R. Cardiovascular autonomic function and baroreflex sensitivity in drug-resistant temporal lobe epilepsy. Epilepsy Behav. 2023;138:109013. https://doi.org/10.1016/j.yebeh.2022.109013. Epub 2022 Dec 14.
100. Noachtar S, Peters AS. Semiology of epileptic seizures: a critical review. Epilepsy Behav. 2009;15(1):2–9. https://doi.org/10.1016/j.yebeh.2009.02.029. Epub 2009 Feb 21.
101. Jan MM, Girvin JP. Seizure semiology: value in identifying seizure origin. Can J Neurol Sci. 2008;35(1):22–30. https://doi.org/10.1017/s0317167100007526.
102. Chen C, Shih YH, Yen DJ, Lirng JF, Guo YC, Yu HY, Yiu CH. Olfactory auras in patients with temporal lobe epilepsy. Epilepsia. 2003;44(2):257–60. https://doi.org/10.1046/j.1528-1157.2003.25902.x.
103. Bien CG, Benninger FO, Urbach H, Schramm J, Kurthen M, Elger CE. Localizing value of epileptic visual auras. Brain. 2000;123(Pt 2):244–53. https://doi.org/10.1093/brain/123.2.244.
104. Biraben A, Taussig D, Thomas P, Even C, Vignal JP, Scarabin JM, Chauvel P. Fear as the main feature of epileptic seizures. J Neurol Neurosurg Psychiatry. 2001;70(2):186–91. https://doi.org/10.1136/jnnp.70.2.186.
105. Oehl B, Schulze-Bonhage A, Lanz M, Brandt A, Altenmüller DM. Occipital lobe epilepsy with fear as leading ictal symptom. Epilepsy Behav. 2012;23(3):379–83. https://doi.org/10.1016/j.yebeh.2011.12.014. Epub 2012 Feb 27.
106. Yaşgüçlükal MA, Makhalova J, Carron R, Bartolomei F. Ictal fear during parietal seizures. Epileptic Disord. 2021;23(5):793–8. https://doi.org/10.1684/epd.2021.1321.

107. Cao Q, Cui T, Wang Q, Li ZM, Fan SH, Xiao ZM, Pan SQ, Zhou Q, Lu ZN, Shao XQ. The localization and lateralization of fear aura and its surgical prognostic value in patients with focal epilepsy. Ann Clin Transl Neurol. 2022;9(8):1116–24. https://doi.org/10.1002/acn3.51607. Epub 2022 Jun 14.
108. Parikh S, Gupta A. Autonomic dysfunction in epilepsy and mitochondrial diseases. Semin Pediatr Neurol. 2013;20(1):31–4. https://doi.org/10.1016/j.spen.2013.01.003.
109. You SM, Jo HJ, Cho BH, Song JY, Kim DY, Hwang YH, Shon YM, Seo DW, Kim IY. Comparing ictal cardiac autonomic changes in patients with frontal lobe epilepsy and temporal lobe epilepsy by ultra-short-term heart rate variability analysis. Medicina (Kaunas). 2021;57(7):666. https://doi.org/10.3390/medicina57070666.
110. Panayiotopoulos CP. Autonomic seizures and autonomic status epilepticus peculiar to childhood: diagnosis and management. Epilepsy Behav. 2004;5(3):286–95. https://doi.org/10.1016/j.yebeh.2004.01.013.
111. Okanishi T, Maegaki Y, Ohno K, Togari H. Underlying neurologic disorders and recurrence rates of status epilepticus in childhood. Brain Dev. 2008;30(10):624–8. https://doi.org/10.1016/j.braindev.2008.02.003. Epub 2008 Mar 24.
112. Specchio N, Trivisano M, Claps D, Battaglia D, Fusco L, Vigevano F. Documentation of autonomic seizures and autonomic status epilepticus with ictal EEG in Panayiotopoulos syndrome. Epilepsy Behav. 2010;19(3):383–93. https://doi.org/10.1016/j.yebeh.2010.06.046. Epub 2010 Aug 24.
113. Panayiotopoulos CP. Panayiotopoulos syndrome: a common and benign childhood epileptic syndrome. London: John Libbey; 2002.
114. Panayiotopoulos CP. Early-onset benign childhood occipital seizure susceptibility syndrome: a syndrome to recognize. Epilepsia. 1999;40(5):621–30. https://doi.org/10.1111/j.1528-1157.1999.tb05565.x.
115. Lada C, Skiadas K, Theodorou V, Loli N, Covanis A. A study of 43 patients with panayiotopoulos syndrome, a common and benign childhood seizure susceptibility. Epilepsia. 2003;44(1):81–8. https://doi.org/10.1046/j.1528-1157.2003.32602.x.
116. Durá-Travé T, Yoldi-Petri ME, Gallinas-Victoriano F. Incidence of epilepsies and epileptic syndromes among children in Navarre, Spain: 2002 through 2005. J Child Neurol. 2008;23(8):878–82. https://doi.org/10.1177/0883073808314898.
117. Panayiotopoulos CP. Vomiting as an ictal manifestation of epileptic seizures and syndromes. J Neurol Neurosurg Psychiatry. 1988;51(11):1448–51. https://doi.org/10.1136/jnnp.51.11.1448.
118. Ferrie C, Caraballo R, Covanis A, Demirbilek V, Dervent A, Kivity S, Koutroumanidis M, Martinovic Z, Oguni H, Verrotti A, Vigevano F, Watanabe K, Yalcin D, Yoshinaga H. Panayiotopoulos syndrome: a consensus view. Dev Med Child Neurol. 2006;48(3):236–40. https://doi.org/10.1017/S0012162206000508.
119. Panayiotopoulos CP, Michael M, Sanders S, Valeta T, Koutroumanidis M. Benign childhood focal epilepsies: assessment of established and newly recognized syndromes. Brain. 2008;131(Pt 9):2264–86. https://doi.org/10.1093/brain/awn162. Epub 2008 Aug 21.
120. Covanis A, Lada C, Skiadas K. Children with Rolandic spikes and ictal vomiting: Rolandic epilepsy or Panayiotopoulos syndrome? Epileptic Disord. 2003;5(3):139–43.
121. Parisi P, Villa MP, Pelliccia A, Rollo VC, Chiarelli F, Verrotti A. Panayiotopoulos syndrome: diagnosis and management. Neurol Sci. 2007;28(2):72–9. https://doi.org/10.1007/s10072-007-0790-4.
122. Caraballo R, Cersósimo R, Fejerman N. Panayiotopoulos syndrome: a prospective study of 192 patients. Epilepsia. 2007;48(6):1054–61. https://doi.org/10.1111/j.1528-1167.2007.01085.x. Epub 2007 Apr 18.
123. Ferrie CD, Grünewald RA. Panayiotopoulos syndrome: a common and benign childhood epilepsy. Lancet. 2001;357(9259):821–3. https://doi.org/10.1016/S0140-6736(00)04192-1.
124. Koutroumanidis M. Panayiotopoulos syndrome. BMJ. 2002;324(7348):1228–9. https://doi.org/10.1136/bmj.324.7348.1228.

125. Specchio N, Trivisano M, Di Ciommo V, Cappelletti S, Masciarelli G, Volkov J, Fusco L, Vigevano F. Panayiotopoulos syndrome: a clinical, EEG, and neuropsychological study of 93 consecutive patients. Epilepsia. 2010;51(10):2098–107. https://doi.org/10.1111/j.1528-1167.2010.02639.x. Epub 2010 Sep 21.
126. Sanders S, Rowlinson S, Manidakis I, Ferrie CD, Koutroumanidis M. The contribution of the EEG technologists in the diagnosis of Panayiotopoulos syndrome (susceptibility to early onset benign childhood autonomic seizures). Seizure. 2004;13(8):565–73. https://doi.org/10.1016/j.seizure.2004.01.006.
127. Taylor I, Berkovic SF, Kivity S, Scheffer IE. Benign occipital epilepsies of childhood: clinical features and genetics. Brain. 2008;131(Pt 9):2287–94. https://doi.org/10.1093/brain/awn138. Epub 2008 Jul 9.
128. Michael M, Tsatsou K, Ferrie CD. Panayiotopoulos syndrome: an important childhood autonomic epilepsy to be differentiated from occipital epilepsy and acute non-epileptic disorders. Brain Dev. 2010;32(1):4–9. https://doi.org/10.1016/j.braindev.2009.03.002. Epub 2009 Apr 21.
129. Berg AT, Coffman K, Gaebler-Spira D. Dysautonomia and functional impairment in rare developmental and epileptic encephalopathies: the other nervous system. Dev Med Child Neurol. 2021;63(12):1433–40. https://doi.org/10.1111/dmcn.14990. Epub 2021 Jul 11.
130. Steffenburg U, Hagberg G, Hagberg B. Epilepsy in a representative series of Rett syndrome. Acta Paediatr. 2001;90:34–9.
131. Neul JL, Kaufmann WE, Glaze DG, Christodoulou J, Clarke AJ, Bahi-Buisson N, Leonard H, Bailey ME, Schanen NC, Zappella M, Renieri A, Huppke P, Percy AK, RettSearch Consortium. Rett syndrome: revised diagnostic criteria and nomenclature. Ann Neurol. 2010;68(6):944–50. https://doi.org/10.1002/ana.22124.
132. Weese-Mayer DE, Lieske SP, Boothby CM, Kenny AS, Bennett HL, Ramirez J-M. Autonomic dysregulation in young girls with Rett syndrome during nighttime in-home recordings. Pediatr Pulmonol. 2008;43:1045–60.
133. Nissenkorn A, Levy-Drummer RS, Bondi O, Renieri A, Villard L, Mari F, Mencarelli MA, Lo Rizzo C, Meloni I, Pineda M, Armstrong J, Clarke A, Bahi-Buisson N, Mejaski BV, Djuric M, Craiu D, Djukic A, Pini G, Bisgaard AM, Melegh B, Vignoli A, Russo S, Anghelescu C, Veneselli E, Hayek J, Ben-Zeev B. Epilepsy in Rett syndrome—lessons from the Rett networked database. Epilepsia. 2015;56(4):569–76. https://doi.org/10.1111/epi.12941. Epub 2015 Mar 19.
134. Glaze DG. Neurophysiology of Rett syndrome. J Child Neurol. 2005;20:740–6.
135. Wolff M, Casse-Perrot C, Dravet C. Severe myoclonic epilepsy of infants (Dravet syndrome): natural history and neuropsychological findings. Epilepsia. 2006;47(Suppl. 2):45–8.
136. Skluzacek JV, Watts KP, Parsy O, Wical B, Camfield P. Dravet syndrome and parent associations: the IDEA League experience with comorbid conditions, mortality, management, adaptation, and grief. Epilepsia. 2011;52:95–101.
137. Delogu AB, Spinelli A, Battaglia D, Dravet C, De Nisco A, Saracino A, Romagnoli C, Lanza GA, Crea F. Electrical and autonomic cardiac function in patients with Dravet syndrome. Epilepsia. 2011;52(Suppl 2):55–8. https://doi.org/10.1111/j.1528-1167.2011.03003.x.
138. Trivisano M, Pavia GC, Ferretti A, Fusco L, Vigevano F, Specchio N. Generalized tonic seizures with autonomic signs are the hallmark of SCN8A developmental and epileptic encephalopathy. Epilepsy Behav. 2019;96:219–23. https://doi.org/10.1016/j.yebeh.2019.03.043. Epub 2019 Jun 4.
139. Pons L, Lesca G, Sanlaville D, Chatron N, Labalme A, Manel V, Arzimanoglou A, de Bellescize J, Lion-François L. Neonatal tremor episodes and hyperekplexia-like presentation at onset in a child with *SCN8A* developmental and epileptic encephalopathy. Epileptic Disord. 2018;20:289–94.
140. Negishi Y, Aoki Y, Itomi K, Yasuda K, Taniguchi H, Ishida A, Arakawa T, Miyamoto S, Nakashima M, Saitsu H, Saitoh S. SCN8A-related developmental and epileptic encepha-

lopathy with ictal asystole requiring cardiac pacemaker implantation. Brain Dev. 2021;43(7):804–8. https://doi.org/10.1016/j.braindev.2021.03.004. Epub 2021 Apr 4.
141. Byard RW. Forensic issues and possible mechanisms of sudden death in Rett syndrome. J Clin Forensic Med. 2006;13(2):96–9. https://doi.org/10.1016/j.jcfm.2005.08.013. Epub 2005 Nov 2.
142. Goswami I, Maguire B, Chau V, Tam EW, Pinchefsky E, Whitney R, Wilson D, Miller SP, Cortez MA. Early transient dysautonomia predicts the risk of infantile epileptic spasm syndrome onset: a prospective cohort study. Front Neurol. 2022;13:1090155. https://doi.org/10.3389/fneur.2022.1090155.
143. Ficker DM, So EL, Shen WK, Annegers JF, O'Brien PC, Cascino GD, Belau PG. Population-based study of the incidence of sudden unexplained death in epilepsy. Neurology. 1998;51(5):1270–4. https://doi.org/10.1212/wnl.51.5.1270.
144. Mazzola L, Rheims S. Ictal and interictal cardiac manifestations in epilepsy. A review of their relation with an altered central control of autonomic functions and with the risk of SUDEP. Front Neurol. 2021;12:642645.
145. Nashef L, So EL, Ryvlin P, Tomson T. Unifying the definitions of sudden unexpected death in epilepsy. Epilepsia. 2012;53(2):227–33. https://doi.org/10.1111/j.1528-1167.2011.03358.x.
146. Harden C, Tomson T, Gloss D, Buchhalter J, Cross JH, Donner E, French JA, Gil-Nagel A, Hesdorffer DC, Smithson WH, Spitz MC, Walczak TS, Sander JW, Ryvlin P. Practice guideline summary: sudden unexpected death in epilepsy incidence rates and risk factors: report of the Guideline Development, Dissemination, and Implementation Subcommittee of the American Academy of Neurology and the American Epilepsy Society. Neurology. 2017;88(17):1674–80. https://doi.org/10.1212/WNL.0000000000003685. Erratum in: Neurology. 2019 Nov 26;93(22):982. Erratum in: Neurology. 2020;94(9):414.
147. Tomson T, Nashef L, Ryvlin P. Sudden unexpected death in epilepsy: current knowledge and future directions. Lancet Neurol. 2008;7:1021–31.
148. Sveinsson O, Andersson T, Carlsson S, Tomson T. The incidence of SUDEP: a nationwide population-based cohort study. Neurology. 2017;89:170–7.
149. Keller AE, Whitney R, Li SA, Pollanen MS, Donner EJ. Incidence of sudden unexpected death in epilepsy in children is similar to adults. Neurology. 2018;91:e107–11.
150. Devinsky O, Bundock E, Hesdorffer D, Donner E, Moseley B, Cihan E, Hussain F, Friedman D. Resolving ambiguities in SUDEP classification. Epilepsia. 2018;59(6):1220–33. https://doi.org/10.1111/epi.14195. Epub 2018 May 23.
151. Ryvlin P, Nashef L, Lhatoo SD, Bateman LM, Bird J, Bleasel A, Boon P, Crespel A, Dworetzky BA, Høgenhaven H, Lerche H, Maillard L, Malter MP, Marchal C, Murthy JMK, Nitsche M, Pataraia E, Rabben T, Rheims S, Sadzot B, Schulze-Bonhage A, Seyal M, So EL, Spitz M, Szucs A, Tan M, Tao JX, Tomson T. Incidence and mechanisms of cardiorespiratory arrests in epilepsy monitoring units (MORTEMUS): a retrospective study. Lancet Neurol. 2013;12(10):966–77. https://doi.org/10.1016/S1474-4422(13)70214-X.
152. Langan Y, Nashef L, Sander JW. Sudden unexpected death in epilepsy: a series of witnessed deaths. J Neurol Neurosurg Psychiatry. 2000;68(2):211–3.
153. Mueller SG, Nei M, Bateman LM, Knowlton R, Laxer KD, Friedman D, Devinsky O, Goldman AM. Brainstem network disruption: a pathway to sudden unexplained death in epilepsy? Hum Brain Mapp. 2018;39(12):4820–30. https://doi.org/10.1002/hbm.24325.
154. Walczak TS, Leppik IE, D'Amelio M, Rarick J, So E, Ahman P, Ruggles K, Cascino GD, Annegers JF, Hauser WA. Incidence and risk factors in sudden unexpected death in epilepsy: a prospective cohort study. Neurology. 2001;56(4):519–25.
155. Sperling MR, Harris A, Nei M, Liporace JD, O'Connor MJ. Mortality after epilepsy surgery. Epilepsia. 2005;46(s11):49–53. https://doi.org/10.1111/j.1528-1167.2005.00410.x.
156. Verducci C, Hussain F, Donner E, Moseley BD, Buchhalter J, Hesdorffer D, Friedman D, Devinsky O. SUDEP in the North American SUDEP Registry: the full spectrum of epilepsies. Neurology. 2019;93(3):e227–36. https://doi.org/10.1212/WNL.0000000000007778. Epub 2019 Jun 19.

157. Hebel JM, Surges R, Stodieck SRG, Lanz M. SUDEP following the second seizure in new-onset epilepsy due to limbic encephalitis. Seizure. 2018;62:124–6.
158. Lhatoo SD, Nei M, Raghavan M, Sperling M, Zonjy B, Lacuey N, Devinsky O. Nonseizure SUDEP: sudden unexpected death in epilepsy without preceding epileptic seizures. Epilepsia. 2016;57(7):1161–8. https://doi.org/10.1111/epi.13419. Epub 2016 May 25.
159. Allen LA, Harper RM, Lhatoo S, Lemieux L, Diehl B. Neuroimaging of sudden unexpected death in epilepsy (SUDEP): insights from structural and resting-state functional MRI studies. Front Neurol. 2019;10:185. https://doi.org/10.3389/fneur.2019.00185.
160. Poh MZ, Loddenkemper T, Reinsberger C, Swenson NC, Goyal S, Madsen JR, Picard RW. Autonomic changes with seizures correlate with postictal EEG suppression. Neurology. 2012;8(23):1868–76. https://doi.org/10.1212/WNL.0b013e318258f7f1.
161. Myers KA, Sivathamboo S, Perucca P. Heart rate variability measurement in epilepsy: How can we move from research to clinical practice? Epilepsia. 2018;59(12):2169–78. https://doi.org/10.1111/epi.14587.
162. Ansakorpi H, Korpelainen JT, Suominen K, Tolonen U, Myllylä VV, Isojärvi JIT. Interictal cardiovascular autonomic responses in patients with temporal lobe epilepsy. Epilepsia. 2000;41(1):42–7. https://doi.org/10.1111/j.1528-1157.2000.tb01503.x.
163. Ferri R, Curzi-Dascalova L, Arzimanoglou A, Bourgeois M, Beaud C, Nunes M, Elia M, Musumeci SA, Tripodi M. Heart rate variability during sleep in children with partial epilepsy. J Sleep Res. 2002;11(2):153–60. https://doi.org/10.1046/j.1365-2869.2002.00283.x.
164. Tomson T, Ericson M, Ihrman C, Lindblad LE. Heart rate variability in patients with epilepsy. Presented in part at the 2nd European Congress of Epileptology, The Hague, September, 1996. Epilepsy Res. 1998;30(1):77–83. https://doi.org/10.1016/S0920-1211(97)00094-6.
165. Devinsky O, Perrine K, Theodore WH. Interictal autonomic nervous system function in patients with epilepsy. Epilepsia. 1994;35(1):199–204. https://doi.org/10.1111/j.1528-1157.1994.tb02933.x.
166. Kolsal E, Serdaroğlu A, Çilsal E, Kula S, Soysal AŞ, Kurt ANÇ, Arhan E. Can heart rate variability in children with epilepsy be used to predict seizures? Seizure. 2014;23(5):357–62. https://doi.org/10.1016/j.seizure.2014.01.025.
167. Ergul Y, Ekici B, Tatli B, Nisli K, Ozmen M. QT and P wave dispersion and heart rate variability in patients with Dravet syndrome. Acta Neurol Belg. 2013;113(2):161–6. https://doi.org/10.1007/s13760-012-0140-z.
168. Page T, Rugg-Gunn FJ. Bitemporal seizure spread and its effect on autonomic dysfunction. Epilepsy Behav. 2018;84:166–72. https://doi.org/10.1016/j.yebeh.2018.03.016.
169. Jeppesen J, Fuglsang-Frederiksen A, Brugada R, Pedersen B, Rubboli G, Johansen P, Beniczky S. Heart rate variability analysis indicates preictal parasympathetic overdrive preceding seizure-induced cardiac dysrhythmias leading to sudden unexpected death in a patient with epilepsy. Epilepsia. 2014;55(7):67. https://doi.org/10.1111/epi.12614.
170. Surges R, Henneberger C, Adjei P, Scott CA, Sander JW, Walker MC. Do alterations in inter-ictal heart rate variability predict sudden unexpected death in epilepsy? Epilepsy Res. 2009;87(2–3):277–80. https://doi.org/10.1016/j.eplepsyres.2009.08.008.
171. Bank AM, Dworetzky BA, Lee JW. Sudden unexpected death in epilepsy in a patient with a cardiac pacemaker. Seizure. 2018;61:38–40.
172. Surges R, Adjei P, Kallis C, Erhuero J, Scott CA, Bell GS, Sander JW, Walker MC. Pathologic cardiac repolarization in pharmacoresistant epilepsy and its potential role in sudden unexpected death in epilepsy: a case-control study. Epilepsia. 2010;51(2):233–42. https://doi.org/10.1111/j.1528-1167.2009.02330.x. Epub 2009 Oct 8.
173. Schuele SU, Bermeo AC, Locatelli E, Burgess RC, Lüders HO. Ictal asystole: a benign condition? Epilepsia. 2008;49:168–71.
174. Chaila E, Bhangu J, Tirupathi S, Delanty N. Ictal bradycardia and asystole associated with intractable epilepsy: a case series. Br J Cardiol. 2010;17:245–8.
175. Sveinsson O, Andersson T, Carlsson S, Tomson T. Circumstances of SUDEP: a nationwide population-based case series. Epilepsia. 2018;59:1074–82.

176. Stecker EC, Reinier K, Uy-Evanado A, Teodorescu C, Chugh H, Gunson K, Jui J, Chugh SS. Relationship between seizure episode and sudden cardiac arrest in patients with epilepsy: a community-based study. Circ Arrhythm Electrophysiol. 2013;6(5):912–6. https://doi.org/10.1161/CIRCEP.113.000544. Epub 2013 Aug 21.
177. Nei M, Ho RT, Abou-Khalil BW, Drislane FW, Liporace J, Romeo A, Sperling MR. EEG and ECG in sudden unexplained death in epilepsy. Epilepsia. 2004;45(4):338–45. https://doi.org/10.1111/j.0013-9580.2004.05503.
178. Bruno E, Biondi A, Richardson MP. Pre-ictal heart rate changes: a systematic review and meta-analysis. Seizure. 2018;55:48–56.
179. Beniczky S, Arbune AA, Jeppesen J, Ryvlin P. Biomarkers of seizure severity derived from wearable devices. Epilepsia. 2020;61(Suppl. 1):S61–6.
180. Sivathamboo S, Constantino TN, Chen Z, Sparks PB, Goldin J, Velakoulis D, Jones NC, Kwan P, Macefield VG, O'Brien TJ, Perucca P. Cardiorespiratory and autonomic function in epileptic seizures: a video-EEG monitoring study. Epilepsy Behav. 2020;111:107271. https://doi.org/10.1016/j.yebeh.2020.107271. Epub 2020 Jul 10.
181. Chouchou F, Bouet R, Pichot V, Catenoix H, Mauguière F, Jung J. The neural bases of ictal tachycardia in temporal lobe seizures. Clin Neurophysiol. 2017;128(9):1810–9. https://doi.org/10.1016/j.clinph.2017.06.033. Epub 2017 Jun 27.
182. Surges R, Jordan A, Elger CE. Ictal modulation of cardiac repolarization, but not of heart rate, is lateralized in mesial temporal lobe epilepsy. PLoS One. 2013;8:e64765.
183. van Westrhenen A, De Cooman T, Lazeron RHC, Van Huffel S, Thijs RD. Ictal autonomic changes as a tool for seizure detection: a systematic review. Clin Auton Res. 2019;29:161–81.
184. Stefanidou M, Carlson C, Friedman D. The relationship between seizure onset zone and ictal tachycardia: an intracranial EEG study. Clin Neurophysiol. 2015;126:2255–60.
185. Opherk C, Coromilas J, Hirsch LJ. Heart rate and EKG changes in 102 seizures: analysis of influencing factors. Epilepsy Res. 2002;52(2):117–27.
186. Pang TD, Nearing BD, Krishnamurthy KB, Olin B, Schachter SC, Verrier RL. Cardiac electrical instability in newly diagnosed/chronic epilepsy tracked by Holter and ECG patch. Neurology. 2019;93(10):450–8.
187. Surges R, Taggart P, Sander JW, Walker MC. Too long or too short? New insights into abnormal cardiac repolarization in people with chronic epilepsy and its potential role in sudden unexpected death. Epilepsia. 2010;51:738–44.
188. Strzelczyk A, Adjei P, Scott CA, Bauer S, Rosenow F, Walker MC, Surges R. Postictal increase in T-wave alternans after generalized tonic-clonic seizures. Epilepsia. 2011;52(11):2112–7. https://doi.org/10.1111/j.1528-1167.2011.03266.x. Epub 2011 Sep 20.
189. Bardai A, Lamberts RJ, Blom MT, Spanjaart AM, Berdowski J, van der Staal SR, Brouwer HJ, Koster RW, Sander JW, Thijs RD, Tan HL. Epilepsy is a risk factor for sudden cardiac arrest in the general population. PLoS One. 2012;7(8):e42749. https://doi.org/10.1371/journal.pone.0042749.
190. Devinsky O, Friedman D, Cheng JY, Moffatt E, Kim A, Tseng ZH. Underestimation of sudden deaths among patients with seizures and epilepsy. Neurology. 2017;89(9):886–92. https://doi.org/10.1212/WNL.0000000000004292.
191. Surges R, Thijs RD, Tan HL, Sander JW. Sudden unexpected death in epilepsy: risk factors and potential pathomechanisms. Nat Rev Neurol. 2009;5:492–504.
192. Rugg-Gunn FJ, Simister RJ, Squirrell M, Holdright DR, Duncan JS. Cardiac arrhythmias in focal epilepsy: a prospective long-term study. Lancet. 2004;364(9452):2212–9. https://doi.org/10.1016/S0140-6736(04)17594-6.
193. Nei M, Mintzer S, Skidmore C, Sperling MR, Ho RT. Heart rate and blood pressure in sudden unexpected death in epilepsy (SUDEP). Epilepsy Res. 2016;122:44–6. https://doi.org/10.1016/j.eplepsyres.2016.02.008.
194. Hampel KG, Jahanbekam A, Elger CE, Surges R. Seizure-related modulation of systemic arterial blood pressure in focal epilepsy. Epilepsia. 2016;57:1709–18.

195. Esmaeili B, Kaffashi F, Theeranaew W, Dabir A, Lhatoo SD, Loparo KA. Post-ictal modulation of baroreflex sensitivity in patients with intractable epilepsy. Front Neurol. 2018;9:793.
196. Nass RD, Hampel KG, Elger CE, Surges R. Blood pressure in seizures and epilepsy. Front Neurol. 2019;10:501. https://doi.org/10.3389/fneur.2019.00501.
197. Liebenthal JA, Wu S, Rose S, Ebersole JS, Tao JX. Association of prone position with sudden unexpected death in epilepsy. Neurology. 2015;84(7):703–9. https://doi.org/10.1212/WNL.0000000000001260.
198. Nashef L, Fish DR, Sander JW, Shorvon SD. Incidence of sudden unexpected death in an adult outpatient cohort with epilepsy at a tertiary referral centre. J Neurol Neurosurg Psychiatry. 1995;58(4):462–4.
199. Lamberts RJ, Thijs RD, Laffan A, Langan Y, Sander JW. Sudden expected death in epilepsy: people with nocturnal seizures may be at highest risk. Epilepsia. 2012;53:253–7.
200. Dlouhy BJ, Gehlbach BK, Kreple CJ, Kawasaki H, Oya H, Buzza C, Granner MA, Welsh MJ, Howard MA, Wemmie JA, Richerson GB. Breathing inhibited when seizures spread to the amygdala and upon amygdala stimulation. J Neurosci. 2015;35(28):10281–9. https://doi.org/10.1523/jneurosci.0888-15.2015.
201. Rhone AE, Kovach CK, Harmata GI, Sullivan AW, Tranel D, Ciliberto MA, Howard MA, Richerson GB, Steinschneider M, Wemmie JA. A human amygdala site that inhibits respiration and elicits apnea in pediatric epilepsy. JCI Insight. 2020;5(6):e134852. https://doi.org/10.1172/jci.insight.134852.
202. Park KJ, Sharma G, Kennedy JD, Seyal M. Potentially high-risk cardiac arrhythmias with focal to bilateral tonic-clonic seizures and generalized tonic-clonic seizures are associated with the duration of periictal hypoxemia. Epilepsia. 2017;58(12):2164–71. https://doi.org/10.1111/epi.13934.
203. Venit EL, Shepard BD, Seyfried TN. Oxygenation prevents sudden death in seizure-prone mice. Epilepsia. 2004;45(8):993–6. https://doi.org/10.1111/j.0013-9580.2004.02304.x.
204. Uteshev VV, Tupal S, Mhaskar Y, Faingold CL. Abnormal serotonin receptor expression in DBA/2 mice associated with susceptibility to sudden death due to respiratory arrest. Epilepsy Res. 2010;88(2–3):183–8. https://doi.org/10.1016/j.eplepsyres.2009.11.004.
205. Tupal S, Faingold CL. Evidence supporting a role of serotonin in modulation of sudden death induced by seizures in DBA/2 mice. Epilepsia. 2006;47(1):21–6. https://doi.org/10.1111/j.1528-1167.2006.00365.x.
206. Faingold CL, Randall M, Kommajosyula SP. Susceptibility to seizure-induced sudden death in DBA/2 mice is altered by adenosine. Epilepsy Res. 2016;124:49–54. https://doi.org/10.1016/j.eplepsyres.2016.05.007.
207. Richerson GB, Buchanan GF. The serotonin axis: shared mechanisms in seizures, depression, and SUDEP. Epilepsia. 2011;52(Suppl 1):28–38. https://doi.org/10.1111/j.1528-1167.2010.02908.x.
208. Bruno E, Richardson MP. Postictal generalized EEG suppression and postictal immobility: what do we know? Epileptic Disord. 2020;22:245–51.
209. Moseley BD, So E, Wirrell EC, Nelson C, Lee RW, Mandrekar J, Britton JW. Characteristics of postictal generalized EEG suppression in children. Epilepsy Res. 2013;106(1–2):123–7. https://doi.org/10.1016/j.eplepsyres.2013.05.007.
210. Tang Y, Xia W, Yan B, Zhao L, An D, Zhou D. Periictal electroclinical characteristics of postictal generalized electroencephalographic suppression after generalized convulsive seizures. Medicine. 2020;99(20):e19940. https://doi.org/10.1097/MD.0000000000019940.
211. Kuo J, Zhao W, Li C-S, Kennedy JD, Seyal M. Postictal immobility and generalized EEG suppression are associated with the severity of respiratory dysfunction. Epilepsia. 2016;57(3):412–7. https://doi.org/10.1111/epi.13312.
212. Critchley HD. Electrodermal responses: what happens in the brain. Neuroscientist. 2002;8(2):132–42. https://doi.org/10.1177/107385840200800209.

213. Sarkis RA, Thome-Souza S, Poh MZ, Llewellyn N, Klehm J, Madsen JR, Picard R, Pennell PB, Dworetzky BA, Loddenkemper T, Reinsberger C. Autonomic changes following generalized tonic clonic seizures: an analysis of adult and pediatric patients with epilepsy. Epilepsy Res. 2015;115:113–8. https://doi.org/10.1016/j.eplepsyres.2015.06.005.
214. Mueller SG, Bateman LM, Laxer KD. Evidence for brainstem network disruption in temporal lobe epilepsy and sudden unexplained death in epilepsy. Neuroimage Clin. 2014;5:208–16. https://doi.org/10.1016/j.nicl.2014.06.010.
215. Allen LA, Vos SB, Kumar R, Ogren JA, Harper RK, Winston GP, Balestrini S, Wandschneider B, Scott A, Ourselin S, Duncan JS, Lhatoo SD, Harper RM, Diehl B. Cerebellar, limbic, and midbrain volume alterations in sudden unexpected death in epilepsy. Epilepsia. 2019;60(4):718–29. https://doi.org/10.1111/epi.14689. Epub 2019 Mar 14.
216. Wandschneider B, Koepp M, Scott C, Micallef C, Balestrini S, Sisodiya SM, Thom M, Harper RM, Sander JW, Vos SB, Duncan JS, Lhatoo S, Diehl B. Structural imaging biomarkers of sudden unexpected death in epilepsy. Brain. 2015;138(Pt 10):2907–19. https://doi.org/10.1093/brain/awv233. Epub 2015 Aug 10.
217. Gigout S, Wierschke C, Dehnicke R. Deisz, different pharmacology of N-desmethylclozapine at human and rat M2 and M4 mAChRs in neocortex, Naunyn Schmiedeberg's. Arch Pharmacol. 2015;388:487–96.
218. Broncel A, Bocian R, Kłos-Wojtczak P, Konopacki J. Medial septal cholinergic mediation of hippocampal theta rhythm induced by vagal nerve stimulation. PLoS One. 2018;13:e0206532.
219. Akyuz E, Polat AK, Eroglu E, Kullu I, Angelopoulou E, Paudel YN. Revisiting the role of neurotransmitters in epilepsy: an updated review. Life Sci. 2021;265:118826.
220. Tupal S, Faingold CL. Fenfluramine, a serotonin-releasing drug, prevents seizure-induced respiratory arrest and is anticonvulsant in the DBA/1 mouse model of SUDEP. Epilepsia. 2019;60:485–94.
221. Patodia S, Somani A, O'Hare M, Venkateswaran R, Liu J, Michalak Z, Ellis M, Scheffer IE, Diehl B, Sisodiya SM, Thom M. The ventrolateral medulla and medullary raphe in sudden unexpected death in epilepsy. Brain. 2018;141(6):1719–33. https://doi.org/10.1093/brain/awy078.
222. Goldman AM, Glasscock E, Yoo J, Chen TT, Klassen TL, Noebels JL. Arrhythmia in heart and brain: KCNQ1 mutations link epilepsy and sudden unexplained death. Sci Transl Med. 2009;1(2):2ra6. https://doi.org/10.1126/scitranslmed.3000289.
223. Li Michael CH, O'Brien Terence J, Todaro M, Powell KL. Acquired cardiac channelopathies in epilepsy: evidence, mechanisms, and clinical significance. Epilepsia. 2019;60:1753–67. https://doi.org/10.1111/epi.16301.
224. Bagnall RD, Crompton DE, Petrovski S, Lam L, Cutmore C, Garry SI, Sadleir LG, Dibbens LM, Cairns A, Kivity S, Afawi Z, Regan BM, Duflou J, Berkovic SF, Scheffer IE, Semsarian C. Exome-based analysis of cardiac arrhythmia, respiratory control, and epilepsy genes in sudden unexpected death in epilepsy. Ann Neurol. 2016;79(4):522–34. https://doi.org/10.1002/ana.24596. Epub 2016 Feb 2.
225. Auerbach DS, Jones J, Clawson BC, Offord J, Lenk GM, Ogiwara I, Yamakawa K, Meisler MH, Parent JM, Isom LL. Altered cardiac electrophysiology and SUDEP in a model of Dravet syndrome. PLoS One. 2013;8(10):e77843. https://doi.org/10.1371/journal.pone.0077843.
226. Frasier CR, Zhang H, Offord J, Dang LT, Auerbach DS, Shi H, Chen C, Goldman AM, Eckhardt LL, Bezzerides VJ, Parent JM, Isom LL. Channelopathy as a SUDEP biomarker in Dravet syndrome patient-derived cardiac myocytes. Stem Cell Rep. 2018;11(3):626–34. https://doi.org/10.1016/j.stemcr.2018.07.012. Epub 2018 Aug 23.
227. Kalume F, Westenbroek RE, Cheah CS, Yu FH, Oakley JC, Scheuer T, Catterall WA. Sudden unexpected death in a mouse model of Dravet syndrome. J Clin Invest. 2013;123:1798–808. https://doi.org/10.1172/JCI66220.

228. Auerbach DS, McNitt S, Gross RA, Zareba W, Dirksen RT, Moss AJ. Genetic biomarkers for the risk of seizures in long QT syndrome. Neurology. 2016;87(16):1660–8. https://doi.org/10.1212/WNL.0000000000003056. Epub 2016 Jul 27. Erratum in: Neurology. 2018;90(24):1127.
229. Coll M, Striano P, Ferrer-Costa C, Campuzano O, Matés J, Del Olmo B, Iglesias A, Pérez-Serra A, Mademont I, Picó F, Oliva A, Brugada R. Targeted next-generation sequencing provides novel clues for associated epilepsy and cardiac conduction disorder/SUDEP. PLoS One. 2017;12(12):e0189618. https://doi.org/10.1371/journal.pone.0189618.
230. Sahly AN, Shevell M, Sadleir LG, Myers KA. SUDEP risk and autonomic dysfunction in genetic epilepsies. Auton Neurosci. 2022;237:102907. https://doi.org/10.1016/j.autneu.2021.102907. Epub 2021 Nov 10.
231. Costagliola G, Orsini A, Coll M, Brugada R, Parisi P, Striano P. The brain-heart interaction in epilepsy: implications for diagnosis, therapy, and SUDEP prevention. Ann Clin Transl Neurol. 2021;8(7):1557–68. https://doi.org/10.1002/acn3.51382. Epub 2021 May 28.
232. Parisi P, Oliva A, Coll Vidal M, Partemi S, Campuzano O, Iglesias A, Pisani D, Pascali VL, Paolino MC, Villa MP, Zara F, Tassinari CA, Striano P, Brugada R. Coexistence of epilepsy and Brugada syndrome in a family with SCN5A mutation. Epilepsy Res. 2013;105(3):415–8. https://doi.org/10.1016/j.eplepsyres.2013.02.024. Epub 2013 Mar 25.
233. Ramachandrannair R, Jack SM. SUDEP: what do adult patients want to know? Epilepsy Behav. 2016;64(Pt A):195–9. https://doi.org/10.1016/j.yebeh.2016.09.022.
234. Ramachandrannair R, Jack SM, Meaney BF, Ronen GM. SUDEP: what do parents want to know? Epilepsy Behav. 2013;29(3):560–4. https://doi.org/10.1016/j.yebeh.2013.09.040.
235. Strzelczyk A, Zschebek G, Bauer S, Baumgartner C, Grond M, Hermsen A, Kieslich M, Krämer G, Kurlemann G, May TW, Mayer T, Neubauer BA, Pfäfflin M, Plecko B, Ryvlin P, Schubert-Bast S, Stefan H, Trinka E, Knake S, Seifart C, Rosenow F. Predictors of and attitudes toward counseling about SUDEP and other epilepsy risk factors among Austrian, German, and Swiss neurologists and neuropediatricians. Epilepsia. 2016;57(4):612–20. https://doi.org/10.1111/epi.13337.
236. Casciato S, Quarato PP, Mascia A, D'Aniello A, Esposito V, Morace R, Pavone L, Di Bonaventura C, Tombini M, Assenza G, Di Gennaro G. Ictal asystole in drug-resistant focal epilepsy: two decades of experience from an epilepsy monitoring unit. Brain Sci. 2020;10(7):443. https://doi.org/10.3390/brainsci10070443.
237. Kohno R, Abe H, Akamatsu N, Benditt DG. Long-term follow-up of ictal asystole in temporal lobe epilepsy: is permanent pacemaker therapy needed? J Cardiovasc Electrophysiol. 2016;27:930–6.
238. Benditt DG, van Dijk G, Thijs RD. Ictal asystole: life-threatening vagal storm or a benign seizure selftermination mechanism? Circ Arrhythm Electrophysiol. 2015;8:11–4.
239. Ruiz-Giménez J, Sánchez-Álvarez JC, Cañadillas-Hidalgo F, Serrano-Castro PJ. Antiepileptic treatment in patients with epilepsy and other comorbidities. Seizure. 2010;19(7):375–82. https://doi.org/10.1016/j.seizure.2010.05.008.
240. Olesen JB, Abildstrøm SZ, Erdal J, Gislason GH, Weeke P, Andersson C, Torp-Pedersen C, Hansen PR. Effects of epilepsy and selected antiepileptic drugs on risk of myocardial infarction, stroke, and death in patients with or without previous stroke: a nationwide cohort study. Pharmacoepidemiol Drug Saf. 2011;20(9):964–71. https://doi.org/10.1002/pds.2186.
241. Kasarskis EJ, Kuo CS, Berger R, Nelson KR. Carbamazepine-induced cardiac dysfunction. Characterization of two distinct clinical syndromes. Arch Intern Med. 1992;152:186–91. https://doi.org/10.1001/archinte.152.1.186.
242. Randazzo DN, Ciccone A, Schweitzer P, Winters SL. Complete atrioventricular block with ventricular asystole following infusion of intravenous phenytoin. J Electrocardiol. 1995;28:157–9. https://doi.org/10.1016/S0022-0736(05)80287-0.
243. Nizam A, Mylavarapu K, Thomas D, Briskin K, Wu B, Saluja D, Wong S. Lacosamide-induced second-degree atrioventricular block in a patient with partial epilepsy. Epilepsia. 2011;52(10):e153–5. https://doi.org/10.1111/j.1528-1167.2011.03212.x. Epub 2011 Jul 29.

244. Chinnasami S, Rathore C, Duncan JS. Sinus node dysfunction: an adverse effect of lacosamide. Epilepsia. 2013;54:e90–3. https://doi.org/10.1111/epi.12108.
245. Degiorgio CM. Atrial flutter/atrial fibrillation associated with lacosamide for partial seizures. Epilepsy Behav. 2010;18:322–4. https://doi.org/10.1016/j.yebeh.2010.04.043.
246. Ryvlin P, Cucherat M, Rheims S. Risk of sudden unexpected death in epilepsy in patients given adjunctive antiepileptic treatment for refractory seizures: a meta-analysis of placebo-controlled randomised trials. Lancet Neurol. 2011;10(11):961–8. https://doi.org/10.1016/S1474-4422(11)70193-4.
247. Sperling MR, Barshow S, Nei M, Asadi-Pooya AA. A reappraisal of mortality after epilepsy surgery. Neurology. 2016;86(21):1938–44. https://doi.org/10.1212/WNL.0000000000002700. Epub 2016 Apr 27.
248. Sperling MR, Feldman H, Kinman J, Liporace JD, O'Connor MJ. Seizure control and mortality in epilepsy. Ann Neurol. 1999;46(1):45–50. https://doi.org/10.1002/1531-8249(199907)46:1<45::aid-ana8>3.0.co;2-i.
249. Salanova V, Markand O, Worth R. Temporal lobe epilepsy surgery: outcome, complications, and late mortality rate in 215 patients. Epilepsia. 2002;43:170–4.
250. Bestawros M, Darbar D, Arain A, Abou-Khalil B, Plummer D, Dupont WD, Raj SR. Ictal asystole and ictal syncope: insights into clinical management. Circ Arrhythm Electrophysiol. 2015;8(1):159–64. https://doi.org/10.1161/CIRCEP.114.001667. Epub 2014 Nov 12.
251. Moseley BD, Ghearing GR, Benarroch EE, Britton JW. Early seizure termination in ictal asystole. Epilepsy Res. 2011;97(1–2):220–4. https://doi.org/10.1016/j.eplepsyres.2011.08.008. Epub 2011 Sep 6.
252. van Westrhenen A, Shmuely S, Surges R, Diehl B, Friedman D, Leijten FSS, van Hoey SJ, Benditt DG, van Dijk JG, Thijs RD. Timing of syncope in ictal asystole as a guide when considering pacemaker implantation. J Cardiovasc Electrophysiol. 2021;32(11):3019–26. https://doi.org/10.1111/jce.15239. Epub 2021 Sep 19.
253. Garamendi I, Acera M, Agundez M, Galbarriatu L, Marinas A, Pomposo I, Valle E, Palma JA, Gomez-Esteban JC. Cardiovascular autonomic and hemodynamic responses to vagus nerve stimulation in drug-resistant epilepsy. Seizure. 2017;45:56–60. https://doi.org/10.1016/j.seizure.2016.11.018. Epub 2016 Dec 2.
254. Sveinsson O, Andersson T, Mattsson P, Carlsson S, Tomson T. Clinical risk factors in SUDEP: a nationwide population-based case-control study. Neurology. 2020;94:e419–29.
255. Ryvlin P, So EL, Gordon CM, Hesdorffer DC, Sperling MR, Devinsky O, Bunker MT, Olin B, Friedman D. Long-term surveillance of SUDEP in drug-resistant epilepsy patients treated with VNS therapy. Epilepsia. 2018;59(3):562–72. https://doi.org/10.1111/epi.14002. Epub 2018 Jan 16.
256. Verrier RL, Nearing BD, Olin B, Boon P, Schachter SC. Baseline elevation and reduction in cardiac electrical instability assessed by quantitative T-wave alternans in patients with drug-resistant epilepsy treated with vagus nerve stimulation in the AspireSR E-36 trial. Epilepsy Behav. 2016;62:85–9.
257. Langan Y, Nashef L, Sander JW. Case-control study of SUDEP. Neurology. 2005;64:1131–3.
258. Maguire MJ, Jackson CF, Marson AG, Nevitt SJ. Treatments for the prevention of sudden unexpected death in epilepsy (SUDEP). Cochrane Database Syst Rev. 2020;4:CD011792.
259. van der Lende M, Hesdorffer DC, Sander JW, Thijs RD. Nocturnal supervision and SUDEP risk at different epilepsy care settings. Neurology. 2018;91:e1508–18.
260. Seyal M, Bateman LM, Li CS. Impact of periictal interventions on respiratory dysfunction, postictal EEG suppression, and postictal immobility. Epilepsia. 2013;54(2):377–82. https://doi.org/10.1111/j.1528-1167.2012.03691.x.
261. Kang JY, Rabiei AH, Myint L, Nei M. Equivocal significance of post-ictal generalized EEG suppression as a marker of SUDEP risk. Seizure. 2017;48:28–32. https://doi.org/10.1016/j.seizure.2017.03.017.

262. Nagai Y, Aram J, Koepp M, Lemieux L, Mula M, Critchley H, Sisodiya S, Cercignani M. Epileptic seizures are reduced by autonomic biofeedback therapy through enhancement of fronto-limbic connectivity: a controlled trial and neuroimaging study. EBioMedicine. 2018;27:112–22.
263. Lee J, Devinsky O. The role of autonomic dysfunction in sudden unexplained death in epilepsy patients. Rev Neurol Dis. 2005;2(2):61–9.
264. Ryvlin P, Ciumas C, Wisniewski I, Beniczky S. Wearable devices for sudden unexpected death in epilepsy prevention. Epilepsia. 2018;59(Suppl. 1):61–6.
265. Rheims S. Wearable devices for seizure detection: is it time to translate into our clinical practice. Rev Neurol. 2020;176:480–4. https://doi.org/10.1016/j.neurol.2019.12.012.
266. Beniczky S, Jeppesen J. Non-electroencephalography-based seizure detection. Curr Opin Neurol. 2019;32:198–204. https://doi.org/10.1097/WCO.0000000000000658.
267. Schuele SU, Widdess-Walsh P, Bermeo A, Lüders HO. Sudden unexplained death in epilepsy: the role of the heart. Clevel Clin J Med. 2007;74(Suppl 1):121.
268. Schuele SU, Bermeo AC, Alexopoulos AV, Burgess RC. Anoxia-ischemia: a mechanism of seizure termination in ictal asystole. Epilepsia. 2010;51(1):170–3. https://doi.org/10.1111/j.1528-1167.2009.02168.x.

Chapter 12
Pathophysiology, Clinical Presentation and Management of Neurogenic Bladder

Giuseppe Pelliccioni, Daniele Castellani, Camilla Rocchi, Valentina Cameriere, Deborah Sabbatini, and Pietro Pelliccioni

12.1 Introduction

The voluntary control of micturition requires complex connections between sympathetic and parasympathetic systems, somatic nerves and different brain areas. The coordination between the bladder, urethra and sphincters is mediated by a complex neural control system in the brain, spinal cord, peripheral ganglia and peripheral nerves. Therefore, lower urinary tract (LUT) dysfunction is present in different neurological diseases [1, 2]. A practical model of bladder dysfunction can be useful for neurological clinical practice and diagnostic workup.

G. Pelliccioni (✉) · V. Cameriere · D. Sabbatini
Neurology Department, IRCCS INRCA-National Institute of Health and Science on Aging, Ancona, Italy
e-mail: g.pelliccioni@inrca.it; v.cameriere@inrca.it; d.sabbatini@inrca.it

D. Castellani
Urology Department, Azienda Ospedaliero-Universitaria Ospedali Riuniti di Ancona, Università Politecnica delle Marche, Ancona, Italy
e-mail: daniele.castellani@ospedaliriuniti.marche.it

C. Rocchi
Neurology Unit, Department of Systems Medicine, Policlinico Tor Vergata, University of Rome "Tor Vergata", Rome, Italy
e-mail: camilla.rocchi@ptvonline.it

P. Pelliccioni
Neurology Clinic, Department of Medicine, Surgery and Neuroscience, University of Siena, Siena, Italy

G. Micieli et al. (eds.), *Autonomic Disorders in Clinical Practice*,
https://doi.org/10.1007/978-3-031-43036-7_12

12.2 Neural Control of Urinary Tract

The bladder and urethra have two primary functions: the storage and the periodic elimination of urine; these activities need neural coordination in the central, somatic and autonomic peripheral nervous systems. The voluntary control of micturition requires complex connections between sympathetic and parasympathetic autonomic nerves, pudendal somatic nerves and many areas in the brain. Parasympathetic preganglionic cholinergic outflow, giving excitatory input to the bladder, arises in the sacral parasympathetic nucleus (SPN), localised in the intermediolateral column from the S2–S4 spinal segments. The parasympathetic fibres then travel through pelvic nerves to intramural bladder ganglia and pelvic plexus, where the postganglionic fibres induce detrusor contraction and urinary flow. The parasympathetic activation of M_3 muscarinic and P2X purinergic receptors is involved in the voiding reflex while nitric oxide transmission mediates inhibition of urethral smooth muscle. The sympathetic system, which plays a primary role in the continence mechanism inhibiting the parasympathetic action, originates from the intermediolateral columns in the T11–L2 spinal cord segments. Preganglionic may synapse on postganglionic in the paravertebral sympathetic chain or pelvic plexus; the hypogastric nerve, conveying sympathetic afferents and efferents, releases noradrenaline (NA) on bladder and urethra. The sympathetic efferents therefore activate β_3-adrenergic inhibitory receptors in the detrusor muscle relaxing the bladder, and α_1-adrenergic excitatory receptors in the bladder neck and urethra allowing the continence and urine storage and preventing retrograde ejaculation. The somatic cholinergic pathway originating from S2-S4 motor neurons in Onuf's nucleus (ON) innervates through pudendal nerves the external urethral sphincter (EUS) and pelvic floor muscles, including external anal sphincter (EAS) (Fig. 12.1). The somatic afferents from the bladder neck and the urethra are conveyed from pudendal nerves to the dorsal horns of the spinal cord in the S2–S4 tract, while the sensation of bladder fullness travels through pelvic and hypogastric nerves to the spinal cord, by means of afferent Aδ-fibres, lightly myelinated, and unmyelinated C fibres, up to the cerebral cortex. While Aδ-fibres respond to active contraction and passive distension, C-fibres are activated only in pathological conditions, in particular in spinal injuries, and they are probably involved in the pathophysiological mechanism underlying detrusor hyperreflexia.

Both bladder and the other functional unit consisting of the bladder neck, urethra and EUS are activated and coordinated by various central neural circuits, involving midbrain periaqueductal grey (PAG), cell groups of the preoptic and caudal hypothalamus, the pontine micturition centre (PMC) and the medial frontal cortex. The PMC is activated during voiding (M-region) and bladder filling (L-region or pontine storage centre), and it appears to initiate and coordinate lower urinary tract function.

The cortical-diencephalic circuitry has three major functions: amplification of bladder contraction to allow complete micturition, control of micturition

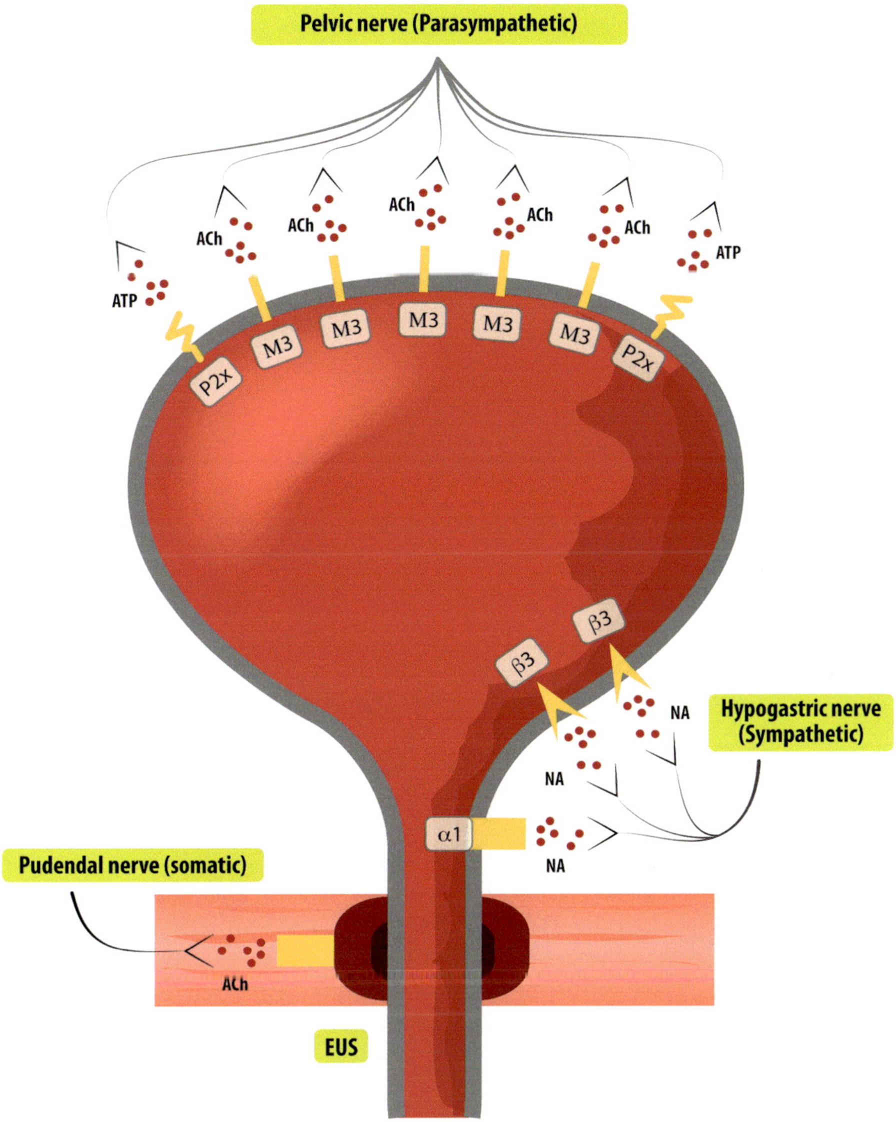

Fig. 12.1 Neurotransmitter mechanisms regulating urinary bladder and EUS function. Distribution of different autonomic and somatic axons. (From Micieli et al. "Disfunzioni Autonomiche" © 2022 Il Pensiero Scientifico Editore with permission)

frequency and coordination of the activity of lower urinary tract muscles. Overlapping between voluntary control and a reflex mechanism is allowed by sympathetic, parasympathetic and somatic peripheral innervation of the bladder and urethra. Higher centres in the CNS induce a modulatory effect over PMC,

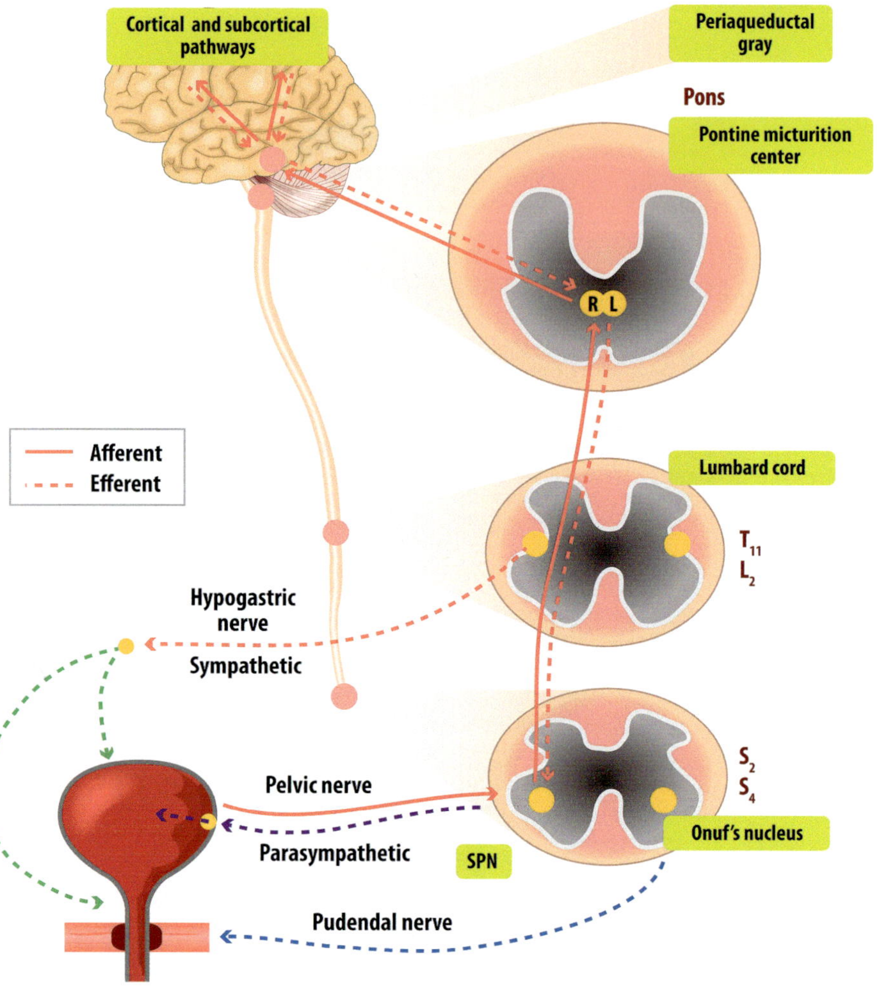

Fig. 12.2 Central and peripheral pathways involved in functional neural control of the urinary tract. (From Micieli et al. "Disfunzioni Autonomiche" © 2022 Il Pensiero Scientifico Editore with permission)

primarily mediated by an inhibitory input. The PMC appears to initiate and coordinate lower urinary tract function, pairing detrusor contraction with inhibition of urethral outlet and sphincter release, while the sacral micturition centre triggers an involuntary reflex detrusor contraction in response to rapid bladder filling. In fact, two distinct voiding reflex pathways exist: a suprasacral reflex that is physiologically active in normal subjects and a sacral reflex which allows voiding in pathological conditions (Fig. 12.2).

12.3 Neurogenic Lower Urinary Tract Disorders

The results of neurological lesions on urinary function can be represented by different voiding dysfunctions on three different levels: the supraspinal (suprapontine) level, the spinal (intrapontine-suprasacral) level, and the sacral and peripheral level [3]. Moreover, there are cases of bladder dysfunction without organic lesions of the urinary tract and with normal patterns in the nervous system's regulation and control [1, 2, 4]. The different clinical, ultrasound and urodynamic features can be explained on the basis of knowledge of the voiding centres (Figs. 12.3 and 12.4).

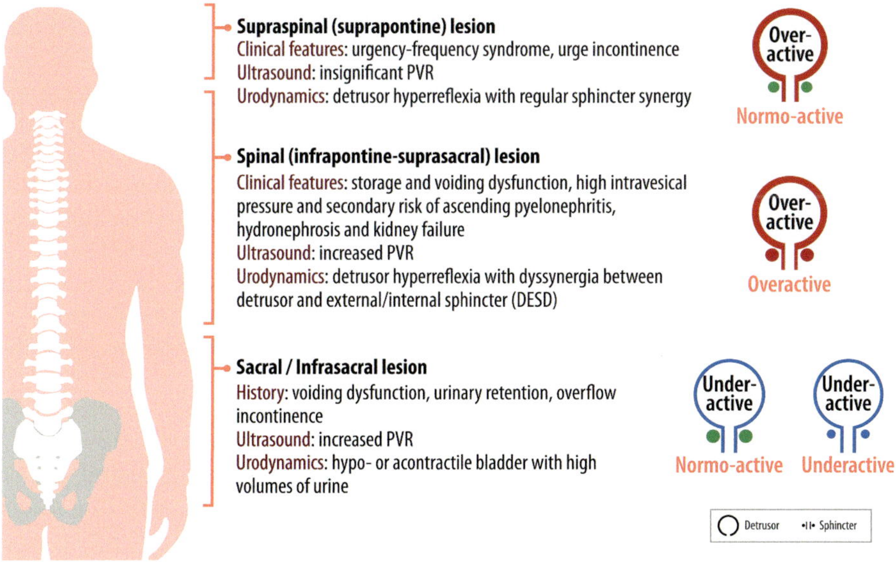

Fig. 12.3 Patterns of LUT dysfunction based on level of neurological disease. (From Micieli et al. "Disfunzioni Autonomiche" © 2022 Il Pensiero Scientifico Editore with permission)

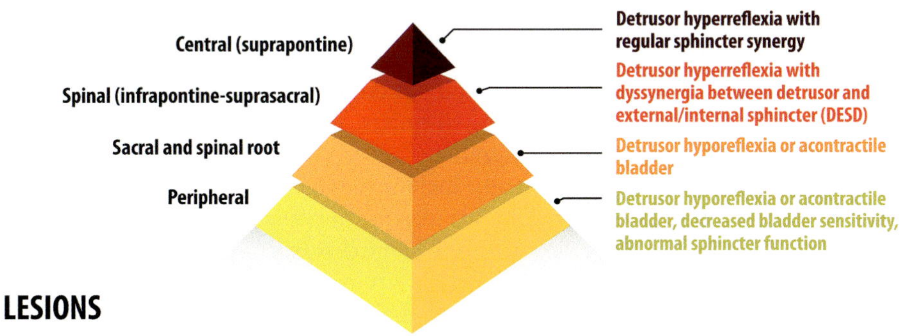

Fig. 12.4 Urodynamic features based on level of neurological disease. (From Micieli et al. "Disfunzioni Autonomiche" © 2022 Il Pensiero Scientifico Editore with permission)

12.3.1 Central Supraspinal Injuries

Patients with supraspinal lesions mainly complain of urinary symptoms characterised by urgency-frequency syndrome and urge incontinence. Cerebrovascular diseases, infantile cerebral palsy, normal pressure hydrocephalus, dementia, intracranial tumours, cranioencephalic trauma, multiple system atrophy (MSA), Parkinson's disease and parkinsonisms [5], multiple sclerosis and other demyelinating disorders, as well as other supraspinal injuries more frequently induce *detrusor hyperreflexia with regular sphincter synergy*, i.e. with a coordinated activity of the external sphincter and bladder neck (Figs. 12.3 and 12.5). In these cases, the cortical inhibition is reduced and it induces uninhibited bladder contractions in response to lower bladder filling volumes, generally much lower (trigger point) than normal bladder capacity, which is about 400 mL.

Uninhibited bladder contractions, especially in the elderly, may also be poorly sustained over time, resulting not only in urgency-frequency syndrome or incontinence but also in incomplete bladder voiding despite the release of external urethral sphincter. This clinical and urodynamic condition, which is common in MSA patients and is the second most common cause of bladder voiding dysfunction in the elderly, is named *detrusor hyperactivity with impaired contractility* (DHIC).

In the presence of relative integrity of the pontine centre, a physiological release of the external urethral sphincter is ensured during bladder contraction. Therefore if a sustained uninhibited contraction is present, the bladder empties efficiently without a significant post-voiding residual volume (PVR). The presence of an elevated PVR suggests DHIC or a preexisting condition of outflow obstruction. It is important to consider that voiding dysfunctions signs and symptoms may differ in relation to the presence of incomplete spinal cord lesions, of associated central and/or peripheral lesions, of drugs use or of urinary outflow obstructions, such as prostate hypertrophy or tumours.

12.3.2 Spinal Injuries (Intrapontine-Suprasacral)

Anatomically, traumatic and non-traumatic spinal cord injuries are defined by level and are classified as cervical, thoracic and lumbosacral. However, when analysing the effects of spinal injuries on voiding disorders, it is preferable to classify these same injuries into suprasacral and sacral.

Suprasacral lesions most frequently include spinal injuries, myelitis, multiple sclerosis, and primary or metastatic bone marrow tumours. As in supraspinal injuries, suprasacral injuries may present urodynamic detrusor hyperreflexia with uninhibited contractions as the bladder reaches its trigger point. More commonly, detrusor hyperreflexia is characterised by a *dyssynergia between detrusor and external sphincter* (DESD), since the pontine centre is no longer able to coordinate the relaxation of the external sphincter during bladder contraction. In the absence of an

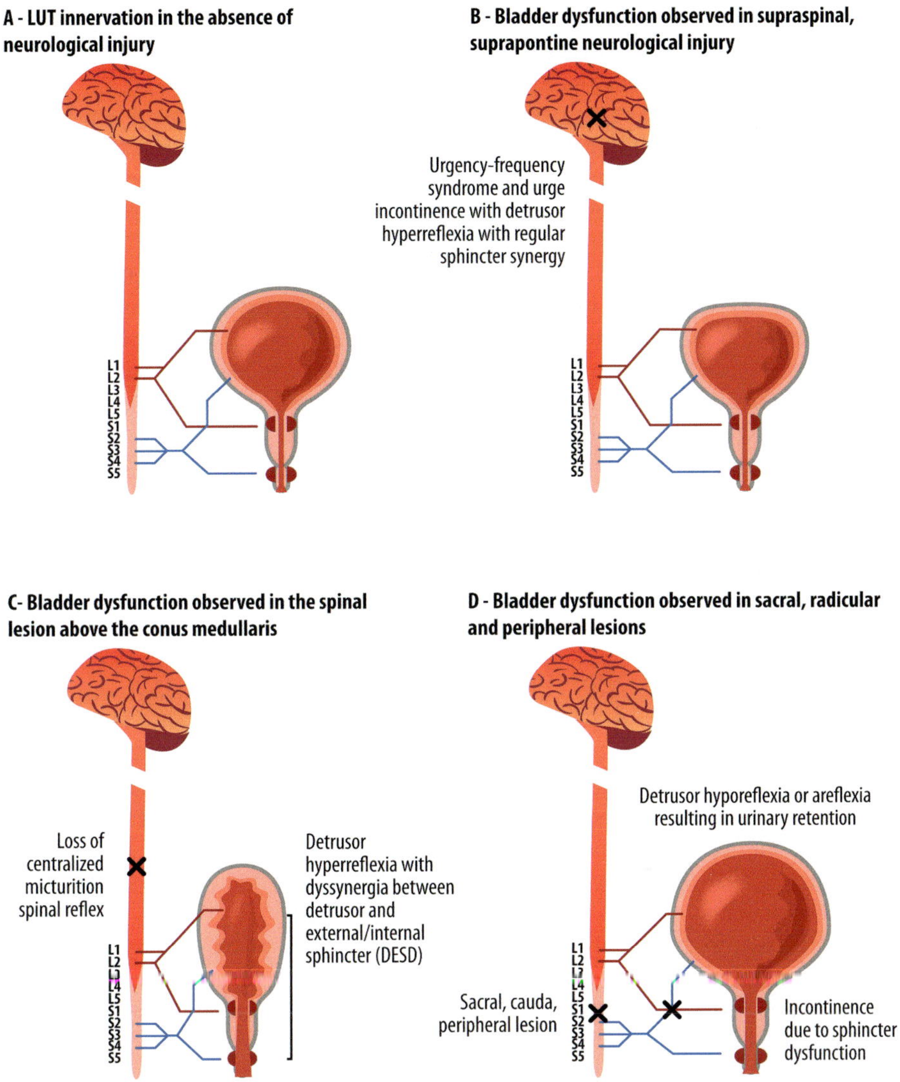

Fig. 12.5 Types of bladder dysfunction typically observed after neurological injury. (From Micieli et al. "Disfunzioni Autonomiche" © 2022 Il Pensiero Scientifico Editore with permission)

input from the pontine centre, uninhibited bladder contractions stimulate a sphincter contraction reflex. DESD should therefore be considered as an exaggerated continence reflex (Figs. 12.3 and 12.5).

In healthy subjects, the continence reflex produces an increase in sphincter activity in order to prevent incontinence in case of excessive bladder filling or increased intra-abdominal pressure. There is not a definite relationship between dyssynergia and lesion level or duration, but the presence of a DESD is certainly more frequent in higher spinal cord lesions than in lower ones. Moreover, it is important to remember that DESD can be associated with a dyssynergia of the internal sphincter or bladder neck during bladder contraction.

In suprasacral lesions, as in supraspinal injuries, different clinical and urodynamic patterns can occur due to variations in the function of the bladder and sphincter related to partial damage or hidden lesions, not detectable by normal imaging techniques but which can sometimes be confirmed by appropriate electrophysiological investigations.

Patients suffering from detrusor hyperreflexia and DESD frequently show increased connective tissue in the bladder wall, especially those suffering from outflow obstruction due to sphincter dyssynergia. Consequences of this phenomenon are high intravesical pressure and the secondary risk of ascending pyelonephritis, hydronephrosis and kidney failure.

Patients with suprasacral lesions and regular bladder sensations usually show urgency-frequency syndrome but may also be incontinent without any awareness.

It must be emphasised that incomplete bladder voiding can exacerbate detrusor hyperreflexia and that an overactive bladder, stimulated by a relevant post-voiding residual volume (PVR), induces additional urgency-frequency symptoms.

12.3.3 Sacral and Spinal Root Injuries

Different types of lesions can involve sacral cord or nerve roots such as trauma, herniated discs, tumours, myelodysplasias, arteriovenous malformations, congenital and acquired lumbar stenosis, and inflammatory processes (arachnoiditis). Trauma is the most frequent cause of conus or cauda equina lesions, followed by L4–L5 and L5–S1 herniated discs that are the cause of cauda equina syndrome in 1–15% of patients.

The damage to the sacral cord or roots is usually responsible for an acontractile bladder with high volumes of urine. However, particularly in patients with incomplete spinal lesions, areflexia may be accompanied by a reduction in bladder compliance resulting in a progressive increase in intravesical pressure during filling. The mechanism by which the disconnected sacral parasympathetic centre induces a decrease in bladder compliance is unclear. In patients with sacral lesions, the external sphincter is often less involved than the detrusor, due to the different positions of the nuclei that provide innervation; the combination of detrusor areflexia with a functionally intact sphincter contributes to bladder overdistention and decompensation (Figs. 12.3 and 12.5). Such patients frequently complain of a sensation of suprapubic fullness, incontinence, and inability to empty the bladder. This clinical picture is caused by urinary retention with overflow incontinence and high post-voiding residual volumes. Furthermore, if bladder sensitivity is relatively normal, a syndrome of increased frequency with the elimination of low amounts of urine, subsequent rapid bladder filling, and new voiding urgency may occur.

12.3.4 *Peripheral Nerve Injuries*

Peripheral lesions show variable urodynamic and clinical findings based on the type of parasympathetic, sympathetic, and/or somatic peripheral injury. Moreover, bladder dysfunction is also frequent in diffuse polyneuropathies involving small calibre fibres, because of bladder widespread autonomic innervation. Dysimmune neuropathies, distal autonomic neuropathies, amyloidosis and diabetes may involve bladder-inducing alterations of detrusor contractility, urinary flow reduction and PVR increase.

Detrusor areflexia is the result of parasympathetic lesions, while sympathetic injury can cause incontinence due to impaired internal urethral sphincter closure. On the other hand, the involvement of motor and/or sensory nerves usually induces chronic bladder overdistension with an increase in post-voiding residual volumes. Patients with exclusive sensory involvement may initially have bladder contractions and normal bladder capacity; however, decreased bladder sensitivity usually leads to chronic overdistention of the bladder itself, with subsequent decompensation and consequent detrusor areflexia (Figs. 12.3 and 12.5).

12.4 Clinical Evaluation

A thorough history and a neurological and urological examination should always be performed in order to diagnose neurogenic pelvic dysfunction and to plan further electrophysiological tests [6, 7]. The examination includes anal sphincter tone, S1–S2 innervated muscle strength (gastrocnemius, gluteal muscles), sensation extending from the soles of the feet to the perianal area, and the presence of anal and bulbocavernosus reflexes.

Medical history:

- Current and past symptoms.
- Family history and neurological and urological risk factors (diabetes mellitus, multiple sclerosis, parkinsonism, encephalitis, cerebrovascular encephalopathy, etc.).
- Previous surgical interventions.
- Pharmacological therapy.
- Cognitive status and evolution of somatic and/or sensory symptoms.
- Bowel: the desire to defecate, rectal tenesmus, pattern and modality of defecation (use of abdominal press, faecal and/or gas incontinence, soiling, etc.).
- Evaluation of lower urinary tract symptoms (investigate both the filling and voiding phases): onset, urinary urgency and frequency, presence and type of incontinence, bladder sensation, the beginning of micturition (use of the abdominal press, strain, Credé manoeuvre, sitting urination), the possible presence of haematuria. Special attention has to be paid to hematuria that requires further investigation to rule out stones and urinary tract cancers. A urinalysis is recommended

in all patients, especially to detect haematuria; treatment of asymptomatic bacteriuria or pyuria is not recommended.

- Completion of the voiding diary at baseline and controls (bladder diaries): number of micturitions, voided volume (information on functional cystometric capacity), episodes of urgency and urinary incontinence. The voiding diary, when compiled for a few days, is a simple and objective method to measure the type of symptoms and their severity. Although not fully validated in neurological patients, three consecutive 24-h bladder diaries are usually reliable tools in daily practice. The number of micturitions, nocturia and episodes of incontinence are thus rapidly evaluated and can be compared with the number and severity of events after the administration of therapy.
- Specific questionnaires for the assessment of urinary symptoms:
  - International Prostate Symptoms Score (IPSS): 8 questions with scores from 0 to 35 (higher score = more symptoms). Validated also in women.
  - Neurogenic Bladder Symptoms Score (NBSS): 25 questions to assess urinary symptoms in neurological patients.
- Evaluation of bowel history: taking a bowel history is also an important step in patient assessment because neurogenic bowel dysfunction may be associated with neuro-urological symptoms. Physicians should ask patients about their defecation habitus, exploring the desire to defecate and rectal sensation, and defecation pattern (e.g. straining or digitation to start defecation and faecal incontinence).
- Evaluation of the sexual sphere: orgasm, dyspareunia, erectile dysfunction, ejaculation, symptoms and sensitivity of the pelvic area. Validated questionnaires: Male Sexual Health Questionnaire, International Index of Erectile Function, Female Sexual Function Index.

12.5 Neurological and Urological Physical Examination

- Comprehensive assessment of lower spinal cord-mediated reflexes and sensitivities (normal/increased/decreased/absent) in accordance with the distribution of dermatomes and cutaneous nerves of the genital, perianal, perineal, and thigh areas. Cremasteric (L1–L2), Patellar (L2–L4), Achilles (S1–S2), Anal (S2–S4), Bulbocavernosus (S2–S4) reflexes.
- Bulbocavernosus reflex: it is a somatic reflex that provides information on the state of the segments of the sacral spinal cord. It can be induced (contractions of the bulbocavernosus muscles and/or external anal sphincter) by painless stimulation (squeezing) of the glans or clitoris. If present, it indicates that the spinal reflex arc (spinal segments S2–S4) with afferent and efferent nerves through the pudendal nerve is intact.
- Assessment of anal sphincter tone (preserved, increased, reduced, absent).

- Rectal exploration: evaluation of prostate volume. Digital rectal examination is the easiest way to assess prostate volume, but the correlation to prostate volume is poor; however, it is sufficient to discriminate between prostate volume above or below 50 mL.
- Palpation of the suprapubic area: the presence of a bladder globe is generally associated with a reduction in the sensation of bladder filling.
- Evaluation of urogenital prolapse.
- Cough test (evaluation of stress incontinence in women), as standardised by the International Continence Society: in supine/lithotomy position with a bladder filling of 200–400 mL. At least four strong coughs with simultaneous visualisation of the external urethral meatus for the presence of leakage. Leakage of fluid/urine from the urethral meatus coincident with or simultaneous to the cough is considered a positive test.

12.5.1 Investigating Lower Urinary Tract Function: Urodynamics

The term *urodynamics* encompasses several investigations, invasive and not, widely used in urological clinical practice as a helpful adjunct to diagnosis. Urodynamic investigations are very useful tests in assessing objectively the function and dysfunction of the LUT. In neurological patients, urodynamics is the cornerstone to provide or confirm diagnosis, to simplify counselling, and to predict and evaluate treatment outcomes. Urodynamics include the following investigations: uroflowmetry, ultrasound measuring of PVR, filling cystometry, pressure-flow study, leak point pressure, electromyography, and triggered tests. There are also advanced tests that are video-urodynamics and ambulatory urodynamics. It must be emphasised that urodynamics has been standardised by the International Continence Society and should be performed according to technical recommendations. Besides, standardised terminology should be used to ensure correct knowledge among practitioners involved in patient care.

12.5.2 Non-invasive Tests: Free Uroflowmetry and Ultrasound Measuring of PVR

Usually, both tests are performed in the same session to provide the first judgement regarding the voiding phase and to screen for bladder outlet obstruction. They are the first steps before planning invasive studies in patients able to void. In free uroflowmetry, patients are asked to come to the outpatient clinic with a "normal" desire to void. Since it is usually difficult to get an adequate and reliable flow in the outpatient clinic, the bladder should be comfortably full and a voided volume of at least

150–200 mL should be obtained. Then, micturition should be performed in privacy, patients should be relaxed and allowed to void in their usual position (standing or sitting) and the test should be repeated at least three times to ensure reproducibility. Soon after voiding, PVR should be assessed. Urine flow is described in terms of flow rate and pattern. The following data are reported:

1. *Flow rate*: volume expelled per unit of time (mL/s)
2. *Maximum flow rate*: maximum measure value of the flow
3. *Voided volume*: total volume expelled (mL)
4. *Average flow rate*: voided volume divided by flow time
5. *Time to the maximum flow*: elapsed time from the onset to the maximum flow

Several nomograms have been developed to relate the maximum flow rate to the voided volume taking sex and age into account. Plotting data in nomograms is helpful to assess bladder outlet obstruction.

- *"Normal" flow pattern* (unobstructed voiding): the curve has a bell shape and the maximum flow is reached within 5 s from the micturition start. The final phase trace usually ends with a rapid decrease from the maximum flow rate. The flow rate differs according to the different voided volumes, but the first and final appearance of the shape is similar. PVR is usually absent or not significant (less than 100–150 mL or <30% of the filled bladder). The bladder should not be overfilled (>400 mL) because the efficiency of the detrusor begins to decrease and the corresponding maximum flow rate becomes lower. The correct bladder filling should be between 200 and 400 mL.
- *Detrusor overactivity flow pattern:* usually, very high maximum flow rates are seen with a very rapid increase in the flow (1–3 s) due to high detrusor contraction velocity.
- *Bladder outlet obstruction flow pattern*: the curve is characterised by a low maximum flow rate and a reduced average flow. The maximum flow rate is reached slower (3–10 s) and the flow decreases slowly giving a flattened bell-shaped (benign prostatic hyperplasia, BPH) or plateau-flattened curve (urethral stricture). The curve may also be intermittent in BPH obstruction due to abdominal straining.
- *Detrusor underactivity flow pattern:* detrusor underactivity is difficult to diagnose with a simple free uroflowmetry because there is a substantial overlap with the obstructed voiding pattern. However, it can be suspected. A low maximum flow rate is present and the time to get the peak flow is usually reached in the second part of the trace. High PVR (>250 mL) is often seen.

Patients suffering from autonomic LUT disorders present in different stages of the disease with a broad spectrum of urodynamics findings that range from an initial phase of detrusor overactivity to a final stage of detrusor underactivity and chronic urinary retention. Therefore, voiding patterns can modify with time from a detrusor overactivity flow pattern at the very beginning to poor flow due to concomitant bladder outlet obstruction and detrusor underactivity in a late stage. Thus, free uroflowmetry and PVR measurement are not enough to understand the disease stage and usually, invasive urodynamics is required to understand the underlying condition and to break the chain of LUT failure and likely subsequent upper tract deterioration (bilateral hydronephrosis and renal failure due to chronic urinary retention).

12.5.3 *Invasive Tests: Filling Cystometry and Pressure-Flow Study*

Non-invasive urodynamic tests are not reliable in assessing the micturition correctly. Free uroflowmetry gives little information about the filling phase and urine flow is a consequence of the interaction between the detrusor contraction (pressure) force and urethral resistance. Unobstructed micturition in males is characterised by high flow and low pressure. Obstructed micturition is characterised by low flow and high pressure, but low flow (with low pressure) is also possible in detrusor underactivity. At the same time, a high flow (with high pressure) is also possible in case of obstructed micturition. Then, measurement of detrusor pressure is required to better understand micturition, particularly in males. A bladder and rectal catheter are required to measure detrusor pressure that is the difference between bladder pressure (bladder catheter) and abdominal pressure (rectal catheter).

Invasive urodynamic investigation (Fig. 12.6) should usually be taken into consideration in neurological patients complaining of LUT symptoms. Indeed, filling cystometry and pressure-flow study are the best tests to reproduce the patient's symptoms and to understand the physiopathology underlying LUT disorders.

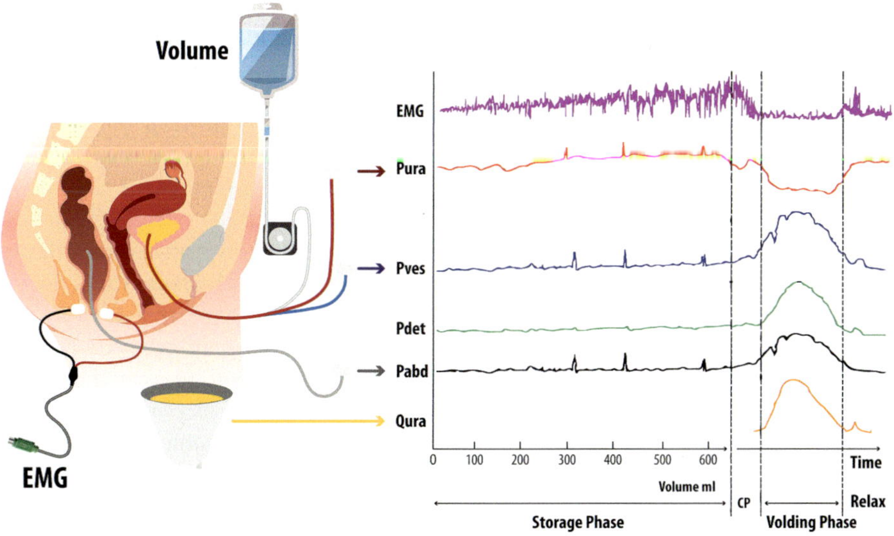

Fig. 12.6 Urodynamic examination. (From Micieli et al. "Disfunzioni Autonomiche" © 2022 Il Pensiero Scientifico Editore with permission)

Invasive urodynamics also enables effective treatment to be given. Filling cystometry assesses the storage phase of micturition, whereas pressure flow studies the voiding phase. It is useful to think about micturition by defining the behaviour of bladder and urethral function as distinct during the storage and voiding phase. The bladder is relaxed with low pressure during filling inside and contracts during voiding. Conversely, the urethra is contracted during filling and relaxed during voiding. This represents the physiological micturition cycle. Then, abnormal function of the bladder and the urethra translates into the failure of their physiological behaviour. However, the bladder cannot be underactive during filling and overactive during voiding, and the urethra cannot be overactive during filling and underactive during voiding. Thus four simple questions help us to understand if bladder and urethral function are "normal" during micturition: (1) Is the bladder relaxed during storage? (2) Is the urethra contracted during storage? (3) Does the bladder contract adequately during voiding? (4) Does the urethra open properly during voiding?

12.5.3.1 Filling Cystometry

Cystometry aims to assess detrusor and urethral function during filling. Bladder filling is usually performed with a sterile 0.9% saline solution at room temperature. The filling velocity is set at 50 mL/min. However, such fast filling in the neurogenic bladder produces artifactual low compliance. Therefore in neurogenic patients filling should commonly start at 10 mL/min. If there is no rise in the detrusor pressure this can be increased to 20–30 mL/min, but if the pressure begins to rise then filling should be stopped for 5–10 min, and then restarted at 10 mL/min. Bladder pressure (*Pves*) and rectal pressure (*Pabd*) are measured by catheters. Bladder contraction is measured as the detrusor pressure (*Pdet*) and by detracting abdominal pressure from intravesical pressure ($Pdet = Pves - Pabd$). A detrusor contraction is present when a pressure change is seen on *Pves* and *Pdet* but not in *Pabd*. A detrusor contraction and an increased abdominal pressure are present in the case of a concomitant increase in *Pves*, *Pabd*, and *Pdet*. Finally, if a rise in pressure is seen only in *Pabd* and *Pves* with no increase in *Pdet* then the rise is only due to increased abdominal pressure. Thus, detrusor function is evaluated by watching the pressure changes, while urethral function is by any fluid leakage. During the filling phase, each desire to void (from first to strong desire; pain sensation) together with urgency and incontinence episodes should be registered and described to assess bladder sensitivity and compliance, and incontinence. This leads to two possible diagnoses: *normal detrusor function with an incompetent urethra* (leaks of filling fluid, urodynamic stress incontinence); *detrusor overactivity with normal* (urgency) *or incompetent urethra* (urodynamic urge-incontinence). However, patients frequently complain of *urgency without any rise in detrusor pressure* (sensory urgency). It is of utmost importance that the urodynamic diagnosis is related to symptoms complaining and the urodynamic findings should be assessed according to the clinical problem. Another important function to evaluate during the filling phase is bladder compliance, which defines the relationship between bladder volume and bladder pressure and is expressed as an increase in bladder volume per centimetre of water increase in pressure (mL/cmH_2O). In a physiologically working lower urinary tract, intravesical pressure should change a little from empty to full. For example, in a bladder with a capacity of 400 mL, the change in pressure from empty to full should be less than 10 cmH_2O, giving normal compliance of greater than 40 mL/cmH_2O. In case of significant bladder fibrosis, compliance may be reduced.

12.5.3.2 Pressure-Flow Study

The pressure-flow study aims to assess the voiding phase. Once the bladder has filled during cystometry and a strong desire to void has been reached, the patient is asked to void in privacy. Care must be ensured to inform to avoid touching the catheters during voiding, as this might cause artefacts. Both detrusor and urethral functions can be defined separately whilst remembering that they work as a single unit. Detrusor activity can be divided as follows:

- Normal: detrusor contracts to empty the bladder with a high flow rate.
- Underactive: detrusor contraction is powerless to empty the bladder and the flow rate is weak, fluctuating, and interrupted.
- Acontractile: no detrusor contraction can be seen during voiding (no change/increase in *Pdet*) and usually patients are not able to void or they void little with an abdominal strain.

During voiding, the urethral outlet is relaxed, allowing the bladder to empty. Even if the urethral sphincter is relaxed there might be a mechanical obstruction such as in the case of benign prostatic enlargement that limits the opening of the prostatic urethra. However, urethral mechanical obstruction may occur at any level from the bladder neck to the external urethral meatus, leading to an increased voiding (i.e. *Pdet*) pressure with, usually, a reduced flow rate (i.e. low *Qmax*). Urethral resistance may be elevated intermittently in case of *urethral overactivity*, which is characterised by intermittent urethral contraction during voiding instead of complete relaxation. In this circumstance, urethral function can be divided into:

- Detrusor-sphincter dyssynergia (DESD): characterised by intermittent contraction of the intrinsic urethral striated muscle during detrusor contraction that produces very high detrusor pressure and an interrupted flow. This condition is typical of neurological patients with high-level (cervical) spinal cord injury.
- Dysfunctional voiding has the same patterns of detrusor-sphincter dyssynergia but is present in patients with intermittent voiding caused by contraction of the pelvic floor muscles.
- Nonrelaxing urethral sphincter obstruction where there is a lack of urethral relaxation during the whole voiding phase, as seen in meningomyelocele patients.

12.5.3.3 Video Urodynamics

Video urodynamics is the integration of pressure/flow study with contemporary cystourethrography with the intent of better understanding LUT function. Video urodynamics should be reserved only for more complex patients who may have concomitant anatomical abnormality (e.g. vesicoureteric reflux) and LUT disorders. This approach is justified not only for the invasiveness of pressure/flow study but also for the radiation exposure. Cystourethrography is usually performed at rest and during filling, couching/straining, and voiding. The following information can be acquired:

- Full bladder, at rest: bladder capacity shape, and outline (e.g. diverticulum and trabeculation), vesicoureteric reflux.
- Strain/cough. Assessment of degree of bladder base descent and bladder neck competence.
- Voiding: speed and extent of the bladder neck opening, calibre, and shape of the urethra, site of any urethral narrowing/dilatation/diverticula, and vesicoureteric reflux.
- Post-voiding: urine residual.

12.5.4 Neurophysiological Evaluation

Extensive neurophysiological investigations should be performed in any patient with LUT and anorectal disorders of suspected central or peripheral neurogenic aetiology [8, 9]. These tests include concentric needle EMG of different pelvic floor muscles, measurement of sacral reflex latency (pudendo-anal or bulbocavernosus reflex), pudendal and anal somatosensory-evoked potentials (SEPs), and motor-evoked potentials (MEPs) from the pelvic floor and EAS muscles by transcranial and lumbosacral magnetic stimulation. Pudendal nerve terminal motor latency (PNTML) has been used in different clinical conditions, but its clinical value has been questioned because the reproducibility, sensitivity, and specificity are uncertain. The recording of a sympathetic skin response (SSR) from the saddle region is useful for testing the lumbosacral autonomic sympathetic system.

Unfortunately, a clinically useful test for evaluating the sacral parasympathetic system, which is crucial for LUT and anorectal functioning, has not been found yet. Tests are usually capable of demonstrating neuropathic lesions and helping to define the specific affected sensory, motor, or autonomic pathway. The severity of lesions can be also assessed, and the underlying mechanisms can be identified. Even when all other functional tests do not show altered findings, the electrophysiological tests can be positive, therefore leading to a surgical or conservative approach and assessing the functional prognosis.

12.5.4.1 Electromyography (EMG)

Needle EMG is the most important neurophysiological technique for evaluating patients with suspected neurogenic aetiology of pelvic floor dysfunction [3]. EMG assessment of pelvic floor, EAS [10] and external urethral sphincter (EUS) is primarily indicated to evaluate:

- the presence of pathological spontaneous activity at rest, fibrillation potentials and positive sharp waves of denervated muscle fibres;
- the presence of collateral reinnervation activity of muscle fibres;
- normal tonic contraction (3–5 Hz) in the EAS, puborectalis muscle and EUS and adequate contraction or relaxation during squeeze or straining;
- recruitment pattern and motor-unit potential (MUP) waveform.

EAS muscle needle EMG examination is the test that is most commonly used to assess the functional state of the pelvic floor and sacral myotomes. EAS is easy to access, its needle evaluation is not very painful and very useful information can be acquired.

When the needle advances in the EAS muscle, the continuous firing of low-threshold MUPs is normally appreciated, and during a brief period of relaxation, the presence of spontaneous activity, fibrillation, or jasper potentials can be recorded.

EMG recordings from the EAS are performed at rest and during squeezing, coughing, and straining that simulate rectal evacuation. In healthy subjects, squeeze and cough increase the MUP recruitment pattern, whereas strain decreases or inhibits MUP firing.

An abnormal EMG pattern may be recorded with surface or needle electrodes during bladder filling or emptying, coughing, or straining. The utility of this technique is to detect a possible dyssynergic functional behaviour, for example the paradoxical contraction of the external urethral sphincter concomitant to the contraction of the detrusor (during the urodynamic test) or a similar inadequate activation of the puborectalis muscle in the attempt to evacuate (constipation from paradoxical contraction of the puborectalis muscle).

12.5.4.2 Sacral Reflexes

Sacral reflexes are motor responses, derived from the pelvic striated floor and sphincter muscles, to electrical stimulation of the dorsal penile or clitoral nerve, perianal skin, bladder neck or proximal urethra. Sacral reflexes evaluate the functional status of the afferent neural fibres of the clitoris or penis, the S2–S4 spinal segments, and the efferent pathways to EAS and bulbocavernosus (BC) muscles. The central circuit at the spinal level is complex and probably involves many sacral interneurons. The motor response in EAS and BC muscles is recorded either with a concentric needle or wire electrodes and can be analysed separately for each side of both muscles. These sacral reflexes, named pudendo-anal and bulbocavernosus reflex, reveal two components with different thresholds at the electrical stimulation:

a first component with a shorter latency of 26–36 ms, probably oligosynaptic, and a second component with a longer latency at about 50–75 ms, typical for a polysynaptic response. The first component is morphologically constant, stable and does not habituate, while the second component or long latency response is not always demonstrable and rapidly habituates. The cutaneous-anal reflex, like the other two reflexes, consists of two or three motor contractions (early response at 5 ms, intermediate at 15 ms and late at about 50 ms) of EAS muscle in response to scratching or pricking the perianal skin. This reflex, which is abolished by transection of the posterior S4 roots, shows marked habituation, is quite variable (35–80 ms) and therefore cannot be used as a diagnostic tool. Vesico-urethral and vesico-anal reflexes are described following stimulation of the bladder neck and mucosa, but their usefulness as a diagnostic tool is considered to be limited.

Recently, a technique for transcutaneous electrical stimulation of the S3 motor root, recording from EAS muscle, has also been described.

A common scheme of sacral evoked responses consists of the anterior electrical stimulation (penile/clitoral) and recording by needle electrode from different pelvic muscles (BC, EAS, and levator ani). Sacral reflexes are useful in different pelvic floor disorders and have been recommended for the assessment of cauda equina and conus medullaris lesions. In the presence of unilateral/asymmetrical lesions of pudendal nerves, sacral roots or lumbosacral plexus, these reflexes may show a reduction of response amplitude and/or increased latencies or a total absence. Only the largest myelinated, fastest fibres convey the neurophysiological signals travelling in the afferent limb of these reflexes. Unfortunately, many disorders of bladder, bowel and sexual function are the result of unmyelinated fibre dysfunction; conduction in these fibres is not tested by these procedures and autonomic and small-fibre neuropathies may not be revealed by these tests.

12.5.4.3 Somatosensory Evoked Potential

Somatosensory evoked potential (SEP) of the pudendal nerve is a method for evaluating the afferent sensory pathway to the parietal cortex and it is used in investigating central and peripheral neurological diseases that affect pelvic floor functional integrity [11]. SEP findings may help in showing lesions in somatosensory pathways, localising them and defining a prognostic value. In a similar way to the other neurophysiological tests, pudendal SEPs may be normal in latency and amplitude also in case of an underlying organic disease. The peripheral electrical stimulation used to obtain a SEP activates predominantly, if not entirely, the large diameter fast-conducting group Ia muscle and group II cutaneous afferent fibres. Loss of dorsal column or lemniscal sensory pathways is invariably associated with abnormal SEPs, indicating that within the spinal cord, the SEPs are mediated predominantly via these tracts. Generally, SEPs are best recorded over the somatosensory cortex and several of their components are widely distributed over the scalp. The pudendal SEPs technique, first described by Haldeman in 1983, depends on the recording by a disk electrode affixed to the scalp of a typical "W-shaped" waveform, as a response that appears with a given latency depending on site stimulation. Although several studies have shown that SEPs can effectively be recorded after dorsal penile and clitoral stimulation, only a few investigations have been published concerning anal somatosensory evoked responses. It is necessary to remind that pudendal SEPs after anal and dorsal penile/clitoral nerve stimulation cannot be considered to produce equivalent results due to separate branches of the pudendal nerve innervating the pelvic region. Therefore, obtaining separate reference values in both sexes for anal and penile/clitoral latencies when evaluating pelvic floor neurophysiology is considered to be relevant. The analogous morphology of pudendal and tibial SEPs might suggest a common neurophysiological mechanism to produce both responses.

The responses are bipolarly recorded using surface electrodes from the scalp, 2 cm behind Cz, referred to as Fz or Fpz (10–20 EEG International System), roughly overlying the sensorimotor cortex for the genital and anal area. Electrical stimulation is performed using a bipolar surface electrode positioned at the anal orifice, at the base of the penis or cranial to the clitoris. The typical recording consists of a series of waves that reflect the sequential activation of neural structures along the somatosensory pathways. A first positive peak can be recorded in normal subjects at about 42 ms using a stimulus intensity of two to four times the sensory threshold. Later negative and positive peaks show a large variability in amplitude between individuals. SEP amplitudes have, however, not been found to differentiate between normal and pathologic responses. SEPs can be used in perineology to confirm and localise sensory abnormalities affecting anal or genitourinary neural pathways. Some authors have already discussed the limitations of pudendal SEPs, showing that sometimes in pathological conditions penile/clitoral SEPs are normal. Pudendal SEPs are considered to be useful in diagnosing impotence associated with spinal cord injury and diabetic neuropathy while in the case of primary erectile dysfunction, their utility is debated.

12.5.4.4 Motor Evoked Potential (MEP)

Conventional electrophysiological methods that activate the descending corticomotoneuronal pathways use the electrical and magnetic stimulation techniques. However, transcranial magnetic stimulation (TMS) has the advantages of being painless and capable of stimulating the more deeply situated nervous structures; electrical stimulation is therefore mainly reserved for intraoperative monitoring. TMS has been commonly used to assess the central and peripheral conduction time to skeletal muscles of the upper and lower limbs, to evaluate the integrity and function of the cortico-spinal pathways. TMS is also applied to study the cortico-spinal pathway to the pelvic floor muscles, including EAS, which is the most common target muscle from which MEPs are recorded, and EUS and PRM, whose recordings are poorly reproducible. The intensity of TMS necessary to obtain an EAS MEP is much higher than the intensity to elicit an MEP in the limbs. This fact can be explained by the cortical representation of the anogenital area that is localised deep within the motor strip in the interhemispheric fissure. This method investigates the motor efferent pathway from the brain and lumbosacral roots to the EAS, allowing us to determine the total conduction time and the lumbosacral latency. Cortical magnetic stimulation is usually performed in two conditions: at rest, with EAS relaxed (MEPs mean latency of about 27 ms), and during facilitation (MEPs mean latency of about 23 ms) due to a voluntary mild contraction of the pelvic floor and EAS muscles. The magnetic stimulation applied over the lower lumbar spine is known to activate the lumbosacral ventral roots at their exit from the vertebral canal. MEPs from lumbosacral magnetic stimulation are obtained only during rest conditions at about 3–6 ms since facilitation does not modify latencies during peripheral nerve stimulation.

Magnetic shocks are delivered by a magnetic simulator; different shapes of coils exist, each of which produces different magnetic field patterns. The coil produces, normally, a peak magnetic field strength of 1.5 T, being placed flat on the scalp, centred on Cz (10–20 I.E.) to stimulate the motor cortex and on the lumbosacral region (L3–L4 interspace) to stimulate the lumbosacral roots. EMG recordings are taken from EAS using a needle electrode placed approximately 1 cm lateral to the anal orifice. The ground electrode is located around the upper portion of the leg. The different types of MEP abnormalities, i.e. responses with decreased amplitude or delayed latency, may imply axonal or demyelinating impairment underlying the different clinical pathological conditions. Corticospinal abnormalities detected by this method in patients with neurogenic bladder and bowel disorders have been reported.

12.5.4.5 Sympathetic Skin Response (SSR)

SSR is a technique that records changes in skin conductance after activation of sweat glands in skin areas rich in eccrine glands (commonly palmar, plantar, and saddle sites) under the neural control of sympathetic cholinergic (sudomotor) fibres. SSR is the only neurophysiological technique directly testing sympathetic fibres. Potentials generated by SSR can be recorded in response to various stimuli; these include electrical peripheral nerve stimulation, acoustic stimuli, and magnetic stimulation of nerves or the brain, although magnetic stimulation lacks specificity in terms of sensory pathways involved. SSR is dependent on the integrity of peripheral sympathetic cholinergic pathways, as it is preserved in selective sympathetic adrenergic failure, and it is absent in pure autonomic failure (PAF) (with sympathetic adrenergic and cholinergic failure) and in pure cholinergic dysautonomia. Different areas in the cerebral cortex and in the brainstem have been proposed as generator sites for the sensory signals of the SSR.

SSRs are recorded from palmar, plantar, and saddle surfaces, both left and right, using surface electrodes. Electrodes are placed on the volar site and on the corresponding area of the dorsal aspect of the hand or foot. For perineum recordings, the active electrode is attached to the perineum (below the scrotum) and the reference electrode to the iliac crest with the ground on the leg. This kind of recording from the perineal region increases the diagnostic sensitivity when evaluating sympathetic function within the thoracolumbar spinal cord. Only a few studies exist regarding the relationship between bladder dysfunction and SSR abnormalities. In particular lack of SSR in bladder neck dyssynergia and in foot following spinal cord injury has been shown.

12.5.4.6 Pudendal Nerve Terminal Motor Latency (PNTML)

Pudendal nerve inferior rectal branches can be evaluated by measuring PNTML, which is the technique most commonly used for assessment in patients with idiopathic neurogenic faecal incontinence. The PNTML technique, first described in 1984 by Kiff and Swash, is determined by recording anal sphincter motor potential evoked by stimulation of the pudendal nerve into the rectum with a special bipolar surface electrode known as St. Mark's electrode. The stimulating electrode is fixed on the tip of a gloved index finger while the two recording electrodes, that pick up the contraction response of EAS, are placed at the base of the finger. On insertion of the finger into the rectum, an electrical stimulation is given near the ischial spine. The pudendal nerve is therefore stimulated as it leaves the pelvis, before branching into the perineal nerve and inferior rectal nerve, which innervate periurethral striated muscle and anal sphincter respectively.

The test owes its popularity to different studies showing abnormal latencies in various clinical situations. In fact, pudendal neuropathy is seen in up to 70% of patients with faecal incontinence, and in more than 50% of patients with sphincter injury. However, PNTML clinical value has been questioned, and two consensus statements, uro-neurological and gastroenterological, did not propose this test for evaluating patients with bladder and bowel dysfunction.

12.6 Management of Neurogenic Lower Urinary Tract Dysfunctions

The goals in neurogenic lower urinary tract dysfunctions are: to promote a regular bladder voiding, to obtain a low-pressure bladder, to achieve and maintain continence, to minimise symptoms and to improve quality of life, to prevent urinary tract infections and to preserve renal function, protecting the upper urinary tract; these are objectives that often require a multidisciplinary approach.

In addition, elderly patients may have concomitant diseases, such as bladder outlet obstruction due to BPH, stress incontinence, and urinary tract infections, which ought to be considered in management.

Management should consider both storage and voiding dysfunctions and determine the severity of symptoms and the risk of upper urinary tract damage [2, 6, 12]. The latter is of utmost importance as renal function impairment can impact survival.

12.6.1 Management and Treatment of Storage Dysfunction

Treatment of lower urinary tract dysfunctions in the neurogenic bladder:

1. Depends on the impact on quality of life
2. Must consider concomitant diseases (BPH obstruction, urinary infections, stress incontinence)
3. Must maintain continence
4. Must protect the upper urinary tract (avoiding chronic retention with bilateral hydroureteronephrosis and kidney failure)

Therefore, when detrusor overactivity is present, treatment should be aimed to convert a high-pressure overactive bladder into a low-pressure bladder, in order to maintain continence, prevent urinary infections and improve quality of life.

Lifestyle changes and bladder voiding strategies:

- Fluid intake reduction, particularly in the evening
- Treatment of constipation
- Timed micturition (every 2–4 h during the day)

Lifestyle interventions and voiding strategies are the first-line non-invasive treatments. Patients should be counselled to reduce fluid intake, particularly in the evening, and to treat constipation. Moreover, a timely voiding every 2–4 h during the day and the use of a double voiding technique may improve bladder emptying, reduce urgency and urge-incontinence episodes, minimising the risk of urinary infection. Older patients may need support from caregivers to carry on these strategies.

The second line of treatment for overactive bladder is pharmacological therapy which is based on the use of antimuscarinic drugs (oxybutynin, trospium, tolterodine, propiverine, darifenacin, solifenacin), that inhibit parasympathetic system, induce a reduction in urgency, micturition frequency and episodes of urge incontinence and increase cystometric capacity. All these drugs are established, effective, and well-tolerated treatments even in long-term use. Treatment must always start at low doses and with a gradual increase only in cases of poor efficacy and without side effects. However, higher doses and a combination of different agents are generally required in neurological patients. These drugs decrease maximum detrusor pressure by 30–40% and increase bladder capacity by 30%.

Antimuscarinics are the most studied drugs for the treatment of urge urinary incontinence and for the urge-frequency syndrome [12]. They are different from each other in pharmacokinetic and pharmacodynamic features, but they are superior to placebo in the treatment of incontinence episodes. Some of the most frequent side effects are xerostomia and constipation; despite the fact that urinary retention is quite rare, PVR should be frequently assessed. Slow-release formulations appear to have a lower incidence of side effects than rapid-release formulations and their pharmacokinetics (poor or absent penetration of the blood-brain barrier) make them more suitable than others for use in elderly patients, avoiding central effects such as confusion. Treatment compliance to antimuscarinics is often low due to possible limited efficacy and to the presence of particularly significant side effects and costs. The antimuscarinic drugs fesoterodine, oxybutynin, propiverine, solifenacin, tolterodine, darifenacin and trospium are recommended with a high grade of recommendation by the European Association of Urology (EAU) guidelines on urinary incontinence [6].

Mirabegron is the first-in-class β3-agonist drug that activates β3 adrenergic receptors located in the bladder wall; these receptors induce relaxation of bladder detrusor smooth muscles. Although being recently approved for overactive bladder therapy, mirabegron seems to lead to greater compliance than antimuscarinics.

Estrogens used topically (vaginally) in postmenopausal women may reduce episodes of urge incontinence, but do not seem to impact stress incontinence.

The third line of treatment uses botulinum toxin type A, which is injected into the detrusor. It is indicated in patients who have had no benefit from antimuscarinic therapy. The 2022 guidelines of the EAU [6] advise, with a high degree of evidence, to propose intravesical botulinum toxin to patients with urge incontinence refractory to conservative therapy. On the other hand, it is important to inform patients treated with this technique about the short duration of response and the risk of inducing detrusor areflexia that needs intermittent catheterization. In fact, botulinum toxin causes a long-lasting chemical bladder denervation (on average 3–6 months) which translates into an increase in bladder capacity, a reduction in bladder pressure and a consequent reduction in episodes of urgency, frequency and urge incontinence. Frequent side effects are represented by urinary infections, hematuria, and urinary retention with possible need for intermittent catheterization.

The therapeutic technique of sacral neuromodulation can also be offered to patients who are refractory to conservative, pharmacological and intradetrusor treatments [13]. Neuromodulation is a technique that consists of the implant of a device that allows a therapeutic modification of the activity of the central, peripheral or autonomic nervous system by means of electrical or pharmacological stimulus. This method is safe, non-destructive and reversible, it does not preclude other therapies, and it shows positive long-term results on quality of life, with the possibility of testing its therapeutic efficacy before performing a permanent implant.

Sacral neuromodulation consists of the implant of a quadripolar electrode connected to a sacral stimulator that is implanted at the level of S3 foramen under local anaesthesia. The 2022 guidelines of the EAU [6] advise, with a high degree of evidence, to propose the sacral neuromodulation technique to patients with overactive bladder and urgency-frequency syndrome or urge incontinence refractory to antimuscarinic therapy.

Surgery to increase bladder capacity can be proposed only when all other conservative therapies have failed. The increase in bladder capacity can be achieved with bladder augmentation surgery using an ileal segment anastomosed with the bladder. At the same time, there is also a reduction in intravesical pressure. This treatment should only be offered as the last treatment in highly motivated patients who accept a possible intermittent self-catheterization in case of post-surgical urinary retention.

In fact, clean intermittent catheterization may become necessary to empty the bladder.

Urinary diversion may be offered as the last treatment when no other therapy was successful, in cases refractory to non-invasive therapies, with the creation of a catheterizable continent stoma, that is unfortunately characterised by high rates of complications. Urinary diversion aims to protect upper urinary tract deterioration (i.e. bilateral hydronephrosis) and renal failure. Continent diversion with a stoma at the umbilicus is the first choice for urinary diversion. This type of diversion is an effective treatment option in neuro-urological patients unable to perform intermittent self-catheterization through the urethra, despite having a high complication rate.

If catheterization is not possible, an incontinent stoma can be constructed using the intestine. In fact, if manual dexterity impairs stoma catheterization, incontinent diversion with a urine-collecting device is indicated. Incontinent diversion is also indicated in patients who are wheelchair-bound or bedridden with untreatable incontinence or in patients with severely compromised upper urinary tract.

12.6.2 Management and Treatment of Voiding Dysfunction

Incomplete bladder voiding can exacerbate detrusor overactivity and make treatments with antimuscarinic drugs and botulinum toxin less effective. The use of intermittent catheterization (IC) significantly improves continence management [14]. Catheterization 4–6 times/day is also recommended to manage complete urinary retention, with a goal of voiding 400–500 mL of urine with each catheterization. The following manoeuvres can be used to facilitate bladder emptying when it is incomplete (bladder expression):

1. Urination with simultaneous Valsalva manoeuvre
2. Urination with simultaneous manual compression of the lower abdomen (Credè manoeuvre)

These manoeuvres can be performed only if there is no increased intravesical pressure and vesicoureteric reflux during storage, due to the risk of upper urinary tract deterioration.

The frequency of catheterization depends on many factors such as bladder volume, fluid intake and post-voiding residual (PVR), and urodynamic factors such as compliance and detrusor pressure. IC, which is used in children with spina bifida and in the elderly with impaired bladder emptying, is also very effective in most patients with multiple sclerosis and, in combination with an oral anticholinergic drug, it is the treatment of choice in spinal cord diseases, where incomplete bladder emptying and detrusor hyperreflexia coexist. The incidence of symptomatic lower urinary tract infections is, fortunately, low despite the fact that bacteriuria is present in 50% of patients performing sterile IC. Patient motivation is essential for the correct use of this technique because they have to develop adequate manual skills. An indwelling catheter to be replaced cyclically or a suprapubic catheter is recommended in patients for whom IC cannot be used; in these cases, there is a greater risk of infections, bladder stones and urethral and bladder neck lesions.

A1-blockers are the first line of pharmacological treatment of voiding dysfunction in men. They are indicated in subjects with moderate/severe symptoms (IPSS >8) and with no response to conservative treatment (reduction of fluid intake, particularly tea, alcohol and coffee, treatment of constipation, use of relaxed and double-voiding techniques, scheduled voiding). They inhibit the effects of endogenous norepinephrine on the smooth muscle cells of the prostate and bladder neck (relaxing effect), with a reduction of bladder neck resistance. The clinical efficacy of the available drugs (alfuzosin, doxazosin, silodosin, tamsulosin, terazosin, naftopidil) is similar and a few weeks are needed before clinical benefit. Clinical effects are represented by a variable reduction in IPSS of 30–40% and an increase in maximum peak flow of 20–25%. Asthenia, anejaculation, orthostatic hypotension, and intraoperative floppy iris syndrome during cataract surgery are the most frequent side effects.

5α-Reductase inhibitors are the second group of drugs used in men with a prostate volume larger than 40 mL. They induce the apoptosis of the prostate gland epithelial cells by inhibiting the conversion of dihydrotestosterone from testosterone and causing a decrease in prostate volume (18–28%) and a concomitant improvement of IPSS and maximum flow rate. Moreover, long-term use of these drugs reduces the risk of acute urinary retention and the need for surgery.

Surgical therapy of benign prostatic hyperplasia remains indicated in the following cases:

1. severe symptoms (IPSS >20),
2. symptoms refractory to medical therapy,
3. absolute indication in the presence of:
   - urinary retention (acute or chronic)
   - bladder diverticula
   - bladder stones
   - recurrent urinary tract infections
   - bilateral hydroureteronephrosis
   - haematuria due to prostatic cause

References

1. Panicker JN, Fowler CJ, Kessler TM. Lower urinary tract dysfunction in the neurological patient: clinical assessment and management. Lancet Neurol. 2015;14(7):720–32.
2. Panicker JN, Sakakibara R. Lower urinary tract and bowel dysfunction in neurologic disease. Continuum (Minneap Minn). 2020;26(1):178–99.
3. Fowler CJ, Brady CM, Frohman EM, Sakakibara R, Stewart JD, editors. Neurologic bladder, bowel, and sexual dysfunction. Amsterdam: Elsevier; 2001.
4. Wyndaele JJ. The management of neurogenic lower urinary tract dysfunction after spinal cord injury. Nat Rev Urol. 2016;13(12):705–14.

5. Sakakibara R, Tateno F, Yamamoto T, Uchiyama T, Yamanishi T. Urological dysfunction in synucleinopathies: epidemiology, pathophysiology and management. Clin Auton Res. 2018;28(1):83–101.
6. EAU guidelines on neuro-urology. Edn presented at the EAU annual congress Amsterdam. 2022. ISBN: 978-94-92671-16-5.
7. Ginsberg DA, Boone TB, Cameron AP, et al. The AUA/SUFU guideline on adult neurogenic lower urinary tract dysfunction: diagnosis and evaluation. J Urol. 2021;206(5):1097–105.
8. Podnar S, Vodusek DB. Protocol for clinical neurophysiologic examination of the pelvic floor. Neurourol Urodyn. 2001;20(6):669–82.
9. Pelliccioni G, Pelliccioni P. Neurophysiology and neurophysiological evaluation of the pelvic floor. In: Martellucci J, editor. Electrical stimulation for pelvic floor disorders. Cham: Springer; 2015.
10. Podnar S, Vodusek DB, Stâlberg E. Standardization of anal sphincter electromyography: normative data. Clin Neurophysiol. 2000;111(12):2200–7.
11. Pelliccioni G, Piloni V, Sabbatini D, Fioravanti P, Scarpino O. Sex differences in pudendal somatosensory evoked potentials. Tech Coloproctol. 2014;18(6):565–9.
12. Ginsberg DA, Boone TB, Cameron AP, et al. The AUA/SUFU guideline on adult neurogenic lower urinary tract dysfunction: treatment and followup. J Urol. 2021;206(5):1106–13.
13. van Ophoven A, Engelberg S, Lilley H, Sievert KD. Systematic literature review and meta-analysis of sacral neuromodulation (SNM) in patients with neurogenic lower urinary tract dysfunction (nLUTD): over 20 years' experience and future directions. Adv Ther. 2021;38(4):1987–2006.
14. Clark C, Haslam C, Malde S, Panicker JN. Urinary catheter management: what neurologists need to know. Pract Neurol. 2021;21(6):504–14.

Chapter 13
Rehabilitation of Neurogenic Lower Urinary Tract Dysfunctions

Donatella Giraudo, Gianluca Ciardi, Vittorio Casati, and Gianfranco Lamberti

13.1 Neurogenic Lower Urinary Tract Dysfunctions (nLUTD)

The rehabilitative treatment of nLUTD (focal diseases such as stroke, spinal cord injuries, neoplastic forms, neural tube defects, spinal cord disease caused by cervical arthritis, pathologies with disseminated lesions such as severe traumatic brain injury, Parkinson's disease, multiple sclerosis, and meningoencephalitis, but also peripheral neuropathies such as diabetic neuropathy) is to date mainly supported by non-comparative studies based on electrical or magnetic stimulation.

13.2 Conservative Treatment

According to international guidelines, conservative treatment in the case of urinary incontinence requires an initial behavioral approach (correct fluid intake in terms of volume, distribution and characteristics), use of a bladder diary, possible training in

D. Giraudo (✉)
Department of Urology, Ospedale San Raffaele Turro, Milan, Italy
e-mail: giraudo.donatella@hsr.it

G. Ciardi · G. Lamberti
Department of Rehabilitative Medicine, AUSL Piacenza, Piacenza, Italy

Degree Course of Physiotherapy, University of Parma, Parma, Italy
e-mail: gianluca.ciardi@unipr.it; g.lamberti2@ausl.pc.it

V. Casati
Department of Rehabilitative Medicine, AUSL Piacenza, Piacenza, Italy
e-mail: v.casati@ausl.pc.it

G. Micieli et al. (eds.), *Autonomic Disorders in Clinical Practice*,
https://doi.org/10.1007/978-3-031-43036-7_13

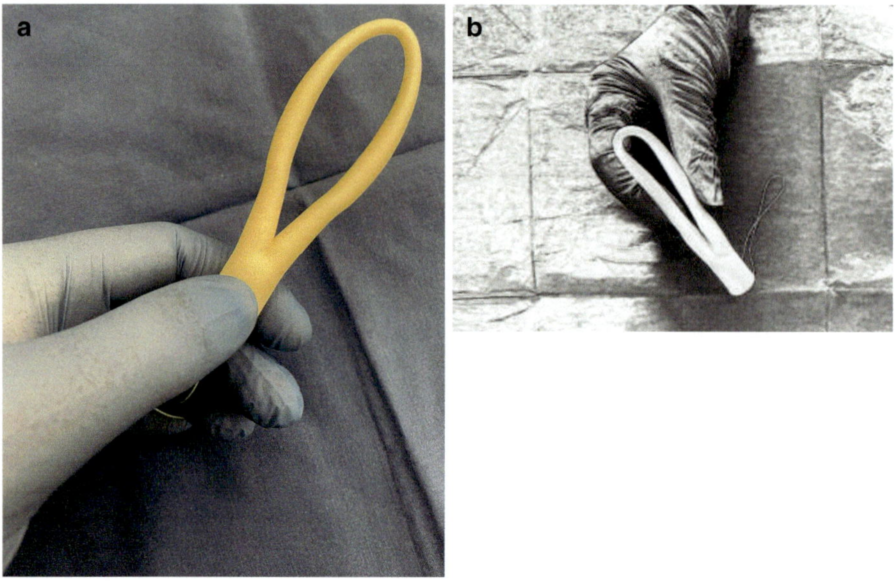

Fig. 13.1 Vaginal device for the complementary treatment of urinary incontinence. (**a**) Before insertion. (**b**) Shape assumed inside the vagina, with an action exerting pressure on the vaginal walls

self-catheterization for complete emptying, where spontaneous urination is present but not adequate to guarantee complete bladder emptying, and the suggestion to use suitable absorbent materials or, in women, urethral or vaginal devices [1] (Fig. 13.1).

13.3 Neuromodulation

Neuromodulation is a technique that modifies its function by stimulating the nerve and inducing a therapeutic response. In addition to the S3 sacral root neuromodulation technique, the use of neuromodulation techniques in rehabilitation, such as PTNS (Percutaneous Tibial Nerve Stimulation), a type of stimulation performed at the level of the posterior tibial nerve using an acupuncture needle, or TTNS (Transcutaneous Tibial Nerve Stimulation) performed using a surface electrode, can be effective and safe in treating neurological lower urinary tract dysfunction. To date, the data in the literature suggest that better-quality studies must be undertaken to obtain definitive conclusions [2–5].

The rationale for the technique is based on the fact that the posterior tibial nerve is a mixed nerve that originates from the L4–S3 roots, thus from the same spinal segments that control the innervation of the bladder and pelvic floor. The posterior tibial nerve trunk is a branch of the sciatic nerve that originates in the popliteal fossa, descends the leg and at the transition to the ankle is positioned posteriorly and below the medial malleolus, before passing through the tarsal tunnel and providing innervation to the calcaneus and the sole through its terminal branches.

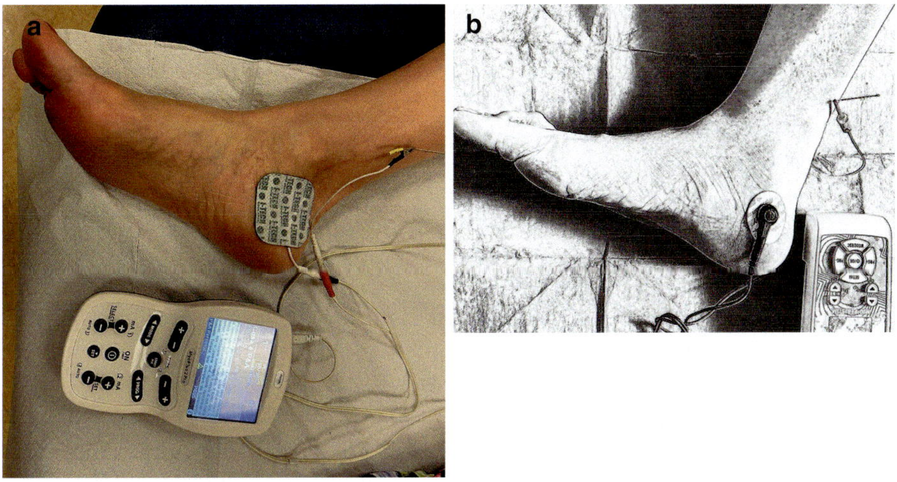

Fig. 13.2 Posterior tibial nerve stimulation. (**a**) Transcutaneous technique (TTNS). (**b**) Percutaneous technique (PTNS)

The mechanism of action of PTNS is based on the assumption that the urinary reflex results typically from the processing of bladder afferents to Onuf's nucleus mediated by spinal interneurons. In turn, the supraspinal centers influence the latter both in an inhibitory and excitatory sense. Stimulation with PTNS, reaching the same spinal cord level, could re-modulate these mechanisms by facilitating inhibitory activity on the detrusor, particularly in the presence of aberrant circuits such as neurogenic detrusor hyperactivity.

The patient can undergo the treatment in a supine position; a 34-gauge acupuncture needle is usually used, positioned 4–5 cm cranially at the medial malleolus and about 2 cm posterior to the tibia; the needle is usually inserted at an angle of 60° and over 2.5–3 cm. The ground electrode is usually placed on the heel (Fig. 13.2).

The pulse is biphasic, with a frequency of 20 Hz and a stimulus duration of 200 μs. The intensity of the stimulus is progressively increased until the fingers start to flex or extend; the duration of the treatment is usually 30 min.

In post-stroke patients, neuromodulating treatment is effective in improving urodynamic tests and bladder diary findings as well as having an effect on the relative impact of neurogenic dysfunction on quality of life [6]. It has proven similarly effective in improving bladder diary data in women with Parkinson's disease [7]; in acute spinal cord injury, a neuromodulating effect on the bladder can be achieved via the autonomic nervous system [8]: treatments are effective in achieving higher cystomanometric capacities, reducing dyssynergia and increasing the volumes determining the sensation of fullness [9].

In patients with Multiple Sclerosis, the combination of neuromodulation and therapeutic pelvic floor exercises can substantially reduce urological symptoms [10, 11]. These combined treatments appear to be more effective than those used in isolation [12].

13.4 Therapeutic Exercises

Therapeutic pelvic floor exercises (with or without biofeedback) may be aimed at reducing detrusor contractions, thereby reducing episodes of urgency and urge incontinence.

Data on the effectiveness of pelvic floor muscle exercise and training almost exclusively concern stress forms of urinary incontinence. There is little data on urge incontinence, although voluntary contraction of the pelvic floor in the event of the urge to urinate shows positive effects comparable to those of drugs and electrostimulation [13]. Unfortunately, to date, it is unclear what number, intensity, and duration of contractions are capable of inhibiting (and for how long) the detrusor [14]; however, the indications for the prescription of therapeutic exercises in female urinary incontinence, whether stress, urge or mixed, even in the elderly, remain strong.

Therapeutic exercises in the event of bladder hyperactivity are effective in people with multiple sclerosis [15, 16], ischaemic stroke [17], and incomplete spinal cord injury [18].

However, as yet there is no reliable information as to the mechanisms of action to explain why therapeutic exercises are effective: experience and empirical observation confirm that it is possible to inhibit the urination stimulus by contracting the perineal or adductor muscles (which in turn are synergic with the elevators of the anus). Few studies have contributed to understanding the mechanism of inhibition of the micturition reflex through the afferent pathway of the reflex itself [19] by increasing detrusor compliance through activation of the perineal-detrusor reflex [20]. Other interpretations of the advantage gained from exercises assume more effective and prolonged voluntary recruitment to control the stimulus until urination [21].

During training, patients are taught to contract their pelvic floor muscles when they experience a sensation of urinary urgency or during those postural changes and increases in intra-abdominal pressure that can generate incontinence episodes.

The rationale for treating patients with urinary urgency symptoms associated with overactive bladder with pelvic floor muscle training is based on the observation that the detrusor muscle can be inhibited by electrically induced pelvic floor muscle contraction [22]. Indeed, it has been shown that electrical stimulation of the anal sphincter activates two reflex mechanisms through the spinal urination center: reflex contraction of the pelvic floor muscles and the anal sphincter and reflex inhibition of detrusor contraction. Shafik's studies on patients with overactive bladder show that contractions of the pelvic floor muscles (Fig. 13.3) lead to the inhibition of detrusor contractile activity and increased urethral pressures and inhibit the urination reflex by preventing the relaxation of the internal sphincter [19].

Functional Magnetic Resonance imaging studies during pelvic floor contractions have demonstrated the activity of the supplementary motor area in the medial wall and the cingulate cortex, insula, posterior parietal cortex, putamen, thalamus, cerebellar vermis, and superior ventral bridge [23] (Fig. 13.4).

It has also been shown that voluntary recruitment of the toes activates brain areas that overlap with the areas responsible for the pelvic floor muscles.

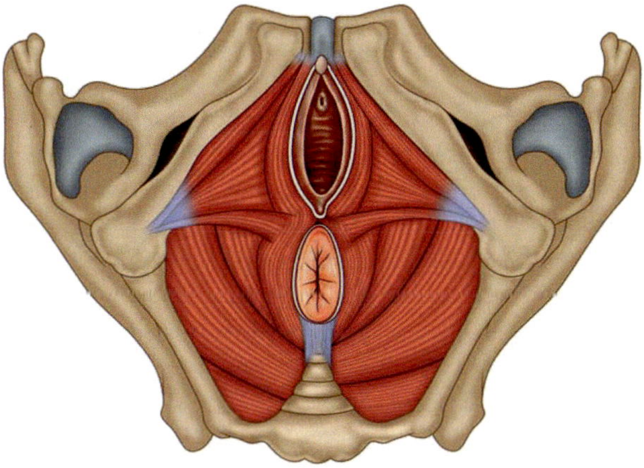

Fig. 13.3 Female pelvic floor muscles: inferior view

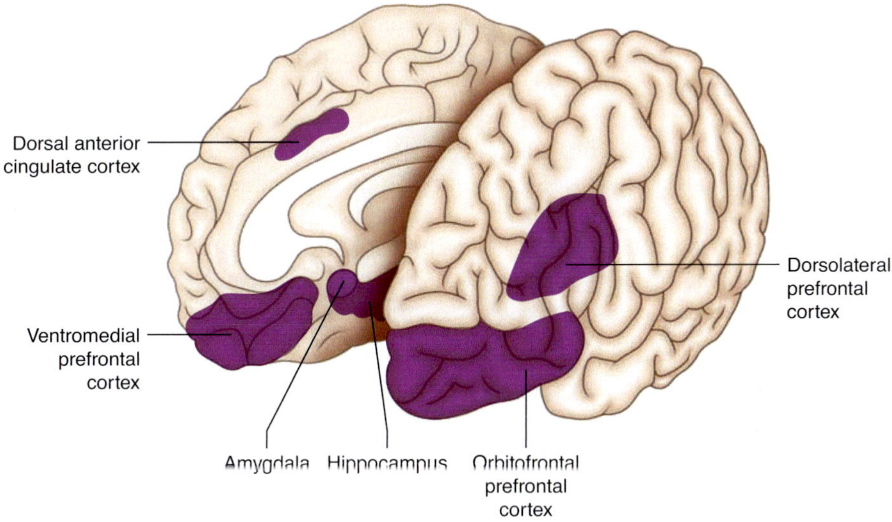

Fig. 13.4 Cortical areas involved in pelvic floor muscles control

Studies using Transcranial Magnetic Stimulation have shown that stimulating the motor efferents of the pelvic floor muscles elicits a simultaneous response to the lower limb muscles, confirming the overlapping of the cortical areas [24, 25].

Finally, it is known that the pelvic floor muscles are activated synergistically with other muscle groups during the performance of functional tasks: this occurs during the activation of the abdominal muscles [26, 27], the gluteal muscles [28, 29], the hip adductors [28] and also the flexors and extensors of the shoulder [30]. It has been shown that synergistic activation of the pelvic floor occurs before activation of the other muscles suggesting that it could be a feed-forward control synergy [26, 31].

Therefore, from all these observations, it is possible to hypothesize a role for therapeutic exercise with the involvement—when possible depending on the person's motor and cognitive condition—of the lower limbs.

There could be two hypotheses on the efficacy of voluntary contraction of the pelvic floor muscles in the inhibition of bladder overactivity: the first suggests that voluntary recruitment at the onset of the urge to urinate is in itself capable of inhibiting detrusor contraction; the second suggests that strength training may lead to permanent morphological changes in the pelvic muscles with a direct effect on urethral closure pressures [32].

However, to date, it is not possible to distinguish precisely how an exercise aimed at the recovery of pure muscle strength (strength training) should be performed, as opposed to endurance training. Generally speaking, strength training involves a low number of repetitions at progressively higher loads, while endurance training involves a high number of repetitions at submaximal loads.

The rationale for strength training is to increase the tone of the pelvic floor muscles, to provide constant "support" to the pelvic organs, keeping them in a correct position [33]; this would also facilitate the automatic increase in motor neuron discharge, which would also allow more effective responses to sudden increases in intra-abdominal pressure [34–36].

In the neurological patient, the most significant difficulty is not only the possible deficit of voluntary recruitment secondary to the neurological damage but also, often, the disturbance of sensation resulting in poor awareness of the pelvic floor itself. Also depending on the neurological damage, the presence of cognitive deficits that impede the correct execution of the exercise, together with motivational deficits, is frequent: in a limited number of clinical experiments, it has been hypothesized that in this case, sensory feedback support can be used to facilitate awareness of the pelvic-perineal area [17].

References

1. Abrams P, Andersson K-E, Apostolidis A, Birder L, Bliss D, Brubaker L, et al. Evaluation and treatment of urinary incontinence, pelvic organ prolapse and faecal incontinence: recommendations of the International Scientific Committee. In: Abrams P, Cardozo L, Wagg A, Wein A, editors. Incontinence: 6th International Consultation on Incontinence, Tokyo, September 2016, vol. 1. 6th ed. Bristol: International Continence Society (ICS) and International Consultation on Urological Diseases (ICUD); 2017.
2. Gross T. Transcutaneous electrical nerve stimulation for treating neurogenic lower urinary tract dysfunction: a systematic review. Eur Urol. 2016;69:1102.
3. Schneider MP, Gross T, Bachmann LM, Blok BF, Castro-Diaz D, Del Popolo G, et al. Tibial nerve stimulation for treating neurogenic lower urinary tract dysfunction: a systematic review. Eur Urol. 2015;68(5):859–67.
4. Booth J. The effectiveness of transcutaneous tibial nerve stimulation (TTNS) for adults with overactive bladder syndrome: a systematic review. Neurourol Urodyn. 2018;37:528–35.
5. Stampas A. Feasibility of self-administered neuromodulation for neurogenic bladder in spinal cord injury. Int Neurourol J. 2019;23:249–54.
6. Guo GY. Effectiveness of neuromuscular electrical stimulation therapy in patients with urinary incontinence after stroke: a randomized sham controlled trial. Medicine. 2018;97:e13702.

7. Araujo TG. Transcutaneous tibial nerve home stimulation for overactive bladder in women with Parkinson's disease: a randomized clinical trial. Neurourol Urodyn. 2021;40:538–45.
8. Stampas A. Bladder neuromodulation in acute spinal cord injury via transcutaneous tibial nerve stimulation: cystometrogram and autonomic nervous system evidence from a randomized control pilot trial. Front Neurosci. 2019;13:119–24.
9. Stampas A, Korupolu R, Zhu L, Smith CP, Gustafson K. Safety, feasibility, and efficacy of transcutaneous tibial nerve stimulation in acute spinal cord injury neurogenic bladder: a randomized control pilot trial. Neuromodulation. 2019;22(6):716–22.
10. McClurg D. Neuromuscular electrical stimulation and the treatment of lower urinary tract dysfunction in multiple sclerosis—a double blind, placebo controlled, randomized clinical trial. Neurourol Urodyn. 2008;27:231–7.
11. Silva Ferreira AP, de Souza Pegorare ABG, Miotto Junior A, Salgado PR, Medola FO, Christofoletti G. A controlled clinical trial on the effects of exercise on lower urinary tract symptoms in women with multiple sclerosis. Am J Phys Med Rehabil. 2019;98(9):777–82.
12. McClurg D. Comparison of pelvic floor muscle training, electromyography biofeedback, and neuromuscular electrical stimulation for bladder dysfunction in people with multiple sclerosis: a randomized pilot study. Neurourol Urodyn. 2006;25:337–42.
13. Arruda RM, Castro RA, Sousa GC, Sartori MG, Baracat EC, Girão MJ. Prospective randomized comparison of oxybutynin, functional electrostimulation, and pelvic floor training for treatment of detrusor overactivity in women. Int Urogynecol J Pelvic Floor Dysfunct. 2008;19(8):1055–61.
14. Dumoulin C, Hay-Smith J, Habée-Séguin GM, Mercier J. Pelvic floor muscle training versus no treatment, or inactive control treatments, for urinary incontinence in women: a short version Cochrane systematic review with meta-analysis. Neurourol Urodyn. 2015;34(4):300–8.
15. McClurg D, Lowe-Strong A, Ashe R. Pelvic floor training for lower urinary tract dysfunction in MS. Nurs Times. 2009;105(7):45–7.
16. Lúcio A, D'ancona CA, Perissinotto MC, McLean L, Damasceno BP, de Moraes Lopes MH. Pelvic floor muscle training with and without electrical stimulation in the treatment of lower urinary tract symptoms in women with multiple sclerosis. J Wound Ostomy Continence Nurs. 2016;43(4):414–9.
17. Shin DC, Shin SH, Lee MM, Lee KJ, Song CH. Pelvic floor muscle training for urinary incontinence in female stroke patients: a randomized, controlled and blinded trial. Clin Rehabil. 2016;30(3):259–67.
18. Vásquez N, Knight SL, Susser J, Gall A, Ellaway PH, Craggs M. Pelvic floor muscle training in spinal cord injury and its impact on neurogenic detrusor over-activity and incontinence. Spinal Cord. 2015;53:887–9.
19. Shafik A, Shafik IA. Overactive bladder inhibition in response to pelvic floor muscle exercises. World J Urol. 2003;20(6):374–7.
20. Mahony DT, Laferte RO, Blais DJ. Integral storage and voiding reflexes. Neurophysiologic concept of continence and micturition. Urology. 1977;9(1):95–106.
21. Goode PS, Burgio KL, Locher JL, Umlauf MG, Lloyd LK, Roth DL. Urodynamic changes associated with behavioral and drug treatment of urge incontinence in older women. J Am Geriatr Soc. 2002;50:808–16.
22. Godec C, Cass AS, Ayala GF. Bladder inhibition with functional electrical stimulation. Urology. 1975;6(6):663–6.
23. Schrum A, Wolff S, van der Horst C, Kuhtz-Buschbeck JP. Motor cortical representation of the pelvic floor muscles. J Urol. 2011;186(1):185–90.
24. Turnbull GK, Hamdy S, Aziz Q, Singh KD, Thompson DG. The cortical topography of human anorectal musculature. Gastroenterology. 1999;117(1):32–9.
25. Brostrøm S. Motor evoked potentials from the pelvic floor. Neurourol Urodyn. 2003;22(7):620–37.
26. Sapsford R, Hodges P, Richardson C, Cooper D, Markwell S, Jull G. Co-activation of the abdominal and pelvic floor muscles during voluntary exercises. Neurourol Urodyn. 2001;20:31–42.

27. Madill SJ, McLean L. Relationship between abdominal and pelvic floor muscle activation and intravaginal pressure during pelvic floor muscle contractions in healthy continent women. Neurourol Urodyn. 2006;25:722–30.
28. Bø K, Stien R. Needle EMG registration of striated urethral wall and pelvic floor muscle activity patterns during cough, valsalva, abdominal, hip adductor, and gluteal muscle contractions in nulliparous healthy females. Neurourol Urodyn. 1994;13:35–41.
29. Peschers U, Vodusek D, Fanger G, Schaer G, DeLancey J, Schussler B. Pelvic muscle activity in nulliparous volunteers. Neurourol Urodyn. 2001;20:269–75.
30. Sjödahl J, Kvist J, Gutke A, Oberg B. The postural response of the pelvic floor muscles during limb movements: a methodological electromyography study in parous women without lumbopelvic pain. Clin Biomech (Bristol, Avon). 2009;24(2):183–9.
31. Hodges PW, Cresswell AG, Thorstensson A. Intra-abdominal pressure response to multidirectional support-surface translation. Gait Posture. 2004;20(2):163–70.
32. Bo K, Fernandes ACNL, Duarte TB, Brito LGO, Ferreira CHJ. Is pelvic floor muscle training effective for symptoms of overactive bladder in women? A systematic review. Physiotherapy. 2020;106:65–76.
33. Madill SJ, Pontbriand-Drolet S, Tang A, Dumoulin C. Effects of PFM rehabilitation on PFM function and morphology in older women. Neurourol Urodyn. 2013;32(8):1086–95.
34. Bø K, Hagen RH, Kvarstein B, Jørgensen J, Larsen S. Pelvic floor muscle exercise for the treatment of female stress urinary incontinence: III. Effects of two different degrees of pelvic floor muscle exercise. Neurourol Urodyn. 1990;9:489–502.
35. Wilson PD, Samarrai TAL, Deakin M, Kolbe E, Brown ADG. An objective assessment of physiotherapy for female genuine stress incontinence. Br J Obstet Gynaecol. 1987;94:575–82.
36. Glavind K, Nøhr S, Walter S. Biofeedback and physiotherapy versus physiotherapy alone in the treatment of genuine stress urinary incontinence. Int Urogynecol J. 1996;7:339–43.

Further Reading

Panicker JN. Neurogenic bladder: epidemiology, diagnosis, and management. Semin Neurol. 2020;40(5):569–79.

de Groat WC, Yoshimura N. Anatomy and physiology of the lower urinary tract. Handb Clin Neurol. 2015;130:61–108.

Fowler CJ, Griffiths D, de Groat WC. The neural control of micturition. Nat Rev Neurosci. 2008;9(6):453–66.

Averbeck MA. Editorial comment: Systematic literature review and meta-analysis of sacral neuromodulation (SNM) in patients with neurogenic lower urinary tract dys-function (nLUTD): over 20 years' experience and future directions. Int Braz J Urol. 2021;47(6):1264–5.

Shafik A. A study of the continence mechanism of the external urethral sphincter with identification of the voluntary urinary inhibition reflex. J Urol. 1999;162(6):1967–71.

Tai C, Shen B, Chen M, Wang J, Liu H, Roppolo JR, de Groat WC. Suppression of bladder overactivity by activation of somatic afferent nerves in the foot. BJU Int. 2011;107(2):303–9.

Reighard J, Jennings HS. Anatomy of the cat. Holt, Rinehart and Winston; 1935.

Onda A, Uchida S, Suzuki H, Hotta H. Stimulus frequency-dependent inhibition of micturition contractions of the urinary bladder by electrical stimulation of afferent Aβ, Aδ, and C fibers in cutaneous branches of the pudendal nerve. J Physiol Sci. 2016;66(6):491–6.

Paquette JP, Paquette JP, Yoo PB. Recruitment of unmyelinated C-fibers mediates the bladder-inhibitory effects of tibial nerve stimulation in a continuous-fill anesthetized rat model. Am J Physiol Renal Physiol. 2019;317(1):F163–71.

Sato A, Sato Y, Schaible HG, Schmidt RF. Types of afferents from the knee joint evoking sympathetic reflexes in cat inferior cardiac nerves. Neurosci Lett. 1983;39(1):71–5.

McPherson A. The effects of somatic stimuli on the bladder in the cat. J Physiol. 1966;185(1): 185–96.

Chapter 14
Erectile Dysfunction

Max Hilz, Ruihao Wang, and David B. Vodušek

14.1 Introduction

This article will focus on the most researched of the male sexual disorders, erectile dysfunction. Other disorders of sexuality, like the most common dysfunction with ageing—male hypogonadism, or the perhaps most prevalent disorder, premature ejaculation will not be discussed and are covered elsewhere [1].

14.2 Definition and Epidemiology of Erectile Dysfunction

In the past, various definitions of Erectile Dysfunction (ED) have been proposed. In 1992, the National Institute of Health (NIH) consensus development conference on impotence defined "Male erectile dysfunction", as the inability to achieve or maintain an erection sufficient for satisfactory sexual performance [2]. In 2015, the fourth International Consultation on Sexual Medicine defined erectile dysfunction as "*consistent or recurrent inability to attain and/or maintain penile erection sufficient for sexual satisfaction*" [3].

The original version of the chapter has been revised. A correction to this chapter can be found at https://doi.org/10.1007/978-3-031-43036-7_20

M. Hilz (✉)
Department of Neurology, University of Erlangen-Nuremberg, Erlangen, Germany

Icahn School of Medicine at Mount Sinai, New York, NY, USA

R. Wang
Department of Neurology, University of Erlangen-Nuremberg, Erlangen, Germany

D. B. Vodušek
Division of Neurology, University Medical Center Ljubljana, Ljubljana, Slovenia

Medical Faculty, University of Ljubljana, Ljubljana, Slovenia

G. Micieli et al. (eds.), *Autonomic Disorders in Clinical Practice*,
https://doi.org/10.1007/978-3-031-43036-7_14

The Massachusetts Male Aging Study found some degree of ED in approximately 52% of the 40–70-year-old men and complete “impotence” in 10% [4]. In 2019, a meta-analysis of population-based studies reported a global ED prevalence of 3–76.5% [5]. ED mainly afflicts men above age 40 and the prevalence of ED increases with age [6]. A follow-up study of 1709 men aged 40–69 years at study entry reported that the annual ED incidence increased from 12.4 cases per 1000 man-years among the 40–49-year-old men to 29.8 and 46.4 cases per 1000 man-years among men aged 50–59, and 60–69 years old [7]. In 2019, Kessler and coworkers reported in their meta-analysis of the global ED prevalence a prevalence of 9.1–49.9% in men below the age of 50 years and 54.9–94.7% in men above the age of 70 years [5]. In men below the age of 40 years, the ED prevalence ranges from 1% to 10% according to a review by Lewis et al. from 2010 [8]. However, the incidence of ED seems to increase: in 1995, ED afflicted approximately 152 million men while 322 million men may experience ED by 2025 [5]. Numerous conditions and risk factors contribute to the increasing incidence of ED, as detailed below [1, 6].

14.3 The Male Genital Response

Conceptually, erection is the normal genital response to (overall) sexual arousal. Physiologically, it is both a reflex mediated chiefly by the lower segments of the sacral spinal cord with preserved afferent and efferent connections, and a brain-induced genital response. This duality is inherent in the normal erection during arousal: it is mediated both by the touch-activated reflex response and the “non-contact” induced activation of brain centres by other sexually relevant stimuli (both externally generated, particularly visual, or internally generated, “psychogenic”) which are importantly shaping the genital responses; both depend on continuous appropriate afferent input.

14.3.1 Central Nervous System Structures Involved in Erectile Function

Sexual arousal is associated with increased neural activity in a complex circuitry of brain areas that includes the inferior right frontal cortex, the inferior temporal cortex, the left anterior cingulate cortex, and the right insula [9–14] (for review see [15]).

In contrast, erection correlates with the activation of a rather limited array of brain regions. According to Ferretti et al., these regions involve the anterior cingulate, insula, amygdala, hypothalamus, and secondary somatosensory cortices [15]. Presentation of sexually stimulating photographs is associated with the activation of the right medial prefrontal cortex, right and left orbitofrontal cortices, insulae, paracentral lobules, right ventral lateral thalamic nucleus, right anterior cingulate cortex, and regions participating in motor imagery and motor responses such as supplementary motor areas and the left ventral premotor area [16]. The early phase of penile tumescence seems to be controlled by frontal, parietal, insular and cingulate cortical areas, while penile tumescence in turn activates somatosensory brain regions [16]. Major control areas of male sexual behaviour are the medial preoptic area and the paraventricular nucleus of the hypothalamus [17–20].

Sensory penile stimulation activates neurons in various supraspinal structures, such as the nucleus paragigantocellularis in the brainstem, the nucleus paraventricularis (PVN), the medial preoptic area (MPOA) in the hypothalamus, and cortical areas [17, 21].

In rats, the paraventricular nucleus of the hypothalamus conveys the pro-erectile effects of oxytocin and apomorphine [22]. There are also androgen receptors in the paraventricular nucleus and the medial preoptic area [17, 23]. The medial nucleus of the amygdala seems to inhibit reflexive erections and support non-contact erections [24].

At the spinal cord level, the thoracolumbar sympathetic (T11–L2) and sacral (S2–S4) parasympathetic centres, and the sacral somatic afferent input and motor centres closely interact and contribute to penile erection. The dorsal grey commissure of L5 –S1 receives afferent impulses not only from the genital region but also from supraspinal areas and connects to the sacral parasympathetic nucleus, and thus seems to contribute to the spinal modulation of erections [21]. Most likely additional spinal areas such as interneurons in the lower thoracic and lumbosacral spinal cord and pro-erectile pathways from the periphery and supraspinal nuclei [17, 25, 26] contribute to this network.

In addition to coordinating erection and ejaculation, the spinal cord also assures the interaction with other pelvic functions, such as inhibition of micturition and defecation, and mediates the contraction of pelvic floor striated muscles with genital stimulation [17].

Sacral preganglionic parasympathetic neurons receive input via adrenergic, dopaminergic, serotonergic, glutamatergic receptors, receptors for prostaglandins, oxytocin, melanocortin, substance P, oestrogen and androgen, to name just a few. Apart from acetylcholine, the neurons synthesise substances such as cholecystokinin, enkephalin, nitric oxide (NO), and somatostatin (for review see [17]). Descending supraspinal pathways from forebrain structures and the nucleus paragigantocellularis in the rostral ventrolateral medulla inhibit pro-erectile spinal reflex responses.

There are androgen receptors in the lumbar and sacral dorsal root ganglia, sacral spinal cord interneurons, spinal neurons, pudendal motoneurons and the major pelvic ganglion. Androgens promote reflexive erections, testosterone and dihydrotestosterone augment reflexive erections in castrated animals [17]. The activity of pudendal motor neurons depends on androgens. Testosterone promotes the synthesis of pro-erectile transmitters such as nitric oxide.

Various peptides contribute to sexual responses such as pro-erectile melanocortin receptor agonists, MT-II and PT-141, with MT-II also enhancing sexual desire [27].

14.3.2 Peripheral Nervous System Structures Involved in Erectile Function

Erection is principally mediated by parasympathetic nerves but sympathetic and somatic nerves also modulate erection [28, 29].

Reflexogenic erection in response to tactile genital stimulation is mediated by impulses from the sacral parasympathetic erection centre at levels S2–S4. Preganglionic parasympathetic fibres travel in the pelvic nerve (nerve splanchnic pelvic) and reach the inferior hypogastric plexus (=pelvic plexus). Via the nervi cavernosi (nervi erigentes), postganglionic parasympathetic fibres convey vascular and trabecular smooth muscle relaxation of the corpora. In spinal cord injury patients with preservation of lower sacral segments reflexogenic erection upon tactile stimulation is preserved [30, 31] (Fig. 14.1).

Sympathetic fibres originate from the intermediolateral column (IML) at the lower thoracic and upper lumbar spinal cord (T11–L2) and from the dorsal grey commissure (DGC) at the levels L1–L2 (Fig. 14.1). Preganglionic fibres travel to the paravertebral sympathetic chain via the ventral root of the spinal nerves and the rami communicantes albi. One part of the sympathetic fibres leave the sympathetic chain and runs within the inferior splanchnic nerves towards the inferior mesenteric plexus and hypogastric nerves. The hypogastric nerves extend to the inferior hypogastric (pelvic) plexus; there, the fibres synapse into postganglionic sympathetic neurons which travel within the cavernous nerves to the genitals and penis [32]. Experimental stimulation of the prevertebral, hypogastric sympathetic fibres provided varying responses that caused controversial interpretations regarding the role of these fibres (for a review see [21]). The hypogastric nerve seems to contain sympathetic fibres with opposing, pro-erectile vasodilating and anti-erectile vasoconstricting functions [21]. Electrical stimulation of sympathetic fibres within the hypogastric plexus results in tumescence [34]; it does seem that there are postganglionic sympathetic neurons with a "*cholinergic*", vasodilating, pro-erectile neurotransmission as well as postganglionic neurons with an "*adrenergic*" transmission activating smooth muscles of the epididymis, vas deferens, seminal vesicles and prostate gland and thus contributing to ejaculation [21]. Another part of the sympathetic fibres reaches the penis after descending within the sympathetic paravertebral chain to the sacral levels S2–S4; from there, postganglionic, unmyelinated fibres run within the pelvic nerve (that also contains the parasympathetic fibres), join the inferior hypogastric plexus (=pelvic plexus), and finally travel within the cavernous nerve to the penis. These

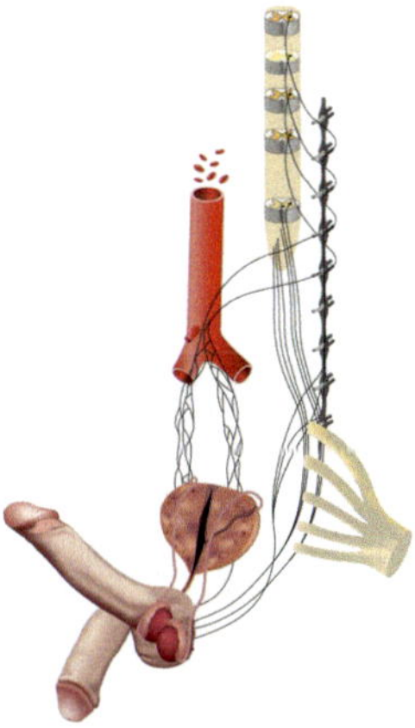

Fig. 14.1 Parasympathetic innervation from S2–S4; sympathetic innervation from T11–L2 via inferior splanchnic nerves, inferior mesenteric plexus, hypogastric nerves to inferior hypogastric (pelvic) plexus, and through sympathetic paravertebral chain to sacral levels S2–S4, to pelvic nerves (also containing parasympathetic fibres), cavernous nerves towards penis. In addition, a portion of the postganglionic sympathetic fibres leaves the paravertebral sympathetic chain and reaches the penis via the pudendal nerve [17, 31] which contains sensory afferent, efferent motor, as well as sympathetic and parasympathetic fibres [32]. (From [33] with permission)

fibres have been considered as "*adrenergic*" and *anti-erectile* mediating vasoconstriction of erectile tissue and detumescence. Other postganglionic sympathetic fibres leave the paravertebral sympathetic chain and reach the penis via the pudendal nerve [17, 31].

The principal somatic peripheral nervous structure relevant for erection is the pudendal nerve. It conveys afferent somatosensory information from the penile, scrotal, and anterior perineal region and therefore contributes to touch-elicited reflexogenic erection, to sensation during brain-mediated psychogenic erection, and mediates afferent impulses during ejaculation. In addition, the pudendal nerve sends motor impulses via the perineal nerve branches to the bulbospongiosus muscles which contract during ejaculation and to the ischiocavernosus muscles which contract during erection and ejaculation. The motor neurons are situated in the Onuf's nucleus located at the sacral spinal cord levels S2–S4 [35].

Moreover, the pudendal nerve carries parasympathetic fibres from the sacral spinal cord and sympathetic fibres from the sacral sympathetic trunk [32].

Due to these complex pathways, patients with sacral spinal cord lesions may still experience psychogenically mediated erections due to preservation of the pro-erectile sympathetic innervation [28]. On the other hand, sympathetic pathway lesions may induce erectile dysfunction [17].

14.3.3 Penile Anatomy and Physiology of Erection

Erection requires the relaxation of smooth muscles of the trabeculae and arterioles in the two dorsal corpora cavernosa and the ventral corpus spongiosum of the penis that also forms the glans. A fibrous capsule, the tunica albuginea, surrounds each corpus cavernosum. The trabeculae are fibrous strands that extend from the inner layer of the tunica albuginea and form lacunar spaces that are lined by vascular endothelium [36]. During the flaccid state of the penis, the cavernosal smooth muscles are contracted and blood is drained from the corpora cavernosa via veins that pass through the tunica albuginea into circumflex veins and the deep dorsal vein. Thus, the lacunar spaces or sinusoids are small during penile flaccidity (Fig. 14.2). Upon relaxation of the smooth muscles, penile arteries dilate and induce an increased arterial influx into the enlarging sinusoids; this increase of the sinusoids causes the

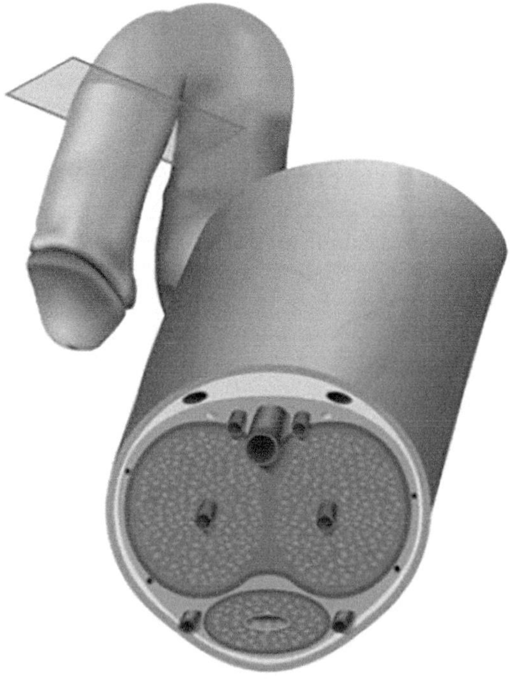

Fig. 14.2 During the flaccid state of the penis, emissary veins drain blood from the narrow lacunar system and leave the corpora cavernosa via wide open gaps in the tunica albuginea towards the circumflex veins that drain blood from the corpus spongiosum, and towards the deep dorsal vein. (From [33] with permission)

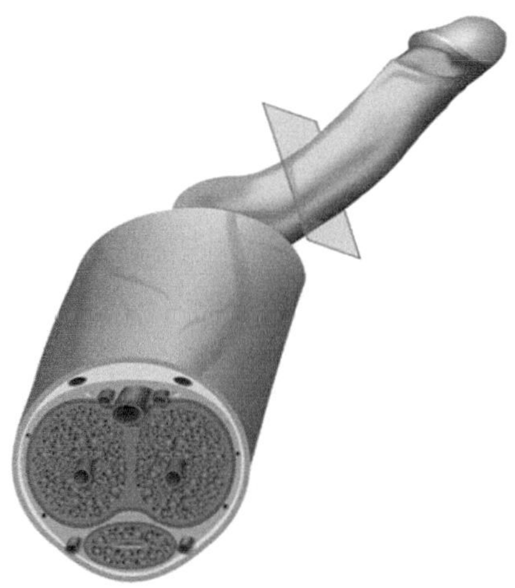

Fig. 14.3 During erection, engorged lacunar spaces compress emissary veins against the tunica albuginea and thus assure that there is no major blood drainage from the corpora cavernosa. Helicine arteries are dilated, circumflex, and cavernosal veins are almost collapsed. (From [33] with permission)

simultaneous passive occlusion of the venous drainage system via passive compression of emissary veins against the tunica albuginea. The three to fourfold dilatation of the small helicine arteries, i.e. serpentine vessels that end directly in the corporal sinusoids, and the reduced venous outflow cause tumescence, i.e. engorgement of the vascular spaces, the sinusoids, and expansion of erectile tissue, while the simultaneous increase in intracavernosal pressure accounts for the penile rigidity [34, 37, 38] (Fig. 14.3). In addition, venous blood drainage is further inhibited by the contraction of the ischiocavernosus muscles [34, 37].

14.3.4 Cellular Mechanisms of Vasodilatation and Erection

It is beyond the scope of this chapter to detail all so far known cellular contributors to penile vasodilatation and erection (for references see, e.g. [1]). However, the dichotomous concept of "adrenergic" and "cholinergic" neurotransmission simplifies the autonomic physiology of erection.

In general, penile erection or flaccidity depends on the amount of intracellular cytoplasmic calcium. Penile flaccidity is due to calcium release from the sarcoplasmic reticulum or intracellular entry from the extracellular milieu which induces myosin-light-chain phosphorylation and subsequent smooth muscle contraction [39]. In contrast, smooth muscle relaxation results when intracellular calcium is pumped back into the sarcoplasmic reticulum or removed towards the extracellular space, i.e. when the intracellular calcium levels decrease [17]. However, smooth muscle contraction may also occur without intracellular calcium increase due to kinases, such as protein kinase C (PKC), tyrosine kinases (TKs) and rho kinase (RhoK) that promote smooth muscle contraction and thus vasoconstriction by

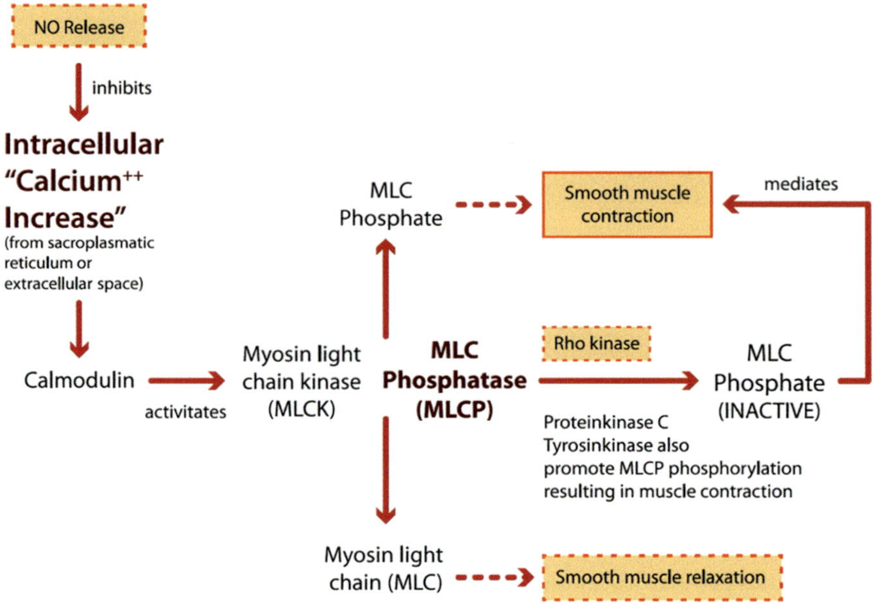

Fig. 14.4 Calcium release from the sarcoplasmic reticulum or Calcium entry from the extracellular milieu increases intracellular Calcium levels which activates myosin-light-chain phosphorylation and thus promotes smooth muscle contraction, a process that assures penile flaccidity. Moreover, kinases, such as protein kinase C (PKC), tyrosine kinases (TKs) and rho kinase (RhoK) promote penile flaccidity without an increase in intracellular calcium levels. The kinases inhibit the myosin-light-chain-phosphatase and thus ensure that there are higher myosin-light-chain-phosphatase levels which in turn mediate smooth muscle contraction (so-called *calcium sensitization*) [39, 40]. (From [33] with permission)

inhibiting the myosin-light-chain-phosphatase which is needed to cleave phosphate from myosin-light-chain-phosphate [39, 40] (Fig. 14.4).

The most important vasodilator is nitric oxide (NO). The majority of parasympathetic cholinergic nerve terminals next to penile small arteries contain vesicular acetylcholine transporter (VAChT) and neuronal nitric oxide synthase (nNOS), i.e. there seems to be a co-localization of acetylcholine and nitric oxide in vasodilation, pro-erectile nerve fibres [39]. NO is the main mediator of erection [17]. There are three nitric oxide synthetases (NOS) that synthesise NO and L-citrulline and H_2O as byproducts from L-arginine and oxygen [41]. Two NO synthetases, the neuronal NOS and endothelial NOS, are located in penile nerves and endothelium, while the inducible NOS (iNOS) is expressed during inflammation [39].

Upon sexual stimulation, parasympathetic fibres mediate the release of NO from cavernous nerve terminals. Nitric oxide activates guanil cyclase in—so far contracted—smooth muscle cells; guanil cyclase increases cyclic guanil monophosphate (cGMP) levels [39]. Cyclic GMP activates protein kinase G (PKG also known as cGMP-dependent protein kinase); PKG lowers intracellular calcium influx, intracellular calcium release, and calcium sensitivity of contractile proteins, e.g. by decreasing rho-kinase activity and by increasing potassium efflux which yields smooth muscle hyperpolarization; as a result, smooth muscle cells relax and penile arteries dilate; the subsequent increase in blood flow expands the trabecular sinusoids and causes endothelial shear stress which—together with neurohumoral factors, e.g., acetylcholine, histamine, and bradykinin—activates endothelial NOS and thus increases release of endothelial NO; the endothelial NO further promotes the relaxing mechanisms initiated by the neuronal NO release, and thus advances tumescence and rigidity [1, 39].

The cGMP that is essential for the cascade which lowers intracellular calcium and calcium sensitivity and thus promotes smooth muscle relaxation and erection is cleaved by specific phosphodiesterases, especially PDE5; the resulting decrease in cGMP levels terminates the vasodilating and relaxing effects of nitric oxide release and the secondary cGMP increase. Consequently, PDE-5 inhibitors maintain high cGMP levels and therefore support erection.

Prostanoids, particularly prostaglandins E1 and E2 synthesised in penile smooth muscle cells and epoprostenol (Prostacyclin [PG I2]) in the vascular endothelium also further smooth muscle relaxation. Prostaglandin E1 does not depend on the endothelium nor nitric oxide and very efficiently relaxes the smooth muscles. The vasodilating effects of Prostaglandin E1 and epoprostenol result from stimulation of adenylate cyclase that converts adenosine triphosphate (ATP) into cyclic adenosine monophosphate (cAMP); elevated cAMP levels again activate protein kinase A (PKA also known as cAMP-dependent protein kinase) and hereby launch the above-mentioned cascade that lowers intracellular calcium levels which triggers smooth muscle relaxation, vasodilation, and erection. This pathway is of therapeutic relevance in patients with ED who no longer produce sufficient amounts of NO, as mentioned below.

In addition, there are other dilators of penile vessels, such as vasoactive intestinal peptide and the endothelium derived hyperpolarization factor (EDHF). Androgens seem to support nitric oxide synthesis while hypoxia, e.g., due to atherosclerosis, compromises NO synthesis and vasodilatation because oxygen is essential for nitric oxide synthesis [1].

14.3.5 Mediators of Penile Vasoconstriction and Detumescence

Release of noradrenaline from adrenergic sympathetic fibres stimulates postsynaptic adrenergic α1 and α2-receptors that induce corporal smooth muscle contraction and arterial vasoconstriction which lead to reduced arterial inflow, sinusoid collapse with subtunical venous decompression and increased venous drainage [42]. In detail, the α1-adrenergic receptor stimulation triggers calcium influx, as well as calcium sensitization via activation of rho kinase, protein kinase C, and tyrosine kinases. Calcium sensitization with myosin light-chain phosphatase phosphorylation and activation of the myosin light-chain kinase shifts the balance between myosin light-chain (MLC) and MLC-phosphate towards the latter and thus promotes smooth muscle contraction, as described above (Fig. 14.4).

While noradrenaline also limits its own further release by stimulating presynaptic α2 adrenergic receptors on sympathetic fibres it also inhibits the NO release from presynaptic "cholinergic" terminals [1, 42]. In contrast, adrenaline release during sexual activity and erection stimulates β-adrenergic receptors. Adrenaline's pro-erectile effect is mediated by β2 receptors that augment cAMP levels and trigger the above-mentioned cAMP-cascade by activating adenylate cyclase [1].

Neuropeptide Y and endothelins also have pro- and anti-erectile effects. The details are beyond the scope of this chapter [1].

In addition to the above mentioned pro-erectile prostanoids, there are also contractile prostanoids such as prostaglandin F2α, thromboxane A2, and prostaglandin E2 in the erectile tissue [43].

Angiotensin II seems to advance penile detumescence while angiotensin II type 1-receptor antagonists decrease contraction and augment intracavernous pressure [1, 44].

14.4 Etiology of Erectile Dysfunction

The cause of ED in an individual patient is often multifactorial and in fact in most cases impossible to define with absolute certainty. In population studies, ED has been associated with risk factors such as increasing age, obesity with dyslipidemia, arterial hypertension, metabolic syndrome, sedentary lifestyle, smoking, alcohol consumption, use of illicit or "recreational" drugs, several therapeutic drugs, as well with chronic diseases of the heart, kidneys, liver, lungs and the nervous system [1, 6]. In the individual patient, the relevant particular causes are sought, as their treatment may improve the patient's health and ED.

Causes of erectile dysfunction are classified as organic, psychogenic, or mixed organic and psychogenic [6] and are discussed below. Organic causes are drug and medication-induced, neurogenic, endocrine, vascular, metabolic, urologic, due to systemic diseases [6].

Drug-induced erectile dysfunction is quite common and important to diagnose since numerous therapeutic drugs as well as illicit or "recreational" drugs, such as nicotine, alcohol, marijuana, heroin, cocaine, amphetamines, benzodiazepines, barbiturates, or opiates including methadone, may significantly compromise erectile function [1, 6] (Table 14.1), and their removal may lead to quick improvement.

Psychotropic drugs including antidepressants, (e.g., amitriptyline, desipramine, doxepin, fluoxetine, imipramine, maprotiline, nortriptyline, paroxetine, protryptiline, sertraline, tranylcypromine, trazodone, trimipramine, venlafaxine) and other psychiatric agents such as phenothiazines, butyrophenones, (e.g. chlorpromazine, clomipramine, clozapine, fluphenazine, haloperidol, lithium, olanzapine,

Table 14.1 Incomplete list of antihypertensives and miscellaneous agents contributing to sexual dysfunction (with permission modified from Hilz 2008 [1])

Antihypertensive agents	Miscellaneous agents	Miscellaneous agents
Alpha-methyldopa	Acetazolamide	Physostigmine
Amiloride	Amiodarone	Primidone
Atenolol	Atropine	Propofol
Benazepril	Baclofen	Ranitidine
Chlorthalidone	Biperiden	Tamoxifen
Clonidine	Carbamazepine	Testosterone
Diltiazem	Cimetidine	**Over-the-counter agents**
Enalapril	Clofibrate	Antihistamines
Guanethidine	Digoxin	Cimetidine
Hydralazine	Disopyramide	Diphenhydramine
Hydrochlorothiazide	Disulfiram	Famotidine
Labetalol	Ethosuximide	Naproxen
Methyldopa	Famotidine	Niacin
Metoprolol	Heparin	Ranitidine
Minoxidil	Indometacin	
Nifedipine	Interferon	
Phenoxybenzamine	Ketamine	
Phentolamine	Ketoconazole	
Pindolol	Levodopa	
Prazosin	Omeprazole	
Propranolol	Oxybutynin	
Reserpine	Phenobarbital	
Spironolactone	Phenytoin	
Verapamil		

risperidone, sulpiride, thioridazine and many others) contribute to ED [1, 6]. The list of drugs that cause or contribute to ED is long and it comprises also antihypertensives such as thiazide diuretics, beta-blockers, calcium antagonists, ACE inhibitors, anticonvulsants, tranquillisers, hypnotics, statins, antiandrogens, antiphlogistic substances, morphines, anticholinergics, histamine H2 receptor antagonists, antiarrhythmics, cytotoxic drugs, gonadotropin antagonists such as estrogens, gonadotropin-releasing hormone-analogues, spironolactone, cimetidine, indomethacin, clofibrate, glycosides, MAO-inhibitors and many other drugs that are constantly prescribed although they interfere with sexual function [1, 6, 45, 46] (for a review see [45]).

Neurogenic causes are many central nervous system disorders (including stroke, multiple sclerosis, neurodegenerative disorders such as Parkinson's disease, multisystem atrophy, Alzheimer's disease, temporal lobe epilepsy, sleep apnea, traumatic brain injuries, encephalitis, intracranial tumours, and spinal cord lesions), and and peripheral nervous system disorders such as cauda equina, nerve root and peripheral nerve lesions, due to trauma or surgery. Among polyneuropathies particularly those which affect autonomic nerve fibres, and especially diabetic neuropathy, may cause erectile dysfunction. Conus medullaris lesions and malformations such as myelomeningocele are often mixed "upper" and "lower" motor neuron lesions and also cause ED [1].

Among endocrine disorders diabetes mellitus is a leading cause of ED, which may even be the first manifestation of diabetes [6] while ED manifests in at least 50% of diabetic men within 10 years after the diagnosis of diabetes [6]. Among other endocrine causes are the decrease in dehydroepiandrosterone-sulfate (DHEA-S), disorders of the hypothalamus, pituitary gland, or gonadal axis, thyroid or adrenal gland disorders, or hormone-active tumours, especially prolactinomas with hyperprolactinemia decreasing testosterone and thus causing ED. In contrast, hypergonadotropic hypogonadism occurs in patients with testicular atrophy, anorchidism, or Klinefelter syndrome. Altered oestrogen metabolism in patients with chronic liver disease, e.g. due to alcohol abuse, may also cause ED [6].

Vascular causes comprise local aortoiliac disorders including aortic aneurysms or stenosis of the aortoiliac arteries as well as arteriosclerosis of penile arteries [1, 6]. Since the diameter of the penile artery is smaller than that of e.g. the proximal left anterior descending coronary artery, ED due to atherosclerosis is likely to manifest years earlier than coronary artery disease. In fact, ED can be considered a predictor of coronary and cardiovascular disease and should trigger a thorough examination and risk assessment of ED patients since their risk of incurring cardiac events in the future is significantly higher than the risk of men without ED [1, 6]. Venous malformation, particularly venous leakage with insufficient closure of emissary veins, may also compromise penile rigidity but the relevance of venous leaks was very likely overestimated in the past [1].

Traumatic, inflammatory, and tumorous causes as well as Peyronie's disease may induce penile changes leading to ED [1].

Surgical (iatrogenic) causes of ED include radical prostate or bladder cancer surgery, but also rectal cancer surgery [47]. There is also a correlation between lower urinary tract symptoms, benign prostate hyperplasia, and the occurrence of ED [1, 48].

Not all psychogenic causes are "psychiatric"—they include performance anxiety, social or religious concerns, a history of sexual abuse, fear of pregnancies, etc. Psychiatric causes include depression, phobias, dementias, psychotic diseases and their treatment, and many others [6].

14.5 Diagnostic Approach in Men with Erectile Dysfunction (Table 14.2)

Many patients are hesitant to report sexual problems. Decent, simple but straightforward questions about the patients' intimate life or difficulties with intercourse may help to create an atmosphere of confidence [49]. A careful medical, sexual, psychiatric; and psychosocial history is needed to evaluate ED [1, 49–51]. In addition, various questionnaires such as the International Index of Erectile Function (IIEF), or the Sexual Health Inventory for Men (SHIM), to name only two easily applied questionnaires, may help to evaluate the severity of ED [1, 6].

Table 14.2 Evaluation of Erectile Dysfunction (with permission modified from Hilz 2008 [1])

History – Medical – Sexual – Psychiatric – Psychosocial – Neurologic – Endocrine	**Clinical examination** – Psychiatric/psychological evaluation – Overall physical examination with emphasis on neurologic examination (also *anal sphincter tone, bulbocavernosus reflex, perianal sensation)* and urological examination (*penis, testicles, secondary sexual characteristics, digital rectal, prostate examination*)
Risk factor evaluation e.g.: – Alcohol – Nicotine – Medication – Illicit drugs – Metabolic syndrome – Diabetes – Dyslipidemia – Arterial hypertension – Cardiac and cardiovascular diseases – Pelvic trauma – Pelvic surgery, or radiation	**Laboratory evaluation** e.g.: – Serum electrolytes – Complete blood cell count – Fasting glucose, hemoglobin A1c – Lipid levels – Renal and hepatic parameters **Endocrine/andrological parameters** e.g.: – Prostate-specific antigen – Total, (free, bio-available) testosterone – Sex hormone-binding globulin – Luteinizing hormone (LH) – Follicle-stimulating hormone (FSH) – Thyroid function assessment – Prolactin
Questionnaires of sexual function e.g.: – International index of erectile function – Sexual health inventory for men	

14.5.1 History

It is important to find out when erectile problems first started, whether they are constant or intermittent, and whether there are other changes in sexual function, e.g. in ejaculation or orgasm, genital pain, changes in sexual desire and orientation or partnership problems [50]. Rigid morning or nocturnal erections, or during sexual thoughts, a sudden beginning or intermittent course of ED might point towards psychogenic causes [6], while a gradual beginning, progressive deterioration and long history of ED are more likely due to an organic aetiology [6].

Common risk factors of ED must be evaluated, for example smoking, hypercholesterolemia or hypertension, cardiovascular diseases, diabetes mellitus, anxiety, depression, alcohol or drug abuse, pre-existing surgeries, trauma or radiation in the pelvic region, neurologic or endocrine disorders, as well as relationship issues, or sexual preferences [1].

14.5.2 (Interdisciplinary) Clinical Examination

An interdisciplinary endocrinological-andrological, psychiatric, neurologic, internal and urological examination may be needed. The 2018, AUA guidelines on ED [51] recommend the physical examination of the abdomen, penis, testicles, secondary sexual characteristics and lower extremity pulses. The neurological evaluation should assess the anal sphincter tone, evaluate the clinically elicited bulbocavernosus reflex, and test for perianal and "saddle" anaesthesia [52].

14.5.3 Cardiovascular Risk Evaluation

According to the Princeton III Consensus Recommendations for the Management of Erectile Dysfunction and Cardiovascular Disease, ED is a marker of an increased risk of cardiovascular disease, independent of other risk predictors as assessed for example with the Framingham Risk Score, such as age, gender, total and high-density lipoprotein cholesterol levels, smoking, systolic blood pressure (BP), or the use of antihypertensives. Particularly, in younger men, up to the age of 60, a diagnosis of ED must be considered a warning sign of possible cardiovascular risk [6, 53]. Since ED frequently is a precursor of cardiovascular disease, particularly coronary artery disease [53], a cardiological work-up is recommended in all men with confirmed ED to rule out or to categorise the cardiovascular risk, particularly the risk of clinically silent coronary artery disease. A resting electrocardiogram (ECG) should be mandatory. Any abnormal finding in the resting ECG should trigger an exercise ECG, particularly in men below 60 years of age [6]. Abnormal results should be followed by further cardiologic examination [6]. The details of the cardiovascular work-up are beyond the scope of this chapter and can be found, e.g. in the Princeton III Consensus Recommendations [53].

Prior to any decision regarding the treatment of ED (sexual intercourse is "hard physical labour"), a detailed cardiovascular work-up may be needed to determine whether the patient is at low, indeterminate (or intermediate), or high cardiovascular risk [1, 54, 55]. High-risk patients are defined as those with unstable or refractory angina, uncontrolled hypertension, severe congestive heart failure (New York Heart Association Class IV), myocardial infarction or cardiovascular accidents within the previous 2 weeks, high-risk arrhythmias, hypertrophic obstructive and other cardiomyopathies and moderate-to-severe valvular disease, particularly aortic stenosis [50, 53–56]. According to the Princeton Consensus statements, high-risk patients should defer sexual activity and must not receive treatment for their sexual dysfunction until their cardiac condition has stabilised [50, 53, 56]. Patients with low cardiovascular risk are those who can usually exercise at modest intensity without symptoms [53]. They may have asymptomatic, controlled hypertension, successful coronary revascularisation, mild valvular disease, left ventricular dysfunction or heart failure New York Heart Association Class I and II without signs of ischemia during exercise testing [50, 54–56]. Low-risk patients can initiate or resume sexual activity and ED treatment, however risk factors and coronary heart disease should be evaluated and follow-up examinations are recommended [50, 54]. Patients with indeterminate risk should first undergo a detailed cardiovascular assessment including, e.g. treadmill testing [56] to reclassify whether the patient is at low or at high risk [54]. The indeterminate-risk patients are those who have mild or moderate stable angina pectoris, suffered a myocardial infarction 2–8 weeks ago without intervention, still need an exercise electrocardiogram, have congestive heart failure NYHA class III, and have complications from noncardiac atherosclerotic diseases such as peripheral artery disease, stroke, or transient ischemic attacks [53]. If an indeterminate-risk patient is reassigned to the high-risk group, the recommendations of the Princeton Consensus Conference again suggest deferral of sexual activity until the cardiac condition is stabilised. Risk factors and coronary heart disease have to be re-assessed in follow-up examinations [50, 54]. Most patients seeking treatment for ED are at low risk and may receive all first-line therapies according to the AUA guidelines on ED [50]. However, during sexual activity, there is an increase in physical exertion with augmented sympathetic activity and elevated blood pressure and heart rate [50, 54]. Therefore, cardiovascular disease patients have a slightly increased risk of myocardial infarction related to sexual activity, independent of the treatment method for ED [50].

14.5.4 Additional Specific Testing Procedures

Additional tests may be needed if patients are not responding to first-line treatment—PDE-5 inhibitors [1, 57].

Intracavernous injection of vasoactive substances, such as prostaglandin E_1, can evaluate cavernous hemodynamics, arterial insufficiency, or venous "leakage" as the substance normally causes a rigid erection within minutes [58]. Prostaglandin E_1 increases cAMP levels in smooth muscle cells and thus causes a decrease in intracellular calcium and smooth muscle relaxation [37]. Prostaglandin E_1 moreover inhibits presynaptic noradrenaline release and thereby promotes cavernosal smooth muscle relaxation [59]. Cavernosal hemodynamics are most likely intact if a small Prostaglandin E_1 dosage yields an erection. In the case of arterial insufficiency high dosages are needed while failure even of high dosages suggests the diagnosis of a "venous leakage". However, prostaglandin E_1-tests may yield inaccurate results while testing of phosphodiesterase type 5 inhibitors at home may provide the same or better information [60].

Colour-coded Doppler and duplex sonography can determine arterial and venous penile function, e.g. after pharmacologically induced erection [61, 62]. Arterial inflow increases during tumescence and systolic velocity, finally reaching a peak while end-diastolic velocity shows negative values upon successful veno-occlusion [62]. Reduced systolic and end-diastolic velocities suggest arterial insufficiency, while end diastolic flow velocities above zero can be seen in patients with veno-occlusive dysfunction [1, 62].

Abnormal ultrasound results may require further invasive arteriography, cavernosometry or cavernosography in patients who might be suitable for vascular reconstructive surgery [63].

If a neurological cause of ED is suspected, neurophysiologic tests may be indicated, particularly in selected patients with suspected peripheral nervous system lesions.

The anal sphincter electromyography shows abnormalities in patients with lesions of the cauda equina, the roots S2–S4 and the pudendal nerve. In acute lesions, it will demonstrate pathological spontaneous activity. In chronic lesions, the area, duration, and number of turns of motor unit potentials will change and allow for differentiation of neuropathic from normal external anal sphincter [64]. Sphincter electromyography has been suggested to distinguish between multiple system atrophy and Parkinson's disease although there is controversy about the differential-diagnostic validity of results [65–67].

Bulbocavernosus reflex testing evaluates afferent pudendal nerve function, spinal S2–S4 segments, and efferent motor nerve fibres as well as the bulbocavernosus muscle or external anal sphincter muscle innervated by these fibres and is useful for the diagnosis of conus medullaris or cauda equina as well as pudendal nerve lesions [67].

Central motor conduction latencies evaluate the conduction from the cerebral cortex along the sacral motor pathway to the pelvic floor and sphincters by means of transcranial magnetic coil stimulation at the vertex and at the L1 level and recording from sphincter and pelvic floor muscles [64, 68]. Subtraction of motor-evoked potential latencies after L1 stimulation and vertex stimulation allows to calculate the central conduction time [68]. Thus, the method assesses lesions of the motor pathway to the pelvic floor and sphincter muscles [35, 64].

Somatosensory evoked potentials after electrical stimulation at the dorsal nerve of the penis or clitoris and recording from the Cz'-Fz positions show a first positive peak (P1 or P40) with an amplitude of 0.5–12 μV and a latency of 41 ± 2.3 ms [65]. The technique is useful for the diagnosis of lesions of large diameter sensory nerve fibres or dorsal column and lemniscal sensory pathways and can be applied, e.g. in patients with perineal sensory deficits or with central demyelination, e.g. due to multiple sclerosis [67]. The method does not evaluate peripheral small nerve fibres or the spinothalamic pathways [1].

The sensitivity of the above "tests of conduction" (of thick myelinated nerve fibres) to diagnose lesions of axonal type (which predominate in clinical practice) is low. The tests are, however, useful in the context of intraoperative monitoring to preserve the uro-ano-genital innervation during spinal surgeries.

The value of penile sympathetic skin response testing is questionable as the sympathetic sudomotor response induced by an arousal stimulus and recorded from the skin of the lateral penis is not always positive and its absence moreover does not necessarily reflect autonomic causes of ED [35, 64].

Quantitative sensory testing of warm, cold and heat pain perception thresholds at the genitalia can be used to evaluate the function and dysfunction of peripheral somatic thinly myelinated A-delta and unmyelinated C-fibres [69, 70]. However, thermal thresholds at the penis require patient cooperation and may vary significantly [71].

Nocturnal penile tumescence and rigidity measurements have been thought to distinguish psychogenic from organic ED [72]. However, sensitivity, specificity, and reproducibility of results is now considered to be low [57, 73].

14.6 Treatment of Erectile Dysfunction

14.6.1 General Aspects

The diagnosis of ED must never trigger a reflex-like prescription of phosphodiesterase type 5 inhibitors but requires a thorough risk assessment including the patient's age, lack of physical exercise, smoking, unhealthy diet, increased alcohol consumption, pre-existing conditions such as hypertension, obesity, metabolic syndrome, prediabetes, dyslipidemia, or sleep apneas to name only a few, and a thorough physical examination with BMI assessment, levels of plasma glucose, plasma lipids, serum creatinine, albumin to creatinine ratio, liver values, haemoglobin A1c, morning levels of total testosterone [53]. In case of testosterone deficiency, i.e. total testosterone levels below 300 ng/dL [51], additional endocrine tests may be needed, such as the assessment of luteinising hormone (LH), follicle-stimulating hormone (FSH), prolactin, thyroid function, and a complete blood count [1, 6, 52].

Lifestyle changes, such as lowering increased body weight, using a healthy diet, exercising regularly, abandoning a sedentary lifestyle and smoking can improve vascular function and erections [1, 30].

The drugs taken by the patient and co-existing diseases must be identified and the issues addressed [50].

Testosterone replacement can be considered—also in combination with PDE5 inhibitors—if the patient has a confirmed decrease in bioavailable testosterone [6, 74].

Psychological components always contribute to and sometimes cause ED and must be addressed, e.g. by patient or couple counselling, psychosexual therapy, cognitive and behaviour therapy [1, 6, 74].

Patients should learn about all treatment options [74] before starting a particular treatment of ED.

14.6.2 *Particular Treatment Possibilities*

14.6.2.1 Oral Pharmacotherapy: Phosphodiesterase Type 5 Inhibitors

Four PDE-5 inhibitors, Sildenafil, Tadalafil, Vardenafil, and Avanafil are currently approved by the respective authorities in the USA [75] and in Europe [74]. PDE-5 inhibitors require sexual stimulation and NO release—as described above—to induce erection [74]. According to the 2018 guidelines of the American Urological Association, the four PDE5 inhibitors seem to have similar efficacy [51]. The efficacy of PDE5 inhibitors is lower in diabetic patients and post-prostatectomy patients with more severe ED than in the general ED population responding to this treatment [51]. Moreover, there are pharmacokinetic differences between the different PDE5-inhibitors.

Sildenafil is available as 25-, 50-, or 100-mg tablets [63]. Erection occurs within 30–60 min after oral ingestion and the serum half-life time is around 4 h [50]. The successful dosage should be taken only once daily [56]. Heavy, high-fat meals may significantly reduce the Sildenafil plasma concentration and delay the time until maximum plasma concentration [56].

Vardenafil is available in 5, 10, and 20 mg doses and is effective within approximately 30 min after administration. However, its efficacy is again reduced by heavy, fatty meals [63]. The mean half-life of Vardenafil and duration of action are again around 4 h. Vardenafil may cause mild QT prolongations and should not be used by patients with prolongation of the electrocardiographic QT interval nor by patients taking class Ia or III antiarrhythmic drugs [1, 50, 56].

Tadalafil is available at 10 and 20 mg doses, induces an erection within 25–30 min, reaches its peak efficacy in approximately 2 h and has a plasma half-life of 17.5 h. Thus, it may still be effective for up to 36 h [63, 76]. Again, only one pill should be taken per day [63]. Food consumption has no relevant effect on the pharmacokinetics and efficacy of Tadalafil. In contrast to Sildenafil and Vardenafil, Tadalafil causes no facial flushing. However, Tadalafil has a higher selectivity for PDE11A than do Sildenafil and Vardenafil; PDE11A is expressed in skeletal muscles; therefore, Tadalafil may induce back pain [76].

Avanafil is available as 50, 100, and 200 mg tablets and reaches peak plasma concentrations already after 30–45 min, erections may even occur after 20 min. Its half-life is 6–17 h. Food delays the absorption of Avanafil. Avanafil may interact with many drugs since its metabolism involves cytochrome P450 (CYP) 3A4. Thus, the drug is contraindicated in patients taking strong inhibitors of CYP3A4, such as ritonavir, itraconazole, or clarithromycin, and its dosage should be reduced in patients on moderate CYP3A4-inhibitors, such as erythromycin, and patients on drugs like fluoxetine may have a reduced clearance of Avanafil [77].

More generalised autonomic system dysfunction with slowing of gastric emptying may delay the onset of action of phosphodiesterase type 5 inhibitors.

The most common side-effects of PDE 5 inhibitors [50, 56] include headache, flushing, dyspepsia, nasal congestion or rhinitis, myalgia and back pain, dizziness, and prolonged erection or priapism (i.e. an erection lasting for more than 4–6 h) [78], and altered colour perception [52]. Sildenafil also has some inhibitory effects on the retinal phosphodiesterase type 6 and may therefore induce visual disturbances with a blue-tinged vision [52]. In patients with retinitis pigmentosa, PDE 5 inhibitors are contraindicated. Since PDE-5 inhibitors lower arterial blood pressure, a baseline blood pressure below 90/50 mmHg is also a contraindication for PDE-5 inhibitors. Due to their hypotensive effect, PDE-5 inhibitors are moreover absolutely contraindicated in patients receiving nitrates or NO-donors such as molsidomine and so called recreational 'poppers' amyl nitrite or amyl nitrate, as the combination causes an unpredictable blood pressure decrease and hypotension [55, 63]. Conversely, acute coronary syndromes should not be treated with nitrates within 24 h after the intake of Sildenafil and Vardenafil, and even for 48 h after Tadalafil intake [52]. The use of PDE5 inhibitors should be reflected with utmost caution in patients with serious cardiovascular diseases, e.g., uncontrolled hypertension and angina, and in patients using alpha-blockers [6]. As mentioned above, ED patients must undergo cardiovascular risk evaluation according to the criteria established by the third Princeton III Consensus Recommendations for the Management of Erectile Dysfunction and Cardiovascular Disease and should only receive PDE-5 inhibitors if they are classified as low-risk patients [74].

Non-arteritic anterior ischaemic optic neuropathy (NAION) is another contraindication for the use of PDE5-inhibitors although a direct association between PDE-5 inhibitor use and NAION has not been established [49].

Patients should also discontinue using PDE-5 inhibitors if there is a sudden decrease or loss of hearing as there have been reports of a temporal association with the use of PDE-5 inhibitors [79].

14.6.2.2 Intracavernous Injections for Patients Not Responding to Oral Treatment

Patients who do not respond to PDE5 inhibitors often benefit from intracavernous prostaglandin E1 (PGE1) injection [1]. Cavernosal injection of 5–40 mcg PGE1 (alprostadil) increases intracellular cAMP levels via adenylate cyclase activation [1, 39] and thus induces erections within 5–15 min. Even in diabetic and cardiovascular ED patients efficacy and satisfaction rates are high.

However, complications may occur including penile pain, prolonged erections, and penile fibrosis that requires discontinuation of injections for several months. Priapism is the most serious acute side effect. In patients with increased risk of priapism, e.g. due to sickle cell anaemia, multiple myeloma, and leukaemia, patients with hypersensitivity to alprostadil, or with bleeding disorders, the cavernosal injections are contraindicated [1]. Patients must know that higher doses may cause arterial hypotension and that there is a risk of prolonged erections or even priapism, i.e. an erection lasting more than 4 h which is an emergency requiring swift treatment to avoid permanent cavernosal tissue damage. While prolonged erections might be treated with oral or intracavernosal application of the β2-adrenergic receptor agonist terbutaline, priapism requires therapeutic blood aspiration under sterile conditions, and in cases of persistent priapism intracavernosal injection of sympathomimetic drugs such as phenylephrine, or even surgery [1]. Priapism therapy must be in the hands of experienced experts since nonischemic, so-called high-flow priapism, e.g. after a perineal trauma, should not be treated with aspiration and sympathomimetic injection [1].

A combination of intracavernosal vasoactive drugs may increase the success rates and reduce side effects since the dosages of the individual drugs can be lowered [1, 6]. Alprostadil (prostaglandin E1) can be combined with papaverine, phentolamine, or vasoactive intestinal polypeptide (VIP). Among the potential side effects are prolonged erections, cavernosal fibrosis, induration, penile deviation, pain, and systemic effects such as peripheral vasodilatation, hypotension, reflex tachycardia, or hepatotoxicity with papaverine application, and tachycardia and orthostatic hypotension with phentolamine application. VIP side effects include decreased blood pressure, tachycardia, or cutaneous flushing [80].

Intraurethral prostaglandin E1 treatment via pellets containing alprostadil (Muse®), the smooth muscle relaxing and vasodilating prostaglandin E1, may also induce erections within 15 min [2, 25]; however, the method is somewhat cumbersome and response rates are not as high as with intracavernosal prostaglandin injection or with PDE5 inhibitors; side-effects include penile or urethral pain and burning, orthostatic hypotension, and syncope [1, 6].

14.6.2.3 Devices

Vacuum erection devices and constrictions rings may induce a sufficient erection in up to 90% [74] but many patients are not satisfied with the method [6] that uses a negative pressure induced by a pump and a cylinder placed over the penis to draw blood into the corpora cavernosa while a constriction ring at the penile base helps maintain the erection [1]. The method is inexpensive and readily available but often causes penile pain and discolouration, inability to ejaculate, bruising and petechiae, numbness, and a cold penis. To prevent tissue damage, constriction rings should be removed within 30 min [81, 82]. The method must not be used in patients with bleeding disorders or on anticoagulant medication [1, 63].

14.6.2.4 Treatment of Vascular Erectile Dysfunction

Penile arterial reconstructive surgery might be useful in patients with pelvic or perineal trauma, or a focal arterial stenosis that is accessible to surgery [35, 50, 74].

Patients with a mild vasculogenic ED might also benefit from low-intensity shockwave therapy. Yet, it is still unclear which of the heterogeneous shockwave generators may yield the most promising results [74].

Venous reconstructive or ligation surgery and venous embolization procedures have been frequently performed in the past in patients with suggested veno-occlusive leakage but are no longer recommended due to poor results [1, 74].

14.6.2.5 Prosthesis

A penile prosthesis is the last option for ED treatment if all other options are unsuccessful.

Malleable, non-inflatable, semi-rigid prosthesis and inflatable two- or three-piece devices are available. Semi-rigid prosthesis might be a solution for older patients with infrequent sexual intercourse [63] while the inflatable devices assure a more ‘natural’ erection [63]. The implantation irreversibly damages the corpus cavernosum tissue and may be associated with haemorrhages, urethral lesions, painful stretching of the tunica albuginea, or penile deviations and erections with a drooping glans due to inadequate size of the implant [35]. Other side effects and complications include infections, erosion, mechanical failure or post-surgical penile shortening, and the need for re-operation and reimplantation [1, 63].

14.7 Conclusion

The awareness of sexual dysfunction and its treatment have significantly improved among physicians and the lay public due to the development of efficient drugs such as PDE-5 inhibitors [1]. However, treatment must never consist of a reflex-like prescription of phosphodiesterase 5 inhibitors.

Any treatment should be preceded by a detailed medical history and a search for prescriptive and entertainment drugs, cardiovascular, metabolic, neurological, and endocrine disorders, particularly diabetes and hypogonadism, for traumatic injuries and surgery [83]. Clinical and laboratory examination should search for cardiovascular, neurological, and endocrine diseases, such as testosterone deficiency, or dyslipidemia, and for psychiatric and psychological conditions of ED, to mention only the main ED causes. Considering the findings, treatment might include lifestyle changes, physical and pelvic floor exercises, weight loss, discontinuation of smoking, and adjustment of medication, for example changes from beta-blockers to angiotensin-converting-enzyme inhibitors in arterial hypertension treatment [1, 82, 83].

All treatment options for poor erection must be discussed with the patient. Always, psychological and psychosexual counselling should be offered to the patient and his partner [35, 83].

While PDE type-5 inhibitors are a first-line therapeutic option, contra-indications must be strictly considered. Intracavernosal injection therapy and vacuum constriction devices may be offered to patients unresponsive to PDE-5 inhibitors [1, 83].

Patients with high or indeterminate cardiovascular risk should refrain from sexual activity and thus ED treatment [1, 83].

References

1. Hilz MJ. Female and male sexual dysfunction. In: Low PA, Benarroch EE, editors. Clinical autonomic disorders. Lippincott Williams & Wilkins (LWW); 2008. p. 657–711.
2. NIH Consensus Conference. Impotence. NIH consensus development panel on impotence. JAMA. 1993;270:83–90.
3. McCabe MP, Sharlip ID, Atalla E, Balon R, Fisher AD, Laumann E, et al. Definitions of sexual dysfunctions in women and men: a consensus statement from the fourth international consultation on sexual medicine 2015. J Sex Med. 2016;13(2):135–43.
4. Feldman HA, Goldstein I, Hatzichristou DG, Krane RJ, McKinlay JB. Impotence and its medical and psychosocial correlates: results of the Massachusetts Male Aging Study. J Urol. 1994;151(1):54–61.
5. Kessler A, Sollie S, Challacombe B, Briggs K, Van Hemelrijck M. The global prevalence of erectile dysfunction: a review. BJU Int. 2019;124:587.
6. Shamloul R, Ghanem H. Erectile dysfunction. Lancet. 2013;381(9861):153–65.
7. Johannes CB, Araujo AB, Feldman HA, Derby CA, Kleinman KP, McKinlay JB. Incidence of erectile dysfunction in men 40 to 69 years old: longitudinal results from the Massachusetts male aging study. J Urol. 2000;163(2):460–3.
8. Lewis RW, Fugl-Meyer KS, Corona G, Hayes RD, Laumann EO, Moreira ED Jr, et al. Definitions/epidemiology/risk factors for sexual dysfunction. J Sex Med. 2010;7(4 Pt 2):1598–607.
9. Arnow BA, Desmond JE, Banner LL, Glover GH, Solomon A, Polan ML, et al. Brain activation and sexual arousal in healthy, heterosexual males. Brain. 2002;125(Pt 5):1014–23.
10. Beauregard M, Levesque J, Bourgouin P. Neural correlates of conscious self-regulation of emotion. J Neurosci. 2001;21(18):RC165.
11. Bocher M, Chisin R, Parag Y, Freedman N, Meir Weil Y, Lester H, et al. Cerebral activation associated with sexual arousal in response to a pornographic clip: a 15O-H2O PET study in heterosexual men. NeuroImage. 2001;14(1 Pt 1):105–17.
12. Hagemann JH, Berding G, Bergh S, Sleep DJ, Knapp WH, Jonas U, et al. Effects of visual sexual stimuli and apomorphine SL on cerebral activity in men with erectile dysfunction. Eur Urol. 2003;43(4):412–20.
13. Hamann S, Herman RA, Nolan CL, Wallen K. Men and women differ in amygdala response to visual sexual stimuli. Nat Neurosci. 2004;7(4):411–6.
14. Redoute J, Stoleru S, Pugeat M, Costes N, Lavenne F, Le Bars D, et al. Brain processing of visual sexual stimuli in treated and untreated hypogonadal patients. Psychoneuroendocrinology. 2005;30(5):461–82.
15. Ferretti A, Caulo M, Del Gratta C, Di Matteo R, Merla A, Montorsi F, et al. Dynamics of male sexual arousal: distinct components of brain activation revealed by fMRI. NeuroImage. 2005;26(4):1086–96.
16. Moulier V, Mouras H, Pelegrini-Issac M, Glutron D, Rouxel R, Grandjean B, et al. Neuroanatomical correlates of penile erection evoked by photographic stimuli in human males. NeuroImage. 2006;33(2):689–99.
17. Giuliano F, Rampin O. Neural control of erection. Physiol Behav. 2004;83(2):189–201.
18. Meisel RL, Sachs BD. The physiology of male sexual behaviour. In: Knobil E, Neill J, editors. The physiology of reproduction. 2nd ed. New York: Raven Press; 1994. p. 3–105.
19. Liu YC, Salamone JD, Sachs BD. Lesions in medial preoptic area and bed nucleus of stria terminalis: differential effects on copulatory behavior and noncontact erection in male rats. J Neurosci. 1997;17(13):5245–53.
20. Liu YC, Salamone JD, Sachs BD. Impaired sexual response after lesions of the paraventricular nucleus of the hypothalamus in male rats. Behav Neurosci. 1997;111(6):1361–7.
21. Giuliano F, Rampin O. Central neural regulation of penile erection. Neurosci Biobehav Rev. 2000;24(5):517–33.

22. Argiolas A, Melis MR, Mauri A, Gessa GL. Paraventricular nucleus lesion prevents yawning and penile erection induced by apomorphine and oxytocin but not by ACTH in rats. Brain Res. 1987;421(1–2):349–52.
23. Greco B, Edwards DA, Zumpe D, Clancy AN. Androgen receptor and mating-induced fos immunoreactivity are co-localized in limbic and midbrain neurons that project to the male rat medial preoptic area. Brain Res. 1998;781(1–2):15–24.
24. Kondo Y, Sachs BD, Sakuma Y. Importance of the medial amygdala in rat penile erection evoked by remote stimuli from estrous females. Behav Brain Res. 1998;91(1–2):215–22.
25. Marson L, Platt KB, McKenna KE. Central nervous system innervation of the penis as revealed by the transneuronal transport of pseudorabies virus. Neuroscience. 1993;55(1):263–80.
26. Sachs BD. The false organic-psychogenic distinction and related problems in the classification of erectile dysfunction. Int J Impot Res. 2003;15(1):72–8.
27. Wessells H, Gralnek D, Dorr R, Hruby VJ, Hadley ME, Levine N. Effect of an alpha-melanocyte stimulating hormone analog on penile erection and sexual desire in men with organic erectile dysfunction. Urology. 2000;56(4):641–6.
28. Comarr AE. Sexual function among patients with spinal cord injury. Semin Urol. 1992;10:74–82.
29. Junemann KP, Persson-Junemann C, Lue TF, Tanagho EA, Alken P. Neurophysiological aspects of penile erection: the role of the sympathetic nervous system. Br J Urol. 1989;64(1):84–92.
30. Neurophysiology BS. In: Kirby RS, Carlson CC, Webster GD, editors. Impotence: diagnosis and management of male erectile dysfunction. Oxford: Butterworth-Heinemann; 1991. p. 27–31.
31. Brackett NL, Bloch WE, Abae M. Neurological anatomy and physiology of sexual function. In: Singer C, Weiner WJ, editors. Sexual dysfunction: a neuro-medical approach. Armonk, NY: Futura Publishing Company, Inc.; 1994.
32. Baader B, Herrmann M. Topography of the pelvic autonomic nervous system and its potential impact on surgical intervention in the pelvis. Clin Anat. 2003;16(2):119–30.
33. Max J. Hilz et al., Disfunzione erettile in Micieli et al. "Disfunzioni Vegetative" © 2022 Il Pensiero Scientifico Editore.
34. Schmidt P, Jünemann KP. Physiologische Grundlagen der Erektion. In: Stief CG, Hartmann U, Höfner K, editors. Erektile dysfunktion, diagnostik und therapie. Berlin: Springer; 1997. p. 188–97.
35. Hilz MJ, Hecht M, Kölsch C. Erektile dysfunktion. Akt Neurol. 2000;27:1–12.
36. Singer C, Weiner WJ. Male sexual dysfunction. Neurologist. 1996;2:119–29.
37. Krane RJ, Goldstein I, Saenz de Tejada I. Impotence. N Engl J Med. 1989;321(24):1648–59.
38. Lue PF. Impotence after prostatectomy. Urol Clin North Am. 1990;40:1347–9.
39. Prieto D. Physiological regulation of penile arteries and veins. Int J Impot Res. 2008;20(1):17–29.
40. Andersson KE. Erectile physiological and pathophysiological pathways involved in erectile dysfunction. J Urol. 2003;170(2 Pt 2):S6–13; discussion S13–4.
41. Moncada S, Higgs EA. The discovery of nitric oxide and its role in vascular biology. Br J Pharmacol. 2006;147(Suppl 1):S193–201.
42. Saenz de Tejada I, Kim N, Lagan I, Krane RJ, Goldstein I. Regulation of adrenergic activity in penile corpus cavernosum. J Urol. 1989;142(4):1117–21.
43. Angulo J, Cuevas P, La Fuente JM, Pomerol JM, Ruiz-Castane E, Puigvert A, et al. Regulation of human penile smooth muscle tone by prostanoid receptors. Br J Pharmacol. 2002;136(1):23–30.
44. Kifor I, Williams GH, Vickers MA, Sullivan MP, Jodbert P, Dluhy RG. Tissue angiotensin II as a modulator of erectile function. I. Angiotensin peptide content, secretion and effects in the corpus cavernosum. J Urol. 1997;157(5):1920–5.
45. Finger WW, Lund M, Slagle MA. Medications that may contribute to sexual disorders. A guide to assessment and treatment in family practice. J Fam Pract. 1997;44(1):33–43.

46. Cirino G, Fusco F, Imbimbo C, Mirone V. Pharmacology of erectile dysfunction in man. Pharmacol Ther. 2006;111(2):400–23.
47. Rees PM, Fowler CJ, Maas CP. Sexual function in men and women with neurological disorders. Lancet. 2007;369(9560):512–25.
48. Calogero AE, Burgio G, Condorelli RA, Cannarella R, La Vignera S. Epidemiology and risk factors of lower urinary tract symptoms/benign prostatic hyperplasia and erectile dysfunction. Aging Male. 2019;22(1):12–9.
49. Rosenberg MT. Diagnosis and management of erectile dysfunction in the primary care setting. Int J Clin Pract. 2007;61(7):1198–208.
50. Montague DK, Jarow JP, Broderick GA, Dmochowski RR, Heaton JPW, Lue TF, et al. The management of erectile dysfunction: an update. Baltimore, MD: American Urological Association, Education and Research, Inc.; 2007.
51. Burnett AL, Nehra A, Breau RH, Culkin DJ, Faraday MM, Hakim LS, et al. Erectile dysfunction: AUA guideline. J Urol. 2018;200(3):633–41.
52. Beckman TJ, Abu-Lebdeh HS, Mynderse LA. Evaluation and medical management of erectile dysfunction. Mayo Clin Proc. 2006;81(3):385–90.
53. Nehra A, Jackson G, Miner M, Billups KL, Burnett AL, Buvat J, et al. The Princeton III consensus recommendations for the management of erectile dysfunction and cardiovascular disease. Mayo Clin Proc. 2012;87(8):766–78.
54. Jackson G, Rosen RC, Kloner RA, Kostis JB. The second Princeton consensus on sexual dysfunction and cardiac risk: new guidelines for sexual medicine. J Sex Med. 2006;3:28–36.
55. Kostis JB, Jackson G, Rosen R, Barrett-Connor E, Billups K, Burnett AL, et al. Sexual dysfunction and cardiac risk (the second Princeton consensus conference). Am J Cardiol. 2005;96(2):313–21.
56. Mikhail N. Management of erectile dysfunction by the primary care physician. Clev Clin J Med. 2006;72:293–311.
57. Jacobsohn K, Wang R. Evaluation and diagnostic testing of erectile dysfunction in the era of phosphodiesterase type 5 inhibitors. Asian J Androl. 2007;9(1):3–7.
58. Hatzichristou D, Rosen RC, Broderick G, Clayton A, Cuzin B, Derogatis L, et al. Clinical evaluation and management strategy for sexual dysfunction in men and women. J Sex Med. 2004;1(1):49–57.
59. Porst H. The rationale for prostaglandin E1 in erectile failure: a survey of worldwide experience. J Urol. 1996;155(3):802–15.
60. Aversa A, Isidori AM, Caprio M, Cerilli M, Frajese V, Fabbri A. Penile pharmacotesting in diagnosing male erectile dysfunction: evidence for lack of accuracy and specificity. Int J Androl. 2002;25(1):6–10.
61. Altinkilic B, Hauck EW, Weidner W. Evaluation of penile perfusion by color-coded duplex sonography in the management of erectile dysfunction. World J Urol. 2004;22(5):361–4.
62. Wilkins CJ, Sriprasad S, Sidhu PS. Colour Doppler ultrasound of the penis. Clin Radiol. 2003;58(7):514–23.
63. Wespes E, Amar E, Hatzichristou D, Hatzimouratidis K, Montorsi F, Pryor J, et al. EAU guidelines on erectile dysfunction: an update. Eur Urol. 2006;49(5):806–15.
64. Podnar S. Comparison of different outlier criteria in quantitative anal sphincter electromyography. Clin Neurophysiol. 2005;116(8):1840–5.
65. Vodusek DB. Anatomy and neurocontrol of the pelvic floor. Digestion. 2004;69(2):87–92.
66. Giladi N, Simon ES, Korczyn AD, Groozman GB, Orlov Y, Shabtai H, et al. Anal sphincter EMG does not distinguish between multiple system atrophy and Parkinson's disease. Muscle Nerve. 2000;23(5):731–4.
67. Lefaucheur JP. Neurophysiological testing in anorectal disorders. Muscle Nerve. 2006;33(3):324–33.
68. Brostrom S. Motor evoked potentials from the pelvic floor. Neurourol Urodyn. 2003;22:620–37.
69. Yarnitsky D, Sprecher E, Vardi Y. Penile thermal sensation. J Urol. 1996;156(2 Pt 1):391–3.

70. Lefaucheur JP, Yiou R, Salomon L, Chopin DK, Abbou CC. Assessment of penile small nerve fiber damage after transurethral resection of the prostate by measurement of penile thermal sensation. J Urol. 2000;164(4):1416–9.
71. Hecht MJ, Neundorfer B, Kiesewetter F, Hilz MJ. Neuropathy is a major contributing factor to diabetic erectile dysfunction. Neurol Res. 2001;23(6):651–4.
72. Hatzichristou DG, Hatzimouratidis K, Ioannides E, Yannakoyorgos K, Dimitriadis G, Kalinderis A. Nocturnal penile tumescence and rigidity monitoring in young potent volunteers: reproducibility, evaluation criteria and the effect of sexual intercourse. J Urol. 1998;159(6):1921–6.
73. Daitch JA, Lakin MM, Montague DK. Nocturnal penile tumescence monitoring. In: Mulcahy JJ, editor. Diagnosis and management of male sexual dysfunction. New York: Igaku-Shoin; 1997. p. 55–73.
74. Salonia A, Bettocchi C, Boeri L, Capogrosso P, Carvalho J, Cilesiz NC, et al. European Association of Urology guidelines on sexual and reproductive health-2021 update: male sexual dysfunction. Eur Urol. 2021;80(3):333–57.
75. Dhaliwal A, Gupta M. PDE5 inhibitors. Treasure Island, FL: StatPearls; 2022.
76. Uckert S, Hedlund P, Andersson KE, Truss MC, Jonas U, Stief CG. Update on phosphodiesterase (PDE) isoenzymes as pharmacologic targets in urology: present and future. Eur Urol. 2006;50(6):1194–207; discussion 207.
77. Avanafil for erectile dysfunction. Aust Prescr. 2019;42(3):113–4.
78. Vilke GM, Harrigan RA, Ufberg JW, Chan TC. Emergency evaluation and treatment of priapism. J Emerg Med. 2004;26(3):325–9.
79. Jankowski JT, Seftel AD, Strohl KP. Erectile dysfunction and sleep related disorders. J Urol. 2008;179(3):837–41.
80. Morice A, Unwin RJ, Sever PS. Vasoactive intestinal peptide causes bronchodilatation and protects against histamine-induced bronchoconstriction in asthmatic subjects. Lancet. 1983;2(8361):1225–7.
81. Kandeel FR, Koussa VK, Swerdloff RS. Male sexual function and its disorders: physiology, pathophysiology, clinical investigation, and treatment. Endocr Rev. 2001;22(3):342–88.
82. Sivalingam S, Hashim H, Schwaibold H. An overview of the diagnosis and treatment of erectile dysfunction. Drugs. 2006;66(18):2339–55.
83. McVary KT. Clinical practice. Erectile dysfunction. N Engl J Med. 2007;357(24):2472–81.

Chapter 15
Autonomic Control of Breathing in Health and Disease

Giuseppe Vita, Andrea Vianello, and Gian Luca Vita

The primary functions of the respiratory system are (1) to provide oxygen (O_2) from the external environment through alveolar ventilation; (2) to supply O_2 to the body's cells via the circulatory system; (3) to maintain acid-base balance; and (4) to remove carbon dioxide (CO_2) produced by cellular metabolism. A neural network, mainly the autonomic nervous system (ANS), plays a major role in generating the rhythmic activity of breathing, regulating airway smooth muscle tone and pulmonary blood flow through a composite interaction of respiration and circulation, and controlling secretions. This chapter discusses the complex anatomical and physiological aspects of respiration and describes both neurological diseases causing altered autonomic control of breathing and respiratory diseases characterised by impaired autonomic control of the airways.

G. Vita (✉)
Neurology, University of Messina, Messina, Italy

Unit of Neurology and Neuromuscular Diseases, Messina University Hospital, Messina, Italy
e-mail: giuseppe.vita@unime.it

A. Vianello
Department of Cardiac, Thoracic and Vascular Sciences, University of Padova, Padova, Italy
e-mail: andrea.vianello@aopd.veneto.it

G. L. Vita
Unit of Neurology, Department of Emergency, P.O. Piemonte, IRCCS Centro Neurolesi "Bonino-Pulejo", Messina, Italy
e-mail: gianluca.vita@irccsme.it

G. Micieli et al. (eds.), *Autonomic Disorders in Clinical Practice*,
https://doi.org/10.1007/978-3-031-43036-7_15

15.1 Brainstem Respiratory Control

Automatic breathing depends on the central pattern generator (CPG) which is located in the lower brainstem and includes functionally and neurochemically distinct cell groups. These rhythmogenic components drive neurons innervating cranial and spinal motor nuclei that control respiratory muscles. Respiratory rhythm generation is made up of three phases, that is active inspiration, post-inspiration (or stage 1 expiration), and passive expiration (or stage 2 expiration), which are under the control of three linked networks of brainstem neurons:

- The pre-Bötzinger complex (pre-BötC), located in the ventrolateral medulla, which drives inspiration. It provides glutamatergic inputs to all pontine and medullary premotor respiratory regions, with neurons expressing neurokinin-1 receptors (NK1R) and somatostatin. It has a relatively low threshold for rhythmicity and is less dependent on neuromodulatory input, reflecting both its role as the "master clock" for breathing-related behaviours and the paramount importance of the inspiratory phase in mammalian breathing.
- The post-inspiratory complex (PiCo) controlling post-inspiration, is located rostral to the pre-BötC. It contains neurons that are rhythmically active in phase with post-inspiration, and stimulation of these neurons resets the rhythm in vitro and in vivo. PiCo fulfils all criteria that define a rhythmogenic network or CPG. PiCo neurons (or at least a subset of them) have a glutamatergic, cholinergic transmitter phenotype. Cholinergic signalling seems to have primarily modulatory functions, whereas, like the pre-BötC, glutamatergic transmission is required for synchronisation of the network.
- The retrotrapezoid nucleus/parafacial respiratory group (RTN/pFRG), located rostral to the pre-BötC and ventral to the PiCo, controls active expiration and plays an important role in central and peripheral chemosensitivity. This region is subdivided into rhythmic lateral (pF_L) and non-rhythmic ventral (pF_V) areas. pFRG is silent at rest and becomes rhythmically active during the stimulation of peripheral chemoreceptors, which also activates adrenergic C1 cells, located in the rostral ventrolateral medulla. It contains glutamatergic neurons, expressing vesicular glutamate transporter (VGLUT2), NK1R, neuromedin B, and pituitary adenylate-cyclase-activating polypeptide (PACAP), and development depends on the transcription factor paired-like homeobox 2B (PHOX2B), a master gene of ANS development.

Organization of the breathing network is consistent with the idea that rhythmic activity emerges from interactions between three coupled oscillators, in which each phase, inspiration, post-inspiration, and active expiration, is generated within the medulla by its own dedicated microcircuit, referred to as the "triple oscillator hypothesis". The dynamic balance between recurrent synaptic excitation, inhibition, and intrinsic bursting properties, i.e., the "rhythmogenic triangle", may control synchronisation within each microcircuit. Mutually inhibitory interactions between the microcircuits may control the temporal sequence of the rhythm generated by the network (Fig. 15.1). This rhythmogenic triangle and multiple other groups of neurons in the brainstem participate in the regulation of respiratory function and other strictly connected and integrated circuits involved in arousal, wake-sleep cycle and cardiovascular function (Table 15.1). Other neural structures are under the developmental control of PHOX2B, such as the locus coeruleus (LC) in the pons, catecholaminergic neurons of the nucleus of the solitary tract (NTS), and the C1 groups in the medulla: all these neurons are also activated by hypercapnia, and participate in the respiratory reflex [1–3].

15.2 Chemosensitivity

Automatic breathing depends on inputs from arterial chemoreceptors, located in the carotid and aortic bodies, which provide information regarding O_2, CO_2, and pH levels in the blood, and central chemoreceptors in the brain, which respond to changes in the partial pressure of carbon dioxide ($PaCO_2$) in their immediate

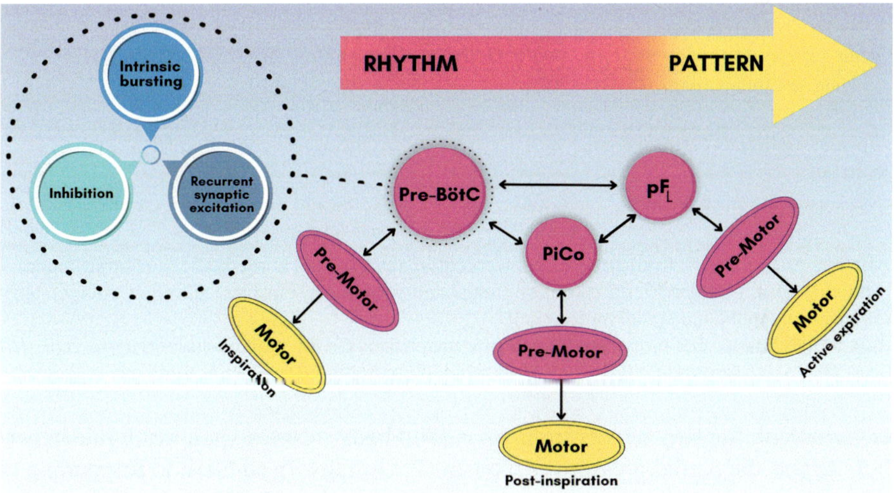

Fig. 15.1 Schematic representation of "triple oscillator hypothesis". According to the triple oscillator hypothesis, each breathing phase is generated by a dedicated microcircuit in the medulla: the pre-Bötzinger complex (pre-BötC) generates inspiration, the post-inspiratory complex (PiCo) generates post-inspiration, and the lateral parafacial region (pF_L) generates active expiration. Each oscillator is coupled by excitatory and inhibitory networks. As shown in the pre-BötC, rhythmicity within each microcircuit is controlled by a dynamic balance between recurrent synaptic excitation, inhibition, and intrinsic bursting properties, making up the rhythmogenic triangle. A gradient of rhythm (pink) and pattern (yellow) generating properties can be independent or interdependent depending on the connectivity between specific rhythm, premotor, and motor elements. The activity of rhythm- and pattern-generating elements can be differentially tuned by various modulatory inputs (i.e., descending synaptic drive from cortex and brainstem, chemo-mechano feedback, neuromodulation) to provide metabolic-, state-, and behaviour-dependent control to breathing

Table 15.1 Neurotransmitter and function of brainstem areas involved in the control of arousal, wake-sleep cycle, cardiovascular, and respiratory functions

Brainstem area	Neurotransmitter	Function
Periaqueductal gray	GABA	REM-off switch
Dorsal raphe nucleus	5-HT, NE	Wake-on, non-REM sleep
Pedunculopontine tegmental nucleus	ACh, L-Glu, GABA	Wake-on, REM-on, ⇧sympathetic, ⇧respiration
Locus coeruleus	NE	Wake-on, REM-off; ⇧sympathetic, ⇧respiration
Nucleus subcoeruleus	L-Glu, GABA	REM-on switch
Parabrachial nuclear complex (lateral)	L-Glu	Hypercapnic arousal, ⇧sympathetic; ⇧ventilation
Parabrachial nuclear complex (medial)	L-Glu	Maintenance of wakefulness
Retrotrapezoid nucleus	L-Glu	CO_2 chemosensitivity
Rostral ventrolateral medulla (incl. C1 area)	L-Glu, Epi	⇧Sympathetic (BP and HR); ⇧arousal and ⇧ventilation in response to hypoxia
Pre-Bötzinger complex	L-Glu	Inspirator pattern generator; promotes arousal
Medullary raphe nuclei (raphe pallidus and obscurus)	5-HT	Wake-on, REM-off, chemosensitivity, ⇧ventilation, airway dilation
Ventral respiratory column	L-Glu, GABA	Inspiratory or expiratory neurons
Nucleus ambiguus (pars compacta)	ACh	Airway control
Nucleus ambiguus (ventrolateral column)	ACh	Cardiovagal control of HR
Nucleus of the solitary tract	L-Glu	Relay and integration of cardiovascular and respiratory reflexes

Afferent circuits derive from arterial chemoreceptors (carotid and aortic bodies), central chemoreceptors (brain), and peripheral receptors (lungs and respiratory muscles). Efferent circuits carry impulses to cranial and spinal motor nuclei
ACh acetylcholine, *BP* blood pressure, *Epi* epinephrine, *GABA* gamma-aminobutyric acid, *HR* heart rate, *5-HT* serotonin, *L-Glu* L-glutamic acid, *NE* norepinephrine, *REM* rapid eye movement

environment. Sensory nerves from the carotid body increase their firing rate hyperbolically as the partial pressure of oxygen (PaO_2) falls. In addition to responding to hypoxia, the carotid body increases its activity linearly as $PaCO_2$ in arterial blood is raised. The carotid body communicates with medullary respiratory neurons through fibres that travel with the carotid sinus nerve, a branch of the glossopharyngeal nerve. Receptors in the respiratory muscles and in the lungs can also affect breathing patterns. These receptors are particularly important when lung function is impaired since they can help maintain tidal volume and ventilation at normal levels.

Hypoxia-activated neurons have also been identified in the pre-BötC, NTS, and C1 sympathoexcitatory areas. The main chemosensitive role of the brainstem depends on the activity of neurons that are intrinsically sensitive to changes in intracellular pH in response to increases in CO_2/hydrogen ions (H^+) levels. These chemosensitive neurons are widely distributed in the brainstem but the highest chemosensitive activity is observed in serotoninergic neurons of the medullary raphe (MR) and glutamatergic neurons of RTN. MR neurons may act as chemodetectors and modulators of the ventilatory response to CO_2 and as modulators of processing of hypoxia-sensitive carotid body afferents in the NTS. RTN neurons are activated by increased $PaCO_2$, via intrinsic proton receptors as well as paracrine signals from astrocytes. These neurons also receive input from peripheral chemoreceptors activated by hypoxia via a relay in the NTS. The lateral area of the hypothalamus contains CO_2/H^+ chemosensitive orexin neurons, and it has been reported that they contribute to the hypercapnic ventilatory response [3, 4].

15.3 Peripheral Pathways

Preganglionic parasympathetic vagal neurons projecting to neurons innervating the tracheal wall are located in the nucleus ambiguus of the medulla, and those of intrapulmonary airways are mainly located in the nucleus ambiguus but also, to a lesser extent, in the dorsal motor nucleus of the vagus nerve. Postganglionic cholinergic neurons induce bronchoconstriction via muscarinic receptors located on the surface of smooth muscle cells. Parasympathetic neurons also induce secretion from exocrine glands and secretory cells of the epithelium, and bronchial smooth muscle relaxation through inhibitory non-adrenergic non-cholinergic (NANC) transmission by nitric oxide (NO) and vasoactive intestinal peptide (VIP). These NANC neurons are located in the myenteric plexus of the oesophagus or are closely associated with the outer striated longitudinal muscle layers. Besides effects on smooth muscle, VIP and NO potently stimulate mucus secretion and are potent vasodilators. In conclusion, vagal innervation of the airways is involved in the cough reflex, mucous production, and control of bronchial diameter; the high incidence of postoperative pneumonia and pulmonary complications may be related to inadvertent transection of the pulmonary vagal nerves during an oesophagectomy [5, 6].

Sympathetic adrenergic nerves play little if any, role in directly regulating smooth muscle tone in the human airways, although they may control constriction of tracheobronchial blood vessels. Circulating noradrenaline induces bronchodilation through activation of β-adrenergic receptors in the airways. Cells bodies of sympathetic neurons are located in the intermediolateral and intercalate nuclei of the thoracic spinal cord. Their function is guided by the hypothalamus, brainstem, and reticular formation. Preganglionic sympathetic neurons project to postganglionic neurons which are located in paravertebral sympathetic chain ganglia (C6–T4). The upper thoracic ganglion is fused with the inferior cervical ganglion and forms the stellate ganglion. Postganglionic sympathetic neurons innervating the lung are derived from the stellate and the thoracic sympathetic chain ganglia T2–T4, whereas those supplying the trachea are derived from the stellate and the superior cervical ganglia. The preganglionic neurotransmitter for the sympathetic nervous system is acetylcholine, whereas the receptors on the postganglionic neurons are of the nicotinic type. The non-adrenergic subpopulation of sympathetic neurons contains VIP and NO [5, 6].

15.4 Interaction Between Respiration and Circulation

The autonomic network involved in breathing plays a major role in the interaction between respiration and circulation. There are three types of cardiorespiratory interactions: (1) respiratory sinus arrhythmia (RSA); (2) cardioventilatory coupling; (3) respiratory stroke volume synchronisation.

RSA, i.e., variability in heart rate (HR) according to the different phases of the respiratory cycle, by which the R–R interval on an ECG shortens during inspiration and extends during expiration, is one of the most studied mechanisms in the complex physiologic cardio-respiratory interactions. The central inspiratory drive inhibits vagal bradycardia, contributing to the increased HR observed during late inspiration. CPG not only drives phrenic nerve efferent activity (driving diaphragmatic inspiration) but also modulates central cardiac vagal outflow, causing rhythmic fluctuations in HR, whereby HR increases during inspiration [7]. The Kölliker-Fuse nucleus, a functionally distinct component of the parabrachial complex, located in the dorsolateral pons of mammals, is active during post-inspiration but is critical for the phasic, not tonic, activity of cardiac vagal motoneurons driving RSA [8]. Furthermore, peripheral feedback mechanisms also operate in RSA. Pulmonary stretch receptors (mechanoreceptors located in the bronchial smooth muscle) are increasingly activated with increasing lung volume, and it has been suggested that pulmonary stretch could, in humans, maintain almost half of the RSA amplitude. Moreover, systemic venous return to the right atrium increases on inspiration and activates atrial stretch receptors, which cause tachycardia and vasodilatation (Bainbridge reflex). However, it must be noted that this latter reflex is less prominent in humans compared to quadrupedal animals. In parallel with increased right atrial venous return, the pulmonary venous return to the left atrium is decreased, reducing left ventricular stroke volume and consequently arterial baroreceptor activity detected at the carotid sinus. This baroreflex response may also reduce vagal efferent activity that drives tachycardia during inspiration [7].

In the case of hypoxia, RSA attenuates. In a conscious dog, during progressive hypoxia lasting approximately 5 min, O_2 saturation of arterial blood decreased from 95% to 73%, and tidal volume and respiratory rate (RR) concomitantly increased from 240 to 800 mL, and from 18 to 24 breaths/min, respectively, while both HR and blood pressure (BP) were augmented [9]. These changes may provide compensatory responses against the threat of hypoxemia. When humans are exposed to acute and progressive hypoxia, the ability to maintain adequate oxygenation of vital organs is essential for survival. To increase oxygen uptake and transport, both ventilation and cardiac output need to increase. Moreover, as diastolic cardiac filling is a major limiting factor of cardiac output when HR is elevated, fluctuations in the heart period such as those with RSA would be disadvantageous for increasing cardiac output. A simultaneous surge in BP is convenient for the redistribution of the blood flow to vital organs. The sympathetic nervous system is mainly activated during peripheral chemo-stimulation with hypoxia, as suggested by the concomitant increase in both HR and BP [9].

Cardioventilatory coupling indicates synchronisation between heartbeat and the onset of inspiration. It is independent of RSA; however, a large RSA amplitude indicates a high degree of cardioventilatory coupling. Its function is mainly unknown, but it has been suggested that oxygen delivery efficiency is enhanced by matching ventilation and perfusion.

Respiratory stroke volume synchronisation is the inverse relationship between left and right cardiac stroke volumes during the respiratory cycle. During inspiration, intrathoracic pressure decreases, allowing air to be drawn into the lungs. At the same time, intra-abdominal pressure increases, and blood flow increases into the large veins in the thoracic cavity. This leads to increases in the filling of the right ventricle and consequently increases in right ventricular stroke volume during inspiration. However, the increased filling of the right ventricle will impede the filling of the left ventricle, as they share a septum and are both located within the pericardial sac. This means that an increase in right ventricular diastolic pressure will transmit to the left ventricle and decrease the filling rate in these low-pressure conditions. Reduced filling of the left ventricle together with a decrease in left cardiac stroke volume during inspiration has been documented. This reciprocal alteration in left cardiac stroke volume along with the respiratory-induced change in HR leads to a near constant cardiac output from the left side of the heart during all phases of the respiratory cycle [7].

In the last decade, the combined cardiovascular, respiratory, and neurophysiological effects of listening to music have been objects of great interest. HR and RR are higher in response to exciting music compared with tranquillising music. During musical frissons (involving shivers and piloerection), both HR and RR increase. Moreover, HR and RR tend to increase in response to music compared with silence, and HR appears to decrease in response to unpleasant music compared with pleasant music. The increase in HR, occurring when listening to exciting music, is associated with a reduction of HR variability (HRV). Music therapy is increasingly used to treat cardiovascular, respiratory, and neurological diseases [10–12]. It has been demonstrated that music induces similar physiological effects in different subjects, contrasting with the common conviction that music appreciation is personal and that cardiovascular reactions to music are secondary to emotional responses [13]. Listening to music increases interpersonal synchronisation on cardiovascular and respiratory rhythms, most likely influencing ANS both directly through the convergence of auditory and vegetative pathways at the level of the reticular formation and indirectly through various cortical and subcortical pathways. However, interpersonal synchronisation is not promoted by all types of music and with the same response. Music with a simpler structure results in greater autonomic group synchronisation, whereas music with a more complex loudness profile disrupts interpersonal synchronism even below the baseline level. Previous music training is not a crucial factor in the occurrence of interpersonal autonomic synchronisation during music listening. In fact, musicians and non-musicians show the same overall pattern of responses. These findings suggest that the use of simple rhythms and melodies during rituals and mass events may be based on the fact that this kind of music has the maximum potential to synchronise bodily rhythms across individuals, hence creating the biological soil for an elevated sense of togetherness [14].

15.5 Multiple System Atrophy

Pathogenetically, multiple system atrophy (MSA) is characterised by abnormal and progressive storage of insoluble aggregates of α-synuclein in neurons and glia. Such pathological features are shared with Parkinson's disease (PD) and dementia with Lewy bodies (DLB). All three diseases are included in the category of α-synucleinopathies. Although pathogenetic mechanisms leading to neurodegeneration are unknown, some experimental findings support the possibility that α-synuclein can propagate like a prion protein. The clinical features of MSA embrace four domains: autonomic dysfunction, levodopa-refractory parkinsonism, cerebellar ataxia, and corticospinal tract dysfunction. It incorporates several neurological entities, in the past believed distinct, such as olivopontocerebellar atrophy, Shy–Drager syndrome, and striatonigral degeneration [15].

Patients with MSA may develop sleep-related respiratory disorders such as obstructive sleep apnoea (OSA) in 15–37% of cases, less common central sleep apnoea (CSA), and stridor, which can all be clinical features that help distinguish MSA from PD and DLB. Neuronal loss in the brainstem nuclei, which modulate breathing and are critical for respiratory rhythmogenesis, is responsible for these disorders, but a combination of different factors may occur. Sudden death, often occurring during sleep, is believed due to either acute bilateral vocal cord adduction leading to asphyxiation and caused by sputum and food inhalation, or ventilatory failure of central origin due to acute dysfunction of brainstem cardiorespiratory drive. It is thought that the normal response to acute ventilatory impairment during sleep is blunted. Sudden death derives from failure to arouse and restart normal breathing, or instability due to autonomic failure. Loss of C1 neurons has been claimed not only to explain orthostatic hypotension but also reduce respiratory chemosensitivity and arousal responses to hypoxia. In this framework, scanty hemodynamic response to apnoea leads to hypotension and death. Moreover, hemodynamic instability caused by dysautonomia may also culminate in sudden death during sleep [16, 17]. Acute respiratory distress may occasionally arise early in MSA and represents a diagnostic challenge [18].

OSA, which can present very early in MSA, may develop because of irregularity in the breathing pattern, causing upper airway obstruction, intermittent hypoxemia, and sleep fragmentation [19]. When 24 patients with probable MSA were followed for a mean of 2.4 years, the first overnight polysomnography revealed OSA in all patients; 13% converted their sleep-disordered breathing from OSA to CSA, whereas 29% of patients had spontaneous improvement. Early development of snoring or stridor may predict rapid progression of impaired breathing in MSA [20].

CSA is characterised by a lack of drive to breathe during sleep, resulting in repetitive periods of hypoventilation and compromised gas exchange. Neurodegeneration of the nucleus ambiguus and the dorsal vagal motor nucleus in the medulla oblongata has been incriminated in the parasympathetic dysfunction in MSA [21]. Disruption of respiratory chemoreceptors, which play a key role in respiratory drive during non-rapid eye movement (NREM) sleep, contributes to CSA as it blunts brain response to $PaCO_2$ inhibiting respiratory drive. CSA, like OSA, may severely impact quality of life (QoL) and is associated with important complications, including frequent night-time awakenings, excessive daytime sleepiness and fatigue, and increased risk of adverse cardiovascular outcomes. Polysomnography (PSG) or video PSG is used to diagnose CSA and OSA.

Laryngeal stridor is very common, up to 70% in MSA patients, and can appear years before motor symptoms. Stridor has been defined as an abnormal, high-pitched, harsh respiration sound, mainly inspiratory, occurring only during sleep or during both sleep and wakefulness and caused by a laryngeal dysfunction leading to narrowing of the rima glottidis. It cannot be confused with regular snoring. Laryngoscopy may help in excluding mechanical lesions or functional vocal cord abnormality due to other neurologic conditions. A recent international conference reached consensus statements for the diagnosis, prognosis, and treatment of stridor in MSA [22]. Damaged brainstem respiratory nuclei and dysfunction of the bulbar and diaphragmatic muscles are associated with an increased risk for stridor. Patients with MSA develop stridor because of impaired vocal cord motion, such as vocal cord abduction/restriction, or paradoxical vocal cord adduction during inspiration [23]. Controversial results have been reported on the prognostic value of stridor, but early occurrence may contribute to shortened survival. The clinical diagnosis of stridor is challenging. The presence of a night-time witness is sometimes necessary as patients are often not aware of it. Video PSG with an audio recording may be very useful.

A tailored treatment of sleep breathing disorders has been suggested in MSA, by using fixed continuous positive airway pressure (CPAP) for isolated OSA or stridor, auto-adjusting CPAP for stridor combined with OSA, and adaptive servo-ventilation for CSA, isolated or in combination with OSA or stridor. Stridor and sleep apnoea disappear, compliance to treatment is good, and survival time increases [24, 25]. Tracheostomy is indicated in severe forms, although is not easily accepted by the patient as it may impair QoL. Like CPAP, tracheostomy may increase survival and reduce the risk of sudden death [17, 22]. A cooperative network of neurologists with pneumologists, otorhinolaryngologists, cardiologists, and experts on sleep medicine, dysphagia rehabilitation, and intensive care is required for the effective cure and care of patients with MSA.

15.6 Diabetes

The cardiovascular system, gastrointestinal tract, and genitourinary tract are involved in the disabling autonomic neuropathy occurring in patients with diabetes [26]. There is evidence supporting the view that diabetic dysautonomia also involves respiratory (chemoreflex) control mechanisms. Chemoreflexes respond acutely to intermittent hypoxia with an increase in sympathetic activity; the subsequent rise in BP initiates a compensatory baroreflex response that attempts to buffer these changes. This mechanism was originally described only for central apnoea, but it is now clear that ANS is highly involved in obstructive apnoea [27]. With chronic exposure to intermittent hypoxia, a sensitization of peripheral chemoreflex occurs. Conversely, the baroreflex may become desensitised: exposure to intermittent hypoxia resets the baroreflex to operate at higher levels of sympathetic activity and BP [28].

OSA is frequent in type 2 diabetic patients. Diabetes and OSA exert a bidirectional influence, with diabetes predisposing to or aggravating OSA, and OSA predisposing to or aggravating diabetes. Moreover, some studies suggest additive or synergistic effects for diabetic complications and a reciprocal enhancement in their impact on hypertension and cardiovascular disease. The presence and severity of OSA may be an additional risk factor for the development of microvascular complications. Intermittent hypoxemia leads to vasoconstriction and increased oxidative stress, resulting in endothelial dysfunction and microvascular impairment. There is also a relation between OSA severity and glucose metabolism alteration. A link between OSA and insulin resistance appears early, prior to impaired glucose tolerance and the onset of diabetes. Despite CPAP being the gold standard for treating patients with OSA, the effect of treatment with CPAP in patients with prediabetes or type 2 diabetes on markers of glucose metabolism has been conflicting. However, a few studies have reported a beneficial effect of CPAP on postprandial/nocturnal glycaemia as well as glycaemic variability. Other studies demonstrated a significant reduction in BP, likely due to a reduction in sympathetic activity. Decreased inflammatory markers, reduced sleepiness, improved QoL, and reduced health-care resource use are other favourable effects [29, 30].

OSA has not been reported to be a risk factor for the incidence of type 1 diabetes. However, in patients with type 1 diabetes, the prevalence of OSA is significantly higher than in the general population (46–52%). Autonomic neuropathy may compromise upper airway reflexes and control of the pharyngeal dilator muscles, predisposing these patients to obstructive events. Parasympathetic derangement in type 1 diabetes results from functional impairment, since it is corrected by oxygen administration, and hypoxia could be the cause [31]. Baseline oxygen saturation and baroreflex sensitivity were reduced whereas the hypercapnic chemoreflex was increased in a cohort of type 1 diabetic patients. The authors postulated that respiratory control alterations might result from a reduced response to hypoxia and lead to compensatory activation of hypercapnic chemoreflex and sympathetic activity. Respiratory control alterations might worsen both autonomic dysfunction and its consequences.

Since they might be functional, they might also be reversible, e.g. by physical activity, breathing control exercises, CPAP [32, 33].

Gestational diabetes mellitus (GDM) is a state of abnormal glucose tolerance typically diagnosed during the second or third trimester and is associated with adverse maternal and foetal outcomes. Several studies have observed an association between OSA and GDM (prevalence of OSA is 30–71% in women with GDM). Women with symptoms of OSA or a diagnosis of OSA have a three-fold increased risk of GDM, but it may be much higher when home PSG is used. The mechanisms underlying this association are likely similar to those linking OSA to type 2 diabetes in the non-pregnant population. In addition to GDM, OSA during pregnancy has been linked to adverse maternal and foetal outcomes, including pre-eclampsia, emergency caesarean-section, premature delivery, low birth weight, and admissions of the newborn to the intensive care unit. Endothelial dysfunction, increased oxidative stress, and sympathetic nervous system overactivity seen in OSA are likely partially responsible for this association. CPAP treatment is safe during pregnancy and is associated with a reduction in BP in a small study of women with hypertension and chronic snoring [30].

15.7 Epilepsy

Patients with epilepsy often have interictal autonomic dysfunction with decreased HRV. Moreover, epilepsy is frequently associated with ictal tachycardia or bradycardia which sometimes precedes the onset of seizures. These cardiac manifestations of seizures have been postulated as possible causes of sudden unexplained death in epilepsy (SUDEP). While sinus tachycardia is the most common cardiac finding during seizures, asystole and malignant tachyarrhythmias may also occur. Seizures can also lead to respiratory dysfunction, including central ictal and obstructive apnoea related to laryngospasm. Available data suggest that there could be underlying autonomic dysfunction, potentially related to genetic, medication, and other factors that might predispose individuals to sudden catastrophic cardiorespiratory dysfunction resulting in SUDEP [34].

Data from the MORTEMUS study, which analysed cardiorespiratory function at the time of death occurring after a convulsive seizure [35], along with data from non-seizure related SUDEP [36], show that tachycardia and tachypnoea precede bradypnoea and bradycardia followed by terminal apnoea and then asystole. These findings suggest that catastrophic autonomic dysregulation may occur due to severe brainstem dysfunction, leading to highly abnormal cardiorespiratory patterns.

Decreased HRV may also correlate with atrophy of specific brainstem regions involved in autonomic control in patients with focal epilepsy [37]. In the same study, a group of patients who subsequently died due to SUDEP had progressive atrophy of these brainstem regions in serial MRI scans prior to death, suggesting a possible link between structural and functional autonomic pathology. Further studies showed that age may affect the degree of sympathetic and parasympathetic activity following seizures [38]. Adults tend to have longer durations of postictal generalised EEG suppression (PGES), which correlate with the degree of sympathetic activation as measured by electrodermal activity. However, after checking for PGES duration, paediatric patients were found to have stronger sympathetic activation as well as greater parasympathetic suppression than adults. These age-dependent findings may correlate with the variable incidence of SUDEP seen in different age groups. Future multicentre studies may yield additional clues regarding the relationship between SUDEP and autonomic dysfunction, possible biomarkers for SUDEP, and effective preventative treatment.

15.8 Chronic Obstructive Pulmonary Disease

Lower HRV, depressed baroreceptor sensitivity, and higher muscle sympathetic nerve activity (MSNA), as an index of increased sympathetic excitation, have been described in patients with chronic obstructive pulmonary disease (COPD). Moreover, supplemental oxygen or the slowing of RR is able to decrease MSNA and enhance baroreceptor sensitivity in patients with COPD [39, 40]. Several studies have identified hypercapnia, physical activity level, muscle function, and circadian rhythm as the major influencing factors of autonomic function, but no definite conclusion could be reached for factors such as dyspnoea, hypoxemia, anxiety, body composition, pulmonary function, age, breathing frequency, ventilatory effort, QoL, and disease severity in COPD patients. No causal relationship was established for such an autonomic impairment, but in many studies, the use of long-acting β_2 agonists was uninterrupted on the day of investigation, and this may have had an effect on some autonomic parameters [41–44].

A possible explanation for the higher sympathetic tone found in patients with COPD is arterial chemoreflex activation. However, a study testing the effect of intermittent hypoxic training (IHT) in patients with mild COPD demonstrated the presence of cardiovascular autonomic abnormalities even if there were no chemoreflex abnormalities. After IHT, baroreflex sensitivity increased up to normal levels and hypercapnic ventilatory response increased as well without changes in hypoxic ventilatory response. However, this study supported the use of IHT as a therapeutic strategy to rebalance early autonomic dysfunction in COPD patients [45]. IHT refers to the discontinuous use of normobaric or hypobaric hypoxia, in an attempt to reproduce some of the key features of altitude acclimatisation, with the ultimate goal of improving sea-level athletic performance. There are two different strategies: (1) providing hypoxia at rest with the primary goal being to stimulate altitude acclimatisation or (2) providing hypoxia during exercise, with the primary goal being to enhance training stimulus.

Taken all together, these findings suggest sympathovagal imbalance as a pathophysiological phenomenon in COPD. Further investigations are needed to clarify this relationship and the therapeutic role of IHT [46].

15.9 Asthma

For more than two decades, literature has discussed the cardiovascular autonomic changes associated with either the pathophysiology of asthma per se or with asthma pharmacotherapy treatment. Adults with asthma have an increase in bronchial sensitivity to cholinergic constrictors and possibly a reduction in sensitivity to adrenergic β_2 bronchodilators. Also, NANC mediators contribute to the pathogenesis of asthma not only by regulating smooth muscle tone in the airways but also by affecting pulmonary blood flow, endothelial permeability, and airway secretions [47]. Moreover, several studies have suggested that the altered autonomic control of airway calibre in asthma might be reflected by a parallel change in HR. This is a controversial topic since some authors found evidence of an increased sympathetic tone and higher levels of circulating catecholamines, while others observed an excessive fall in systolic BP on standing and an excessive rise in diastolic BP in response to a sustained handgrip test, and still others increased cardiac vagal activity [48].

Two randomised controlled trials found that asthma symptoms and pulmonary function improved, and airway inflammation and medication use were reduced after 10 weeks of HRV biofeedback (HRVB) daily practice. HRVB is a non-pharmacological intervention used for its regulatory effects on autonomic cardiac regulation by increasing HRV and restoring cardiac vagal control [49]. IHT, used in COPD, could also be a valid treatment for asthma. Finally, recent evidence suggests that certain neurotransmitters/neuropeptides, including those involved in autonomic control of breathing, which play a role in the pathogenesis of asthma, may represent new therapeutic targets [50].

15.10 Congenital Central Hypoventilation Syndrome

Congenital central hypoventilation syndrome (CCHS; MIM# 209880) is a rare neurological disorder characterised by the deficient autonomic control of breathing, due to the malfunctioning of PHOX2B-mediated regulation of autonomic respiratory control and chemosensitivity. The hallmark of the disease is alveolar hypoventilation caused by a reduced or absent ventilatory response to hypoxia and hypercapnia [51]. CCHS has been reported for many years with the term Ondine's curse or syndrome. Ondine's curse is one of the most fascinating mythical tales in the field of medicine. The nymph Ondine was an immortal water spirit who became human after falling in love with a man, marrying him, and having a baby. In one of the versions of the tale, when she caught her husband sleeping with another woman, she cursed him to remain awake in order to control his own breathing. During the nineteenth century, the rare syndrome characterised by loss of autonomic breath control, while voluntary respiration remains intact, was named "Ondine's curse". Moreover, acquired Ondine syndrome has been reported due to bulbar poliomyelitis, brainstem trauma vascular disease or tumours, CSA, and other conditions [52].

CCHS generally presents in newborns, but late onset has been reported in childhood or even adulthood. The disease may also involve a spectrum of non-respiratory symptoms, such as seizures and other conditions reflecting a more global ANS dysfunction, including cardiac arrhythmias and congenital heart disease, ocular disorders (strabismus, pupillary abnormalities, convergence insufficiency), aganglionic megacolon Hirschsprung's disease and neural crest tumours. It is transmitted with an autosomal dominant trait with variable expressivity and incomplete penetrance. Different mutations of the *PHOX2B* gene have been reported, in-frame triplet duplications of different lengths are the most frequent but heterozygous missense, nonsense, and frameshift mutations have also been reported. The respiratory phenotype in CCHS is mainly due to developmental defects in brainstem RTN, a structure that integrates peripheral and central chemoreception, and that is missing in the Phox2b/+7 alanine knock-in mouse model of CCHS. Defects in other areas, such as LC, have been reported in post-mortem brains of CCHS patients. The variable phenotypes observed in CCHS individuals carrying the same mutation also suggest the involvement of modifier genes of expressivity [53].

Patients with CCHS usually have no overt clinical signs of hypoventilation, do not feel any sensation of dyspnoea, hypoxia, or hypercapnia, and do not increase RR or effort in response to hypoxia. The classical pattern is a reduction in the RR and in the amplitude of airflow and tidal volume. Alveolar hypoventilation with low or absent ventilatory responses to hypercapnia and hypoxia is more severe during NREM sleep than during wakefulness. Central apnoea can be observed. Neurocognitive deficits have been reported in CCHS children, with both primary developmental damage and chronic episodes of hypoxia contributing to the neurological phenotype.

Since CCHS can be lethal without adequate treatment, immediate tailored respiratory care is required, including CPAP, intubation, tracheostomy, mechanical ventilation, and intensive monitoring. Oxygen supplementation may produce variable results, sometimes increasing hypercapnia. CCHS commonly requires lifelong ventilatory support during sleep in all patients, but approximately one-third of them need continuous assisted respiration when awake. Full-time ventilatory-dependent patients may benefit from diaphragmatic pacing, an alternative mode of ventilation that affords mobility and a more normal lifestyle [51].

15.11 Familial Dysautonomia

Familial dysautonomia (Riley-Day syndrome), a rare debilitating genetic disorder present since birth, affects the development and survival of sensory, and autonomic neurons. Neuronal degeneration progresses throughout life. Affected individuals have impaired pain and temperature sensation, gait ataxia, absent deep reflexes, optic neuropathy, reduced tear production, gastrointestinal dysfunction with dysphagia, and frequent aspiration. Respiratory disorders include recurrent pneumonia leading to restrictive and obstructive lung disease, chemoreflex failure, and sleep-disordered breathing (noisy breathing, snoring, stridor, OSA, and CSA), to various degrees, which occur in almost all paediatric and adult patients. OSA events are more frequent in adults, whereas CSA events are more severe and frequent in children. They, together with blood pressure instability, lead to an increased risk of sudden death. In response to hypoxia, patients develop paradoxical hypoventilation, hypotension, bradycardia, and, which potentially, leads to death. Impaired ventilatory control due to chemoreflex failure acquires special relevance during sleep when conscious control of respiration withdraws. The disease is inherited in an autosomal recessive manner, due to a mutation in the IkB kinase-associated protein gene (*IKBKAP*). This produces a deficiency of the protein IKAP (ELP-1). Despite advances in clinical care and increased life expectancy, respiratory disease remains a significant cause of morbidity and mortality [54, 55].

Children with familial dysautonomia have been monitored during both day and night. Selective shortening of inspiratory time produced an overall increase in respiratory frequency with higher daytime respiratory variability versus controls, suggesting alterations in central rhythm-generating circuits that may contribute to the heightened risk for sudden death. Overall heart rate was increased, and variability was reduced. Time and frequency domain measures of autonomic tone indicated lower parasympathetic drive. These results suggest withdrawal of vagal, rather than sympathetic tone, as a cause for the sustained increase and dramatic lability in respiration and heart rates that characterise this disorder [56].

Recommendations for the evaluation of respiratory disorders in familial dysautonomia comprise clinical interview and examination, radiological evaluation by chest x-ray and CT, dysphagia evaluation, gastroesophageal reflux evaluation, sputum cultures, bronchoscopy, laryngoscopy, spirometry with quantitative measurements of peak cough flow, and home or in-laboratory PSG. Management of respiratory disorders includes prevention of aspiration, airway mucus clearance and chest physical therapy, home pulse oximetry, prevention and treatment of respiratory infections with vaccinations, special precautions during high altitude or airflight travel, empiric anti-acid reflux treatment, CPAP, nocturnal oxygen supplementation, and tracheostomy [54].

References

1. Benarroch EE. Brainstem integration of arousal, sleep, cardiovascular, and respiratory control. Neurology. 2018;91(21):958–66.
2. Ramirez JM, Baertsch N. Defining the rhythmogenic elements of mammalian breathing. Physiology (Bethesda). 2018;33(5):302–16.
3. Di Lascio S, Benfante R, Cardani S, Fornasari D. Research advances on therapeutic approaches to congenital central hypoventilation syndrome (CCHS). Front Neurosci. 2021;14:615666.
4. Benarroch EE. Brainstem respiratory control: substrates of respiratory failure of multiple system atrophy. Mov Disord. 2007;22(2):155–61.
5. van der Velden VH, Hulsmann AR. Autonomic innervation of human airways: structure, function, and pathophysiology in asthma. Neuroimmunomodulation. 1999;6(3):145–59.

6. Audrit KJ, Delventhal L, Aydin Ö, Nassenstein C. The nervous system of airways and its remodeling in inflammatory lung diseases. Cell Tissue Res. 2017;367(3):571–90.
7. Elstad M, O'Callaghan EL, Smith AJ, Ben-Tal A, Ramchandra R. Cardiorespiratory interactions in humans and animals: rhythms for life. Am J Physiol Heart Circ Physiol. 2018;315(1):H6–H17.
8. Farmer DG, Dutschmann M, Paton JF, Pickering AE, McAllen RM. Brainstem sources of cardiac vagal tone and respiratory sinus arrhythmia. J Physiol. 2016;594(24):7249–65.
9. Yasuma F, Hayano J. Respiratory sinus arrhythmia: why does the heartbeat synchronize with respiratory rhythm? Chest. 2004;125(2):683–90.
10. Koelsch S, Jäncke L. Music and the heart. Eur Heart J. 2015;36(44):3043–9.
11. Barnish J, Atkinson RA, Barran SM, Barnish MS. Potential benefit of singing for people with Parkinson's disease: a systematic review. J Parkinsons Dis. 2016;6(3):473–84.
12. Huang J, Yuan X, Zhang N, Qiu H, Chen X. Music therapy in adults with COPD. Respir Care. 2021;66(3):501–9.
13. Bernardi L, Porta C, Casucci G, Balsamo R, Bernardi NF, Fogari R, Sleight P. Dynamic interactions between musical, cardiovascular, and cerebral rhythms in humans. Circulation. 2009;119(25):3171–80.
14. Bernardi NF, Codrons E, di Leo R, Vandoni M, Cavallaro F, Vita G, Bernardi L. Increase in synchronization of autonomic rhythms between individuals when listening to music. Front Physiol. 2017;8:785.
15. Koga S, Dickson DW. Recent advances in neuropathology, biomarkers and therapeutic approach of multiple system atrophy. J Neurol Neurosurg Psychiatry. 2018;89(2):175–84.
16. Shimohata T, Aizawa N, Nakayama H, Taniguchi H, Ohshima Y, Okumura H, Takahashi T, Yokoseki A, Inoue M, Nishizawa M. Mechanisms and prevention of sudden death in multiple system atrophy. Parkinsonism Relat Disord. 2016;30:1–6.
17. Ralls F, Cutchen L. Respiratory and sleep-related complications of multiple system atrophy. Curr Opin Pulm Med. 2020;26(6):615–22.
18. Glass GA, Josephs KA, Ahlskog JE. Respiratory insufficiency as the primary presenting symptom of multiple-system atrophy. Arch Neurol. 2006;63(7):978–81.
19. Nakayama H, Hokari S, Ohshima Y, Matsuto T, Shimohata T. Breathing irregularity is independently associated with the severity of obstructive sleep apnea in patients with multiple system atrophy. J Clin Sleep Med. 2018;14(10):1661–7.
20. Ohshima Y, Nakayama H, Matsuyama N, Hokari S, Sakagami T, Sato T, Koya T, Takahashi T, Kikuchi T, Nishizawa M, Shimohata T. Natural course and potential prognostic factors for sleep-disordered breathing in multiple system atrophy. Sleep Med. 2017;34:13–7.
21. Suzuki M, Nakamura T, Hirayama M, Ueda M, Imai E, Harada Y, Katsuno M. Relationship between cardiac parasympathetic dysfunction and the anteroposterior diameter of the medulla oblongata in multiple system atrophy. Clin Auton Res. 2020;30(3):231–8.
22. Cortelli P, Calandra-Buonaura G, Benarroch EE, Giannini G, Iranzo A, Low PA, Martinelli P, Provini F, Quinn N, Tolosa E, Wenning GK, Abbruzzese G, Bower P, Alfonsi E, Ghorayeb I, Ozawa T, Pacchetti C, Pozzi NG, Vicini C, Antonini A, Bhatia KP, Bonavita J, Kaufmann H, Pellecchia MT, Pizzorni N, Schindler A, Tison F, Vignatelli L, Meissner WG. Stridor in multiple system atrophy: consensus statement on diagnosis, prognosis, and treatment. Neurology. 2019;93(14):630–9.
23. Warnecke T, Vogel A, Ahring S, Gruber D, Heinze HJ, Dziewas R, Ebersbach G, Gandor F. The shaking palsy of the larynx-potential biomarker for multiple system atrophy: a pilot study and literature review. Front Neurol. 2019;10:241.
24. Rekik S, Martin F, Dodet P, Redolfi S, Leu-Semenescu S, Corvol JC, Grabli D, Arnulf I. Stridor combined with other sleep breathing disorders in multiple system atrophy: a tailored treatment? Sleep Med. 2018;42:53–60.
25. Silvestri R. Sleep-disordered breathing in multiple system atrophy: pathophysiology and new insights for diagnosis and treatment. J Clin Sleep Med. 2018;14(10):1641–2.
26. Cernea S, Raz I. Management of diabetic neuropathy. Metabolism. 2021;123:154867.

27. Spicuzza L, Bernardi L, Calciati A, Di Maria GU. Autonomic modulation of heart rate during obstructive versus central apneas in patients with sleep-disordered breathing. Am J Respir Crit Care Med. 2003;167(6):902–10.
28. Freet CS, Stoner JF, Tang X. Baroreflex and chemoreflex controls of sympathetic activity following intermittent hypoxia. Auton Neurosci. 2013;174(1–2):8–14.
29. Greco C, Spallone V. Obstructive sleep apnoea syndrome and diabetes. Fortuitous association or interaction? Curr Diabetes Rev. 2015;12(2):129–55.
30. Reutrakul S, Mokhlesi B. Obstructive sleep apnea and diabetes: a state of the art review. Chest. 2017;152(5):1070–86.
31. Bernardi L, Rosengård-Bärlund M, Sandelin A, Mäkinen VP, Forsblom C, Groop PH, FinnDiane Study Group. Short-term oxygen administration restores blunted baroreflex sensitivity in patients with type 1 diabetes. Diabetologia. 2011;54(8):2164–73.
32. Bernardi L, Bianchi L. Integrated cardio-respiratory control: insight in diabetes. Curr Diab Rep. 2016;16(11):107.
33. Bianchi L, Porta C, Rinaldi A, Gazzaruso C, Fratino P, DeCata P, Protti P, Paltro R, Bernardi L. Integrated cardiovascular/respiratory control in type 1 diabetes evidences functional imbalance: possible role of hypoxia. Int J Cardiol. 2017;244:254–9.
34. Sevcencu C, Struijk JJ. Autonomic alterations and cardiac changes in epilepsy. Epilepsia. 2010;51(5):725–37.
35. Ryvlin P, Nashef L, Lhatoo SD, Bateman LM, Bird J, Bleasel A, Boon P, Crespel A, Dworetzky BA, Høgenhaven H, Lerche H, Maillard L, Malter MP, Marchal C, Murthy JM, Nitsche M, Pataraia E, Rabben T, Rheims S, Sadzot B, Schulze-Bonhage A, Seyal M, So EL, Spitz M, Szucs A, Tan M, Tao JX, Tomson T. Incidence and mechanisms of cardiorespiratory arrests in epilepsy monitoring units (MORTEMUS): a retrospective study. Lancet Neurol. 2013;12(10):966–77.
36. Lhatoo SD, Nei M, Raghavan M, Sperling M, Zonjy B, Lacuey N, Devinsky O. Nonseizure SUDEP: sudden unexpected death in epilepsy without preceding epileptic seizures. Epilepsia. 2016;57(7):1161–8.
37. Mueller SG, Nei M, Bateman LM, Knowlton R, Laxer KD, Friedman D, Devinsky O, Goldman AM. Brainstem network disruption: a pathway to sudden unexplained death in epilepsy? Hum Brain Mapp. 2018;39(12):4820–30.
38. Barot N, Nei M. Autonomic aspects of sudden unexpected death in epilepsy (SUDEP). Clin Auton Res. 2019;29(2):151–60.
39. Heindl S, Lehnert M, Criée CP, Hasenfuss G, Andreas S. Marked sympathetic activation in patients with chronic respiratory failure. Am J Respir Crit Care Med. 2001;164(4):597–601.
40. Raupach T, Bahr F, Herrmann P, Luethje L, Heusser K, Hasenfuss G, Bernardi L, Andreas S. Slow breathing reduces sympathoexcitation in COPD. Eur Respir J. 2008;32(2):387–92.
41. Camillo CA, Pitta F, Possani HV, Barbosa MV, Marques DS, Cavalheri V, Probst VS, Brunetto AF. Heart rate variability and disease characteristics in patients with COPD. Lung. 2008;186(6):393–401.
42. van Gestel AJ, Kohler M, Steier J, Teschler S, Russi EW, Teschler H. Cardiac autonomic dysfunction and health-related quality of life in patients with chronic obstructive pulmonary disease. Respirology. 2011;16(6):939–46.
43. Mohammed J, Meeus M, Derom E, Da Silva H, Calders P. Evidence for autonomic function and its influencing factors in subjects with COPD: a systematic review. Respir Care. 2015;60(12):1841–51.
44. Rasheedy D, Taha HM. Cardiac autonomic neuropathy: the hidden cardiovascular comorbidity in elderly patients with chronic obstructive pulmonary disease attending primary care settings. Geriatr Gerontol Int. 2016;16(3):329–35.
45. Haider T, Casucci G, Linser T, Faulhaber M, Gatterer H, Ott G, Linser A, Ehrenburg I, Tkatchouk E, Burtscher M, Bernardi L. Interval hypoxic training improves autonomic cardiovascular and respiratory control in patients with mild chronic obstructive pulmonary disease. J Hypertens. 2009;27(8):1648–54.

46. Vogtel M, Michels A. Role of intermittent hypoxia in the treatment of bronchial asthma and chronic obstructive pulmonary disease. Curr Opin Allergy Clin Immunol. 2010;10(3):206–13.
47. Jartti T. Asthma, asthma medication and autonomic nervous system dysfunction. Clin Physiol. 2001;21(2):260–9.
48. Lewis MJ, Short AL, Lewis KE. Autonomic nervous system control of the cardiovascular and respiratory systems in asthma. Respir Med. 2006;100(10):1688–705.
49. Fournié C, Chouchou F, Dalleau G, Caderby T, Cabrera Q, Verkindt C. Heart rate variability biofeedback in chronic disease management: a systematic review. Complement Ther Med. 2021;60:102750.
50. Pavón-Romero GF, Serrano-Pérez NH, García-Sánchez L, Ramírez-Jiménez F, Terán LM. Neuroimmune pathophysiology in asthma. Front Cell Dev Biol. 2021;9:663535.
51. Trang H, Samuels M, Ceccherini I, Frerick M, Garcia-Teresa MA, Peters J, Schoeber J, Migdal M, Markstrom A, Ottonello G, Piumelli R, Estevao MH, Senecic-Cala I, Gnidovec-Strazisar B, Pfleger A, Porto-Abal R, Katz-Salamon M. Guidelines for diagnosis and management of congenital central hypoventilation syndrome. Orphanet J Rare Dis. 2020;15(1):252.
52. Demartini Z, Maranha Gatto LA, Koppe GL, Francisco AN, Guerios EE. Ondine's curse: myth meets reality. Sleep Med X. 2020;2:100012.
53. Di Lascio S, Benfante R, Cardani S, Fornasari D. Advances in the molecular biology and pathogenesis of congenital central hypoventilation syndrome—implications for new therapeutic targets. Exp Opin Orphan Drugs. 2018;6:719–31.
54. Kazachkov M, Palma JA, Norcliffe-Kaufmann L, Bar-Aluma BE, Spalink CL, Barnes EP, Amoroso NE, Balou SM, Bess S, Chopra A, Condos R, Efrati O, Fitzgerald K, Fridman D, Goldenberg RM, Goldhaber A, Kaufman DA, Kothare SV, Levine J, Levy J, Lubinsky AS, Maayan C, Moy LC, Rivera PJ, Rodriguez AJ, Sokol G, Sloane MF, Tan T, Kaufmann H. Respiratory care in familial dysautonomia: systematic review and expert consensus recommendations. Respir Med. 2018;141:37–46.
55. Palma JA, Gileles-Hillel A, Norcliffe-Kaufmann L, Kaufmann H. Chemoreflex failure and sleep-disordered breathing in familial dysautonomia: implications for sudden death during sleep. Auton Neurosci. 2019;218:10–5.
56. Carroll MS, Kenny AS, Patwari PP, Ramirez JM, Weese-Mayer DE. Respiratory and cardiovascular indicators of autonomic nervous system dysregulation in familial dysautonomia. Pediatr Pulmonol. 2012;47(7):682–91.

Chapter 16
Neuropathic Pain

Camilla Rocchi, Massimiliano Valeriani, and Rita Di Leo

16.1 Introduction

Neuropathic pain is one of the most frequent symptoms in neurological clinical practice. It is caused by a lesion or disease of the somatosensory nervous system. The neurologist often deals with neuropathic pain conditions associated with diseases such as diabetic peripheral neuropathy, which is the most frequent cause of neuropathic pain, non-diabetic neuropathies, post-herpetic neuralgia, craniofacial pain, radiculopathies, traumatic nerve lesions, central post-stroke pain, spinal cord injuries and multiple sclerosis [1].

16.2 Pathophysiology

Neuropathic pain is often classified as central or peripheral depending on the site of injury causing the pain. However, it can be considered as a manifestation of different processes in the central and peripheral nervous system that cause sensitisation of both systems (Fig. 16.1). Central sensitisation refers to the increased arousal and reduced inhibition of central nervous system pathways that are associated with neuropathic

C. Rocchi (✉)
Neurology Unit, Policlinico Tor Vergata, Rome, Italy
e-mail: camilla.rocchi@ptvonline.it

M. Valeriani
Department of Neuroscience, Pediatric Hospital Bambino Gesù, IRCCS, Rome, Italy
e-mail: massimiliano.valeriani@opbg.net

R. Di Leo
Neurology Unit, San Giovanni e Paolo Hospital, Venice, Italy
e-mail: rita.dileo@aulss3.veneto.it

G. Micieli et al. (eds.), *Autonomic Disorders in Clinical Practice*,
https://doi.org/10.1007/978-3-031-43036-7_16

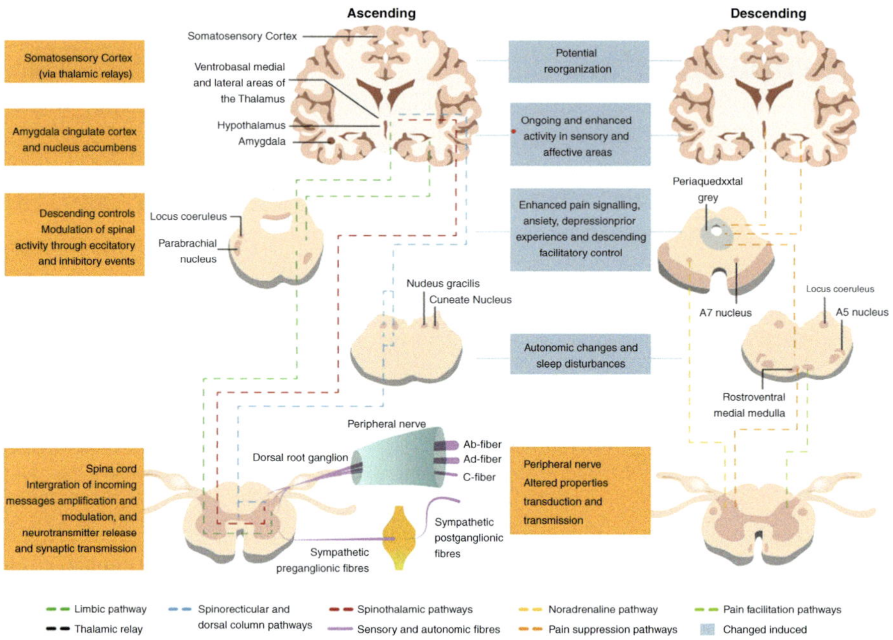

Fig. 16.1 Central and peripheral sensitisation

pain. Repeated input from C-fibres results in increased excitability of the spinal cord. In addition, lesions at the level of the central nervous system can alter sensory processing. At the level of the peripheral nervous system, ectopic neuronal activity has been reported at the level of primary afferents and the dorsal root ganglion, which appears to be mainly related to dysregulation of the synthesis or functioning of sodium channels (mainly tetrodotoxin-resistant channels), although it appears that potassium channels may be involved. The role of the sodium channel Nav1.7 has received particular interest, as mutations in the SCN9A gene encoding this channel cause both congenital insensitivity to pain and erythromelalgia. Evidence is mixed regarding the role of other SCN9A sequence variants [2]. Blocking axon potentials with sodium channel blockers has been the action for which some anti-epileptic drugs such as carbamazepine and oxcarbazepine are used in neuropathic pain. On the other hand, the α2δ1 subunit of N-type calcium channels on C-fibres in the superficial dorsal horn of the spinal cord is the mechanical target of gabapentinoids. γ-aminobutyric acid (GABA) is involved in neuropathic pain, but GABA and GABA transporter antagonist drugs have not shown efficacy in neuropathic pain [3]. Peripheral nerve injury also induces overexpression of several receptor proteins, including the vanilloid receptor (TRPV1), a membrane receptor activated by temperatures >42 °C and capsaicin, which is found on subtypes of peripheral nociceptive endings and is physiologically activated by noxious heat. After nerve injury, TRPV1 is overexpressed in C-fibres and hypo-expressed in injured nerve fibres. Other causes of peripheral sensitisation include increased reactivity to inflammatory mediators released by injured cells and sprouting of sympathetic neurons in the dorsal root ganglion [4].

16.3 Diagnosis

The diagnosis of neuropathic pain requires clinical and instrumental assessment as a single symptom or diagnostic test is not always sufficient to identify neuropathic pain. In fact, in most patients with neuropathic pain, different types of pain may coexist. This makes a careful history and neurological physical examination extremely important in patients being evaluated for neuropathic pain. Neuropathic pain is defined as pain caused by a lesion or disease of the somatosensory nervous system [5]. The neuropathic pain interest group (NeuPSIG) of the International Association for the Study of Pain (IASP) has proposed a grading system, according to which the presence of signs or symptoms alone is not sufficient for the definitive diagnosis of neuropathic pain, which requires confirmatory instrumental examinations [6]. In cases of chronic neuropathic pain, it is important to include the evaluation of psychological comorbidities, sleep disturbances, problems related to work or personal life, and expectations regarding therapy. Occasionally, conditions such as anxiety or depression may cause exaggerated responses to pain (or change the perception of pain itself) [3]. In general, the intensity, quality, duration, location of symptoms, and distribution of pain should be established. A complete neurological examination can often establish the metameric or non-metameric distribution of pain, the site of injury, and the quality of neuropathic pain. The examiner should first apply sensory stimuli to an unaffected area and then to the area affected by the pain. Patients should be instructed to state whether the second stimulus was the same as the first, and if not, whether it was more or less intense and whether the type and intensity of pain changed. The different sensory modalities that should be tested include pinprick, touch, temperature, vibration, and proprioception. Pinprick, light touch, and temperature sensations are carried by small myelin and unmyelinated fibres and ascend the spinothalamic pathway. Vibratory sensitivity and proprioception are transported by large myelin fibres and ascend in the dorsal columns [2, 7].

16.4 Neuropathic Pain Screening

16.4.1 Self-Assessment Scales

- Numerical rating scale—NRS [8, 9]

- It is a one-dimensional quantitative 11-point pain rating scale; the scale requires the operator to ask the subject to select the number that best describes the intensity of his or her pain, from 0 to 10, at that precise moment.
- VAS (visual analogue scale) [10]
- It is the visual representation of the magnitude of pain that the subject subjectively feels. The SEA is represented by a line 10 cm long in the original validated version. One end indicates the absence of pain and corresponds to 0, the other

end indicates the worst pain imaginable and corresponds to 10. The scale is filled in manually by the patient who is asked to draw a mark on the line representing the perceived pain.

- Verbal rating scale—VRS [11]
- It is based on the subject's choice of six verbal descriptive indicators of pain (no pain—very mild pain—mild pain—moderate pain—severe pain—very severe pain). The patient defines pain verbally, using the adjective they consider most appropriate out of a proposed set.

16.4.2 Instrumental Examinations for the Diagnosis of Neuropathic Pain

For the definitive diagnosis of neuropathic pain, instrumental examinations must document the presence of lesion or disease of the somatosensory system' [5].

Although it is an examination that provides subjective data and although it can be considered as an extension of the neurological objective examination, the Quantitative Sensory Testing (QST) should be mentioned first. This is an in-depth study of the various modalities of somatosensory sensitivity using a number of instruments, such as Von Frey filaments for mechanical somatosensory sensitivity or a thermode for thermal and thermo-dural somatosensory sensitivity. The QST allows an extremely precise definition of the patient's pain characteristics and somatosensory abilities, which is often sufficient to arrive at a diagnosis. The main limitations are that such a detailed study takes quite a long time and, above all, requires the cooperation of the patient [12].

A major role in the diagnosis of neuropathic pain is played by neurophysiological techniques. Among these, those that can be defined as 'standard methods' should first be considered: nerve conduction velocity study, somatosensory evoked potentials, and trigeminal reflexes. Based on electrical stimulation of large-calibre myelin fibres (A beta), these techniques provide information on the function of the non-nociceptive somatosensory system. Currently, neurophysiological techniques are also available for the selective study of the nociceptive somatosensory system: laser-evoked potentials (LEPs) and caloric contact stimulation-evoked potentials (CHEPs). With regard to LEPs, these responses are evoked by a radiant caloric stimulus delivered via a laser beam. The most commonly used laser stimulators in clinical practice are the CO_2 and neodymium (YAP) lasers. Laser stimuli cause a heating of the superficial layers of the epidermis, which selectively stimulates the free endings of nociceptors, while the non-nociceptive receptors, located deeper down, are not activated. When the intensity of the laser stimulus is above the pain threshold, the subject experiences a painful but tolerable stinging sensation. Although it has been demonstrated using microneurography that at this intensity small myelin fibres (A delta) and unmyelinated fibres (C) are activated, the responses evoked at the scalp level are generated exclusively by the A delta input [13]. If, on the other hand, the intensity of the laser stimulus is kept below the pain threshold, so that the subject only perceives a sensation of diffuse heat, only the thermoreceptors and their amyelin afferents (C) are activated. The potentials evoked with this type of stimulation are therefore generated by the C input. It must be emphasised, however, that due to the low skin density of C thermoreceptors, LEPs from C fibres can only be reliably obtained by stimulating the face or midline, whereas, unfortunately, normative values have not been obtained by stimulating the limbs [14]. Another neurophysiological technique that allows the selective assessment of nociceptive afferents is CHEPs. In this case, skin heating is obtained by contact with a thermode. The possibility of studying A-delta fibres with CHEPs is substantially superimposed on that with LEPs, however, it is not possible to record evoked potentials from C-fibres. Stimulation with thermode has the advantage that it does not cause any burns on the skin, whereas laser stimuli can leave an erythema on the skin, which, however, resolves in 24–48 h. Among the neurophysiological techniques for studying nociceptive afferents, mention should be made of microneurography, which, however, requires considerable expertise and has an almost exclusive application in the field of research.

The diagnostic technique that is considered the 'gold standard' for diagnosing small somatosensory fibres disease is the punch skin biopsy study. By means of a punch biopsy, the reduction of intraepidermal C-fibres can be assessed. This method can provide information on both thermo-painful and vegetative somatosensory afferents [15].

Finally, when faced with a patient in whom there is a suspicion of neuropathic pain, the possibility of demonstrating the presence of a lesion or disease of the somatosensory system by means of MRI should be considered, which is particularly useful in the case of compression of peripheral or central nerve structures.

16.5 Symptoms

Typically, neuropathic pain has both positive and negative sensory symptoms and signs (Fig. 16.2) [1]. Positive symptoms are assumed to represent excessive activity in a sensory pathway caused by a lower threshold or high excitability. Negative signs and symptoms are experienced as decreased or absent sensation and are due to a loss of sensory function.

16.5.1 Positive Symptoms

Tingling (pins and needles)
Sudden or stabbing
Pulling or tightening
Burning

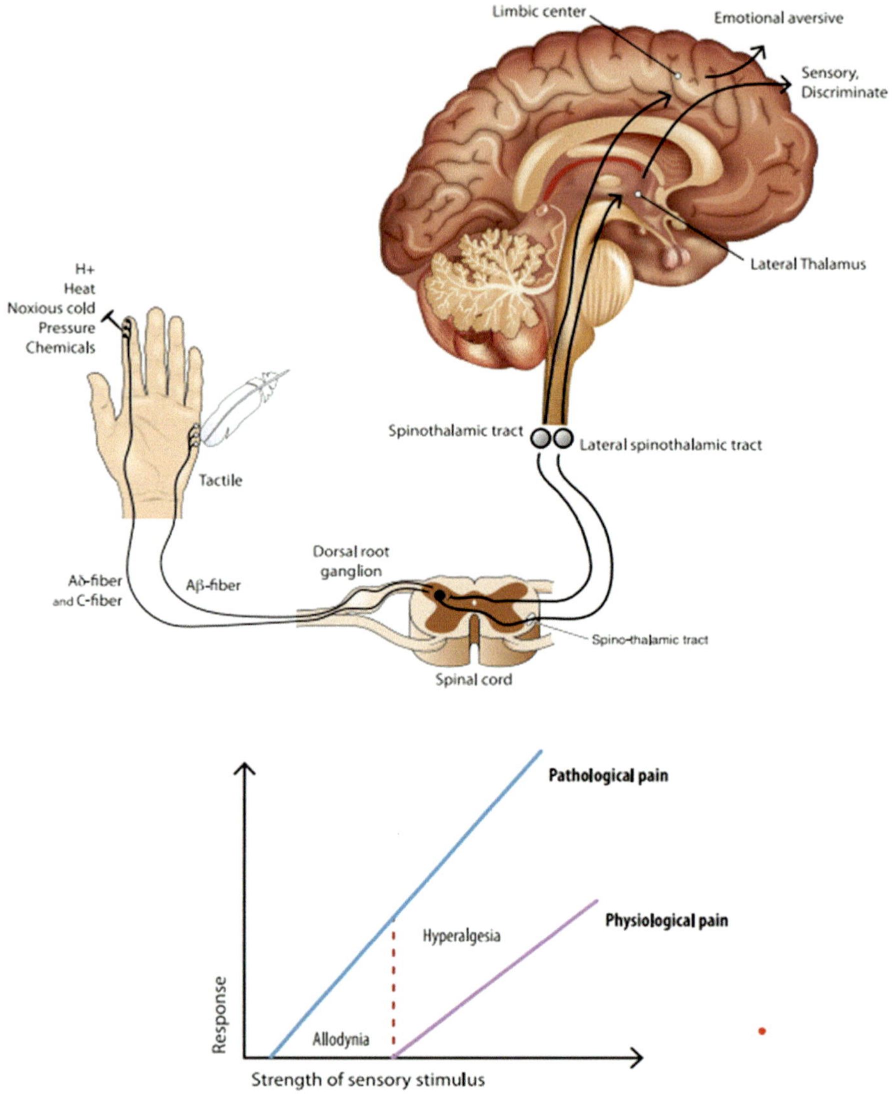

Fig. 16.2 Anatomical-functional correlates of pain responses

Prickling
Electric shock-like

16.5.2 Negative Symptoms

Numbness
Sensory loss
Feeling of wearing socks or gloves all the time

Neuropathic pain is characterised by peculiar clinical aspects that can be revealed by objective examination and includes:

- Paresthesia: an abnormal sensation, (typically spontaneous, may be provoked)
- Hyperesthesia: increased sensitivity to a stimulation
- Hyperalgesia: increased response to a painful stimulus
- Allodynia: painful response to a nonpainful stimulus
- Hypoesthesia: reduced sensitivity to stimulation
- Hypoalgesia: reduction of pain in response to a painful stimulus
- Analgesia: loss of pain sensation
- Anaesthesia: loss of sensation

16.6 Classification of Neuropathic Pain

Neuropathic pain is traditionally classified according to the underlying pathology. In the new ICD11 classification [6] neuropathic pain is primarily organised into peripheral and central neuropathic pain according to the location of the lesion or disease in the peripheral or central somatosensory nervous system (Fig. 16.3).

16.6.1 Chronic Peripheral Neuropathic Pain (Table 16.1)

Chronic peripheral neuropathic pain is caused by an injury or disease of the peripheral somatosensory nervous system.

16.6.1.1 Trigeminal Neuralgia

Trigeminal neuralgia is a manifestation of orofacial neuropathic pain limited to one or more branches of the trigeminal nerve. The pain is recurrent, arises and regresses paroxysmally, and is triggered by innocuous stimuli (such as chewing or talking). It is typically likened to an electric shock or described as a stab wound. Some patients

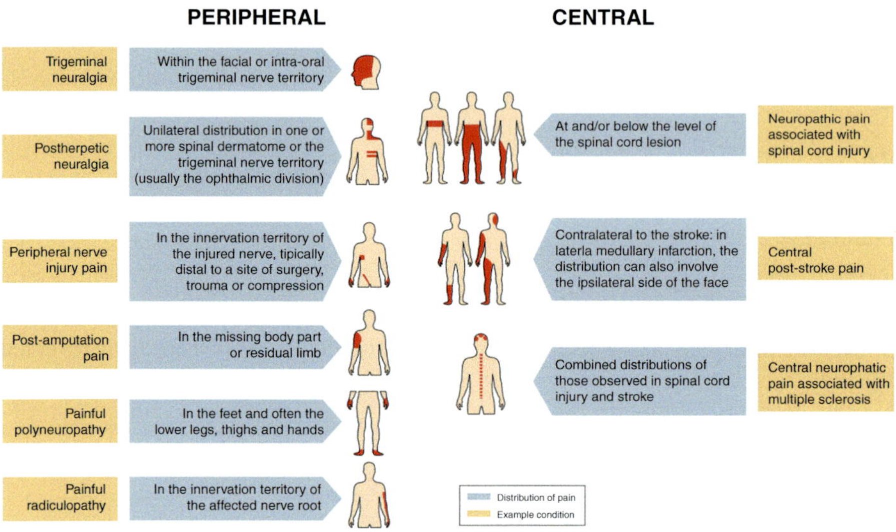

Fig. 16.3 Peripheral and central neuropathic pain

Table 16.1 Causes of chronic peripheral neuropathic pain

Diabetic polyneuropathy, painful diabetic neuropathy, diabetic amyotrophy
Polyneuropathy associated with monoclonal gammopathy
Chemotherapy-induced polyneuropathy (taxanes, oxaliplatin, vincristine, thalidomide, bortezomib)
Idiopathic small-fibre polyneuropathy
Post-herpetic neuralgia
Trigeminal neuralgia
Neuropathy associated with metabolic syndrome
Human immunodeficiency virus (HIV)-associated polyneuropathy
Hereditary sensory and autonomic neuropathies
Polyneuropathy associated with Sjögren's syndrome
Pyridoxine toxicity (vitamin B6)
Radiculopathies
Inflammatory neuropathies (acute and chronic inflammatory demyelinating polyneuropathy)
Post-traumatic neuropathy
Coeliac neuropathy
Alcoholic and other toxic neuropathies
Immunoglobulin light chain and hereditary amyloidotic neuropathies
Neuropathies from nutritional deficiencies
Complex regional pain syndrome
Phantom limb pain

experience continuous pain between these painful paroxysmal episodes. Diagnosis includes idiopathic trigeminal neuralgia, neuralgia produced by vascular compression of the trigeminal nerve, and secondary neuralgia caused by a tumour or cyst in the pontocerebellar angle or multiple sclerosis [16].

16.6.1.2 Chronic Neuropathic Pain After Peripheral Nerve Injury

Chronic neuropathic pain after peripheral nerve injury is persistent or recurrent neuropathic pain caused by a peripheral nerve injury. A history of plausible nerve injury with a temporal relationship between the onset of pain and the injury and the distribution of pain in the innervation territory of a peripheral nerve is required for diagnosis. The formation of a neuroma can cause pain at the site of injury [3].

16.6.1.3 Post-herpetic Neuralgia

Post-herpetic neuralgia is defined as pain that persists for ≥3 months after the onset or recovery of herpes zoster. The innervation territory of the first branch (ophthalmic branch) of the trigeminal nerve and the thoracic dermatomes are the sites most frequently affected by chronic post-herpetic pain. Post-herpetic neuralgia may present in continuity with the acute pain associated with the rash or develop after a pain-free interval. Negative and positive sensory symptoms or signs must be compatible with the innervation territory of the affected cranial nerve or peripheral dermatomes [3].

16.6.1.4 Painful Polyneuropathy

Chronic pain occurs in polyneuropathies caused by metabolic, autoimmune, familial, or infectious diseases, secondary to environmental or occupational toxin exposure, or treatment with a neurotoxic drug. Chronic pain also occurs in polyneuropathies of unknown aetiology. Pain may be the initial symptom of a neuropathy or develop in the course of the disease. Negative and positive sensory symptoms must be compatible with the anatomical distribution pattern of the polyneuropathy [3].

16.6.1.5 Painful Radiculopathy

Chronic painful radiculopathy is persistent or recurrent pain caused by an injury or disease involving the cervical, thoracic, lumbar, or sacral nerve roots. The most frequent causes are degenerative changes in the spinal column, including ligaments and intervertebral discs. Painful radiculopathy may also result from trauma, neoplastic meningitis, infection, ischemic or hemorrhagic injury, or iatrogenic injury, for example during injection therapy or surgery. Pain may be spontaneous, but is typically exacerbated or provoked by assuming or maintaining a certain body position or during movement. Negative or positive sensory symptoms must be compatible with the innervation territory of the nerve root(s) affected [3].

16.6.2 *Central Chronic Neuropathic Pain (Table 16.2)*

16.6.2.1 Chronic Neuropathic Pain Associated with a Spinal Cord Injury

Chronic neuropathic pain associated with a spinal cord injury is caused by a lesion or disease of the somatosensory pathways in the spinal cord. Pain may be spontaneous or evoked, as an increased response to a painful stimulus (hyperalgesia) or a painful response to a normally non-painful stimulus (allodynia). Diagnosis requires a history of spinal cord injury or disease and a plausible neuroanatomical distribution of pain, i.e. pain must be felt either in the dermatomes at or below the level of the lesion in the areas affected by sensory disturbances [6].

16.6.2.2 Chronic Central Neuropathic Pain Associated with Brain Injury

Chronic central neuropathic pain associated with brain injury is caused by a lesion or disease of the somatosensory cortex or brain regions or pathways connected to the somatosensory cortex. A history of trauma or brain pathology with a temporal relationship between pain onset and site of injury with somatotopic pain distribution is required for diagnosis [6].

16.6.2.3 Chronic Central Post-Stroke Pain

Chronic central post-stroke pain is caused by a cerebrovascular lesion, infarction, or haemorrhage, of the brain or brainstem. Pain may be spontaneous or evoked, as an increased response to a painful stimulus (hyperalgesia) or a painful response to a normally non-painful stimulus (allodynia). The diagnosis of central post-stroke pain requires a history of stroke and a neuroanatomically compatible distribution with the site of the stroke, so pain is felt in the region of the body represented by the central nerve structures affected by the stroke and may be localised to an entire hemisoma or a smaller body region [6].

Table 16.2 Causes of chronic central neuropathic pain

Spinal cord injuries
Stroke
Compressive myelopathy
Multiple sclerosis
Syringomyelia

16.6.2.4 Chronic Central Neuropathic Pain Caused by Multiple Sclerosis

Chronic central neuropathic pain in multiple sclerosis is caused by a lesion of somatosensory brain regions or pathways connected to these regions. Pain may be spontaneous or evoked, as an increased response to a painful stimulus (hyperalgesia) or a painful response to a normally non-painful stimulus (allodynia). Diagnosis requires a history of multiple sclerosis and a neuroanatomically plausible distribution of pain. Negative or positive sensory symptoms or signs indicating brain or spinal cord involvement must be present in the area of the body affected by the pain [6].

16.7 Neuropathic Pain Therapy

Neuropathic pain is difficult to treat and patients often have to try several pharmacological agents alone or in combination before a significant level of pain relief is achieved. Each drug should be tried at the maximum tolerated dose for 6–8 weeks before discontinuing therapy or combining it with a new drug. Particular care must be taken during dose titration to minimise the risk of side effects and at the same time any reduction [17].

16.7.1 First-Line Therapy of Neuropathic Pain

16.7.1.1 α2δ Calcium Channel Agonists

The analgesic effect of gabapentin and pregabalin is mainly related to a decrease in central sensitisation and nociceptive transmission through action on the alpha-2-delta subunit of voltage-dependent calcium channels located in the dorsal horns of the spinal cord, causing inhibition of these channels and a modulation of neurotransmitter release. Gabapentin can be started at a daily dose of 900 mg/day divided into three doses, although it is often started at a lower dose. The dosage is titrated according to clinical response up to a maximum of 3600 mg/day.

Gabapentin is generally well tolerated and is often the first drug to be used in the treatment of painful neuropathy due to its limited drug interactions, easy titration, and good tolerability. The most common causes of treatment discontinuation are sedation or ineffectiveness. Other common side effects include dizziness, peripheral oedema, weight gain, and asthenia. Gabapentin has a plasma half-life of 5–9 h, does not bind to plasma proteins, and is excreted virtually unchanged in the urine. The dosage must be adjusted according to creatinine clearance. The initial dose of pregabalin is 150 mg daily (75 mg 2 times or 50 mg 3 times daily), which can be increased to a dose of 300 mg daily after 1 or 2 weeks to a maximum dose of 600 mg/day. However, daily doses above 300 mg are not necessarily more effective and are associated with a higher rate of side effects. The dosage of pregabalin must also be adjusted in patients with renal insufficiency [18].

16.7.1.2 Tricyclic Antidepressants

The efficacy of tricyclic antidepressants (TCAs) is mainly established in diabetic PPN and postherpetic neuralgia. Their analgesic efficacy is independent of their antidepressant effect. They also act as histamine and muscarinic cholinergic receptor antagonists, producing a characteristic side-effect profile. The most common anticholinergic side effects are dry mouth, constipation, blurred vision, orthostatic hypotension, urinary retention, cognitive disturbances, central (drowsiness and sedation), and metabolic (weight gain). For these reasons, particular care must be taken in elderly patients or those with pre-existing cognitive or vegetative dysfunction as they may be more susceptible to anticholinergic side effects. The two tricyclic antidepressants most commonly used for painful polyneuropathy are amitriptyline and nortriptyline. Nortriptyline has fewer anticholinergic effects and induces less sedation. TCAs should be started at a low dose (10–mg) at bedtime, increased by 10–25 mg daily every 7–14 days up to a maximum dose of 75–150 mg/day, although many patients can achieve pain relief at lower doses [19].

16.7.1.3 Serotonin-Noradrenaline Reuptake Inhibitors

The efficacy of the serotonin and norepinephrine reuptake inhibitors (SNRIs) duloxetine and venlafaxine has been established mainly in diabetic PPN6-7. Nausea is the most common adverse effect; other side effects include dry mouth, constipation, reduced appetite, diarrhoea, sedation, and dizziness and treatment discontinuation reported in clinical trials ranges from 15% to 20%. There are rare reports of increased plasma glucose, liver enzymes, or blood pressure; therefore duloxetine is contraindicated in patients with severe hepatic dysfunction or unstable hypertension. The main side effects of venlafaxine are gastrointestinal disturbances, increased sweating is also a frequent effect. However, increased blood pressure and significant ECG changes have been described in 5% of diabetic PPN patients. Adequate doses of duloxetine are between 60 and 120 mg with no clear superiority of 120 mg (but no additional benefit has been seen from taking dosages above 60 mg/day), to avoid nausea treatment should be started at 30 mg daily and then titrated up to 60 mg/day after 1 week. The initial dose of venlafaxine extended-release is 37.5 or 75 mg once daily and should be increased over the course of 2–4 weeks to 150 or 225 mg daily [20].

16.7.2 First-Line Therapy for Trigeminal Neuralgia

The first-line treatment for trigeminal neuralgia is sodium channel blockers, carbamazepine, or oxcarbazepine. The two drugs have the same mechanism of action, i.e. blockade of voltage-dependent sodium channels. Treatment recommendations are generally the same in classic or secondary idiopathic trigeminal neuralgia. In general, sodium channel blockers are effective in most patients with trigeminal neuralgia. However, side effects of carbamazepine including dizziness, drowsiness, skin rash, and tremor are frequent. Oxcarbazepine may be preferred for its better tolerability compared to carbamazepine. Of the two drugs, carbamazepine has a higher discontinuation rate due to side effects, with the exception of hyponatremia, for which discontinuation has only occurred with oxcarbazepine [21].

16.7.3 Second-Line Therapy for Neuropathic Pain

16.7.3.1 Opioid Analgesics

Opioids are widely used for pain management and inhibit nociceptive transmission through presynaptic and postsynaptic μ-opioid receptors. Tramadol is a μ-opioid agonist, but it also exerts effects that may contribute to its analgesic properties in neuropathic pain, including inhibition of serotonin and noradrenaline reuptake [17, 22].

16.7.3.2 Lidocaine and Capsaicin

Lidocaine and capsaicin are recommended as second-line drugs in patients with peripheral neuropathic pain. Lidocaine patches that block voltage-dependent sodium channels locally reduce ectopic nerve discharges. Capsaicin is a potent agonist of the vanilloid receptor (TRPV1) [23].

16.7.4 Third-Line Therapy

16.7.4.1 Strong Opioid Analgesics

Oxycodone and morphine are two strong opioids recommended as third-line due to their complexity of control and monitoring and their potential negative side effects from drug abuse [24].

16.7.4.2 Botulinum Toxin Type A

Botulinum toxin type A (BTX-A) is a potent neurotoxin commonly used to treat spasticity, based on its ability to inhibit synaptic exocytosis and thus neural transmission. Subcutaneous injection of BTX-A is effective in patients with focal peripheral neuropathic pain and allodynia. It is indicated as a third-line treatment in refractory cases of localised peripheral neuropathic pain [25].

16.7.5 Other Therapies

16.7.5.1 α-Lipoic Acid

α-Lipoic acid is an antioxidant that has shown benefit on the symptoms of patients with painful diabetic polyneuropathy. It is most commonly used as adjunctive therapy or as a second-line agent. It may also be suggested to patients who are averse to conventional pharmacotherapy and prefer a nutraceutical option [26].

First-line therapy

Drug	Dosage	Minimum treatment period	Side effects	Precautions
Calcium channel blockers $\alpha 2\delta$				
Gabapentin	100–300 mg 1 or 3 times/day from holder up to 3600 mg/day	5–10 weeks (2 weeks with maximum dosage)	Sedation, dizziness, weight gain, oedema	Reduce the dose in patients with renal insufficiency
Pregabalin	50 mg 3 times/day or 75 mg 2 times/day, up to times to 300–600 mg/day	4 weeks	Sedation, dizziness, weight gain, oedema	Reduce the dose in patients with renal insufficiency risk of dependence and tolerance
Tricyclic antidepressants				
Amitriptyline Nortriptyline	10–25 mg at night before bedtime, up to 150 mg/day	6–8 weeks (2 weeks with the maximum dose)	Sedation, anticholinergic effects (dry mouth, blurred vision, constipation, urinary retention), cardiac conduction disturbances	Caution in patients with heart rhythm disorders, risk of serotonergic syndrome
Serotonin-noradrenaline reuptake inhibitors (SNRIs)				

Drug	Dosage	Minimum treatment period	Side effects	Precautions
Duloxetine	30 mg once daily from titrated up to 60 mg 1 or 2 times/day	4 weeks	Nausea, increased sweating, increased BP	Risk of serotonergic syndromes
Venlafaxine	Venlafaxine immediate-release 75 mg 2 or 3 times daily, titrated up to 225 mg/day Venlafaxine extended-release 37.5 mg or 75 mg 1 time/day, titrated up to 225 mg 1 time/day	4–6 weeks	Nausea, increased sweating, increased BP	Hepatic dysfunction; immediate-release venlafaxine is associated with withdrawal syndrome
First-line therapy for trigeminal neuralgia				
Carbamazepine Oxcarbazepine	200–400 mg/day up to 1200 mg/day 300–1800 mg/day		Drowsiness, dizziness, rash, tremor Drowsiness, dizziness, dose-dependent hyponatremia	Start with reduced dosage in elderly patients
Second-line therapy				
Opioid analgesics				
Tramadol	50 mg 1 or 2 times/day, titration every 3–7 days from 50 to 100 mg. Maximum dose 400 mg/day 300 mg/day in patients over 75 years of age	4 weeks	Nausea, vomiting, constipation, dizziness, drowsiness	Reduce the dose in patients with renal insufficiency. Contraindicated in patients with a history of substance abuse Contraindicated in patients with epilepsy.
Topical therapy				
Topical lidocaine	1–3 patches at 5% for up to 12 h Lidocaine 5% cream	3 weeks	Erythema or skin rash	Not effective in central neuropathic pain Indicated in localised neuropathic pain

Capsaicin 8%			Initial increase in pain erythema pressure increase secondary to the initial pain	None Indicated in localised neuropathic pain

Third-line therapy

Strong opioid analgesics				
Morphine Oxycodone	10–120 mg/day 10–120 mg/day	4 weeks	Nausea, vomiting, constipation, dizziness, drowsiness	Contraindicated in patients with a history of substance abuse (narcotics?) Contraindicated in patients with epilepsy.
Botulinum toxin type A				
Botulinum toxin type A	25–300 IU diluted in 0.9% saline solution		Pain at the inoculation site	Indicated in localised peripheral neuropathic pain

References

1. Zilliox LA. Neuropathic pain. Continuum (Minneap Minn). 2017;23:512–32. https://doi.org/10.1212/CON.0000000000000462.
2. Cazzato D, Lauria G. Small fibre neuropathy. Curr Opin Neurol. 2017;30:490–9. https://doi.org/10.1097/WCO.0000000000000472.
3. Peltier AC, Wood D. Management of neuropathic pain in polyneuropathy. Continuum (Minneap Minn). 2020;26:1299–322. https://doi.org/10.1212/CON.0000000000000928.
4. Attal N. Neuropathic pain: mechanisms, therapeutic approach, and interpretation of clinical trials. Continuum (Minneap Minn). 2012;18:161–75. https://doi.org/10.1212/01.CON.0000411564.41709.2D.
5. Finnerup NB, Haroutounian S, Kamerman P, et al. Neuropathic pain: an updated grading system for research and clinical practice. Pain. 2016;157:1599–606. https://doi.org/10.1097/J.PAIN.0000000000000492.
6. Scholz J, Finnerup NB, Attal N, et al. The IASP classification of chronic pain for ICD-11: chronic neuropathic pain. Pain. 2019;160:53. https://doi.org/10.1097/J.PAIN.0000000000001365.
7. Devigili G, Cazzato D, Lauria G. Clinical diagnosis and management of small fibre neuropathy: an update on best practice. Expert Rev Neurother. 2020;20:967. https://doi.org/10.1080/14737175.2020.1794825.
8. Downie WW, Leatham PA, Rhind VM, et al. Studies with pain rating scales. Ann Rheum Dis. 1978;37:378–81. https://doi.org/10.1136/ARD.37.4.378.
9. Grossi E, Borghi C, Cerchiari EL, et al. Analogue chromatic continuous scale (ACCS): a new method for pain assessment. Clin Exp Rheumatol. 1983;1:337–40. https://pubmed.ncbi.nlm.nih.gov/6681150/. Accessed 26 Apr 2022.

10. Graphic representation of pain. https://pubmed.ncbi.nlm.nih.gov/1026900/. Accessed 26 Apr 2022.
11. Keele KD. The pain chart. Lancet. 1948;2:6–8. https://doi.org/10.1016/S0140-6736(48)91787-5.
12. Rolke R, Baron R, Maier C, et al. Quantitative sensory testing in the German Research Network on Neuropathic Pain (DFNS): standardised protocol and reference values. Pain. 2006;123:231–43. https://doi.org/10.1016/J.PAIN.2006.01.041.
13. Nerve fibre discharges, cerebral potentials and sensations induced by CO2 laser stimulation. https://pubmed.ncbi.nlm.nih.gov/6330009/. Accessed 26 Apr 2022.
14. Valeriani M, Truini A, le Pera D, et al. Laser evoked potential recording from intracerebral deep electrodes. Clin Neurophysiol. 2009;120:790–5. https://doi.org/10.1016/J.CLINPH.2009.02.162.
15. Nolano M, Provitera V, Caporaso G, et al. Cutaneous innervation of the human face as assessed by skin biopsy. J Anat. 2013;222:161. https://doi.org/10.1111/JOA.12001.
16. Cruccu G, Finnerup NB, Jensen TS, et al. Trigeminal neuralgia: new classification and diagnostic grading for practice and research. Neurology. 2016;87:220–8. https://doi.org/10.1212/WNL.0000000000002840.
17. Attal N, Cruccu G, Baron R, et al. EFNS guidelines on the pharmacological treatment of neuropathic pain: 2010 revision. Eur J Neurol. 2010;17:1113-e88. https://doi.org/10.1111/J.1468-1331.2010.02999.X.
18. Bockbrader HN, Wesche D, Miller R, et al. A comparison of the pharmacokinetics and pharmacodynamics of pregabalin and gabapentin. Clin Pharmacokinet. 2010;49:661–9. https://doi.org/10.2165/11536200-000000000-00000.
19. Vrethem M, Boivie J, Arnqvist H, et al. A comparison of amitriptyline and maprotiline in the treatment of painful polyneuropathy in diabetics and nondiabetics. Clin J Pain. 1997;13:313–23. https://doi.org/10.1097/00002508-199712000-00009.
20. Gahimer J, Wernicke J, Yalcin I, et al. A retrospective pooled analysis of duloxetine safety in 23,983 subjects. Curr Med Res Opin. 2007;23:175–84. https://doi.org/10.1185/030079906X162719.
21. Cruccu G, Gronseth G, Alksne J, et al. AAN-EFNS guidelines on trigeminal neuralgia management. Eur J Neurol. 2008;15:1013–28. https://doi.org/10.1111/J.1468-1331.2008.02185.X.
22. Finnerup NB, Attal N, Haroutounian S, et al. Pharmacotherapy for neuropathic pain in adults: a systematic review and meta-analysis. Lancet Neurol. 2015;14:162–73. https://doi.org/10.1016/S1474-4422(14)70251-0.
23. Derry S, Rice ASC, Cole P, et al. Topical capsaicin (high concentration) for chronic neuropathic pain in adults. Cochrane Database Syst Rev. 2017;1:CD007393. https://doi.org/10.1002/14651858.CD007393.PUB4.
24. Umukoro NN, Aruldhas BW, Rossos R, et al. Pharmacogenomics of oxycodone: a narrative literature review. Pharmacogenomics. 2021;22:275–90. https://doi.org/10.2217/PGS-2020-0143.
25. Egeo G, Fofi L, Barbanti P. Botulinum neurotoxin for the treatment of neuropathic pain. Front Neurol. 2020;11 https://doi.org/10.3389/FNEUR.2020.00716.
26. Ziegler D, Ametov A, Barinov A, et al. Oral treatment with alpha-lipoic acid improves symptomatic diabetic polyneuropathy: the SYDNEY 2 trial. Diabetes Care. 2006;29:2365–70. https://doi.org/10.2337/DC06-1216.

Chapter 17
Pupillary and Lacrimation Alterations

Marcello Romano, Rita Di Leo, Davide Mascarella, Giulia Pierangeli, and Alessandra Rufa

17.1 Neuroanatomical and Physiological Substrates

The ocular structures innervated by the autonomic nervous system are the iris muscles, the ciliary muscle, the smooth muscles of the eyelids, the choroidal and conjunctival blood vessels, and the lacrimal gland. The diameter of the pupil can vary from 1 to 5 mm depending on lighting conditions and response to nearby stimuli. The dimensions vary linearly with age, the diameter being greatest at the age of 20 years and decreasing thereafter at a rate of approximately 0.04 mm/year. Due to in-depth neuroanatomical and functional knowledge, the clinical examination of the pupils: size, shape, and response to light and near, is considered an indicator of optic nerve conduction, brainstem integrity, vigilance, and coma.

Pupillary responses also provide information on the function of both the sympathetic and parasympathetic branches of the autonomic nervous system. The parasympathetic nervous system causes mydriasis in response to light and near stimuli. The sympathetic nervous system causes mydriasis in response to a variety of both physiological (wakefulness) and pathological (pain) factors [1].

M. Romano (✉)
Unit of Neurology and Stroke Unit, AOOR Villa Sofia Cervello, Palermo, Italy

R. Di Leo
UOC of Neurology, S. Giovanni e Paolo Hospital, Venice, Italy

D. Mascarella · G. Pierangeli
Department of Biomedical and Neuromotor Sciences DIBINEM, IRCCS Institute of Neurological Sciences of Bologna ISNB, University of Bologna, Bologna, Italy
e-mail: davide.mascarella@studio.unibo.it; giulia.pierangeli@unibo.it

A. Rufa
Department of Medical and Surgical Sciences and Neuroscience, University of Siena, Siena, Italy
e-mail: rufa@unisi.it

G. Micieli et al. (eds.), *Autonomic Disorders in Clinical Practice*,
https://doi.org/10.1007/978-3-031-43036-7_17

17.1.1 Miosis: Pupillary Constriction and Parasympathetic Pathway

17.1.1.1 Pupillary Reflex to Light

Intrinsically photosensitive rods, cones, and photoreceptors (with melanopsin chromophore) contribute to the pupillary reflex to light [2]. The afferent arm of the pupillary reflex to light follows the afferent arm of the visual pathway to the posterior portion of the optic tract, in part running with the nasal fibers that cross in the chiasma. The pupillary fibers exit in the posterior third of the optic tract and pass within the brachium of the superior colliculus to the pretectal nucleus, located in the midbrain near the superior colliculus. Thus, in response to the light stimulus, the retinal ganglion cells activate the ipsilateral pretectal nucleus (olivary nucleus). The axons originating from each pretectal nucleus innervate both the ipsilateral and contralateral Edinger-Westphal nucleus (EWN) (the contralateral is reached through cross-fibers that cross the posterior commissure in the dorsal midbrain). The contralateral Edinger-Westphal nucleus receives more innervation than the ipsilateral, therefore direct light in one eye will cause constriction of the ipsilateral pupil (direct response) and the contralateral pupil (consensual response). Both direct and consensual responses occur relatively quickly (reflex latency varies from 200 to 500 ms). During activation of the parasympathetic system, pupil constriction occurs, while the dilator muscle is inhibited. When the light is removed from the eye and the Edinger-Westphal neurons stop their discharge, the pre-ganglionic sympathetic fibers are no longer inhibited, their discharge frequency increases, and the tone of the dilator muscle increases (mydriasis).

17.1.1.2 Pupillary Reflex for Near

The triad accommodation-convergence-miosis is not a true reflex but rather a synkinesis or association of three functional activities that aim to maintain focus and singular vision of an object placed at a close distance. In fact, convergence, accommodation, and miosis can occur separately [3]. The afferent pathway of this reflex runs with the visual pathway to the striate cortex. From the striate cortex, information is sent to other regions, including the frontal ocular fields that communicate with the oculomotor and other midbrain nuclei including the raphe interpositus nucleus, superior colliculus, and mesencephalic reticular formation, via the internal capsule. The near reflex triad employs the same common final pupillomotor pathway as the light reflex, including the Edinger-Westphal nuclei and the ciliary bodies, but the parasympathetic neurons mediating the near reflex at the midbrain level are more numerous than those involved in the pupillary light reflex at a ratio of 30:1.

17.1.1.3 Common Parasympathetic Pupillomotor Pathway via Cholinergic Input

The pupillary sphincter contracts in response to light stimulation or the fixation of a nearby target [4]. Both stimuli cause miosis by activating the efferent pupillomotor pathway consisting of two neurons. The *first-order neuron* of the pathway is located in the ipsilateral Edinger-Westphal cholinergic nucleus in the superior mesencephalon. The parasympathetic preganglionic fibers run anteriorly through the red nuclei, joining other fibers of the oculomotor nuclear complex and exiting the midbrain emerging as the third cranial nerve in the interpeduncular fossa. In the subarachnoid space, the parasympathetic fibers lie superficially within the oculomotor nerve near the posterior communicating artery. In the cavernous sinus, the fibers are more scattered and closer to the bony wall. At the orbital level, the fibers join the inferior division of the oculomotor nerve before terminating in the ciliary ganglion. The **ciliary ganglion** houses the *second-order neurons* of the parasympathetic pathway and is located within the muscular cone between the lateral rectus muscle and the optic nerve. Acetylcholine (ACh) is the neurotransmitter of ciliary neurons that have muscarinic receptors. The parasympathetic postganglionic fibers emerging from the ciliary ganglion pass through the temporal sclera forming the *short posterior ciliary nerves* and passing into the suprachoroidal space: only 3–5% of these neurons terminate diffusely in the iris sphincter muscle; the rest terminate in the ciliary muscle and control accommodation. The iris sphincter muscle has circular fibers, which surround the edge of the pupil and contain no-muscarinic choline-receptors (mainly M3). Parasympathetic stimulation causes pupillary constriction (miosis), thus decreasing retinal illumination and reducing chromatic and spherical aberrations. It also causes contraction of the ciliary muscle, allowing the eye to focus on nearby objects (accommodation), and contributes to the reabsorption of aqueous from the trabecular meshwork (Fig. 17.1).

17.1.2 Mydriasis: Pupillary Dilation and Sympathetic Pathway

Pupil dilation is achieved by the *noradrenergic* stimulation of the *pupil dilator muscle by* the sympathetic nervous system, which is a three-neuron system [1, 3, 5, 6]. The **neurons first-order sympathetic fibers are** located in the paraventricular and arcuate nuclei of the ipsilateral hypothalamus and descend without crossing through the brainstem and upper spinal cord to synapse on **second-order neurons** of Budge's cilium-spinal center at C8–T1 (sometimes T2). Second-order preganglionic sympathetic fibers then emerge from the spinal cord into the ventral roots (mainly T1) and cross the upper thorax into the pulmonary apex and subclavian artery, where they adhere to the common carotid artery. The second-order axons synapse on the **third-order neurons** of the superior cervical ganglion (stellate ganglion), adjacent to the carotid bulb. This synapse mediates acetylcholine and type II nicotinic receptors. Third-order axons innervate the tarsal muscles of Müller (both

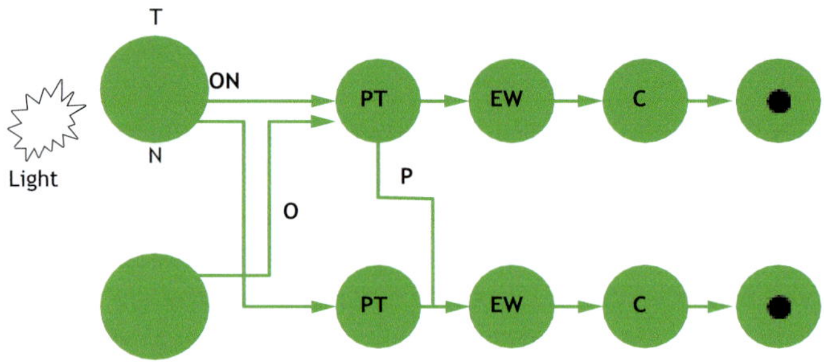

Fig. 17.1 Pupillary miosis. Light and near reflex. The light stimulus from the retina via the optic nerve reaches the pre-tectal nucleus. Fibers from the temporal retina reach the ipsilateral nucleus (direct pathway); fibers from the nasal retina decussate in the chiasma and reach the contralateral nucleus. Some fibers from the pretectal nucleus decussate in the posterior commissure and reach the contralateral Edinger Westphal nucleus. From here the parasympathetic pathway runs into the nerve trunk of the third cranial nerve and reaches the ciliary ganglion. The postganglionic parasympathetic fibers reach the peripheral effectors from whose stimulus pupillary constriction results. *T* temporal, *N* nasal, *ON* optic nerve, *OT* optic tract, *OC* optic chiasm, *PTN* pretectal nucleus, *PC* posterior commissure, *EWN* Edinger Westphal nucleus, *CG* ciliary ganglion

superior and inferior), the pupillary dilator, and the sweat glands of the face. The postganglionic fibers that innervate the pupillary dilator and the superior and inferior tarsal muscles form a plexus in the adventitia of the internal carotid artery and ascend through the foramen lacerum into the middle cranial fossa where they lie in close relation to the trigeminal ganglion. They pass through the cavernous sinus, where they are near the homolateral abducens nerve, and then follow the ophthalmic artery towards the orbit through the superior orbital fissure and join the *long ciliary nerve* (a branch of the ophthalmic division of the trigeminal nerve) and the *short ciliary nerves* (which derive from the ciliary ganglion). Third-order neurons synapse with muscle fibers using *epinephrine and norepinephrine* and 1-adrenergic receptors as mediators. Third-order neurons of the superior cervical ganglion that innervate the facial sweat glands send their axons along the external carotid artery [7].

17.1.3 Tearing

The parasympathetic preganglionic fibers originate in the pons (lacrimal nucleus of the VII cn), then leave the pons with the motor fibers of the facial nerve and enter the internal auditory canal, passing through the geniculate ganglion of the facial nerve without making synapses. They leave the ganglion with the great petrous nerve, at whose level are joined by the deep petrous nerve, composed of postganglionic sympathetic fibers from the carotid plexus, together the two nerves form the **Vidian nerve** (pterygoid canal nerve). The Vidian nerve enters the pterygopalatine ganglion, where the parasympathetic fibers enter the synapse. The pterygopalatine ganglion (also called the sphenopalatine ganglion) resides in the upper portion of the pterygopalatine fossa. The second-order axons leave the ganglion with the maxillary branch of the trigeminal nerve, pass into the zygomatic nerve, and then form a branch communicating with the lacrimal nerve. Another pathway bypasses the zygomatic nerve and reaches the gland directly. The parasympathetic fibers innervating the lacrimal gland are secretomotor and thus cause increased secretion. Sympathetic fibers innervate the blood vessels of the gland and cause vasoconstriction by decreasing the secretion production of the lacrimal gland. The sympathetic fibers of the zygomatic nerve also branch into the lower eyelid to innervate the Müller muscle of the lower eyelid [8].

17.2 Physiological and Pharmacological Testing of Pupillary Function

Most clinical information is detected by pupil observation and recording of the response to light and accommodation. Detectable changes at the objective examination are reported in the specific sections. The recording of pupil diameter, standardization of stimuli, and measurement of responses have enabled greater diagnostic sensitivity and specificity and are indispensable for research purposes. Flash photography has proven useful in diagnosis, especially in diabetes.

Infrared video pupillography allows for accurate and repeatable dynamic pupil measurements and recording of light response and near and psychosensory reflexes. The latest equipment uses an infrared video camera with subsequent image analysis with dedicated software. Recently, an iPhone application, the *sensitometer* test for evaluating the pupillary reflex to light, has been developed. Various factors must be considered when assessing the pupil, e.g. the pupil diameter in the dark is influenced by age. Older people have smaller pupils. Bremner et al. developed a formula to estimate the expected pupil diameter versus age in a cohort of 315 subjects. Genetic factors, background, and accommodation can also influence pupil diameter.

The observation and quantification of responses to physiological tests can be supplemented with specific pharmacological tests for the detection of damage to sympathetic or parasympathetic innervation. At least 24–48 h must elapse between pharmacological tests.

17.2.1 Evaluation of Sympathetic Innervation in the Myopic Pupil

The test with the greatest sensitivity in the assessment of suspected Horner's syndrome is the dynamic recording of the pupil response to light and noise, possibly assisted by pharmacological tests.

The light response of the pupil follows a specific waveform in healthy subjects. After about 250 ms the pupil constricts rapidly and reaches maximum miosis about 1 s later. The re-dilation of the pupil when the light goes out has two phases. An early, rapid phase that reflects the fall of the para-sympathetic drive to the sphincter. A late, slower phase that appears to be due to sympathetic activation of the dilator muscle. An increase in redilation lag indicates sympathetic damage. In the case of unilateral damage, evaluation of the difference in pupil diameter measured on two photographs taken 5 and 15 s after the light is switched off may be sufficient. In bilateral forms it is necessary to obtain the absolute value of the redilation lag. Studies with adrenergic receptor antagonists have shown that the time required for 75% pupil redilation (T3/4) reflects the function of the peripheral sympathetic drive. The latter can also be activated by a psychosensory stimulus by evoking a *startled response* with a sudden noise.

17.2.2 Pharmacological Tests Useful in Cases of Unilateral Myosis

In the case of unilateral myosis, pharmacological tests are aimed at identifying whether there is damage to the sympathetic pathway and, in the case of nerve damage, can provide us with localizing information about the damage, i.e., the level at which the sympathetic pathway has been damaged [9, 10].

17.2.2.1 Apraclonidine 0.5–1%

Apraclonidine is an adrenergic agonist with a predominant α_2 effect and weaker α_1 agonist activity, currently used for its α_2 effect in the treatment of glaucoma. The adrenergic α_2 receptors are located both pre-synaptically and post-synaptically; activation of receptors located on presynaptic sympathetic terminals inhibits the release of noradrenaline, leading to a reduction in pupil diameter in the healthy eye; whereas receptors α_2 located on the ciliated epithelium and trabecular meshwork mediate a reduction in intraocular pressure through a reduction in aqueous flow.

In the healthy eye, therefore, apraclonidine's effect is mainly related to the α_2 activity. Whereas the minor α_1 effect manifests itself exclusively as conjunctival vasoconstriction and mydriasis that is often imperceptible because it is balanced by the presynaptic α_2 effect (i.e., inhibition of noradrenaline release and miosis).

However, in patients with Bernard-Horner syndrome (BHS), there is a sympathetic adrenergic pathway lesion, which causes a reduction of sympathetic outflow and a depletion of noradrenaline levels at the target tissue. In this condition, 36–48 h after the sympathetic damage, postganglionic alpha receptors in the ocular and accessory tissues are upregulated, with predominant upregulation of α_1 receptors in the pupil dilator muscle. Hence, in a patient with BHS, the instillation of apraclonidine eye drops induces marked mydriasis in the affected eye, whereas no change or weak myosis is observed in the healthy eye, thus leading to a **reversal of anisocoria**. For example, in a patient with suspected left BHS due to unilateral miosis, a drop of apraclonidine (0.5–1%) is administered into both eyes; the patient is re-evaluated after at least 60 min in order to avoid false negatives (pharmacological effect may be observable even earlier). The test is considered positive if the left eye shows pronounced mydriasis, while the right eye has a weak or absent reaction to the eye drop, thus demonstrating a reversal of the anisocoria.

Therefore, one would expect apraclonidine to have a relevant clinical effect exclusively in Horner's syndromes secondary to third-order sympathetic neuron damage. In fact, it appears to have an equal mydriatic effect in BHS secondary to lesions of the first and second neurons of the sympathetic pathway, making it the pharmacological gold standard for the diagnosis of BHS. Some concerns have been raised, however, following the description of apraclonidine post-administration drowsiness in children under the age of 6 months, and its use is now only recommended in adults [11–14].

17.2.2.2 Cocaine 4–10%

Cocaine is a tropane alkaloid with a sympathomimetic effect mediated by inhibition of noradrenaline reuptake at the synaptic cleft. The instillation of cocaine in eye drops at 4–10% has historically been considered the gold standard for the diagnosis of BHS. In the healthy eye, in fact, the reduction of noradrenergic reuptake causes an accumulation of the neurotransmitter at the target tissue, thus inducing a pupil diameter dilation of at least 2 mm on average. A Horner's pupil, on the other hand, is unable to respond to cocaine administration due to sympathetic denervation. The test is considered positive if, after administration of eye drops in both pupils, the pupil suspected of sympathetic injury does not respond (or minimally responds), while the contralateral pupil shows a normal response (dilation of at least 2 mm). Due to the side effects of apraclonidine in children, the 4–10% cocaine test is still the diagnostic gold standard in this age group [15].

17.2.2.3 Hydroxyamphetamine 0.5–1%

Unlike cocaine and apraclonidine, which are useful in diagnosing Bernard-Horner syndrome, hydroxy amphetamine is useful in distinguishing a central from a peripheral BHS. Its ocular pharmacological activity results in the release of noradrenaline from the post-synaptic terminal and the ensuing mydriasis. In the context of a peripheral lesion (i.e., third-order sympathetic neuron damage), administration of a 0.5% solution of hydroxy amphetamine does not induce any clinically appreciable response, due to peripheral denervation. Whereas in the case of a central and preganglionic lesion (first- and second-order neurons, respectively), the post-ganglionic sympathetic termination is intact and therefore a marked mydriasis follows the administration of the drug, possibly even more pronounced than the appreciable mydriasis in the healthy eye due to denervation hypersensitivity [9, 16].

17.2.2.4 Phenylephrine 1–2%

It is a sympathomimetic drug, acting as an α_1 agonist, and used as a mydriatic in ophthalmology for dilating the healthy pupil in concentrations ranging from 2.5% to 10%. At higher dilutions (1–2%) it can be a viable alternative to hydroxy amphetamine in the localization of the lesion in patients with BHS. On the basis of the principle of denervation hypersensitivity, a BHS caused by a postganglionic lesion (third-order neuron) responds to conjunctival instillation of phenylephrine diluted 1% with a mydriatic response; the pupil of a patient with BHS caused by a central (first order neuron) lesion shows no response, and in lesions of the second-order neuron a minimal dilatory response can be observed. Administration of phenylephrine at this concentration also shows no appreciable change in the healthy pupil. A comparison study between phenylephrine 1% and hydroxy amphetamine 1% showed overlapping results in the localizing usefulness of these drug tests in patients diagnosed with BHS (sensitivity and specificity of 81% and 100% for phenylephrine and 93% and 83% for hydroxy amphetamine, respectively). These localizing tests obviously have limitations: the reliability of the response depends on the extent of the post-detection hyper-sensitivity phenomenon. It may therefore be complex to distinguish a pre-ganglionic lesion from a partial post-ganglionic lesion. In addition, false positives and false negatives may depend on the variability of corneal drug penetration and age-related phenylephrine sensitivity (dilatory response increases on average by 0.23 mm/decade after the age of 20) (Table 17.1) [10, 11].

17.2.3 Pharmacological Tests Useful in Cases of Unilateral Mydriasis

In the case of unilateral mydriasis, mechanical damage must initially be ruled out by slit-lamp assessment. In the absence of mechanical damage, the presence or absence of a parasympathetic outflow deficit must be investigated. In this case, the main test used involves pilocarpine at two different dosages [17].

17.2.3.1 Pilocarpine

It is a parasympathomimetic drug, often classified as a complete or partial muscarinic agonist, capable of inducing a contraction of the pupil sphincter muscle and is currently used in the treatment of glaucoma and xerostomia.

Table 17.1 Pharmacological tests for suspected Bernard Horner syndrome

Drug	Apraclonidine 0.5–1%	Cocaine 4–10%	Hydroxy amphetamine 0.5%	Phenylephrine 1%
Mechanism of action	Adrenergic agonist 2, reduces noradrenaline release In the lesion, effect 1 from denervation hypersensitivity prevails	Noradrenaline reuptake blockade	Releases stored noradrenaline	Receptor agonist 1 at muscle level pupil dilator
Effect				
Normal pupil	Does not dilate	Dilate	Dilate	Does not dilate
Preganglionic injury (I, II neurons)	Dilate	Does not dilate	Dilate	Does not dilate
Postganglionic lesion (third neuron)	Dilate	Does not dilate	Does not dilate	Dilate

In the case of anisocoria due to unilateral mydriasis, the first stage of the pharmacological test involves the instillation of a drop of pilocarpine eye drops diluted to 0.1%. This concentration is only capable of inducing miosis in the case of denervation hypersensitivity, a condition typically associated with Adie's tonic pupil. In this case, there is postganglionic damage at the level of the ciliary ganglion itself or the short ciliary nerves, and consequent receptor *upregulation* leads to high sensitivity. The 0.1% pilocarpine test is considered positive if the involved eye responds with a significantly greater sphincter muscle contraction than the contralateral eye.

This test has several limitations: there is inter-individual variability, it cannot be performed acutely as the latency for the development of hypersensitivity is days or weeks, and only 80% of cases of Adie's tonic pupil show the phenomenon of denervation hypersensitivity. In cases of acute onset disorder, the slit-lamp assessment may instead show an asymmetrical arrangement of the iris trabeculae (sectorial paralysis), which is very sensitive and specific for acute postganglionic damage.

In the event that the mydriatic eye has not responded to the administration of pilocarpine 0.1%, we proceed to the second stage of the pharmacological test, i.e., the use of pilocarpine 1%. If there is no response to this dosage, the most likely diagnostic hypothesis is a pharmacological muscarinic blockade. Whereas a positive response (miosis) indicates probable pre-ganglionic damage of the sympathetic pathway and thus possible oculomotor nerve damage [18, 19] (Fig. 17.2).

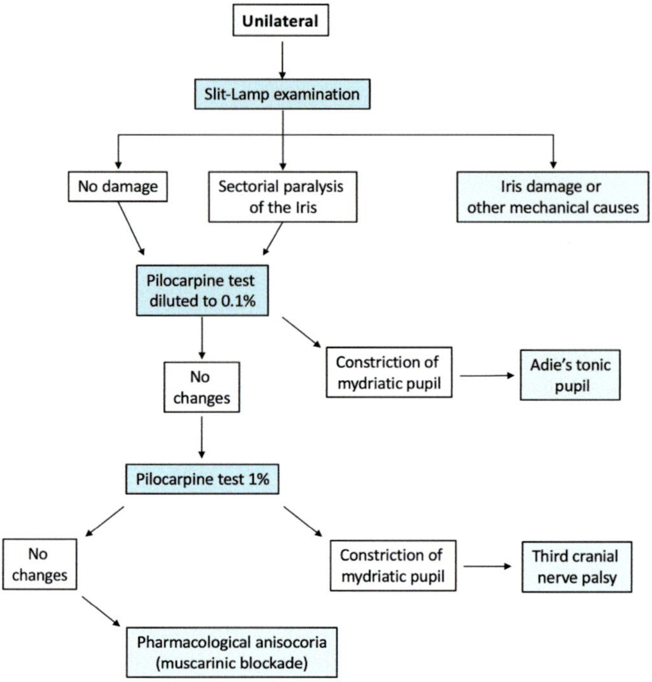

Fig. 17.2 Assessment of the mydriatic pupil

17.3 Tear Function Test

17.3.1 Schirmer's Test

Developed by the German ophthalmologist Otto Schirmer in 1903, it is a quantitative test for assessing the secretory capacity of the lacrimal glands in the suspicion of both lacrimal hyperfunction and hypofunction. Currently, it is mainly used in suspected tear hypofunction (Sjogren's syndrome, keratoconjunctivitis).

The test is based on the principle of capillarity, which allows the aqueous component of the tear film to travel along the Schirmer strips for a distance proportional to the secretory capacity of the glands, in a defined time.

It is a minimally invasive test that can assess both the basal tear function (by the main lacrimal gland) and the reflex tear function (tear production following an irritative stimulus, by the accessory lacrimal glands). The Schirmer's test can also be performed either without local anesthesia or with a local anesthetic in order to minimize the irritative stimulus of the streak and allow an exclusive assessment of basal lacrimation.

The test is carried out simultaneously in both eyes, the patient is asked to look upwards, and then the two Schirmer strips (of sterile absorbent paper 5 mm × 35 mm), folded to form an angle of approximately 90°, are placed between the conjunctiva and the lower eyelid rime. The patient is then asked to keep their eyes closed for a period of 5 min, after which they can open their eyes and look upward to allow the strip to be removed. The distance traveled by the aqueous component due to capillary action along the Schirmer's millimeter strip is then observed.

Commonly accepted results state that a test is considered normal if the distance traveled is greater than or equal to 10 mm; it is considered pathological when the distance is less than 5 mm. Between 10 and 5 mm the result is considered inconclusive. However, there is no universal agreement on the methods and cut-offs for interpreting the test and these may vary depending on the experience of the center.

Several studies have compared the test under different conditions, depending on the position and state of opening/closing the eyes, whether (or not) anesthetic was used, and the time the test was performed, without producing definitive results. The isolated positivity of the test can be influenced by many factors (age, hydration status, emotions) and does not have a diagnostic value, but when included in a broader diagnostic algorithm, the test can be of great value in confirming a suspicion of impaired tear secretion [20].

17.3.2 *Tear Breakup Time (BUT) or Tear Film Break-Up Test*

It is a qualitative test that assesses the time between the blink and the moment when the first breakpoint (dry spot) of the tear film covering the eye appears.

It is carried out using a dye (fluorescein) instilled into the eye; then the patient is asked to blink (to distribute the dye) and position themselves comfortably to be exposed to the slit lamp with cobalt blue filter light. The patient is then asked to stop blinking during observation under the lamp, and the time between the last blink and the appearance of the first tear film breakpoint is timed. The test is repeated three times per eye and the results are then averaged. It is considered positive if the elapsed time is less than 10 s.

There is also a non-invasive method (Non-Invasive tear Breakup Time, NIBUT), which involves the use of instruments capable of projecting a grid or concentric circles onto the patient's cornea, that shows a distortion of the projected image following the interruption of the tear film. It is a useful test to identify any condition of deficiency in the aqueous production of the tear film [21].

17.4 Monocular Mydriasis

Monocular mydriasis results from the interruption of parasympathetic input to the pupillary sphincter. Anisocoria should be maximized in bright ambient light when the other eye narrows and the affected eye fails to do so. Mydriasis may be due to damage of the oculomotor nerve before synapse on the ciliary ganglion, damage to the ciliary ganglion or its axons on their way to the pupillary sphincter, pharmacological dilatation of the pupil or damage to the sphincter itself. The first step is to assess the presence of third nerve palsy with a careful examination of the elevator of the eyelid, the inferior rectus, the medial rectus, the superior rectus, and the inferior oblique function.

Common causes of third nerve palsy include compression (aneurysmal or otherwise) and microvascular ischemia. It is important to note that most cases of aneurysmal compression are painful. The third nerve is more resistant to trauma than the fourth and sixth cranial nerves. Traumatic paralysis of the third nerve is therefore unlikely to occur with mild cranial trauma or in isolation without accompanying paralysis of the fourth and sixth nerves. Midbrain lesions (e.g. infarction, hemorrhage) occur frequently but rarely in neurological isolation. Nuclear paralysis of the third nerve causes hyposthenia of the ipsilateral inferior rectus, oblique inferior rectus, and medial rectus; bilateral hyposthenia of the elevator of the eyelid; and contralateral or bilateral hyposthenia of the superior rectus.

Damage to the ciliary ganglion or its axons results in a mydriatic pupil referred to as the 'tonic pupil' due to its slow constriction and lazy redilation. The pupil is often irregular with sectoral hypokinesia or vermiform movements that may not be seen with the naked eye but are often easily visible with the aid of a slit lamp. These pupils constrict better to near visual stimuli than to light stimuli; this is presumably due to the 30:1 ratio of the parasympathetic fibers mediating the near reflex to those mediating the pupillary reflex to light and, therefore, their relative preservation in the face of injury. Cholinergic hypersensitivity of the pupillary sphincter develops 1–2 weeks after ciliary ganglion lesions. To test hypersensitivity, diluted pilocarpine (a direct cholinergic agonist) is used.

Tonic pupils are mostly benign and idiopathic (Adie's pupil), but history and examination should consider findings indicative of giant cell arteritis, generalized dysautonomia, orbital inflammation (sarcoid), neoplasia, Guillain-Barré syndrome, or trauma. Adie pupils are generally monocular, observed in female patients, and isolated, although they may be accompanied by loss of deep tendon reflexes of the lower extremity, in which case the term Holmes-Adie syndrome is used.

Pharmacological dilation of the pupils may result from the administration of sympathomimetics (e.g. phenylephrine) or anticholinergics (e.g. tropicamide eye drops, ipratropium nebulizers, involuntary scopolamine transmission from ear patches to the eye). The patient should also be questioned about any source of iris trauma, surgical or accidental, that may have caused an irregular mydriatic pupil [22] (Table 17.2).

Table 17.2 Unilateral mydriasis approach

- Assess the clinical evidence of third nerve palsy and note any slight dissociation
- Assess an irregular pupil margin (if compatible with the tonic pupil, it should narrow to 0.125% pilocarpine)
- If there is no evidence of third nerve palsy or tonic pupil, administer two drops of pilocarpine 2%; if there is no constriction, mydriasis is pharmacological

17.4.1 Tonic Pupil

Linked to damage of the ciliary ganglion or short ciliary nerves with aberrant regeneration of the accommodative fibers. Initially, there is an isolated internal ophthalmoplegia characterized by a fixed, dilated pupil with loss of accommodation, later there is a mydriasis with little or no reaction to light but a slow constriction to prolonged near strain (near light dissociation). There is segmental sphincter paralysis with cholinergic hypersensitivity of the denervated muscles. Paresis of accommodation.

Adie's tonic pupil is a common but idiopathic pupillary phenomenon. The typical presentation is an isolated larger anisocoria in light. Patients often present with acute awareness of the dilated pupil. It may be unilateral or bilateral, more common in women between 20 and 40 years of age, and may be associated with altered corneal sensation and reduced or absent patellar and Achilles reflexes (Holmes-Adie syndrome). With time the dysfunction of the ciliary muscle improves and the pupil becomes progressively myopic (old Adie's pic-cola). The pupillary reflex to light typically does not recover and may worsen. Patients with unilateral Adie tend to develop a tonic pupil in the contralateral eye. Although most tonic pupils in Adie are unilateral, bilateral involvement may develop at a frequency of 4% per year. Rarely, it may be associated with a chronic vagal co-involvement cough. History and objective examination differentiate secondary forms of tonic pupils from idiopathic Adie (Table 17.3).

17.4.2 Pharmacological or Toxic Mydriasis

A careful history is necessary for patients who inadvertently or intentionally expose themselves to agents that may affect pupil size (glaucoma therapy, topical cycloplegic treatment for uveitis). Pharmacologically induced pupillary abnormalities may produce a large pupil from increased sympathetic tone with stimulation of dilation (ocular decongestants, adrenergic inhalants in Intensive Care Units) or reduced parasympathetic tone with sphincter blockade (belladonna alkaloids, scopolamine patches, anticholinergic inhalants, topical gentamycin, lidocaine injections into the orbit). Small pupils may indicate reduced sympathetic tone or increased parasympathetic stimulation (pilocarpine drops in glaucoma, anticholinesterases such as flea collars or insecticides). Pharmacological adrenergic mydriasis (phenylephrine) produces pallor, residual conjunctival vessels, and retracted upper eyelid from sympathetic stimulation. Exposure to anticholinesterases may cause pupillary miosis [23].

Table 17.3 Causes of tonic pupils

Local ganglion or ciliary nerve injury (ocular or orbital)
• Infections: campylobacter, diphtheria, choroiditis, herpes simplex, herpes zoster, measles, influenza, parvovirus, whooping cough, scarlet fever, chickenpox, hepatitis, syphilis (bilaterally dilated pupils fixed to both light and close-up strain), sinusitis, post-morbid vaccination
• Inflammations: iritis, uveitis, rheumatoid arthritis, sarcoidosis, endometriosis
• Ischemia: orbital vasculitis, lymphomatous granulomatosis, migraine, giant cell arteritis (bilateral mydriasis, asymmetric, rare), polyarteritis nodosa, orbital or choroidal tumors
• Local anesthesia: lower tooth block, retrobulbar alcohol injection
• Surgery: cataract, cryotherapy, retinal, strabismus, orbital, diathermy, deep keratoplasty
• Laser therapy
• Toxicity: chinine, trichloroethylene
• Non-surgical trauma: ciliary plexus, orbital floor fracture, retrobulbar hemorrhage, short ciliary nerve damage
Neuropathic
• Vegetative or peripheral neuropathies: amyloidosis, diabetes, alcoholic, familial dysautonomia, hereditary (CMT or Charcot Marie Tooth), Guillan Barré, Fisher syndrome, CIDP or chronic demyelinating polyradiculonevritis, acute sensorimotor polyneuropathies with tonic pupils and abduction deficit with polyarteritis nodosa
• Pandisautonomia
• PAF
• Multi-System Atrophy
• Ross syndrome with tonic pupil, segmental hyporeflexia, and anhidrosis
• Segmental facial anhidrosis and tonic pupils with preserved tendon reflexes
• Sjogren's syndrome
Fibromuscular dysplasia
• Paraneoplastics: Eaton Lambert syndrome, carcinomatosis neuropathy
• Congenital neuroblastoma with Hirschprung's disease and central hypoventilatory syndrome
• Unilateral Adie in a patient with small cell lung cancer and anti-Hu antibodies
• Following oculomotor nerve palsy
• Following bone marrow transplantation
• Adie's tonic pupillary syndrome

17.4.3 Drugs and Environmental Agents Associated with Mydriasis

17.4.3.1 Topical Parasympatholytics

- Atropine
- Cyclopentolate (Cyclogyl)
- Scopolamine
- Tropicamide (Mydriacyl)
- Gentamicin
- Glycopyrrolate
- Lidocaine gel introduced into the eye
- Ipratropium bromide (anticholinergic) in aerosol administered through a loose-fitting mask

17.4.3.2 Topical Sympathomimetics

- Apraclonidine (adrenergic agonist)
- Dexamethasone
- Epinephrine
- Phenylepinephrine
- Cocaine (e.g. nasal topical travels in the conjunctival sac)
- Eye decongestants (tetrahydrozoline hydrochloride, pheniramine maleate, chlorferinamide maleate, and nefazoline)
- Pesticides in flea collars

17.4.3.3 Local and Systemic Agents

- Airway anesthetic agents (phenylephrine/lidocaine spray)
- Amphetamines
- Atropine (systemic)
- Benzotropin
- Barracuda meat
- Football
- Cocaine
- Diphenhydramine
- Epinephrine
- Fenfluramine/Norfluramine
- Glutethimide
- Ipratropium (systemic)
- Levodopa
- Lidocaine (e.g. orbital injection, anterior chamber injection)
- Lysergic acid diethylamide
- Magnesium
- Nalorphine
- Propantheline bromide (Pro-Banthine)
- Scopolamine methylbromide, scopolamine transdermal patches
- Selective serotonin reuptake inhibitors (SSRIs)
- Thiopental
- Tricyclic antidepressants

17.4.3.4 Other

- Bulb siderosis/iron mydriasis—iron-containing intraocular foreign body
- Viscoelastic hypromellose in cataract surgery
- Alkaloids (Alkaloid belladonna)
- Common *stramonium* (*Datura stramonium*)
- Blue belladonna or European nightshade (*Solanum dulcamara*)

- Deadly nightshade (*Atropa belladonna*)
- Henbane (*Hyoscyamus niger*)
- Moonflower (*Datura wrightii* or *D. meteloides*)
- Other Datura species (*D. suaveolans* [angel's trumpet], aurea, candida, sanguine, *stramonium*, *wrightii*)
- *Brugmansia arborea* (also known as angel's trumpet)

17.4.4 Drugs and Environmental Agents Associated with Miosis

17.4.4.1 Topical Parasympathomimetics (Cholinergics)

- Aceclidine
- Carbachol
- Methacholine (Mecholyl)
- Organophosphate esters
- Pilocarpine
- Physostigmine (hexamine)

17.4.4.2 Topical Sympatholytics (Anti-adrenergic)

- Adrenergic blockers
- Thymoxamine hydrochloride
- Dapiprazole (RevEyes)
- Dibenzilin (haemoxybenzamine)
- Phentolamine (Regitine)
- Tolazoline (Priscoline)
- Guanethidine
- Timolol with epinephrine

17.4.4.3 Local and Systemic Agents

- Chlorpromazine
- Heroin
- Lidocaine (extradural anesthesia)
- Marijuana
- Methadone
- Morphine and other narcotics
- Phenothiazines

17.4.4.4 Other

- Antifleas collar (anticholinesterase)
- Pyrethrin and piperonyl butoxide insecticides (anticholinesterases)

17.5 Monocular Myosis (Horner's Syndrome)

Pathological miosis typically results from the denervation of the sympathetic input to the pupil dilator. Therefore, anisocoria will be maximized under low ambient light conditions when the denervated eye fails to dilate and the other eye dilates maximally. Careful observation may reveal slow dilatation after a light stimulus has been removed from the affected pupil; this is referred to as dilation delay.

The sympathetic fibers run together with those that innervate Müller's tarsal muscles and, up to the carotid bifurcation, the fibers that provide sudomotor function to the facial sweat glands. Complete, incomplete, or partial Horner's syndrome may occur.

A complete Horner's syndrome, which includes mild homo-lateral ptosis, miosis, and facial anhidrosis, results from damage to the sympathetic pathway proximal to the divergence of the sympathetic fibers that irrigate the facial sweat glands (adherent to the external carotid artery) and those that innervate the pupillary sphincter and tarsal muscles (both adherent to the internal carotid artery, with those that innervate the tarsus leaving the internal carotid more distally). Horner's syndrome may be incomplete, even if the lesion is proximal.

Some patients with Horner's syndrome have accompanying features that are absent from the classical triad but can be useful clues in cases of partial Horner's syndrome. Among the most important are conjunctival injection due to vasodilatation resulting from decreased sympathetic tone and decreased intraocular pressure compared to the other eye, resulting from decreased aqueous humor production from part of the ciliary body, a process stimulated by the sympathetic nervous system (Table 17.4).

First-order neurons originate in the hypothalamus. The most common site for first-order neuronal injury is in the dorsolateral medulla; this is a common component of Wallenberg syndrome. Rostral spinal cord lesions are found in Budge's ciliospinal nucleus, particularly in patients with Brown-Séquard syndrome.

Table 17.4 Horner's syndrome

- First-order Horner's syndrome (accompanied by ipsilateral ptosis and anhidrosis of the ipsilateral face and body)
- Second-order Horner's syndrome (accompanied by ipsilateral ptosis and ipsilateral facial anhidrosis)
- Third-order Horner's syndrome (accompanied by ipsilateral ptosis of the upper and lower eyelids without anhidrosis)

The second-order neuron is often damaged by thoracic neoplasms; the classic association is with Pancoast tumor in the lung apex, but any pathology at this site (e.g. aneurysm, sarcoidosis) may be responsible. The common carotid artery is a less frequent site of injury. The third-order neuron ascending the carotid artery is prone to injury in the context of carotid dissection. With this differential diagnosis in mind, a targeted examination should be performed in detail, both clinically and radiographically. The typical radiographic profile includes an MRI of the brain and cervical spine with contrast medium (which may, in some institutions, be registered for imaging of the pulmonary apex; a CT scan of the thorax with contrast medium may be performed otherwise) and an MRA angiogram of the head and neck (including the great vessels). Rare cases of Horner's syndrome are associated with idiopathic headache syndromes, including the vegetative trigeminal headache family, idiopathic Raeder's paratrigeminal syndrome, and migraine with vegetative features.

17.6 Dissociation of Reflection in Light and Near

The near-light dissociation (Table 17.5) is seen when the pupils shrink better upon effort for near gaze than upon presentation of bright light. The opposite condition is not expected because the fibers mediating the triad (accommodation-convergence-miosis) are much more numerous than those mediating the light reflex, so the system is inherently less susceptible to damage. In addition, the fibers of the pupillary reflex to light are anatomically more susceptible to structural damage than the fibers of the near-field diffuse supranuclear reflex. Dissociation occurs from lesions typically located in the dorsal mesencephalon, ciliary ganglion, and optic nerves.

Dorsal midbrain syndrome. Lesions affecting the posterior communication present with mild to near dissociation, retraction of the upper eyelids, vertical gaze paralysis, convergence retraction nystagmus.

Ciliary ganglion lesions. Ganglionopathies often present with a light-near dissociation. This discrepancy is due to the greater number of neurons dedicated to light than to the light-near response at the level of the ciliary ganglion, which is the opposite of what occurs in the EWN (Edinger-Westphal Nucleus).

Table 17.5 Light-near dissociation

	Causes
Dorsal mesencephalic syndrome	Stroke, pineal tumors, hydrocephalus, encephalitis, TAU-synucleinopathies, multiple sclerosis, Wernicke's encephalopathy, sarcoidosis, neuroborreliosis
Ciliary ganglionopathies	Tonic pupil, Argyll Robinson
Optic nerve disorders or amaurosis	Demyelinating, ischaemic autoimmune, infectious traumatic genetic neuritis

Diseases of the optic nerve. Injuries at any level of the limb affected by the light reflex lead to a slow constriction of the pupil to bright light, but a consensual constriction is preserved at the nearby stimuli. When one eye cannot perceive light at all, the pupil is called amaurotic (no reaction to light irradiated ipsilaterally), but the consensual reflex is preserved when light is irradiated on the intact optic nerve of the other eye.

17.7 Bilateral Myosis

Bilaterally small pupils may result from bilateral sympathetic denervation of the pupil dilator, from factors causing parasympathetic tone to predominate over sympathetic tone, or from chronic reinnervation:

- Parasympathetic excess
  - Sedative drugs
  - Cholinergic agonists (e.g. pilocarpine)
- Sympatolysis
  - Diencephalic lesions
  - Lesions of the pontine segment
  - Bilateral peripheral Horner's syndrome
- Chronic ganglionopathies
  - Argyll Robertson pupil
  - Chronic tonic pupils

17.8 Bilateral Mydriasis

Bilaterally large pupils are observed when the sympathetic input to the iris exceeds the parasympathetic input for:

- Increased sympathetic innervation of the pupil dilator (e.g. iatrogenic drugs such as phenylephrine and tricyclics, and recreational antidepressants such as cocaine)
- Decreased parasympathetic innervation of the pupil sphincter
- Loss of supranuclear input to both Edinger-Westphal nuclei
- Severe bilateral blindness
- Defects of the final common path:
  - Edinger-Westphal core
  - Third cranial nerve palsy
  - Ciliary ganglion (tonic pupils, 10% are bilateral: acute tonic pupil, Miller Fisher syndrome, diabetes mellite)

- Neuromuscular junction (iatrogenic anticholinergics such as tropicamide drops used for dilatation, scopolamine contamination from anti-emetic patches, or ipratropium sulfate in the eye rather than in the airways, botulism, which prevents the release of acetylcholine from the ciliary ganglion neuron, and never myasthenia gravis)
- Injury of the iris due to sphincter rupture or surgical trauma

17.9 Acute/Subacute Generalized Autonomic Dysfunction

Pandisautonomy may occur acutely/subacutely with the involvement of peripheral sensory and motor fibers. A parasympathetic dysfunction results in relative mydriasis in response to light stimulus and reduced reflex constriction with or without a tonic pupil. A sympathetic dysfunction involves relative mydriasis in the dark with slowed dilation and reduced reflex constriction triggered by unexpected events as occurs in Horner's syndrome. Some forms may have an exclusive orthosympathetic or parasympathetic involvement. In some cases, in addition to an increase in CSF proteins, antibodies directed against the ganglionic acetylcholine receptor subunit alfa-3 can be detected.

17.9.1 Pure Autonomic Failure

In the Pure autonomic failure description, the subjects had iris atrophy and anisocoria. In later reports, Horner's syndrome has been described; however, pupillary function is normal in most subjects.

17.9.2 Diabetes Mellitus

Most commonly a myotatic pupil is observed, particularly in the dark with a normal light reflex; rarely a dilated pupil with altered light reflexes suggests that the sympathetic innervation of the iris is more susceptible than the parasympathetic innervation. The response in mydriasis to direct sympathomimetic agents is related to denervation hypersensitivity. Retinopathy and laser photocoagulation attenuate the activity of the affected branch of the photomotor reflex.

17.9.3 *Amyloidosis*

Pupillary abnormalities in the course of the various forms of amyloidosis are generally associated with other signs of dysautonomia and are characterized by a parasympathetic deficit due to the deposition of amyloid deposits in the ciliary ganglion. A bilateral slowing of pupil dilation indicates an orthosympathetic deficit due to the deposition of amyloid in the cervical orthosympathetic chain.

17.9.4 *Paraneoplastic Syndromes*

Several pupillary alterations in paraneoplastic syndromes have been described: bilateral tonic pupil in Lambert Eaton syndrome, tonic pupil with hypersensitivity to pilocarpine in subjects with neuroblastoma and neuronopathy with anti-Hu positive antibodies, bilateral Horner's syndrome during anti-Hu positive demyelinating neuropathy.

17.9.5 *Sjogren's Syndrome*

Unilateral or bilateral tonic pupil, usually with light-vessel dissociation.

17.9.6 *Family Dysautonomia (HSAN Type III)*

Familial dysautonomia or Riley-Day syndrome presents at the ocular level with alacrimia, corneal hypoesthesia, corneal ulcerations, and corneal cataracts. Pupillary abnormalities are characterized by an exaggerated response in miosis to methacholine (2.5%) or pilocarpine (0.1–0.125%).

17.9.7 *Dopamine-Hydroxylase Deficiency*

This hereditary disorder is characterized by the inability to transform dopamine into norepinephrine, resulting in an ortho-sympathetic deficit. The pupils are myopic with a normal reaction to light and hypersensitivity to epinephrine and phenylephrine [24].

17.9.8 Ross Syndrome

The clinical criteria for the diagnosis of Ross syndrome are tonic pupil, hypoareflexia, and segmental anhidrosis with or without compensatory hyperhidrosis. In one-third of subjects, the tonic pupil is the onset symptom [25].

17.10 Lacrimal Gland Disorders

17.10.1 Lacrimation Disorders

Disorders that disrupt the neural control of lacrimation can be divided into three types: hypo lacrimation, excessive lacrimation or epiphora, and inappropriate lacrimation [26].

17.10.1.1 Hypolacrimation

Keratoconjunctivitis sicca is a condition of reduced tear production:

- Clinical manifestations include chronic conjunctivitis with injection, discomfort, and photophobia
- Paradoxically epiphora
- Afferent inputs for reflex tearing are predominantly carried by the ophthalmic division of the trigeminal nerve
- Significant hypo lacrimation may result from deafferentation of the tear reflex in severe trigeminal neuropathy
- Lesions of the pontine angle of the petrous stronghold or of the Meckel cord may damage the trigeminal nerve and the neighboring parasympathetic lamina fibers traveling in the intermediate nerve or in the superficial petrous large nerve, with lacrimal reduction by combined damage of the afferent and efferent branches of the lacrimal reflex
- Lesions of the trunk involving the facial nucleus often produce loss of lacrimation from involvement of the superior salivary nucleus
- Peripheral facial palsy may be associated with ipsilateral loss of the tear reflex when the lesion is proximal to both the cerebellum-pontine angle and the petrous base. The secretomotor fibers for lachrymation and salivation exit the brainstem, the intermediate nerve that lies between the motor trunk of the facial nerve and the cochlear vestibular nerve, sic-as they cross the angle cerebellum-pontine and the internal auditory meatus. Injuries in this area (e.g. tumors) can produce hearing loss, vestibular damage, facial paralysis, reduced salivation, impaired taste, and a dry eye on the side of the lesion

- Lesions involving the floor of the cranial fossa media near Gasser's ganglion may damage the tear fibers in the superficial great petrous nerve with ipsilateral tear deficiency
- Finding altered tear secretion on the side of an acquired abducens nerve palsy is of significant locative value indicating that the lesion is in the middle cranial fossa (usually extradural)
- Lesions of the sphenopalatine ganglion may cause pain and hypoesthesia in the cheek (supply area of the maxillary branch of the trigeminal nerve) with reduced lacrimation and dry eyes on the same side
- Damage to the temporal zygomatic nerve can also cause temporal denervation of the lacrimal gland by traumafacial involving the posterior orbital lateral wall or tumors, especially metastases, in the same region

17.10.1.2 Hyperlacrimation

- Excessive afferent **triggers** of the tear reflex
- **Overstimulation** of parasympathetic efferent fibers
- **Pseudobulbar palsy**
- **Meningitis and encephalitis**
- **SUNCT** (Short-lasting Unilateral Neuralgiform Headache): A neuralgic syndrome characterized by moderately severe, strictly unilateral attacks of stinging or stabbing pain confined to the orbital and periorbital regions and associated with a lacrimation cessation. Attacks last from 10–120 s with symptomatic periods that may last from days to months. **SUNA** syndrome (Short-lasting Unilateral Neuralgiform Headache Attacks with Cranial Autonomic Symptoms) characterized by short-lasting unilateral neuralgic pain with cranial vegetative signs is similar to SUNCT. Patients may have cranial vegetative symptoms in addition to conjunctival injection and lacrimation (e.g. nasal blockage, rhinorrhea, eyelid edema, sweating or facial flushing) or only one of these symptoms (conjunctival injection or lacrimation) may be present. The etiology of these clinical pictures is unknown.
- **Sphenopalatine neuralgia (Sluder's neuralgia)**, a syndrome of nasal pain accompanied by ipsilateral hyper lacrimation, rhinorrhea, salivation, photophobia, and hemifacial redness (old name for **cluster headache**)
- Certain drugs can induce tearing by irritating the corneal epithelium or by direct parasympathomimetic action (**pilocarpine or methacholine**)

17.10.1.3 Inappropriate Tearing

The **taste-lacrimal reflex** commonly known as **crocodile tears (Bogorad's syndrome)** results from an abnormal tear gland innervation that causes profuse and inappropriate tearing in response to stimulation of the taste buds. The term crocodile tears derives from the idea that the crocodile will cry on a man's head after it has devoured the body and finished eating the head as well. Most commonly, this phenomenon occurs unilaterally in the eye on the side of a facial paresis.

The **taste-lacrimal reflex may be congenital** and often associated with congenital abduction paralysis of the eye. In congenital cases chewing or sucking movements may evoke tearing. The reflex may also be acquired in the early stages of facial paresis, without facial paresis, or as a result of facial paresis. The mechanism **of** cases occurring at the onset of facial **paresis** is probably by **ephaptic transmission between afferent and efferent vegetative neurons in the proximal trunk of the facial nerve**. When this reflex occurs after facial paralysis or sectioning of the large superficial petrous nerve it is thought that **collateral axons** originate from the glossopharyngeal preganglionic nucleus, where the tympanic branch forms an anastomosis with the larger superficial petrous nerve. These sprouts reinnervate the sphenopalatine ganglion and lacrimal gland and become collateral to healthy fibers that normally innervate the otic ganglion and parotid gland. Salivary axons may then bypass a superficial petrous nerve that has been cut.

17.10.2 Generalized Disorders of Autonomic Function Involving Tearing

Riley-Day syndrome (familial dysautonomia) is characterized by:

- Autonomic instability
- Pain
- Altered taste sensation
- Fever
- Crisis
- Vomiting attacks
- Often associated with severe dryness of the eyes, corneal anesthesia, and corneal ulceration
- Crying elicits a reduced amount of tears in these patients
- However, a local dose of methacholine produces copious tears suggesting denervation hypersensitivity of the lacrimal glands
- There is often miosis to dilute pilocarpine solutions indicating cholinergic denervation hypersensitivity
- This rare disorder is found quite exclusively in persons of Ashkenazi Jewish descent with responsibility for the gene on chromosome 9q31-33
- Is an autosomal recessive form of inheritance

Multisystem atrophy (Shy Drager syndrome) is characterized by:

- Orthostatic hypotension
- Anhydrosis
- Urinary incontinence
- Impotence

- Often associated with extrapyramidal signs

Common eye characteristics include:

- Anisocoria
- Iris atrophy
- Convergence deficit
- Nystagmus

Pupillary abnormalities from sympathetic or parasympathetic ocular insufficiency include:

- Alternating Horner's syndrome
- Mydriasis
- Cholinergic hypersensitivity
- Reduced lacrimation
- Corneal hypoesthesia

Diffuse vegetative neuropathies:

- Idiopathic, paraneoplastic, or autoimmune
- Pan-autonomic dysfunction often associated with mydriasis, poor or absent constriction to light and near stimulus, irregularity of pupillary margins
- By parasympathetic and sympathetic postganglionic denervation with denervation hypersensitivity

Systemic amyloidosis:

- Amyloid deposits in the eyelids, extraocular muscles, ocular adnexa, and vitreous gel
- Pupillary hypo-reactivity, asymmetrical or non-reactive pupils, light dissociation, near reaction, tonic pupils
- Parasympathetic deficit from amyloid deposition in the cingulate ganglion

Diabetes:

- Myosis particularly in the darkness
- The more frequent occurrence of a small pupil with poor light reflex gives rise to a greater susceptibility to damage of the sympathetic inner iris
- Denervation hypersensitivity with exaggerated mydriatic response to direct sympathomimetic agents

Miller Fisher variant of Guillan-Barré syndrome:

- Dilated, poorly reactive, or non-reactive pupils suggest ciliary ganglion involvement
- Pharmacological tests indicate both parasympathetic postganglionic blockade and sympathetic involvement

Eaton Lambert myasthenic syndrome:

- Abnormal pupillary response to light

- Reduced reflex tear production
- Sympathetic and parasympathetic denervation hypersensitivity

17.11 Local Autonomic Symptoms in Primary Headaches

Some primary headaches may be associated with local autonomic symptoms including pupillary symptoms. This occurs almost in all of patients with trigeminal autonomic cephalalgias (TACs) but can also occur in migraine patients.

17.11.1 Trigeminal Autonomic Cephalalgias (TACs)

It is a group of primary headaches characterized by the presence of strictly lateralized headache attacks associated with autonomic cranial symptoms ipsilateral to the pain. Cluster headache, paroxysmal migraine, continuous hemicrania, Short-lasting Unilateral Neuralgiform Headache Attacks with Conjunctival Tearing (SUNCT), and Short-lasting Unilateral Neuralgiform Headache Attacks with Cranial Autonomic Symptoms (SUNA) belong to the TACs.

The pathophysiology of TACs is still the subject of debate. All the pathophysiological models proposed must be able to explain the strict unilaterality of pain in these syndromes. Therefore, much emphasis has always been placed on a possible peripheral (and therefore trigeminal) genesis of pain [27].

However, there is further evidence supporting a possible central genesis, including the temporal characteristics of attacks such as, for example, the link with the circadian rhythm in Cluster headache, or even the absence of peripheral triggers as, for example, occurs in trigeminal neuralgia.

The relationship between pain and autonomic manifestation in TACs is a complex topic, which is not fully clarified and therefore of great scientific interest. Between 3% and 7% of patients with Cluster headaches do not present vegetative manifestations during attacks. Furthermore, occasionally patients with TACs may present episodes characterized exclusively by autonomic manifestations in the absence of pain, in part suggesting a separate genesis of the two manifestations [28].

Our current understanding of these conditions allows us to assume involvement on three levels:

- **Trigeminal-vascular system**: Consisting of the peripheral trigeminal afferents that terminate at the level of the trigeminal-cervical complex formed by the close connection between the caudal nucleus of the trigeminal and the neurons of the posterior horns of the muscle at the C1–C2 level. This represents the first true relay station of the pathway as well as the point of contact between the periphery and the central nervous system, particularly the cortico-subcortical areas that constitute the *central pain network* [29, 30].

- **Autonomic nervous system**: Involves, among other central structures, the *superior salivatory nucleus* and its efferences directed towards the lacrimal glands and nasal cavities, mediated by the facial nerve, the great petrous nerve, and the pterygopalatine ganglion. There is a close correlation between the trigeminal-vascular system and the autonomic system, to such an extent that it can be considered a single circuit called trigeminal-autonomic. The afferent arm is represented by the trigeminal pathway and the efferent arm by the facial pathway and the activation of this circuit may result in parasympathetic hyperfunction (lacrimation, nasal management, rhinorrhea) and reduction of the sympathetic tone that seems to be more correlated with ocular symptoms (miosis, ptosis) [31].
- **Hypothalamus**: Considered one of the possible headache attack triggers in the central genesis theories of TACs. In addition to clinical notions, the strongest evidence supporting a hypo-thalamic role is provided by functional neuroimaging studies in which activation of the posterior hypothalamus during attacks of all TACs was demonstrated. However, it appears that other nuclei connected to the central autonomic nervous system network (Central Autonomic Network) may play an important role, such as the paraventricular nucleus and the suprachiasmatic nucleus, which is responsible for circadian regulation [32].

17.11.2 Classification [33]

The International Headache Classification (ICHD-3) defines TACs according to the following criteria.

17.11.2.1 Cluster Headache

Attacks of severe, strictly unilateral pain which is orbital, supraorbital, temporal, or any combination of these sites, lasting 15–180 min and occurring from once every other day to eight times a day. The pain is associated with ipsilateral signs such as conjunctival injection, lacrimation, nasal congestion, rhinorrhea, forehead, and facial sweating, miosis, ptosis and/or eyelid edema, and/or with restlessness or agitation.

Diagnostic criteria:

A. At least five attacks fulfilling criteria B–D.
B. Pain of severe or very severe intensity, unilateral, in the orbital, supraorbital, and/or temporal site, lasting 15–180 min (if untreated).
C. Either or both of the following:

   1. At least one of the following symptoms or signs ipsilateral to the headache:

      – Conjunctival injection and/or lacrimation
      – Nasal congestion and/or rhinorrhea

- Eyelid edema
- Facial and forehead sweating
- Miosis and/or ptosis

2. Feeling of restlessness or agitation.

D. The frequency of attacks is between 1 every 2 days and 8 a day.
E. Not better accounted for by any other ICHD-3 diagnosis.

17.11.2.2 Paroxysmal Hemicrania

Attacks of severe, strictly unilateral pain which is orbital, supraorbital, temporal, or any combination of these sites, lasting 2–30 min, occurring several or many times a day. The attacks are usually associated with ipsilateral conjunctival injection, lacrimation, nasal congestion, rhinorrhea, forehead and facial sweating, miosis, ptosis, and/or eyelid edema. The attacks respond absolutely to indomethacin.Diagnostic criteria:

A. At least 20 attacks fulfilling criteria B–E.
B. Severe unilateral orbital, supraorbital, and/or temporal pain lasting 2–30 min.
C. Either or both of the following:

1. Headache is accompanied by at least one of the following symptoms or signs ipsilateral to the pain:

- Conjunctival injection and/or lacrimation
- Nasal congestion and/or rhinorrhea
- Eyelid edema
- Forehead and facial sweating
- Miosis and/or ptosis

2. A feeling of restlessness or agitation.

D. The frequency of attacks is >5 per day.
E. Attacks are prevented completely by therapeutic doses of indomethacin.
F. Not better accounted for by any other ICHD-3 diagnosis.

17.11.2.3 Unilateral Neuralgiform Headache Attacks of Short Duration (Short-Lasting Unilateral Neuralgiform Headache Attacks)

Attacks of moderate or severe, strictly unilateral head pain, lasting from seconds to minutes, occurring at least once a day and usually associated with prominent tearing and redness of the ipsilateral eye.

Diagnostic criteria:

A. At least 20 bindings that meet criteria B–D.

B. Moderate or severe unilateral head pain, with orbital, supraorbital, temporal, and/or other trigeminal distribution, lasting 1–600 s, manifesting as a single stab, series of stabs, or in a saw-tooth pattern.
C. At least one of the following five cranial autonomic signs or symptoms, ipsilateral to pain:
    1. Conjunctival injection and/or lacrimation
    2. Nasal congestion and/or rhinorrhea
    3. Eyelid edema
    4. Forehead and facial sweating
    5. Miosis and/or ptosis
D. The frequency of attacks is at least 1 per day.
E. Not better accounted for by any other ICHD-3 diagnosis.

This syndrome is in turn divided into SUNCT if there is both conjunctival injection and lacrimation or SUNA if only one of the two is present.

17.11.2.4 Hemicrania Continua

Persistent, strictly unilateral headache, associated with ipsilateral conjunctival injection, lacrimation, nasal congestion, rhinorrhoea, forehead, and facial sweating, miosis, ptosis and/or eyelid edema, and/or with restlessness and agitation. The attacks respond completely to treatment with indomethacin.

Diagnostic criteria:

A. Unilateral headache fulfilling criteria B–D.
B. Present for >3 months with exacerbations of moderate or greater intensity.
C. Either or both of the following:
    1. At least one of the following signs or symptoms ipsilateral to the headache:
        – Conjunctival injection and/or lacrimation
        – Nasal congestion and/or rhinorrhea
        – Eyelid edema
        – Forehead and facial sweating
        – Miosis and/or ptosis
    2. Sense of restlessness or agitation, or aggravation of pain with movement.
D. Complete remission with adequate doses of indomethacin.
E. Not better accounted for by any other ICHD-3 diagnosis.

17.11.2.5 Migraine

It is a complex and disabling neurological disorder, characterized by recurrent headache episodes and many other clinical manifestations.

The current international headache classification (ICHD-3) divides migraine into:

- ***Migraine without aura*** is defined as:

  A. At least five attacks fulfilling criteria B–D
  B. Headache attacks lasting 4–72 h (untreated or unsuccessfully treated)
  C. Headache has at least two of the following four characteristics:

     1. Unilateral localization
     2. Pain of pulsating quality
     3. Moderate or severe pain intensity
     4. Aggravation by or causing avoidance of routine physical activity (e.g. walking, climbing stairs)

  D. Headache is associated with at least one of the following conditions:

     1. Presence of nausea and/or vomiting
     2. Presence of photophobia and phonophobia

  E. Not better accounted for by another ICHD-3 diagnosis.

- ***Migraine with aura***, itself defined by the following criteria:

  A. At least two attacks fulfilling criteria B and C.
  B. One or more of the following fully reversible aura symptoms:

     1. Visual
     2. Sensory
     3. Speech/language
     4. Motor
     5. Brainstem
     6. Retinal

  C. At least three of the following six characteristics:

     1. At least one symptom of the aura develops gradually within 5 min
     2. Two or more aura symptoms occur in succession
     3. Each individual aura symptom lasts 5–60 min
     4. At least one symptom of the aura is unilateral
     5. At least one symptom of the aura is positive
     6. The aura is accompanied, or followed within 60 min, by a headache

  D. Not better accounted for by another ICHD-3 diagnosis.

This classification, however, does not extensively consider the multiphasic and evolutionary nature of the migraine attack with its four phases: *prodromal phase, aura, headache, and postprodromal phase.* During all these phases, migraine patients may experience complex symptoms, which are not limited to pain but involve sensory processes as well as central and peripheral autonomic pathways.

In the *prodromal phase* (present inconstantly in about 70% of migraine sufferers), patients may recognize numerous manifestations as 'premonitory' of a migraine attack. These symptoms are indicative of neuronal activation at several levels; the most frequent are **hypothalamic** symptoms (increased appetite, drowsiness, yawning, changes in body temperature), **gastrointestinal** symptoms (constipation, diarrhea), and **cognitive** symptoms (concentration difficulties, irritability) [34].

The aura, described by the criteria listed above, precedes the migraine attack and is typically characterized by positive symptomatology, reflecting the *cortical spreading depolarization* process. The most common symptomatology is visual, which finds its most peculiar expression in the presence of bright, predominantly colorless geometric shapes with gradual extension from the point of fixation to the external edge of the hemi-visual field (e.g., Forthergill's fortification spectrum). In order of frequency, sensory symptoms (gradually progressing paresthesias), speech changes, motor manifestations, and others, may also be present [35].

In the ***headache phase***, in addition to the typical pain, symptoms related to autonomic manifestations of the migraine attack are commonly observed, in particular **nausea and vomiting** (included in the diagnostic criteria). Furthermore, migraine patients may experience a parade of symptoms termed *cranial autonomic symptoms* that include *periorbital edema*, *conjunctival injection*, *lacrimation*, *rhinorrhoea*, *nasal congestion* and appear to be secondary to parasympathetic activation through the seventh and eighth cranial nerves. These symptoms are commonly considered distinctive features suggestive of the diagnosis of trigeminal-autonomic cephalalgias (TACs), however, they are present in up to 30% of migraine patients and can cause diagnostic errors and delays [36, 37].

Pupillary changes during a migraine attack have often been described. These are currently much debated and rarely counted within the *cranial autonomic symptoms*. During the migraine attack, anisocoria may be present with an altered pupillary diameter (not necessarily ipsilateral to the headache or other *cranial autonomic symptoms)* that is described mainly as unilateral mydriasis and to a lesser extent as miosis, often associated with ptosis. In addition, a higher prevalence of Adie's tonic pupil has been described in migraine patients [38].

The ***postdrome phase*** is the period between the end of the headache phase and the perception of complete well-being. It is present in 81% of migrainous patients [39] and it is composed of at least one non-headache symptom. Postdrome symptoms can be clustered in *neuropsychiatric* (concentration difficulties, mood changes, insomnia, or sleepiness), *gastrointestinal* (*constipation, nausea, food craving*), *sensory* (*light sensitivity, thirst*), *and general symptoms* (*tiredness, yawning*). Although the role of brainstem noradrenergic mechanisms and cortical spreading depolarization has been suggested, the pathophysiology of the postdrome phase is still unclear [40, 41].

References

1. McDougal DH, Gamlin PD. Autonomic control of the eye. Eye Compr Physiol. 2015;5(1):439–73.
2. May P, Sun W, Wright NF, Erichsen JT. Pupillary light reflex circuits in the macaque monkey: the preganglionic Edinger-Westphal nucleus. Brain Struct Funct. 2020;225:403–25.
3. Gamlin Paul DR. Subcortical neural circuits for ocular accommodation and vergence in primates. Ophthal Physiol Opt. 1999;19(2):81–9.
4. Kelbsch C, Strasser T, Chen Y, et al. Standards in pupillography. Front Neurol. 2019;10:129.
5. Khan Z, Bollu PC. Horner syndrome. In: StatPearls. StatPearls Publishing; 2018.
6. Morales J, Brown SM, Abdul-Rahim AS, Crosson CE. Ocular. J Neuroophthalmol. 2010;30(1):7–11.
7. Almog Y, Gepstein R, Kesler A. Diagnostic value of imaging in Horner syndrome in adults. J Neuroophthalmol. 2010;30(1):7–11.
8. Biousse V, Touboul PJ, D'Anglejan-Chatillon J, Lévy C, Schaison M, Bousser MG. Ophthalmologic manifestations of internal carotid artery dissection. Am J Ophthalmol. 1998;126(4):565–77.
9. Ludwig PE, Jessu R, Czyz CN. Physiology, eye. In: StatPearls. Treasure Island, FL: StatPearls Publishing; 2022.
10. Miller N, Kanagalingam S. Horner syndrome: clinical perspectives. Eye Brain. 2015;7:35–46.
11. Smit DP. Pharmacological testing in Horner's syndrome—a new paradigm. S Afr Med J. 2010;100(11):738–40.
12. Bremner F. Apraclonidine is better than cocaine for detection of Horner syndrome. Front Neurol. 2019;10:55.
13. Koc F. The sensitivity and specificity of 0.5% apraclonidine in the diagnosis of oculosympathetic paresis. Br J Ophthalmol. 2005;89(11):1442–4.
14. Nguyen MTB, Farahvash A, Zhang A, Micieli JA. Apraclonidine for the pharmacologic confirmation of acute Horner syndrome. J Neurol Sci. 2020;419:117190.
15. Martin GC, Aymard P-A, Denier C, et al. Usefulness of cocaine drops in investigating infant anisocoria. Eur J Paediatr Neurol. 2017;21(6):852–7.
16. Danesh-Meyer HV. The correlation of phenylephrine 1% with hydroxyamphetamine 1% in Horner's syndrome. Br J Ophthalmol. 2004;88(4):592–3.
17. Pronin AN, Wang Q, Slepak VZ. Teaching an old drug new tricks: agonism, antagonism, and biased signaling of pilocarpine through M3 muscarinic acetylcholine receptor. Mol Pharmacol. 2017;92(5):601–12.
18. Yoo Y-J, Hwang J-M, Yang HK. Dilute pilocarpine test for diagnosis of Adie's tonic pupil. Sci Rep. 2021;11:10089.
19. Rivero Rodríguez D, Scherle Matamoros C, Pernas SY. Adie pupil. Pilocarpine test. Med Clín (Engl Ed). 2018;151(4):170.
20. Cho P, Yap M. Schirmer test. I. A review. Optom Vis Sci. 1993;70(2):152–6.
21. Sweeney DF, Millar TJ, Raju SR. Tear film stability: a review. Exp Eye Res. 2013;117:28–38.
22. Bouffard MA. The pupil. Continuum (Minneap Minn). 2019;25:1194–214.
23. Brazis PW, Lee AG. In: Low A, Benarroch EE, editors. Clinical autonomic disorders. Philadelphia: Lippincott Williams & Wilkins; 2008. p. 588–606.
24. Bremner FD, Smith SE. Pupil abnormalities in selected autonomic neuropathies. J Neuroophthalmol. 2006;26(3):209–19.
25. Lamotte G, Sandroni P, Cutsforth-Gregory JK, et al. Clinical presentation and autonomic profile in Ross syndrome. J Neurol. 2021;268(10):3852–60.
26. Brazis PW, Lee AG. In: Low A, Benarroch EE, editors. Clinical autonomic disorders. Philadelphia: Lippincott Williams & Wilkins; 2008. p. 606–9.
27. Benarroch EE. The central autonomic network: functional organization, dysfunction, and perspective. Mayo Clin Proc. 1993;68(10):988–1001.

28. Leone M, Bussone G. Pathophysiology of trigeminal autonomic cephalalgias. Lancet Neurol. 2009;8(8):755–64.
29. Cortelli P, Pierangeli G. Chronic pain-autonomic interactions. Neurol Sci. 2003;24(S2):s68–70.
30. Guo S, Petersen AS, Schytz HW, et al. Cranial parasympathetic activation induces autonomic symptoms but no cluster headache attacks. Cephalalgia. 2018;38(8):1418–28.
31. Drummond PD. Autonomic disturbances in cluster headache. Brain. 1988;111(5):1199–209.
32. May A, Burstein R. Hypothalamic regulation of headache and migraine. Cephalalgia. 2019;39(13):1710–9.
33. Headache Classification Committee of the International Headache Society (IHS). The International Classification of Headache Disorders, 3rd edition. Cephalalgia. 2018;38(1):1–211.
34. Cortelli P, Pierangeli G. Hypothalamus and headaches. Neurol Sci. 2007;28(S2):S198–202.
35. Danno D, Wolf J, Ishizaki K, Kikui S, Yoshikawa H, Takeshima T. Cranial autonomic symptoms of migraine in Japan: prospective study of 373 migraine patients at a Tertiary Headache Center. Headache. 2020;60(8):1592–600.
36. Sharav Y, Katsarava Z, Charles A. Facial presentations of primary headache disorders. Cephalalgia. 2017;37(7):714–9.
37. de Coo IF, Wilbrink LA, Haan J. Symptomatic trigeminal autonomic cephalalgias. Curr Pain Headache Rep. 2015;19(8):39.
38. Burish MJ, Rozen TD. Trigeminal autonomic cephalalgias. Neurol Clin. 2019;37(4):847–69.
39. Giffin NJ, Lipton RB, Silberstein SD, Olesen J, Goadsby PJ. The migraine postdrome: an electronic diary study. Neurology. 2016;87(3):309–13. https://doi.org/10.1212/WNL.0000000000002789. Epub 2016 Jun 22.
40. Goadsby PJ, Lambert GA, Lance JW. The mechanism of cerebrovascular vasoconstriction in response to locus coeruleus stimulation. Brain Res. 1985;326(2):213–7. https://doi.org/10.1016/0006-8993(85)90030-7.
41. Bose P, Karsan N, Goadsby PJ. The migraine postdrome. Continuum (Minneap Minn). 2018;24(4, Headache):1023–31. https://doi.org/10.1212/CON.0000000000000626.

Chapter 18
Sweating Disorders

Rita Di Leo and Camilla Rocchi

18.1 Introduction

The autonomic nervous system maintains the internal body temperature at the relatively constant value of 37 °C. Thermoregulation requires an exact balance between the systems that generate and dissipate heat. Eccrine sweating is the main mechanism of heat loss and is essential to thermoregulation in humans.

18.2 Physiology

The regulation of body temperature involves several neural systems. The center of thermoregulation is the preoptic area of the anterior hypothalamus, which establishes a set point of 37 °C for core body temperature. The thermoreceptors in this area detect and respond to the slightest changes in core body temperature and receive and integrate input from cutaneous, visceral, and spinal receptors. The afferent pathway of thermoregulation ascends in the spinal-thalamic tract to the brainstem reticular formation, the thalamus, and the hypothalamus. Hypothalamic heat-sensitive neurons activate the efferent sudomotor pathway, which descends through the brainstem and the thoracic spinal cord where it connects with the preganglionic neurons of the sympathetic system in the intermediate-lateral column and, subsequently, with ganglionic neurons that, via cholinergic amyelinic C-fibers, innervate the sweat glands of the skin.

R. Di Leo (✉)
Neurology Unit, San Giovanni e Paolo Hospital, AULSS3 Serenissima, Venice, Italy

C. Rocchi
Neurology Unit, Policlinico Tor Vergata, Rome, Italy

G. Micieli et al. (eds.), *Autonomic Disorders in Clinical Practice*,
https://doi.org/10.1007/978-3-031-43036-7_18

Activation of the sweat glands is mainly mediated by acetylcholine acting through M3-type muscarinic receptors. Activation of these receptors triggers an increase in intracellular calcium concentration, which rises the permeability of potassium and chloride channels and initiates the release of an isotonic precursor fluid from the secretory cells. Other co-transmitters, such as the vasoactive intestinal polypeptide, cause vasodilation, which subsequently promotes sweating. The sympathetic fibers innervate 2–4 million eccrine sweat glands distributed over the body surface. The highest density of eccrine sweat glands associated with thermoregulation is found on the forehead, followed by the upper limbs, trunk and finally the lower limbs. The palms of the hands and soles of the feet have a high density of sweat glands (from 600 to 700 glands/cm^2), which are, however, mainly dedicated to emotional sweating rather than thermoregulation. The skin arterioles also receive copious sympathetic innervation mediated by adrenergic receptors and local non-adrenergic mediators. When body temperature exceeds the hypothalamic set point, the sympathetic system generates a generalized response consisting of sweating, vasodilation and hyperpnea restoring thermal homeostasis. Any lesion along this pathway, central or peripheral, can cause a sweating disturbance. Sweating and/or thermoregulation disorders are manifested by increased vs. reduced/absent sweating (hyperhidrosis vs. hypo/anhidrosis).

There are different degrees of hyperhidrosis: it ranges from excessive sweating that can interfere with work and social activities and leads to psychological discomfort for the subject to massive sweating that can determine severe dehydration and dysionia (Table 18.1)

The reduction in sweating can be generalized or localized (hypohidrosis) and in some diseases progresses to anhidrosis; its distribution can guide us in the differential diagnosis of the underlying pathologies.

Reduced or absent sweating results in the body's difficulty/impossibility to dissipate heat with the consequent risk of developing hyperthermia under environmental or pathological conditions, which if not promptly recognized is life-threatening [1].

18.2.1 Essential Generalized Hyperhidrosis

Essential generalized hyperhidrosis is diffused throughout the body, but mainly involves those parts where there is a greater density of sweat glands, it may already present at low temperatures or at the beginning of exercise. Primary focal hyperhidrosis affects the palms of the hands, soles of the feet, armpits, and sometimes the craniofacial region, it is not related to thermoregulation, it can be exacerbated by the emotional state, environmental temperature, and exercise.

Table 18.1 Causes of hyperhidrosis

Generalized

Generalized essential hyperhidrosis

Secondary to diseases of the central nervous system
- Family dysautonomia
- Shapiro's syndrome (episodic hypothermia with hyperhidrosis)
- Secondary to diseases of the central and peripheral nervous system
- Familial fatal insomnia
- Parkinson's disease
- Morvan's fibrillary chorea
- Post-traumatic or post-hemorrhagic

Secondary to systemic diseases
- Infections
- Metabolic: thyrotoxicosis, diabetes mellitus, hypopituitarism, menopause
- Neoplasms: pheochromocytoma, lymphoma, leukemia, carcinoid, renal cell cancer, Castleman disease
- Night sweats: tuberculosis, lymphoma, endocarditis, diabetes mellitus, acromegaly, opiate withdrawal, alcohol
- Obstructive apnea, Prinzmetal's angina

Drug-related: neuroleptic malignant syndrome, serotonergic syndrome.

Focal

Essential focal hyperhidrosis: palmoplantar, axillary, craniofacial.

Secondary to diseases of the central nervous system
- Autonomic hyperactivity
- Cerebral infarction
- Spinal cord injury autonomic dysreflexia
- Post-traumatic syringomyelia
- Sweating triggered by the cold
- Olfactory hyperhidrosis
- Chiari malformation type I

Associated with diseases of the peripheral nervous system
- Autonomic neuropathy
- Dermatomeric due to irritation of a nerve trunk

Craniofacial pathologies
- Gustatory/olfactory perspiration
- Tear sweating
- Harlequin syndrome

Associated with dermatological pathologies
- Pretibial myxedema
- POEMS (polyneuropathy, endocrinopathy, monoclonal plasma cell gammopathy, skin lesions)

Drugs
- Antidepressants: tricyclics, serotonin reuptake inhibitors (SNRIs), selective serotonin reuptake inhibitors
- Anticholinesterases: pyridostigmine
- Muscarinic receptor agonists: pilocarpine, bethanechol
- Opioids
- Proton pump inhibitors

18.2.2 Parkinson's Disease

Sweating disorders are common in Parkinson's disease. They may manifest as hypohidrosis but more frequently hyperhidrosis is reported, which is one of the non-motor signs that begin in the first decade of the disease. Episodes of diaphoresis accompany the off states and dyskinesias. The pathophysiological mechanism appears to be central and peripheral. The treatment for focal forms is botulinum toxin. In some studies, deep brain stimulation of the subthalamic nucleus seems to reduce hyperhidrosis [2].

18.2.3 Sweating Triggered by the Cold

It is a rare disorder characterized by profuse sweating in a cold environment caused by a mutation in the gene coding for the cytokine receptor (CRLF1). The pathogenesis is not fully known. It has been shown in vitro that CRLF1 is involved in the differentiation of a nerve terminal from noradrenergic to cholinergic. During development, the induction of sweating is defined by cholinergic and catecholaminergic neurotransmission, while the maintenance of secretory function is ensured by cholinergic transmission. A role in the abnormal sweating response in CISS (cold-induced sweating syndrome) may be related to an impairment of temperature control in the hypothalamus and preoptic area [3].

18.2.4 Gustatory Sweating

Gustatory sweating is characterized by facial redness and sweating following gustatory stimulation as a result of aberrant reinnervation of the sweat glands that are physiologically innervated by the sympathetic by the parasympathetic fibers that physiologically innervate the salivary glands. Causes include damage to the auriculotemporal nerve circuit (Frey's syndrome) as a result of trauma, surgery or following an alteration of the autonomic nervous system in the course of neuropathies such as diabetic neuropathy [4].

18.2.5 Paroxysmal Autonomic Hyperactivity

It is characterized by an autonomic storm due to an injury to both the central and peripheral nervous system.

Sweating is one of the symptoms of hyperactivity of the sympathetic autonomic nervous system (Tables 18.2 and 18.3).

Table 18.2 Clinical signs of paroxysmal autonomic hyperactivity

Signs of sympathetic hyperactivity	Signs of parasympathetic hyperactivity
Tachycardia	Bradycardia
Hyperhidrosis	Flushing
Hypertension	Hypotension
Mydriasis	Miosis
Skin pallor and piloerection	Increased bronchial secretions
Hyperthermia	
Muscle rigidity	

Table 18.3 Causes of paroxysmal sympathetic autonomic hyperactivity

- Head trauma
- Global cerebral ischemia-anoxia
- Subarachnoid hemorrhage from ruptured aneurysm
- Brain hemorrhage (especially for diencephalic or ponto-mesencephalic involvement)
- Insular ischemic stroke
- Temporal lobe epilepsy
- Acute bacterial meningitis
- Viral encephalitis
- Cerebral malaria
- Autoimmune encephalitis
- Fat embolism cerebral embolism
- Toxic encephalopathies (e.g., serotonergic syndrome, neuroleptic malignant syndrome, alcohol withdrawal, cocaine overdose)
- Cervical and thoracic spinal cord trauma above T5 as part of dysreflexia
- Guillain-Barré syndrome

18.3 Hypo/Anhidrosis (Table 18.4)

18.3.1 α Synucleinopathies

In α-synucleinopathies, multisystem atrophy is characterized by diffuse anhidrosis, whereas in Parkinson's disease the sweating deficit affects the distal districts of the lower limbs and in dementia with Lewy bodies there is an intermediate picture between the two (Fig. 18.1).

Table 18.4 Causes of hypo/anhidrosis

Central nervous system disorders
• Multisystem atrophy
• Lewy body dementia
• Parkinson's disease
• Ischemic/hemorrhagic stroke
• Multiple sclerosis
• Myelopathies
Peripheral nervous system disorders
• Isolated autonomic failure
• Autonomic autoimmune ganglionopathy
Autonomic neuropathies
• Diabetic neuropathy
• Paraneoplastic neuropathy
• Amyloid neuropathy
• Lepromatous neuropathy
• Hereditary neuropathies
• Sjögren's syndrome
• Ross syndrome
• Harlequin syndrome
• Fabry disease
• Idiopathic chronic anhidrosis
Dermatological pathologies
• Skin lesions
• Systemic sclerosis
• Agenesis of the sweat glands
Iatrogenic causes
• Drugs
• Sympathectomy
• Surgery
Drugs
• Anticholinergics: glycopyrrolate, atropine, cyproheptadine, doxepin
• Tricyclic antidepressants: amitriptyline
• Antihistamines: diphenhydramine
• Bladder relaxants: oxybutynin, tolterodine
• Antipsychotics and antiemetics: chlorpromazine, clozapine, quetiapine
• Carbonic anhydrase inhibitors
• Antiepileptics: topiramate, zonisamide
• Antihypertensives with central adrenergic action: clonidine
• Hypothalamic receptor agonists μ: fentanyl, morphine, oxycodone, hydrocodone
• Presynaptic acetylcholine release inhibitors: botulinum toxin

18.3.2 Ross Syndrome

Ross syndrome is characterized by hyporeflexia, tonic pupil, and segmental anhidrosis with compensatory hyperhidrosis. Another clinical characteristic is intolerance to heat and exercise manifested by hyperthermia and transient loss of consciousness, tachycardia, dry skin, and gastrointestinal symptoms [5].

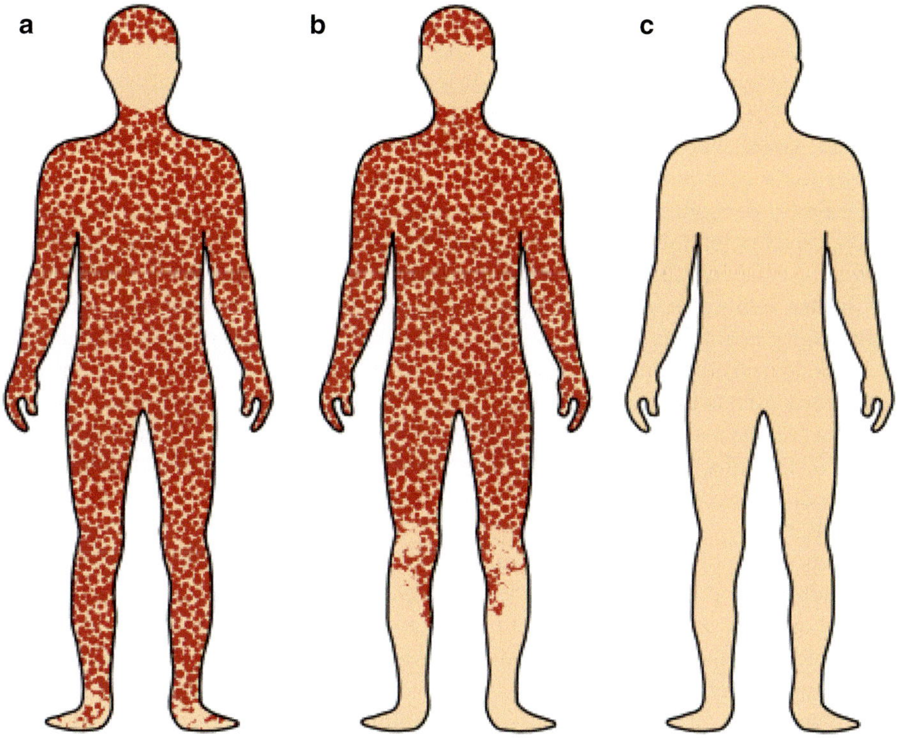

Fig. 18.1 Thermoregulatory sweat patterns in synucleinopathies: (**a**) Parkinson's disease, (**b**) Lewy body disease, (**c**) multiple system atrophy

Table 18.5 Sweating assessment questionnaires

• Compass 31
• Hyperhidrosis severity scale

18.4 Diagnosis

A meticulous anamnesis, which is also carried out with the help of self-assessment questionnaires (Table 18.5) or administered directly, gives an idea of the extent of the sweating disorder and whether it is associated with other symptoms of central, peripheral or autonomic nervous system involvement. A careful objective examination allows the state of the skin to be assessed, which in the presence of both hypo- and anhidrosis may show specific lesions [6].

In addition to the anamnesis and objective examination, the diagnosis is based on colorimetric methods to assess the distribution of sweating.

Dynamic sweating test: Allows to study the integrity of the central and peripheral sympathetic autonomic system, without being able to distinguish between a preganglionic and a postganglionic lesion. It is performed in a room under controlled conditions of humidity and temperature. The patient, in which both external and internal temperature is monitored, is sprinkled with a powder whose color changes in the areas where the subject sweats. It is necessary to raise the body temperature by about 1° for 35–65 min, increasing the temperature of the room. Using a digital camera, sweat maps are made. The advantage of this technique is that visually it allows the localization of the sweating disorder to be assessed, the limitations are the need for dedicated equipment and the long pre-production and execution times, so it is an examination that remains limited to selected cases [7]. Both isolated autonomic insufficiency and autoimmune autonomic ganglionopathy are characterized by diffuse anhidrosis, which may improve in dysimmune forms following immunomodulatory treatment. In neuropathies the distribution of anhidrosis is length dependent as for positive and negative somatic symptoms. In complete myelopathies anhidrosis affects the part of the body below the lesion. In radiculopathies and isolated nerve lesions it follows the dermatomeric distribution and the innervation territory of the affected nerve, respectively. In some conditions, both congenital and acquired, of incomplete hypo/anhidrosis, areas of hyperhidrosis can also occur (Fig. 18.2).

Study of the direct and indirect quantitative axon sudomotor reflex: This allows the study of the postganglionic sympathetic cholinergic system using acetylcholine iontophoresis as a stimulus to sweat production. A colorimetric powder is then used to characterize the number, size and percentage area of the total area occupied by the sweat droplets [8].

Cutaneous sympathetic response is a neurophysiological technique to study the cholinergic sympathetic by recording changes in potential at the skin level of the

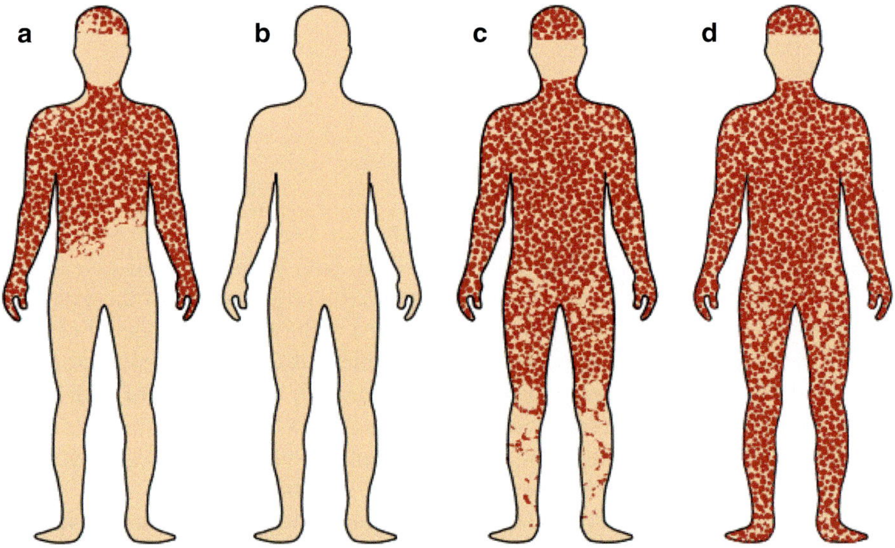

Fig. 18.2 Thermoregulatory sweat patterns: (**a**) regional/widespread, (**b**) global, (**c**) length-dependent, (**d**) normal

forehead or limbs at rest and after electrical stimulus, emotional or breath changes. The advantage is the easy execution with the instrumentation used for the neurophysiological study. The limitations are several: it is a test that does not allow discrimination between preganglionic and postganglionic lesions, it is habit-forming, the response is influenced by the subject's age and is altered for pathologies affecting both the central and peripheral nervous system.

Skin biopsy: allows the morphological study of small fibers through "intraepidermal fiber density", to quantify and characterize the sudomotor, pilomotor, vasomotor and intraepidermal sweat glands. It can be performed remotely to assess the evolution of the pathology and responses to therapy. Limitations: it is still a minimally invasive method and requires a laboratory equipped to process and read the biopsies [9].

Sudoscan®: an apparatus that allows the measurement of electrochemical skin conductance by means of reverse iontophoresis and chronoamperometry on the hands and feet. Electrochemical skin conductance appears to assess small fiber function through the study of postganglionic sympathetic cholinergic and intraepidermal fiber density.

18.5 Hyperhidrosis Therapy

The treatment of idiopathic focal hyperhidrosis refers to several strategies (Tables 18.6, 18.7, and 18.8).

Topical therapy makes use of drugs with anti-perspirant, astringent and anticholinergic activity. They are effective in mild forms and have a short duration of action. The drugs used in the treatment of hyperhidrosis (Table 18.7) are employed with an 'off-label' indication, exploiting the systemic anticholinergic activity or central sympatholytic activity or anxiolytic action.

18.5.1 Botulinum Toxin

The use of onabotulinum toxin A in the treatment of axillary hyperhidrosis has been approved since 2001. Since then, it has been widely used in the treatment of focal hyperhidrosis [10].

Table 18.6 Hyperhidrosis therapy

Topical therapy
Medical therapy
Botulinum toxin
Iontophoresis
Surgical therapy
Others: biofeedback and psychotherapy

Table 18.7 Drugs used to treat hyperhidrosis

Anticholinergics
• Glycopyrrolate bromide
• Propantheline bromide
• Methantheline bromide
• Atropine
• Oxyphencyclimine
• Phenoxybenzamine
Sympatholytic
• Clonidine
• Benzodiazepines

Table 18.8 Surgical therapy

• Thoracic sympathectomy
• Excision of axillary tissue
• Axillary cavity liposuction

References

1. Coon EA, Cheshire WP. FAAN sweating disorders. Continuum (Minneap Minn). 2020;26(1):116–37.
2. Niemann N, Billnitzer A, Jankovic J. Parkinson's disease and skin. Parkinsonism Relat Disord. 2021;82:61–76.
3. Di Leo R, Nolano M, Boman H, et al. Central and peripheral autonomic failure in cold-induced sweating syndrome type 1. Neurology. 2010;75(17):1567–9.
4. Dunbar EM, Singer TW, Singer K, Knight H, Lanska D, Okun MS. Under- standing gustatory sweating. What have we learned from Lucia Frey and her predecessors? Clin Auton Res. 2002;12(3):179–84.
5. Nolano M, Provitera V, Perretti A, et al. Ross syndrome: a rare or a misknown disorder of thermoregulation? A skin innervation study on 12 subjects. Brain. 2006;129(8):2119–31.
6. Pierangeli G, Turrini A, Giannini G, et al. Translation and linguistic validation of the Composite Autonomic Symptom Score COMPASS 31. Neurol Sci. 2015;36(10):1897–902.
7. Illigens BMW, Gibbons CH. Sweat testing to evaluate autonomic function. Clin Auton Res. 2009;19(2):79–87.
8. Novak P. Electrochemical skin conductance correlates with skin nerve fiber density. Front Aging Neurosci. 2016;8:199.
9. Nolano M, Tozza S, Caporaso G, Provitera V. Contribution of skin biopsy in peripheral neuropathies. Brain Sci. 2020;10:989.
10. Hosp C, Naumann MK, Hamm H. Botulinum toxin treatment of autonomic disorders: focal hyperhidrosis and sialorrhea. Semin Neurol. 2016;36(1):20–8.

Chapter 19
Autonomic Dysfunction Due to Toxic Agents and Drugs

Carlo Alessandro Locatelli, Davide Lonati, Azzurra Schicchi, and Valeria Margherita Petrolini

19.1 Introduction

Acute poisoning/intoxication and adverse effects of drugs often cause autonomic dysfunction. Overall, causative agents (i.e. chemicals, drugs, substances of abuse, natural toxins) are a very large group of molecules that, with different exposures and modalities, can cause clinical problems of varying severity. Adverse effects of therapeutic treatments are also a potential cause of major autonomic dysfunction (e.g., bradycardia/tachycardia, urinary retention, paralytic ileus, postural hypotension), sometimes not easy to diagnose. Diagnostic-therapeutic aspects, moreover, are complicated when the potentially causative agents are multiple and/or cause interactions, as it often is in the case of poisonings and multidrug treatments.

Alterations in autonomic systems are usually more severe and prolonged in acute poisonings (exposure to larger amounts of molecules), but agents with high toxicological potency (e.g., natural toxins such as botulinum and tetanus toxins) can cause major autonomic dysfunction even for small-dose exposure. Autonomic dysfunction, however, may appear late as consequence of severe intoxication even when it involves poisons that are not primarily neurotoxic [1, 2]. In some cases, moreover, autonomic changes are not caused directly by the poisonous agent, but by withdrawal from substances of abuse or drugs (Table 19.1) [3].

C. A. Locatelli (✉) · D. Lonati · A. Schicchi · V. M. Petrolini
Toxicology Unit, Pavia Poison Control Centre-National Toxicology Information Centre, Laboratories of Clinical and Experimental Toxicology, Research Hospital of Pavia, Istituti Clinici Scientifici Maugeri, Pavia, Italy
e-mail: carlo.locatelli@icsmaugeri.it; davide.lonati@icsmaugeri.it; azzurra.schicchi@icsmaugeri.it; valeria.petrolini@icsmaugeri.it

G. Micieli et al. (eds.), *Autonomic Disorders in Clinical Practice*,
https://doi.org/10.1007/978-3-031-43036-7_19

Table 19.1 Main typical toxicological syndromes (toxidromes) with autonomic dysfunction, and causative agents (non-exhaustive list) (modified and adapted from [4])

	Anticholinergic syndrome (atropine, scopolamine, tricyclic antidepressants)	Cholinergic syndrome (organophosphorus insecticides)	Sympathomimetic syndrome (cocaine, amphetamine)	Serotonin toxicity (SSRI)	Neuroleptic malignant syndrome	Ethanol and sedative-hypnotic syndrome (ethanol, barbiturates, benzodiazepines)	Opioids syndrome (heroin, morphine, methadone, oxycodone, fentanyl, clonidine)	Withdrawal from ethanol or sedative-hypnotics	Withdrawal from opioids
Signs/symptoms									
BP	–/↑	Indifferent	↑	↑	↑/↓	↓	↓	↑	↑
P	↑	↓/↑/±	↑	↑	↑	↓	↓	↑	↑
RR	±	↓/↑/±	↑	–/↑	±/↓	↓	↓	↑	–
T°C	↑	±	↑	–/↑	↑	↓	↓	↑	–
Mental status	Delirium/agitation	From normal to depressed	Agitation	From normal to agitated delirium	Confusion, delirium, coma	Coma	Coma	Agitation, disoriented, hallucination	Normal, anxious
Pupils	Mydriasis	Indifferent	↑	–/↑	–/↓	±	Pinpoint miosis	↑	↑
Peristalsis	↓/Absent	↑	–/↑	↑	±	↓	Reduced/absent	↑	↑
Diaphoresis	Absent	↑	↑	↑	↑	Indifferent	Indifferent	↑	↑
Other	Xerostomia, urinary retention	Salivation, lacrimation, bronchorrhea, urinary incontinence, diarrhea, fasciculations, paralysis	Tremor, seizures	Clonus, tremor, seizures	Lead-pipe muscular rigidity, tremor, pallor, urinary incontinence bradykinesia	Hyporeflexia hypotonia, ataxia	Hyporeflexia	Tremor, seizures	Rhinorrhea, piloerection, yawning, vomiting diarrhea
Antidote	Physostigmine	Atropine/oxime			Bromocriptine/ dantrolene	Flumazenil	Naloxone		

BP blood pressure, *P* pulse, *RR* respiratory rate, *T* °C body temperature, ↑ increase, ↓ decrease, – unmodified, ± variable

Most of the new psychoactive substances (NPS), which today account for a major portion of the consumption of substances of abuse, also result in significant autonomic dysfunction. Some families of these molecules (phenethylamines, piperazines, tryptamines) show different effects and receptor affinities for norepinephrine, dopaminergic and serotonergic systems [5, 6]. In general, the novel psychoactive and stimulant substances of abuse cause amine release, inhibition of biogenic amine reuptake, and inhibition of monoamine-oxidase. Newer hallucinogens tend to be direct agonists of serotonin receptors, and entactogens cause serotonin release. The manipulation of parts of the chemical structures of these substances alters the molecule's ability to cross the blood–brain barrier, enter the cells, stimulate or inhibit receptors, resist enzymatic degradation, and affect cellular transporters [7, 8].

This chapter reports some clinical pictures of autonomic dysfunction related to chemicals/drugs/substances of abuse that can be correlated with one or more causative agents, namely:

- Poisoning characterized by "typical toxic syndromes" with autonomic dysfunction
- Intoxications/adverse effects to drugs causing major autonomic dysfunction (e.g., serotonergic syndrome and neuroleptic malignant syndrome)
- Intoxications from natural toxins characterized by major vegetative dysfunction (e.g., botulism).

19.2 Diagnostic Process in Toxic Autonomic Dysfunctions

Knowledge and evaluation of the pharmaco-toxicological effects of toxic agents can facilitate the clinical-toxicological diagnostic process, especially when the medical history is unknown: provided it is not a case of poisoning due to a combination of many molecules with different effects!

Schematically, the autonomic dysfunctions of many substances (drugs, substances of abuse, natural toxins, etc.) can be framed into anticholinergic, parasympathomimetic, sympatholytic, and sympathomimetic effects (Table 19.1). However, these effects cannot always be totally framed in these four main groups, as some of the group-specific effects may be modified in cases of intoxication, for example, in relation to the dose taken or by the simultaneous presence of more than one syndrome and more than one molecule.

Based on the main involvement of the sympathetic, parasympathetic, serotoninergic, and opioid systems, the main clinical-toxicological syndromes are defined as

- Sympathomimetic
- Sympatholytic
- Anticholinergic

These major syndromes can in turn be subdivided into sub-syndromes, based on the prevalence of stimulation/inhibition of different receptors and neurological pathways: the signs/symptoms of the major subtypes of sympathomimetic syndrome (Table 19.2) and cholinergic syndrome (Table 19.3) are given.

Table 19.2 Main signs/symptoms of sympathomimetic syndrome subtypes and examples of causative agents

Causal agents (examples)	Alpha-adrenergic syndrome	Beta-adrenergic syndrome	Mixed sympathomimetic syndrome (alpha- and beta-adrenergic)
• Phenylpropanolamine • Phenylephrine	• Hypertension • Reflex bradycardia • Dilated pupils		
• Salbutamol • Metaproterenol • Theophylline • Caffeine		• Vasodilation • Hypotension • Tachycardia	
• Cocaine • Amphetamines • Phenethylamines • Piperazine • Tryptamine			• Hypertension • Tachycardia • Dilated pupils • Sweaty skin (but with dry mucous membranes) • Tremors • Nystagmus • Seizures

Table 19.3 Main signs/symptoms in cholinergic syndrome subtypes with examples of causative agents

Causal agents (examples)	Nicotinic syndrome	Muscarinic syndrome	Mixed cholinergic syndrome (muscarinic and nicotinic)
• Nicotine • Succinylcholine	• Tachycardia followed by bradycardia • Muscle fasciculation followed by paralysis • Dilated pupils		
• Bethanechol		• Bradycardia • Miosis • Sweating • Salivation • Bronchorrhea • Pulmonary edema • Increased peristalsis • Urinary incontinence	
• Organophosphates insecticides • Carbamate insecticides • Physostigmine			• Fasciculations followed by muscle weakness and paralysis • Bradycardia • Miosis • Sweaty skin • Increased peristalsis

In the nicotinic syndrome, stimulation of nicotinic receptors at the autonomic ganglia and neuromuscular plaques results in the activation of both the sympathetic and parasympathetic systems, with unpredictable or biphasic results. Initial tachycardia may be followed by bradycardia, and initial muscle fasciculations may be followed by paralysis (e.g., nicotine, succinylcholine[1]).

Muscarinic receptors are found in the effector organs of the parasympathetic system, and they generally mediate major secretory functions. Their stimulation results in bradycardia, miosis, sweating, hyperperistalsis, bronchorrhea, bronchial constriction, wheezing, excessive salivation, and urinary incontinence (e.g., bethanechol).

In contrast, when both nicotinic and muscarinic receptors are stimulated, mixed effects are observed. Pupils are usually miotic, skin is sweaty, and peristaltic activity is increased. Fasciculations are manifestation of nicotinic stimulation of the neuromuscular junction and may evolve into muscle weakness or paralysis.

Autonomic dysfunctions also occur as a result of intoxication by agents that do not act directly on the sympathetic and parasympathetic systems, but in various ways manage to involve them or cause overlapping and confounding effects. These agents may include the following syndromes:

- Opioid
- Hypnotics/sedatives
- Serotonin toxicity
- Botulism

One of the aspects that provides better insight into possible autonomic effects in the early stages of the patient's clinical examination is the assessment of pupil size, its changes, and eye movements [9]. In fact, pupil size is affected by several drugs or chemical agents that act on the autonomic nervous system (examples in Table 19.4).

Numerous drugs and toxic agents cause horizontal nystagmus: among these, the most commonly implicated are barbiturates, ethanol, carbamazepine, phenytoin and also some natural toxins such as that inoculated by the African American scorpion. Phencyclidine, on the other hand, can cause horizontal, vertical and even rotatory nystagmus.

Hippus (pupillary athetosis), characterized by rhythmic contractions and modification of pupil size, can be caused by various hallucinogens, aconitine, and by seizures caused by numerous drugs and agents active on both the parasympathetic and sympathetic systems.

The most typical ocular effect of botulism is mydriasis associated with eyelid ptosis and unconjugated gaze, due to the toxic effects on the neurons innervating the eye muscles.

Somewhat more complex is the toxicity of methanol (through the formation of the metabolite formic acid) and of some chloroquine-like antimalarials: visual

[1] Depolarizing neuromuscular blocker acting on nicotinic receptors in skeletal muscle.

Table 19.4 Common pharmaco-toxicological causes of miosis and mydriasis

Miosis[a]	Mydriasis
Sympatholytic agents • Opioids • Clonidine • Phenothiazines • Tetryzoline • Oxymetazoline • Valproic acid	Sympathomimetic agents • Amphetamines and derivatives • Cocaine • Dopamine • LSD • IMAO • (Nicotine[b])
Cholinergic agents • Organophosphates insecticides • Carbamate insecticides • Physostigmine • Nicotine • Pilocarpine	Anticholinergic agents • Atropine and other anticholinergics • Tricyclic antidepressants • Antihistamines • Glutethimide • Carbamazepine
Other • GHB/GBL	Other • Botulism • Methanol[c]

[a] The most common differential diagnoses with non-toxicologic causes include stroke, pontine infarction, and subarachnoid hemorrhage
[b] Commonly causes miosis, but in some cases also results in mydriasis
[c] Direct neurotoxicity

acuity problems and papilledema are due to toxic effects on the retina and, in the case of methanol, are often associated with mydriasis.

A particular alteration is synesthesia (e.g., seeing sounds, hearing colors): this effect does not depend on a toxic mechanism of action on the eye but rather on the hallucinations and central nervous system alterations caused by serotonergic hallucinogens such as LSD.

19.3 "Typical Toxic Syndromes" Characterized by Autonomic Dysfunction

"Typical syndromes" in clinical toxicology are characterized by a constellation of signs and symptoms associated with a category of poisons/toxic agents. The clinical features of the main typical syndromes of neurological interest in "classic" presentations are shown in Table 19.1. Unfortunately, however, many poisons/toxic agents that are often the cause of intoxication do not cause a typical syndrome (e.g., carbon monoxide). It should also be considered that (1) clinical manifestations may be variable from what is reported in Table 19.1 (partial forms and whips), especially when more than one toxic agent is involved or when the toxic agents (drugs, animal/vegetal poisons) contain more than one toxin, (2) the signs and symptoms present at a given time may change after a few minutes, (e.g., new clinical condition caused by a second agent or other variables).

In some cases, the presence of unexpected combinations of signs/symptoms is extremely important and useful in identifying the cause of intoxication: examples include dissociation between pairs of autonomic alterations that are typically co-present:

- Increased heart rate associated with hypotension may characterize intoxication by tricyclic antidepressants and phenothiazines
- Decreased heart rate associated with increased blood pressure may characterize ergotamine alkaloid intoxication.

The ex-adjuvantibus use of antidotes may also allow the clarification of doubts generated by a typical syndrome shared by more than one toxic agent: failure to respond to adequate naloxone administration, for example, may lead to the distinction between an opioid syndrome and a gamma-hydroxybutyrate (GHB) syndrome.

Identification of a typical syndrome allows the rapid identification of a specific toxic agent or class of agents. In clinical practice, however, not all patients present with all the signs and symptoms of a typical syndrome. Of course, mixed exposure to multiple agents can also complicate or compromise the clinical identification of the typical syndrome. A further complication concerning the diagnostic aspect is the fact that some drugs, although belonging to the one class of agents that causes a typical syndrome, may cause different toxic effects. Examples are some drugs often involved in cases of poisoning:

- Meperidine and tramadol: do not cause miosis despite both being opioids
- Phenothiazines: because of concomitant $\alpha 1$-antagonism, they can often cause miosis despite having predominantly anticholinergic effects (and thus mydriasis would be expected).

Cholinergic syndrome and anticholinergic syndrome are described in this section.

19.3.1 Cholinergic Syndrome

Acetylcholine (Ach), a neurotransmitter released by cholinergic nerve endings, activates two main types of receptors, centrally and peripherally: nicotinic and muscarinic (there are five subtypes for each). Nicotinic receptors are found in the CNS (mainly in the spinal cord), in the ganglia of the autonomic systems (both sympathetic and parasympathetic), in the adrenal medulla, and in the skeletal neuromuscular plates, where they mediate muscle contraction. Muscarinic receptors are present in the CNS (especially in the brain), in the parasympathetic innervated postganglionic effector organs, and in many sweat glands [10].

The neurotransmitter acetylcholine transmits impulses to synapses in the CNS and autonomic nervous system, between nerves and muscles. Acetylcholinesterase present in synapses hydrolyses acetylcholine released for impulse transmission into choline and acetate. Inhibition of this enzyme results in prolonged and uncoordinated stimulation of nerves and muscles.

Clinically, cholinergic syndrome is mainly characterized by hyperstimulation of muscarinic and nicotinic receptors by acetylcholine. The patient may present with convulsions, vomiting, diarrhea, bradycardia/tachycardia, profuse sweating, and muscle fasciculations. When the causative toxic agent is potent, the patient may deteriorate abruptly due to significant bronchial hypersecretion (sialorrhea and bronchorrhea) associated with bronchospasm. Typical symptomatology may occur with varying degrees of severity and may require the rapid administration of antidotes (especially atropine).

Many xenobiotics (drugs, natural toxins such as snake and spider venoms, mushrooms, and plants) produce hyperstimulation of acetylcholine receptors (direct agonists), others reduce receptor stimulation by preventing acetylcholine from activating them (antagonism) (Table 19.5). Their effect is generally reversible but can be lethal when the dose of the xenobiotic is high or when diagnosis and treatment are implemented late.

Table 19.5 Agents acting on cholinergic neurotransmission (non-exhaustive list)

Cholinergic or cholinomimetics	Cholinolytics
Determine Ach release • α2-Adrenergic receptor antagonists[a] • Aminopyridine • Black widow's venom • Carbachol • Guanidine	Direct nicotinic antagonists • α-Bungarotoxin[b] • Nondepolarizing muscle blockers
Anticholinesterase agents • Donepezil • Edrophonium • *N*-methylcarbamates • Organophosphorus insecticides • Physostigmine • Rivastigmine	Indirect nicotinic antagonists • Galantamine • Physostigmine • Tacrine
Direct nicotinic agonists • Carbachol • Coniine • Cytisine • Nicotine • Succinylcholine[c] • Varenicline	Direct muscarinic antagonists • Atropine • Scopolamine • Tricyclic antidepressants • Antihistamines • Orphenadrine • Phenothiazines • Benztropine • Clozapine • Cyclobenzaprine • Procainamide • Trihexyphenidyl
Indirect nicotinic agonists • Chlorpromazine • Ethanol • Ketamine • Local anesthetics • Phencyclidine • Volatile anesthetics	Ach-release inhibitors • Botulinum toxin • α2-Adrenergic receptor agonists[d] • Crotalid venom

Table 19.5 (continued)

Cholinergic or cholinomimetics	Cholinolytics
Direct muscarinic agonists • Arecoline • Bethanechol • Carbachol • Methacholine • Muscarine • Pilocarpine	

[a] The antagonism of these receptors increases the ACh release at parasympathetic endings
[b] Elapid neurotoxins
[c] Depolarizing muscle blockers
[d] The stimulation of presynaptic α2-adrenergic receptors on parasympathetic terminals prevents Ach release

Many chemicals/drugs and natural toxins affect the cholinergic nervous system: different mechanisms of action correspond to different predominant clinical effects. The following are some examples:

- Botulinum toxins, some snake neurotoxins, and β-neurotoxins from elapids prevent the release of Ach from peripheral nerve endings. This causes ptosis, weakness, and respiratory failure. Hypermagnesemia also inhibits Ach release, probably by inhibiting Ca^{2+} influx into nerve endings [10, 11]. Black widow venom causes Ach release through the opening of neuronal Ca^{2+} channels, resulting in muscle cramps and sweating [4, 12].
- Toxic agents that activate nicotinic receptors stimulate sympathetic and parasympathetic postganglionic neurons, skeletal muscle endplates, the adrenal medulla, and/or CNS neurons. Prolonged depolarization of the receptor causes decreased responses to receptor occupancy [13]. Therefore, in nicotine (agonist) poisoning, hypertension, tachycardia, vomiting, diarrhea, muscle fasciculations, and convulsions occur, followed by hypotension, brady-dysrhythmia, paralysis, and coma. Typically, succinylcholine (neuromuscular blocker) first stimulates and then blocks muscle activity through prolonged depolarization of nicotinic receptors.
- Xenobiotics that instead block nicotinic receptors in skeletal neuromuscular junctions (direct nicotinic antagonists, such as tubocurarine and atracurium) cause weakness and paralysis. The α-neurotoxins of elapid venom (α-bungarotoxin) directly antagonize nicotinic receptors at the neuromuscular plate, causing ptosis, muscle weakness, and respiratory failure due to paralysis [4, 14].
- However, nicotinic receptor functions are also modulated by several xenobiotics that either do not bind to the Ach-binding site, or do not only bind to the Ach-binding site, but also bind to other allosteric sites. Physostigmine, tacrine, and galantamine, for example, in addition to inhibiting acetylcholinesterase, bind to

a non-competitive allosteric activator site on nicotinic receptors to enhance channel opening and ion conductance. Various other xenobiotics (e.g., chlorpromazine, phencyclidine, ketamine, local anesthetics) bind to one or more non-competitive negative allosteric sites on nicotinic receptors to inhibit inward ion fluxes without directly affecting Ach binding [15].

- Peripheral muscarinic agonists are in hundreds, and produce bradycardia, miosis, salivation, lacrimation, vomiting, diarrhea, bronchospasm, bronchorrhea, and urination. Central muscarinic agonists produce sedation, extrapyramidal dystonia, rigidity, coma, and seizures.
- Blockade of muscarinic receptors causes the "typical anticholinergic syndrome," which is an "antimuscarinic syndrome" [16]. Peripheral effects include mydriasis, anhidrosis, tachycardia, and urinary retention, while central effects include confusion, agitation, myoclonus, tremor, abnormal movement and speech, hallucinations, and coma [4].

The effects of some toxic agents (pesticides, mushrooms) responsible for cholinergic syndrome most frequently encountered in clinical practice are reported as follows.

19.3.1.1 Intoxication by Acetylcholinesterase Inhibitors: Organophosphorus Insecticides

Organophosphorus insecticides (OP) and carbamate insecticides, as well as nerve agents (chemical weapons, warfare, and terrorism agents), cause toxic effects by covalently binding to the enzyme acetylcholinesterase and causing its inhibition/blockage [17]. The inhibition persists until the inhibitor is hydrolytically cleaved by the enzyme: this can range from minutes to weeks. Toxic effects due to this inhibition become evident when enzyme activity is inhibited by about 50%, with symptoms, including nausea and vomiting, increased salivation and sweating, blurred vision, weakness, and chest pain. When enzyme inhibition is 50–80%, seizures appear: inhibition above 80% is rapidly fatal, mainly from respiratory failure.

The picture of severe acute OP intoxication is the only clinical situation in which such a potent and complete inhibition of acetylcholinesterase occurs, with clinically important effects on different types of cholinergic receptor: there are no spontaneous diseases capable of causing such important effects on the cholinergic system.

The effects of acetylcholinesterase inhibition can affect the entire nervous system (sympathetic, parasympathetic autonomic ganglia, effector organs, neuromuscular junctions, brain, and spinal cord), causing various and very potent signs (Table 19.6) of nicotinic and muscarinic cholinergic hyperstimulation [17, 18]:

- Overstimulation of postganglionic muscarinic receptors (SNPs) of the peripheral nervous system, which are present in the secretory glands and smooth muscle of organs such as lungs, gastrointestinal tract, eye, and bladder. The signs/symptoms related to these receptors are typical and obvious: miosis, lacrimation, profuse sweating, sialorrhea, decreased visual acuity, nausea, vomiting, abdominal

Table 19.6 Main clinical effects mediated by different cholinergic receptors (muscarinic, nicotinic, and central) in acute OP intoxication

Cholinergic fibers	Parasympathetic postganglionic	Sympathetic and parasympathetic preganglionic	Neuromuscular junction	Central nervous system (CNS)
Receptor	Muscarinic	Nicotinic	Nicotinic	Muscarinic and nicotinic
Clinical manifestations	Miosis Lacrimation Hyperhidrosis Sialorrhea Bronchorrhea Pulmonary edema Vomiting Diarrhea Abdominal pain Bradycardia Hypotension	Pallor Mydriasis Tachycardia Hypertension Hyperglycemia	Muscle spasms Fasciculations Hyposthenia Flaccid paralysis	Anxiety Agitation Confusion Tremors Respiratory and circulatory depression Convulsions Hypothermia Coma

pain, diarrhea, urinary incontinence, but especially increased bronchial secretions that can lead to massive pulmonary edema, bronchospasm, cough, dyspnea, and bradycardia (masked in the early phase by the ganglionic nicotinic effect responsible for tachycardia)

- Overstimulation of nicotinic receptors at neuromuscular junctions causes muscle weakness, fasciculations, and paralysis
- At the level of nicotinic receptors in the sympathetic and parasympathetic ganglia, stimulation of both autonomic systems occurs, which cause tachycardia and hypertension
- Overstimulation of muscarinic and nicotinic receptors in the CNS causes agitation, confusion, anxiety, restlessness, ataxia, dizziness, headache, asthenia, drowsiness, seizures, and coma with which a reduction of respiratory rate of bulbar origin may be associated.

The lethality of these agents in the early stages of poisonings is related to the blockage of respiratory exchanges with flooding of the lungs, bronchospasm, and respiratory paralysis.

OP intoxication is a major toxicological emergency worldwide. Accidental or intentional poisoning by various OPs (e.g., dimethoate, malathion, chlorpyrifos, methidathion, diazinon) is quite frequent: these agents have also sometimes been involved in homicidal poisonings.

The diagnosis of OP poisoning is based on the recognition of the typical syndrome and the finding of low levels of cholinesterase in plasma and/or in red blood cells. The determination of plasma pseudo-cholinesterase is the only laboratory test available in a suitable time for the clinical emergency. Because of their similarity to synaptic cholinesterases, intra-erythrocyte cholinesterases are a useful index for monitoring the response to treatments with antidotes.

The treatment of these poisonings is based, in addition to the decontamination measures (cutaneous and/or gastrointestinal depending on the mode of exposure), on symptomatic treatment and support of vital functions, and on two antidotes: (a) atropine, which immediately and completely counteracts the muscarinic receptor hyperstimulation, and (b) oximes, which accelerates the reactivation of the acetylcholinesterase enzyme blocked by OPs. Therefore, the following antidotes are employed:

- Atropine: is the muscarinic receptor antagonist used to block the hyperstimulation caused by the excess of acetylcholine accumulating in the synapse (no longer metabolized). The goal of this antidote is to allow respiratory exchanges by mainly counteracting the effects of cholinergic hypertonus on the respiratory system (lung flooding and bronchospasm). In most severe cases, this is achieved by continuous intravenous infusion of very high doses of atropine (1–5 mg i.v., repeatable every 3–5 min) with the goal of achieving total disappearance of bronchial secretions. The maintenance dose/h is usually 10–20% of the starter dose, or in the range of 0.02–0.08 mg/kg/h. In very severe cases, more than 500/1000 mg/day of atropine (up to 0.5–2.4 mg/kg/h) has been required [19]. In children (age <12 years), doses between 0.01 and 0.05 mg/kg are expected to be repeated every 10–30 min. In contrast, atropine has no effect on the nicotinic receptors.
- Cholinesterase reactivators such as oximes (e.g., pralidoxime): after the control of muscarinic hyperstimulation has been achieved by administering antidotal doses of atropine, the administration of pralidoxime is needed. This antidote is capable of breaking down the bond between OP and acetylcholinesterase, counteracting its inhibition, and thus counteracting the nicotinic toxic effects: it is thus able to reactivate function in skeletal muscle and to interfere with some of the sympathetic responses to cholinergic hyperstimulation [17]. Pralidoxime (200 mg bottles of freeze-dried active ingredient) is administered by slow intravenous administration of a bolus dose of 1000–2000 mg followed by a maintenance dose of 500 mg/h. In children, slow intravenous administration of a bolus dose of 20–40 mg/kg (up to a maximum of 1 g) is followed by a maintenance dose of 10/mg/kg/h.
- Benzodiazepines are useful for rapid control of excitatory effects on the central nervous system.

Nerve Agents

In March 1995, mass poisoning occurred because of the terrorist attack with the release of the nerve agent sarin in the Tokyo subway [20]. More than 5000 people required medical evaluation and treatment in several hospitals of the metropolitan area affected by the attack: there were 11 dead. Exposure to sarin had also caused several deaths and hundreds of injuries in Matsumoto, Japan, in June 1994 [21, 22]. Sarin was also used in actions during the Syrian civil war [23]; more recently, other nerve agents (novichok) have also been used in attacks. In fact, nerve agents are one of the feared weapons in the hospital preparedness for terrorist attacks, and the clinic and treatment of their effects should be well known to all emergency workers in the national health systems.

19.3.1.2 Cholinergic Syndrome Secondary to Mushroom Ingestion

The main mushrooms responsible for this short-incubation syndrome (latency between ingestion and symptoms of less than 4 h) are *Clitocybe dealbata*, *C. rivulosa*, *C. claviceps*, *C. inversa*, and *Inocybe patouillardi*. All Clitocybe have a centrally depressed cap; on the lower face the lamellae decorate to the upper part of the stem, which is full and fleshy. Clitocybe can be confused with *Cantarellus cibarius* (edible mushroom).

Poisoning by *C. dealbata* (and similar species) causes an early syndrome due to muscarine and its isomers: the increase of the parasympathetic cholinergic effects is due to these toxins. Symptoms appear after a very short incubation period of 30 min to 2 h after ingestion. The clinical picture is characterized by peripheral cholinergic hypertonus with profuse sweating (the prominent symptom), sialorrhea, nasal, lacrimal, and bronchial hypersecretion, miosis, visual disturbances, and abdominal colic with vomiting and diarrhea. Sometimes a state of euphoria, paresthesia, tremor, and vasomotor disturbances occur. Rarely, excitation of the central nervous system appears with delirium and hallucinations.

Treatment is based on the usual methods of gastrointestinal decontamination. All cholinergic signs promptly regress after administration of atropine, but in lower doses than those required in OP poisoning: the usual dose in adults is 0.5–1 mg intravenously, repeatable if necessary.

19.3.2 Anticholinergic (Antimuscarinic) Syndrome

Anticholinergic syndrome can be central and/or peripheral depending on the permeabilities of the blood–brain barrier to the toxic agent: the two forms may be present simultaneously or individually [9]. Some agents (tertiary compounds) are able to pass the blood–brain barrier and thus cause central effects, others only have peripheral effects (quaternary compounds). Examples of tertiary amines are atropine, belladonna, hyoscyamine, and scopolamine; quaternary amines are anisotropine, ipratropium bromide, and isopropamide.

Receptor blockade and the resulting clinical effects may vary in severity (dose- and potency-related) and duration (toxicokinetic).

The main classes of drugs with anticholinergic effects are belladonna alkaloids, gastrointestinal and genitourinary antispasmodics, antihistamines, antiparkinsonian agents, neuroleptics, and tricyclic antidepressants [9]. Anticholinergic manifestations are also caused by many plants and mushrooms (Table 19.7).

Table 19.7 Examples of drugs, plants, and mushrooms with anticholinergic effect

Drugs	Plants	Mushrooms
Antispastic	*Atropa belladonna*	*Amanita muscaria*
Antihistamines	*Datura metel*	*Amanita pantherina*
Antiparkinsonian drugs	*Datura stramonium*	
Neuroleptics	*Mandragora officinarum*	
Tricyclic antidepressants	*Solanum dulcamara*	
Scopolamine	*Solanum nigrum*	
Atropine		
Ipratropium bromide		

Table 19.8 Signs/symptoms of peripheral and central anticholinergic syndrome

Peripheral anticholinergic syndrome	Central anticholinergic syndrome
• Warm, dry skin • Skin reddening due to peripheral vasodilatation • Hyperthermia • Blockage of sweating • Neuromuscular hyperactivity • Xerostomia from blockage of salivary secretions • Blockage of bronchiolar secretions • Mydriasis, with poor reactivity to light and disturbance of accommodation • Tachycardia due to blockade of vagal effects on muscarinic receptors located at the atrial sinus node • Slight increase in blood pressure • Inhibition of gastric emptying • Blockage of intestinal peristalsis • Urinary retention by inhibition of ureteral and bladder contractility	• Psychomotor agitation • Delirium • Visual and auditory hallucinations • Confusion • Short-term memory loss • Tremors • Hyperactivity • Non-finalized motor activity (myoclonus, choreoathetosis) • Dysarthria • Incoherent speech • Seizures • Coma

Anticholinergic agents block the action of acetylcholine through competitive binding to muscarinic and nicotinic receptors, which differ in their sensitivity to different agents. The receptor blockade and clinical effects are dose dependent: low levels of anticholinergics result in reduced salivary and bronchial secretions and sweating, while at higher levels mydriasis, disturbance of accommodation, and tachycardia occur. At even higher doses, urinary retention, blockage of peristalsis, gastric atony, and major neurological manifestations are observed.

Anticholinergic syndrome is characterized by a set of signs and symptoms that may involve different organs (Table 19.8): agents that do not cross the blood–cerebral barrier (e.g., joscine *N*-butyl-bromide, ipratropium bromide) cause a peripheral anticholinergic syndrome, while those that do cross it (e.g., atropine, tricyclic antidepressants) cause the syndrome both centrally and peripherally.

The diagnosis is based on a positive history of exposure to substances with anticholinergic properties and on the presence of typical clinical manifestations.

Physostigmine (or eserine) salicylate is the effective antidote of choice for the treatment of central anticholinergic syndrome. It is a short half-life, nonselective cholinesterase inhibitor drug that can cross the blood–brain barrier. It should be administered slowly intravenously, monitoring the patient until the clinical picture resolves. Regression of symptoms occurs in approximately 3–8 min after administration, and the duration of effect is 30–90 min. The half-life is 15–40 min.

Adverse effects such as bradycardia, nausea, vomiting, sialorrhea, diarrhea, bronchorrhea, bronchospasm, and fasciculations (which characterize the cholinergic syndrome) may occur if administration is too rapid and/or in an overdose and/or in the absence of a severe cholinergic blockade.

Neostigmine, on the other hand, is a quaternary amine and is, therefore, unable to cross the blood–brain barrier: however, it has proven to be more effective than physostigmine in treating peripheral anticholinergic effects. The time of action is 7–11 min, while the duration of effects is 1–2 h.

Benzodiazepines are the drug of choice for the treatment of tremors and muscle fasciculations, while they are generally ineffective in resolving agitation/excitement, hallucinatory phenomena, and seizures. There is now ample evidence that these symptoms are much better controlled by physostigmine (acting on the mechanism of action that leads to toxicity), an antidote that often reduces the need to intubate the patient and shortens the time of resolution of clinical manifestations. Unfortunately, the drug is not always available, but should be, in all emergency departments.

Cardiotoxicity is a relevant aspect of the anticholinergic syndrome: anticholinergics are the most frequent drugs that cause tachycardia, sometimes sinus, and are often also associated with evident electrocardiographic alterations (blocks, interval lengthening, supraventricular, and ventricular arrhythmias), which are the main causes of lethality in these severe intoxications.

19.3.2.1 Tricyclic Antidepressants

Although the clinical use of tricyclic antidepressants (TAD) has been considerably reduced after the introduction of non cyclic antidepressants, they remain drugs that often cause poisoning and hospitalization [9]. TADs cause significant reuptake inhibition of some important neurotransmitters (Table 19.9): pharmaceutical formulations are in drops and tablets, sometimes also combined with other molecules.

Tricyclic antidepressants are weak bases that, at therapeutic doses, are rapidly absorbed and undergo an important hepatic first-pass effect that reduces their bioavailability. At toxic doses there is an increase in the gastric ionized portion, which, combined with the appearance of the anticholinergic effect of the gradually absorbed portions, slows the rate of absorption. Saturation of hepatic metabolic sites also proportionally reduces the first-pass effect, increasing bioavailability. In summary, as it is always the case, toxicokinetic differs from pharmacokinetic.

TADs have high protein binding and high volume of distribution [9]: concentrations in tissues, including myocardium, are tens/hundreds of times higher than those in plasma. In the liver, they are metabolized (mainly by the CYP2D6 subunit) into metabolites that are still active and have a prolonged half-life: in addition to the

Table 19.9 Inhibition of neurotransmitters reuptake by TAD

TAD	Neurotransmitter reuptake inhibition		
	Noradrenaline	Serotonin	Dopamine
Amitriptyline	+	+	
Amoxapine	+		+
Clomipramine	+	+	
Desipramine	+		
Doxepin	+	+	
Imipramine	+	+	
Maprotiline	+		
Nortriptyline	+		
Protriptyline	+		
Trimipramine	+	+	

urinary route, TADs are also excreted in part by the biliary route, and thus have an important entero-hepatic recirculation.

TADs have multiple mechanisms of action, particularly in the autonomic nervous system:

- At the presynaptic level they inhibit the reuptake of neurotransmitters such as norepinephrine, serotonin, and dopamine (Table 19.9)
- Exert inhibitory effects on M1 muscarinic receptors, resulting in anticholinergic symptoms
- At the peripheral level they inhibit α-1 receptors present in vessels: this explains the hypotension caused by these drugs
- They exert an inhibitory effect on H1 receptors and chlorine channels linked to GABA-receptors in the central nervous system
- At cardiac level they interact with
  - Sodium channels, resulting in lengthening of phase 0 of the action potential
  - Potassium channels, with lengthening of the repolarization time

The latter alterations lead to a widening of the QRS complex (>100 ms) and a lengthening of the QT interval on the electrocardiogram.

The clinical manifestations of acute TAD intoxication occur starting 30–40 min after ingestion but may also be delayed due to factors that slow down the absorption of the drug (e.g., ingestion of sustained-release formulations). Symptoms can be categorized into three main problems: (a) central anticholinergic syndrome, (b) cardiotoxic effects, and (c) seizures. The clinical manifestations may coexist or occur separately and depend both on the dose taken and on the susceptibility of the patient. Central anticholinergic syndrome (Table 19.8) manifests with sedation, agitation, confusion, hallucination, delirium, seizures, coma, mydriasis, decreased secretions with skin dryness and xerostomia, blockage of peristalsis, urinary retention with possible bladder globe, and tachycardia. Muscle tremors and myoclonus are present.

The toxicity of TADs on the cardiovascular system is due to the effect of these molecules at three levels:

1. Alteration of the autonomic system (inhibition of neurotransmitter reuptake and inhibition of muscarinic receptors)
2. Alteration of cardiac ion homeostasis (blockade of sodium and potassium channels)
3. Alteration of vasoregulation (inhibition of $\alpha 1$ receptors).

Electrocardiographic changes can be various: tachycardia, QRS complex enlargement, QT tract lengthening, right bundle branch block, and ST-segment abnormality. The presence of tachycardia increases the risk of arrhythmias because it increases the number of blocked/susceptible sodium channels in the unit of time. The torsade-des-pointes secondary to QT prolongation is an exceptional event in TAD poisonings, as bradycardia is rarely present.

Seizures may occur in severe intoxications, and seem to depend both on the increased concentration of excitatory neurotransmitters (norepinephrine and serotonin) at the synaptic level, and on the inhibitory effect on GABA-receptor-associated chlorine channels. Seizures may be recurrent or persistent. Together with myoclonus due to the anticholinergic effect and blockage of sweating, they can lead to hyperthermia, rhabdomyolysis, and brain damage. The mortality is due to ventricular arrhythmias, intractable cardiogenic shock, and status epilepticus with hyperthermia.

The blood level of TAD must be evaluated by considering the sum of the concentrations of TAD molecules and their active metabolites. A level up to 300 ng/mL for almost all TADs is considered therapeutic; concentrations above 1000 ng/mL are to be considered very dangerous and predictive of major toxic manifestations, such as seizures and ventricular arrhythmias. Regarding these major complications, enlargement of QRS-complex (>100 ms) has been found to have the same prognostic value as the blood concentration. Therefore, where urgent analytical determination of TAD and its active metabolites on blood is not available, monitoring of the QRS complex can be used as an indicator of toxicity. Urine determination of TAD by enzyme immunoassay has no prognostic value, as it is not quantitative, is positive even for therapeutic doses, and does not allow a temporal relationship with intake.

TAD-poisoned patients require continuous multiparametric monitoring. In the cases of massive ingestions of tablet (especially for extended-release formulations, e.g., clomipramine), gastric lavage after several hours is also indicated, and sometimes it is necessary to complete the decontamination procedure with a decontaminating gastroscopy.

Physostigmine (a reversible acetylcholinesterase inhibitor) can resolve the central anticholinergic syndrome. Sodium bicarbonate, on the other hand, is indicated for the treatment of arrhythmias due to poisoning by drugs that block the sodium channel, such as TADs. Sodium bicarbonate appears to act both by altering blood pH (alkalemia) and by supplying sodium. In fact, 90% of sodium channel blockade occurs through the ionized portion of TAD, and alkalemia increases the nonionized portion of the drug. When alkalemia is obtained, TAD dissociates more rapidly from the channel binding sites and is distributed more to deep tissues, because of the increased liposolubility. Increased sodium intake also increases the ability of Na+ to pass through the channel. The recommended dose of sodium bicarbonate is 1–3 mEq/kg, to be repeated or followed by continuous infusion. The goal of this treatment is to achieve a blood pH between 7.45 and 7.55. Blood pH and electrolyte must be monitored during the treatment, with reference to potassium, whose reduction may exacerbate the effects on repolarization due to potassium channel blockade.

19.3.2.2 Anticholinergic Mushrooms Syndrome (e.g., *Amanita muscaria*, *A. pantherina*)

Amanita muscaria and *A. pantherina* mushrooms are easily found in coniferous forests and can be confused with the Caesar's mushroom (*Amanita cesarea*) in the early stage of development. *Amanita muscaria* is a mushroom with a globular cap whose color ranges from a striking red to yellow or orange, with scattered white "flakes" (scales), and with white gills and white spores under the cap; the stem is white with a white ring; the flesh is white. It is the classic mushroom of cartoons and comic, which perhaps explain how children (but sometimes also adults) are led to believe that it cannot be a poisonous mushroom. The *Amanita muscaria* has had a religious use, particularly in Asia, where it has been used in a sacred, hallucinogenic ritual drink called "soma" for over 4000 years.

Amanita muscaria poisoning has a short incubation time, and the clinical effects occur early (generally, within 4 h) after the poisonous mushroom ingestion. The toxins, present in varying amounts, are muscarine, muscazone, but above all some muscimol and ibotenic acid (and its derivatives); the latter appear to be the main culprits of the toxic syndrome. These chemicals have GABAergic and glutamatergic effects (agonist to glutamate and GABA receptors).

Amanita muscaria and *A. pantherina* poisonings sometimes result in convulsions and coma (rarely fatal) but generally, despite the alarming and impressive symptomatology, when properly treated, there is complete recovery within 24 h.

Symptoms, which appear 30 min to 4 h after ingestion of the mushroom, are partly nonspecific (malaise, dizziness, heartburn, nausea, and vomiting), somnolence, dizziness, ataxia, alternating with excitatory effects on the central nervous system such as confusion, agitation, delirium, hallucinations, tremors, myoclonic movements, and more rarely seizures. Mydriasis and contraction of diuresis are present. There usually follows a period of resolution with drowsiness (or coma) and polyuria, from which the poisoned patient recovers after a few hours without neurological sequelae and without memory of the toxic episode. In the most severe cases, death may occur during coma due to respiratory paralysis.

The treatment is based on gastric lavage, administration of activated charcoal followed by saline catharsis and repeated administrations of activated charcoal.

Benzodiazepines are indicated to control agitation and seizures. When neurological signs are severe, the use of physostigmine (antidote of choice in central anticholinergic syndrome) may be effective resolving them.

19.4 Serotonin Toxicity or Serotonin Syndrome (SS)

Serotonin (5-hydroxytryptamine, 5-HT) is an indole-alkylamine found widely throughout living nature (animals and plants). In humans, the serotonergic system is extremely diverse, with 14 receptor subtypes organized into 7 classes. All receptor classes are coupled to G-proteins except for 5-HT3, which is a ligand-dependent ion channel [4]. Serotonin is involved in the regulation of multiple functions: mood, emotions, learning, memory, personality, affection, appetite, aggression, thermoregulation, sexual activity, pain perception, sleep induction, and other fundamental functions. Serotonin is not essential for any of these processes but modulates their quality and magnitude.

Experimentally, 5-HT shows effects on the cardiovascular and peripheral nervous systems, such as in vasoconstriction or vasodilation. 5-HT1B receptor agonists (e.g., sumatriptan) can cause coronary vasoconstriction.

Serotonin does not cross the blood–brain barrier but is synthesized in the CNS from the amino acid l-tryptophan. Serotonin is metabolized preferentially by MAOs. Cocaine and indirectly acting sympathomimetics, particularly amphetamines, cause the release of 5-HT. The 5-HT reuptake inhibitors include amphetamines, cocaine, various antidepressants, meperidine, tramadol, dextromethorphan, and the two antiepileptics carbamazepine and lamotrigine (Table 19.10). Trazodone and nefazodone act primarily as 5-HT2 receptor antagonists, but they are also weak reuptake inhibitors both undergo metabolism to m-chlorophenylpiperazine (mCPP), which activates most 5-HT receptors, particularly the 5-HT2C receptors.

Serotonin syndrome (SS), or serotonin toxicity, is characterized by a series of clinical manifestations, of varying intensity, caused by substances that can increase serotonergic stimulation at various sites. It was first described in patients whose therapy with MAOIs was combined with other drugs capable of enhancing serotonergic activity. SS is the most common serious adverse effect associated with taking serotonergic antidepressants. The pathophysiological mechanism is not yet fully elucidated but includes overstimulation of 5-HT1A and 5-HT2A receptors.

The most frequent causes of SS are some drugs, including selective serotonin reuptake inhibitor (SSRIs), monoamine oxidase inhibitors (MAOIs), lithium, and substances of abuse such as cocaine and methylenedioxymethamphetamine (MDMA) (Table 19.10). In addition to overdose cases, the SS frequently appears in patients taking drugs active on the serotonergic system and/or combinations of antidepressants [24].

The SS manifests rapidly, usually within 24 h after an overdose or an increase in the assumed dose, and is characterized by confusion, muscle rigidity and

Table 19.10 Agents that may cause serotonergic syndrome

Serotonin precursors
- L-Tryptophan (dietary supplements)

Direct serotonin agonists
- Triptans (almotriptan, rizatriptan, sumatriptan)
- Lysergic acid diethylamide (LSD),
- Ergotamine e derivatives
- Opioids (fentanyl and meperidine)
- Antidepressants/mood stabilizers (mirtazapine, trazodone, lithium)

Substances that enhance serotonin release
- Amphetamine ed ecstasy
- Cocaine
- Dextromethorphan
- Fenfluramine
- Levodopa
- Carbidopa

Substances that block serotonin reuptake
- SSRI e SNRI (citalopram, escitalopram, fluoxetine, fluvoxamine, paroxetine, sertraline, duloxetine, venlafaxine)
- Atomoxetine
- Tricyclic antidepressants (e.g. amitriptyline, clomipramine, imipramine)
- Amphetamine and derivatives
- Cocaine
- Ecstasy
- Bupropion (indirect effect)
- Metoclopramide
- Some opioids (tramadol, tapentadol, pethidine, meperidine, methadone pentazocine, dextromethorphan)
- Valproate
- Carbamazepine
- Sibutramine (SNRI)
- Milnacipran (SNRI)

Substances that inhibit serotonin metabolism
- Monoamine oxidase inhibitors (MAO-A and non-selective MAO: selegiline, linezolid, hypericum)
- Harmin and harmaline (Ayahuasca, psychoactive substance)
- Methylene blue
- Isoniazid

5HT3 antagonist
- Ondansetron, granisetron
- Antihistamines: chlorphenamine
- Hypericum (*Hypericum perforatum*)

Other substances that increase serotonin toxicity by an unspecified mechanism
- Second-generation antipsychotics (e.g., quetiapine, risperidone, olanzapine, clozapine, aripiprazole)
- Buspirone
- Lithium
- *S*-adenosylmethionine
- Ginseng

myoclonus (especially in the lower limbs), sweating, autonomic instability, and hyperthermia (Table 19.11). If hyperthermia is severe and untreated, hypotension, rhabdomyolysis, coagulopathy, cardiac and renal failure, brain damage, and death may occur. Permanent neurological sequelae are possible as consequence of severe intoxications.

The diagnosis is basically clinical [25, 26] in relation to a history of taking one or more serotonergic agents and the presence of characteristic signs and symptoms: the most commonly used diagnostic criteria are given in Table 19.12.

The criteria initially established by Sternbach [27] were based on side effects at therapeutic doses of SSRIs in a small number of patients; those reviewed by Radomski et al. also refer only to cases of adverse effects during therapy. Those who have been called "Hunter's criteria" by Dunkley et al. [29], on the other hand, refer mainly to much larger case series of acute intoxications.

The differential diagnosis includes withdrawal from sedative-hypnotic drugs or ethanol (delirium tremens), heatstroke, thyrotoxicosis, meningitis/encephalitis, and other infections. Neuroleptic malignant syndrome (especially when in a nonsevere form) enters into the differential diagnosis if the patient is also being treated with neuroleptics.

Table 19.11 Signs and symptoms on neuromuscular and autonomic systems in mild, moderate, and severe serotonin toxicity

	Neuromuscular system	Autonomic system	Other
Mild	Akathisia Hyperreflexia Inducible clonus	Diarrhea Tachycardia Hypertension	Insomnia Anxiety
Moderate	Sustained clonus Myoclonus Tremors	Hyperthermia Sweating Mydriasis	Agitation
Severe	Respiratory failure Rigidity Rhabdomyolysis	Severe hyperthermia	Confusion Stupor

Table 19.12 Diagnostic criteria for SS proposed by Sternbach, Radomski et al. and Dunkley et al. (adapted from [25, 26])

Sternbach H [27]	Radomski et al. [28]	Dunkley et al. [29]
Assumption of a serotoninergic agent, or addiction or increased dose of a serotonergic drug in a previous treatment regimen, associated with the occurrence of at least three of the following signs/symptoms	Assumption of an agent, or addiction or increased dose of a serotonergic drug to a previous treatment regimen, associated with the occurrence of at least four of the following major symptoms or three major plus two minor ones	Presence of a serotonergic drug/agent and one or more of the following groups of signs/symptoms

(continued)

Table 19.12 (continued)

Sternbach H [27]	Radomski et al. [28]		Dunkley et al. [29]
• Altered mental status (confusion, hypomania) • Agitation • Myoclonus • Hyperreflexia • Diaphoresis • Shivering • Tremors • Diarrhea • Incoordination • Hyperthermia	*Major symptoms*	*Minor symptoms*	• Spontaneous clonus • Inducible clonus AND [agitation OR diaphoresis] • Ocular clonus AND [agitation OR diaphoresis] • Tremors AND hyperreflexia • Hypertonus AND hyperthermia >38 °C AND [ocular clonus OR inducible clonus]
	Mental status manifestations		
	• Impairment of consciousness • Agitation • Coma	• Restlessness • Insomnia	
	Neurological signs/symptoms		
	• Myoclonus • Shivering • Tremors • Rigidity	• Incoordination • Mydriasis • Akathisia • Hyperreflexia	
	Autonomic manifestations		
	• Hyperthermia • Sweating	• Tachycardia • Tachypnea/dyspnea • Diarrhea • Hypertension/hypotension	
Other causes (e.g. infectious, metabolic or endocrine, substance abuse or withdrawal) must have been excluded. No neuroleptic drugs must have been started (or their dose increased) prior to the onset of signs and symptoms.	Clinical features must not have been present in the underlying psychiatric disorder before treatment with a serotonergic drug/agent was started. Other causes (e.g. infectious, metabolic, endocrine, substance abuse or withdrawal) must have been excluded. Neuroleptic drugs must not have been started (or their dose increased) prior to the onset of signs and symptoms		

In addition to symptomatic and supportive treatments, the therapy includes rapid and immediate external cooling by evaporation (sponging and warm ventilation), rehydration, and control of agitation and convulsions (benzodiazepines). In some cases, cyproheptadine (nonspecific 5-HT1A and 5-HT2 receptor antagonist; initial dose of 12 mg orally, followed by 4 mg every hour for 3–4 doses) and/or intravenous chlorpromazine (25–50 mg) have proved effective.

19.4.1 Serotonergic Antidepressants

The main serotonergic (or atypical, or second-generation) antidepressant drugs are reported in Table 19.13.

This group of antidepressants differs from traditional monoamine oxidase inhibitors (MAOIs) and tricyclic antidepressants (TADs) in its more selective pharmacological activity and markedly different toxicological behavior, corresponding to less severe clinical pictures of acute poisoning than MAOIs and TADs. However, serotonergic antidepressants are a heterogeneous group of molecules that differ in chemical structure, mechanism of action, pharmacokinetic characteristics, and toxicity profile [30].

When taken in therapeutic doses, the peak of concentration is reached after 4–8 h. SSRIs have high protein binding, ranging from 77% for fluvoxamine to more than 90% for other agents. The volume of distribution is high for most of these molecules. The high number of active metabolites substantially increases both the duration of therapeutic effect (norfluoxetine, a metabolite of fluoxetine, has a half-life of 7 days) and possible drug–drug interactions.

Most serotonergic antidepressants cause CNS depression. None of the drugs in this category have significant anticholinergic effects. Some molecules, however (such as bupropion, also used in smoking cessation therapies), have excitatory effects that may lead to seizures. Overdose and/or interaction between SSRIs or with other types of antidepressants (MAOIs) can lead to the development of serotonin syndrome.

Table 19.13 Main serotonergic and atypical antidepressants

Selective serotonin reuptake inhibitors (SSRI) • Citalopram • Escitalopram • Fluoxetine • Fluvoxamine • Paroxetine • Sertraline
Serotonin and noradrenaline reuptake inhibitors (SNRI) • Duloxetine • Venlafaxine
SSRI with alpha1-adrenergic antagonists • Trazodone
Serotonin reuptake inhibitors/partial receptor agonists • VortioxetinePresynaptic serotonin (5-HT2–5-HT3) and norepinephrine releaser • Mirtazapine
Norepinephrine/dopamine reuptake inhibitors • Bupropion

SSRIs have low affinity for cardiac sodium, calcium, and potassium channels, and, therefore, cardiotoxicity and the ability to induce conduction alterations are less frequent and less severe than those of TADs [30] exceptions, of course, are massive overdoses and mixed intoxications.

Citalopram and its enantiomer escitalopram, fluoxetine, trazodone, and venlafaxine are the serotonergic antidepressants that show greater ability to induce cardiotoxicity. Most of the effects that occur following acute overdose represent a direct extension of the drug's activity at therapeutic doses. Serotonergic overstimulation is predominant and nonselective. The clinical picture includes gastrointestinal symptoms (nausea, vomiting), central effects (ataxia, sedation, agitation, tremors, seizures, coma), and cardiotoxic effects represented by sinus tachycardia and QRS complex widening or QT prolongation.

Trazodone and mirtazapine also produce peripheral alpha-adrenergic blockade that may induce hypotension.

Treatment of patients with acute serotonergic antidepressant poisoning is mostly symptomatic and supportive. Depending on the time elapsed since intake and the drug formulations (e.g., extended-release formulations), patients must undergo gastrointestinal decontamination as indicated for TADs. To date, there are no specific antidotes available for this type of poisoning. The techniques for enhanced elimination (dialysis, hemoperfusion, repeated dose activated charcoal) are ineffective due to the high volumes of distribution and degree of protein binding. Benzodiazepines are indicated in agitation and seizures, while sodium bicarbonate is used to treat the cardiotoxic effects.

The analytical determination of serotonergic antidepressants is not part of the normal toxicological screening tests available in emergency departments but may be carried out in specialized laboratories in severe poisonings whenever a differential diagnosis is needed.

19.5 Neuroleptic Malignant Syndrome (NMS)

Hyperthermia ($T > 38$ °C) is a common manifestation of toxicity (Table 19.14) and can be related to exposure to different xenobiotics/drugs/substances of abuse in relation to different toxic syndromes (e.g., malignant hyperthermia, serotonin toxicity, neuroleptic malignant syndrome) [31].

When hyperthermia reaches life-threatening levels ($T > 41.1$ °C), damage can occur to many organs causing cerebral edema, ARDS, myocardial ischemia/stunning, arrhythmias, extensive rhabdomyolysis, liver damage, acute myoglobinuric renal damage, and coagulopathy. Therefore, it must be identified and corrected immediately.

Neuroleptic malignant syndrome (NMS) is an uncommon idiosyncratic response to neuroleptics (0.02–1.5% of patients), but represents a life-threatening neurological emergency: it can occur even with withdrawal of dopamine agonists, for example, in patients with Parkinson's disease [32]. The main and distinctive clinical

Table 19.14 Toxicological causes (substances, interactions, and adverse effects to drugs) of severe and life-threatening hyperthermia

• Anticholinergics (atropine, antihistamines) • MAOIs • Serotonin syndrome • Neuroleptic malignant syndrome • Anesthetic malignant hyperthermia	• Agents that uncouple oxidative phosphorylation (e.g. dinitrophenols, amiodarone, buprenorphine, salicylates, indomethacin) • Thyrotoxicosis • Sympathomimetics (e.g. cocaine, amphetamines) • Phencyclidine • Ethanol withdrawal • Abstinence from sedative-hypnotics

Table 19.15 Characteristic of the NMS (neuroleptic malignant syndrome)

Tetrad characterizing NMS[a]	
Muscular rigidity and motor symptoms	• Muscular rigidity described as "lead-pipe" (increased muscle tone with resistance to passive movement) due to involvement of the dopaminergic basal ganglia • Tremor may overlap (cogwheel rigidity) • Extrapyramidal movement disorders (tremor, bradykinesia, akinesia, hypomimia, festinating gait) are also possible
Altered mental status	• Confusion • Delirium • Stupor, coma • Catatonic agitation at onset (less frequent)
Hyperthermia	• Typically, above 38 °C (may exceed 41 °C) (fever may be absent in some cases)
Autonomic dysfunction	• Respiratory failure • Cardiac arrhythmias (tachycardia) • Hypertension or hypotension • Diaphoresis • Sialorrhea • Pallor • Urinary incontinence

[a] Mental status changes and rigidity usually preceded the development of hyperthermia and autonomic instability

manifestations include neuromotor symptoms, muscle rigidity, altered mental status, hyperthermia, and autonomic dysfunction (Table 19.15) [33]: these are closely related effects resulting from the blockade of nigrostriatal D2 receptors by neuroleptics. The presence of autonomic dysfunction (hypertension, tachycardia, tachypnea, sweating, urinary incontinence) is one of the diagnostic criteria: reversible dilated myocardiopathy (Takotsubo myocardiopathy) has also been reported [34, 35]. In some cases, moreover, peripheral mechanisms causing altered mitochondrial function of skeletal muscle may also be involved [36].

When the patient is being treated with drugs that can cause both SS and NMS, the differential diagnosis may not be straightforward [37]. SS has some common features to NMS, such as alterations in consciousness, autonomic instability, and changes in muscle tone that may lead to the development of hyperthermia. However, the drugs involved, the pathophysiological mechanism and the course are different. The development of NMS involves the blockade of CNS dopaminergic neurons, while SS results from the overstimulation of serotonergic neurons. The clinical picture of SS develops within a few hours of exposure to the causative agent, whereas NMS is characterized by a latency of days or weeks and may continue for many days after discontinuation of the causative drug. Patients with SS are most likely to manifest agitation, hyperactivity, ocular or generalized clonus, tremors, shivering and hyperreflexia, while patients with NMS usually show bradykinesia and muscle rigidity.

The cornerstones of the treatment of NMS are recognizing the condition as an emergency, ensuring good supportive care (e.g., admission to intensive care unit, supplemental oxygen, assisted ventilation when needed), and immediately withdrawing the drug that caused the disease. Fluids and alkaline diuresis (in some cases dialysis) are essential to prevent acute myoglobinuric renal injury due to rhabdomyolysis. When NMS occurs after discontinuation of a dopamine agonist (e.g., levodopa), the drug must be resumed immediately. NMS hyperthermia is multifactorial in origin and requires aggressive treatment: when elevated (>41 °C), it requires aggressive treatments such as ice water immersion, or (although less effective) the use of active cooling blankets, ice pack placement or other techniques. Continuous monitoring of biochemical and instrumental parameters is needed. Benzodiazepines are the first-line therapy when patients are agitated or restless: they mitigate the sympathetic hyperactivity by facilitating GABA-mediated chloride transport.

Specific treatment with centrally acting dopamine receptor agonists (e.g., bromocriptine) and, in the case of marked stiffness, with a peripheral muscle relaxant such as dantrolene, is often necessary.

Bromocriptine is used to reverse striatal D_2 antagonism related to antipsychotics. In patients with moderate to severe NMS it is administered orally or via nasogastric tube at dosages between 2.5 and 10 mg three to four times daily. Dopaminergic agents are obviously associated with exacerbation of the underlying psychiatric illness.

Dantrolene, a drug that reduces skeletal muscle activity by inhibiting ryanodine receptor type 1 calcium release channels, is essential in malignant hyperthermia. However, its use in NMS (dose of 50–100 mg/day by mouth/nasogastric tube, or 2–3 mg/kg/day by intravenous infusion) is controversial and not recommended as a routine treatment since muscle rigidity is mainly a centrally mediated process.

19.5.1 Antipsychotics/Neuroleptics

The "positive symptoms" of schizophrenia result from excessive dopaminergic signaling in the mesolimbic and mesocortical pathways. There are at least five subtypes of dopamine receptors (D_1–D_5): schizophrenia principally involves the D_2 receptor and, consequently, antipsychotic drugs have been developed based on their predominant antagonism of D_2 neurotransmission. Some antipsychotic drugs (e.g., promethazine, haloperidol, droperidol) are also used as antiemetics.

Antipsychotics are classified according to structure and pharmacologic profile into different classes (e.g., benzamides, benzothiazoles, benzisoxazoles, butyrophenones, dibenzodiazepines, dibenzoxazepines, dibenzothiazepines, diphenylbutylpiperidines, dihydroindolones, phenothiazines, quinolinones and thioxanthene derivatives): this classification, however, is of little clinical use. Classification according to receptor effect profile is more useful as antipsychotics, in addition to their antagonism through different binding profiles at the D_2 receptor, interfere to varying degrees with other receptors, including muscarinic, histamine H_1 and α-adrenergic receptors (Table 19.16). The extent to which these receptors are blocked at toxic doses may predict the toxic effects in poisonings.

The latest generation of antipsychotics, the so-called atypical, cause fewer extrapyramidal adverse effects and appear to be effective also against the negative symptoms (e.g., absence of emotion, poor language and communication functions,

Table 19.16 Receptor affinity (apart from dopaminergic receptors) of neuroleptics, and their clinical effects[a]

	α1-Adrenergic antagonism	Muscarinic antagonism	Fast sodium channels blockade	Delayed rectifier potassium channels blockade	Usual dose in adult (mg/die)
Clinical effects	Hypotension	Central and peripheral anticholinergic effects	QRS complex widening, myocardial depression	QT interval prolongation, torsade de pointes	
Typical antipsychotics					
Chlorpromazine	+++	++	++	++	200–2000
Promethazine	–	++	+	–	25–200
Fluphenazine	–	–	+	+	25–20
Haloperidol	–	–	+	++	1–100
Droperidol			++	++	2–10
Loxapine	+++	++	++	+	60–100
Mesoridazine	+++	+++	+++	++	150–400
Perphenazine	+	–	+	++	10–30
Pimozide	+	–	+	++	2–10
Thioridazine	+++	+++	+++	+++	150–300
Trifluoperazine	+	–	+	++	1–40
Atypical antipsychotics					
Aripiprazole	++	–	–	–	10–30
Clozapine	+++	+++	–	+	100–900
Olanzapine	++	+++	–	–	5–20
Paliperidone	++	–	–	+	3–12
Quetiapine	+++	+++	+	+/–	150–750
Risperidone	++	–	–	–	4–16
Ziprasidone	++	–	–	+++	60–160

[a] Modified from [38]

inability to concentrate, lack of pleasure and motivation) and the neurocognitive deficits of schizophrenia. They also have a lower propensity to cause tardive dyskinesia in prolonged treatments.

The toxicity of neuroleptics is often the result of an extended pharmacological action and manifests itself mainly through neurological and cardiovascular changes. Knowledge of the different affinity levels of individual antipsychotic for D_2 receptors and for other receptors can be useful in predicting adverse effects at therapeutic doses and in predicting toxic effects in case of overdose (Table 19.16):

- High α1-adrenergic antagonism (e.g., phenothiazines, clozapine, olanzapine, risperidone, ziprasidone, sertindole): this effect cause orthostatic hypotension, reflex tachycardia, miosis, and nasal congestion
- High binding affinity to histamine H_1 receptors (e.g., phenothiazines, clozapine, olanzapine, loxapine, and quetiapine): this results in central depression, increased appetite, and hypotension
- High binding affinity to M_1 muscarinic receptors (e.g., phenothiazines, clozapine, olanzapine) causes central and peripheral anticholinergic effects (e.g., agitation, blurred vision, delirium, dry skin and mucous membranes, hallucinations, hypertension, ileus, mydriasis, tachycardia, urinary retention)
- Ability to block norepinephrine reuptake and to antagonize the GABA-A receptor may be partly responsible for the pro-convulsant activity of some drugs (e.g., clozapine, loxapine)
- Sialorrhea, a unique feature of clozapine, is probably mediated by its partial agonism on M_1 and M_4 receptors.

The new class of atypical antipsychotics, also referred to as "dopaminergic system stabilizers" (e.g., aripiprazole) includes drugs that act as partial agonists of the D_2 receptors: they reduce dopaminergic neurotransmission when it is excessive, and enhance it when it is reduced, bringing it back to normal levels. They provide antipsychotic effects by minimizing the adverse effects of excessive D_2 receptor antagonism.

The pharmacokinetic of antipsychotics is complex, and although parameters are similar for classes of agents, substantial interindividual variability exists. All antipsychotics are eliminated primarily through hepatic metabolism. Metabolites are generally active and further metabolized in the liver and then excreted in urine or bile. The large interindividual variability in the biotransformation of antipsychotics results in substantial differences in plasma concentrations at fixed therapeutic doses. The half-life is usually between 18 and 40 hours, and allows a single daily administration for many drugs. "Depot" preparations have half-lives between 7 and 21 days.

The most common sign in acute intoxication is central nervous system depression. Anticholinergic manifestations and miosis may be present. Seizures are uncommon and occur more easily in individuals with one or more risk factors (organic brain disease, epilepsy, taking poly-drugs or high doses of the drug). Although the acute extrapyramidal syndrome with typical dyskinesias is often an idiosyncratic reaction to therapeutic doses of antipsychotics, it can also occur in overdoses. Extrapyramidal effects may be the first sign in children after accidental ingestion. Orthostatic hypotension and sinus tachycardia are common: however, electrocardiographic changes also include:

- Prolongation/widening of PR, QRS and QT intervals
- T-wave and U-wave alterations (e.g., inversion)
- ST-segment depression; atrioventricular, fascicular, intraventricular and branch conduction disturbances
- Supraventricular and ventricular tachyarrhythmias.

The treatment of a patient with an antipsychotic overdose relies on supportive treatment, often in an intensive setting, due to the need of continuous monitoring and support of vital functions. Gastrointestinal decontamination and activated charcoal administration are necessary for patients who present within a few hours of an overdose: in addition, since many antipsychotics exist in sustained-release preparations and have significant antimuscarinic activity (which slows gastric emptying), removal of tablets from the stomach by decontaminative gastroscopy followed by whole bowel irrigation is indicated in selected cases.

Hypotension, often due to peripheral α-adrenergic blockade, occurs more frequently with older antipsychotics and may require the use of direct agonists (noradrenaline, phenylephrine). The widening of the QRS complex involves the use of sodium bicarbonate (1–2 mEq/kg) as first-line therapy until a blood pH of no more than 7.5 is reached: a careful monitoring is required to avoid hypokalemia (risk of increasing the QT interval prolongation). Lidocaine (1–2 mg/kg, followed by continuous infusion) is the second-line antiarrhythmic. Sinus tachycardia related to anticholinergic activity does not usually require specific treatment: when necessary, esmolol is the indicated short-acting β-adrenergic antagonist. Seizures are treated with benzodiazepines (lorazepam, diazepam), while phenobarbital is the second-line therapy. Physostigmine (0.5 mg every 3–5 min) is the safe and more effective treatment of central antimuscarinic syndrome (e.g., agitated delirium). The treatment of NMS is reported in the previous paragraph.

19.6 Botulism Poisoning

Botulism is a life-threatening intoxication caused by botulinum toxin produced by *Clostridium botulinum* and other clostridia species. Toxigenic clostridia are anaerobic gram-positive bacteria whose distribution is ubiquitous.

To date, seven types of immunologically distinct serotypes of botulinum toxins (BoNTs) have been identified, named with the letters of the alphabet (from A to G), which include dozens of subtypes. BoNTs are internalized within peripheral cholinergic terminals and cross into the cytosol blocking peripheral neuroexocytosis, thus causing flaccid paralysis. More specifically, the internalization of the toxin at the presynaptic junction cause damage to the SNAP receptor proteins (SNAREs), whose primary role is to mediate vesicles transport and modulate their fusion to the presynaptic membrane producing exocytosis of neurotransmitters from the neurons [39].

The serotypes causing human intoxication are, in order of frequency, serotypes A, B, E and, rarely, F. Serotype G has never been associated with cases of intoxication in humans or animals. Considerable amino acid sequence variability has been found among toxins of the same serotype, and several isoforms have been identified.

Botulinum poisoning can occur in several ways and different forms of botulism are distinguished: foodborne, intestinal (infant and adult), wound, iatrogenic, and inhalation. Some authors identify a sixth form called "botulism of unknown origin". The most frequent form of botulism is foodborne; however, the epidemiological characteristics of intoxication vary widely from country to country. The foodborne form and the infant intestinal form of botulism are considered in this chapter [40].

The route of exposure may affect the latency between the exposure and the onset of the typical neurological syndrome. In general, the rapidity of onset of symptoms is inversely proportional to the amount and load of toxin absorbed by the body. Furthermore, depending on the route of exposure, the causative agent may enter the body as a *Clostridium* producer of neurotoxin (e.g., in intestinal and wound forms) or as a preformed toxin (e.g., in the foodborne form).

Regardless of the route and mode of exposure, clinical neurological manifestations are common to all forms of botulism and are caused by the toxin (produced in situ or preformed).

Clinically, it manifests as an acute descending paralysis involving mainly the muscles innervated by the cranial nerves and, among them, especially the ocular and pharyngeal muscles.

The paralysis is symmetrical and extends with variable rapidity in the cranio-caudal direction. Symptoms of autonomic dysfunction (mydriasis, difficulty in accommodation, xerostomia, constipation, urinary retention, and hemodynamic instability) are often associated. In the foodborne form, neurological symptoms may be preceded by gastrointestinal symptoms (vomiting and diarrhea): these symptoms may be absent or mild enough to be underestimated by the patient who, therefore, does not resort to medical evaluation. Typically, intoxication presents itself in apyretic patient with intact sensorium. The natural history of the disease is characterized by complete recovery and restitutio ad integrum of the neurological structures involved. In severe cases, death may occur due to respiratory failure or infectious complications related to prolonged ventilatory support [41].

The treatment aims to prevent the internalization of the toxin at the presynaptic junction and the subsequent damage to the SNAP receptor proteins (SNAREs). In case of "intestinal" or "wound" forms of botulism, additional treatments aimed to the in-situ reduction of toxin production may be considered.

Experimental data and clinical experience show that the most severe form of foodborne botulism in humans is caused by type A toxin, which causes most patients to require respiratory support. In relation to incubation time, however, type E botulism has shorter incubation periods than type B.

Botulism is not a contagious infectious disease and does not require isolation. However, certain precautions are necessary for clinical management. An outbreak of two cases of infant botulism in which hospital transmission of *Clostridium butyricum* type E occurred is reported in the scientific literature, emphasizing the importance of limiting the spread of spores to avoid nosocomial transmission of intoxication. The same procedures for preventing hospital transmission in *Clostridium difficile* colitis can be used for this purpose.

Botulism poisoning can occur in epidemic outbreaks with the potential involvement of many people and represents a real public health emergency. Early diagnosis and rapid identification of potentially affected foodstuffs (especially of industrial production) are of paramount importance to prevent the spread of the epidemic. To this end, botulism is a compulsorily notifiable disease.

In the first half of the twentieth century, the mortality rate was about 60%, whereas it is now around 5–15%. The decrease in mortality is mainly attributed to improved resuscitation techniques that allow respiratory function to be sustained until recovery (in absence of infectious complications), but also to the early administration of the antitoxin. In the absence of complications, botulinum intoxication has a favorable outcome.

19.6.1 Foodborne Botulism

The clinical syndrome of foodborne botulism (that is the more frequent form) is characterized by signs and symptoms attributable to the blockade of cholinergic transmission at the level of autonomic synapses and neuromuscular junctions [40, 41].

The time between the exposure to the toxins and the onset of symptoms is highly variable. In foodborne poisoning, the latency varies from a few hours to 15 days, but usually the first gastroenteric and/or neurological symptoms appear after 12–72 h. Neurological symptoms involve the muscles innervated by cranial nerves at an early stage, probably due to high innervation and vascularization. Frequently, the first detectable signs on clinical examination are ocular with diplopia, inability to accommodate, mydriasis including fixed mydriasis, bilateral ptosis, and ophthalmoplegia. The patient presents amimic, with an intact sensorium and apyretic. Clinical manifestations may then include dysphagia, dysphonia, dysarthria, associated with mucosal dryness due to autonomic involvement. Paralysis of the pharyngeal and masticatory muscles can cause, in the early stages, marked feeding difficulties that can lead to aspiration of food material resulting in ab-ingestis pneumonia, which is the most feared complication of the first stage. Progressive symmetrical paralysis may subsequently involve the limbs and respiratory muscles, leading to marked respiratory failure. The onset of respiratory failure can be attributed either to upper airway obstruction due to hypotonia of the pharyngeal muscles or to diaphragmatic paralysis. Respiratory support of patients requiring orotracheal intubation lasts on average of 4–8 weeks, although in some cases patients may require respiratory assistance for up to 7–8 months.

Neurological symptoms may be preceded by the appearance of gastroenteric symptoms (vomiting, diarrhea, abdominal pain). According to some studies, such symptoms are absent in 30% of cases. The gastroenteric syndrome may be followed by constipation (in about 70% of cases), sometimes obstinate, and urinary retention (bladder globe) due to bladder paralysis may be present. Impairment of cardiovascular autonomic control with orthostatic hypotension and heart rhythm instability is common. Sensory alterations are generally not present. Recovery and restitutio ad integrum of the involved neurological structures occurs slowly, with formation of new synaptic buttons that "sprout" [sprouting] from the blocked neuron endplate and vicariate its function in the first phase of recovery, being then eliminated following reactivation of the original neuromuscular junction. Autonomic dysfunction with postural hypotension, changing in resting heart rate, and urinary retention may persist longer in some patients.

The diagnosis of botulism is mainly based on clinical criteria and medical anamnesis. The role of the laboratory is crucial in confirming the diagnosis and identifying the serotype of toxin involved, as well as in establishing with certainty the source of intoxication. The diagnosis of botulism necessitates the exclusion of other common diseases that may manifest in a similar manner; these include acute demyelinating disorders such as Guillain-Barré syndrome in its descending form (Miller-Fisher), acute cerebrovascular events, and myasthenia gravis. Other conditions that enter the differential diagnosis are poliomyelitis, post-diphtheria paralysis, Lambert-Eaton syndrome, intoxication by other chemical agents (methanol, atropine, magnesium) and tick paralysis. In approximately 10% of patients with suspected botulism, the diagnosis of Guillain-Barré syndrome is made at the end of the diagnostic process. In typical cases, the diagnosis may be easy, but in the early stages the nuanced symptomatology may lead the patient not to seek emergency services immediately: sometimes the first medical visit is with otolaryngologists (because of the appearance of dysphonia or dysphagia), ophthalmologists (diplopia), and neurologists. It is likely that many mild cases go undiagnosed: it is, therefore, a medical picture that can present considerable diagnostic difficulties, but for which early diagnosis can be crucial to the patient's prognosis. Botulism must be considered in all patients presenting acute muscle weakness, particularly regarding the eye or oropharynx, not associated with fever or sensory changes.

The specific treatment of botulism poisoning is the administration of the antitoxin consisting of antibody fragments, which bind the circulating toxins and prevent their interiorization in the neurons. The efficacy of the antitoxin in preventing the progression of paralysis is supported by animal studies and some retrospective studies demonstrating its efficacy in humans. Currently available preparations are equine-derived and differ widely in dosage (indicated by the manufacturer) and in specificity toward different serotypes of toxin. Some evidence in the literature suggest that, being antitoxin a heterologous serum, its administration must be carefully monitored and is most effective if carried out within the first 24 h. Adverse effects of the treatment are reported in about 9% of patients, and severe anaphylactic reactions in 1.9%.

19.7 Conclusions

Many acute intoxications, in addition to the examples given in this chapter, are characterized by several autonomic dysfunctions. On the other hand, the variability of clinical-toxicological diseases is extremely wide. It is for this reason that the World Health Organization, since 1950s, has identified specific roles and functions in Poison Control Centres (PCC), specialized public health services "… charged with providing specialized and expert advice on the diagnosis, prognosis, and treatment of intoxication, as well as on the prevention of intoxication in humans" (EEC Resolution 1990). PCCs provide specialist medical advice on toxicological issues to the NHS through trained/specialized medical doctors, 24 h a day, 7 days a week. They ensure unique expertise in healthcare, and the first operational form of telemedicine.

Analytical tests capable of identifying and quantifying causative agents are not yet sufficiently available also in developed countries. These tests are essential for many diagnostic and prognostic aspects, for the identification of the most appropriate monitoring, as well as for the appropriate use of antidotes and/or other treatments. In all cases, however, the availability of analytical tests, both qualitative and quantitative, cannot be separated from the clinical evaluation of the case: numerous factors, in fact, such as mode and time elapsed since intake, metabolic pathways (e.g., active metabolites), kinetic and dynamic interferences, as well as the applied treatments, may condition the significance of analytical tests. For these reasons, the referring PCC can intercept the analytical needs of the individual case, activate laboratories capable of performing the necessary toxicological tests, and then interpret the results.

Antidotes are drugs that can improve the prognosis *quoad vitam* or *quoad functionem* of poisoned patients. Therefore, they often play a decisive role in the management of the intoxicated patient, even when used in contexts of multidrug treatments and together with other supportive treatments. Some antidotes are commonly used in clinical practice, and their therapeutic effects and side effects are widely known (e.g., naloxone, flumazenil); others are rarely used and their availability is scarce, although in some cases they are true life-saving drugs. The appropriate use of antidotes, data on their efficacy, indications and contraindications, and the correct dosage for the individual case are an essential part of the PCC specialist advice.

The autonomic dysfunctions of the typical syndromes reported in this chapter are generally counteracted very effectively by the antidotes that have been reported: more precise indications are related to the symptoms presented by the individual patient and are the subject of the specialist consultation that must be referred to in all cases of intoxication.

References

1. Rahman SS, Kadakia S, Balsam L, Rubinstein S. Autonomic dysfunction as a delayed sequelae of acute ethylene glycol ingestion. A case report and review of the literature. J Med Toxicol. 2012;8:124–9. https://doi.org/10.1007/s13181-011-0195-x.
2. Madan K, Sharma PK, Makharia G, Poojary G, Deepak KK. Autonomic dysfunction due to lead poisoning. Auton Neurosci. 2007;132(1–2):103–6. https://doi.org/10.1016/j.autneu.2006.10.002. Epub 2006 Nov 21.
3. Karol DE, Muzyk AJ, Preud'homme XA. A case of delirium, motor disturbances, and autonomic dysfunction due to baclofen and tizanidine withdrawal: a review of the literature. Gen Hosp Psychiatry. 2011;33(1):84.e1–2. https://doi.org/10.1016/j.genhosppsych.2010.10.003. Epub 2010 Nov 13.
4. Curry SC, O'Connor AD, Graeme KA, Min Kang A. Chap. 13: Neurotransmitters and neuromodulators. In: Nelson LS, Howland MA, Lewin NA, Smith SW, Goldfrank LR, Hoffman RS, Flomenbaum NE, editors. Goldfrank's toxicologic emergencies. 11th ed. McGraw-Hill Education; 2019. p. 203–35.
5. King A, Dimovska M, Bisoski L. Sympathomimetic toxidromes and other pharmacological causes of acute hypertension. Curr Hypertens Rep. 2018;20(1):8. https://doi.org/10.1007/s11906-018-0807-9.
6. Locatelli CA, Lonati D, Petrolini VM. New drugs of abuse and cardiovascular function. In: Govoni S, Politi P, Vanoli E, editors. Brain and heart dynamics. Cham: Springer; 2020. First online 30 Apr 2020. https://doi.org/10.1007/978-3-319-90305-7_55-1.
7. Hill SL, Thomas SH. Clinical toxicology of newer recreational drugs. Clin Toxicol (Phila). 2011;49(8):705–19. https://doi.org/10.3109/15563650.2011.615318.
8. Locatelli CA, Petrolini VM, Lonati D, Cirronis M, Crevani M, Schicchi A, Maida F, Micieli G. Neurotoxicological emergencies. In: Micieli G, et al., editors. Decision algorithms for emergency neurology. Springer Nature; 2020. ISBN: 978-3-030-51275-0.
9. Olson KR. Poisoning and drug overdose. 7th ed. McGraw-Hill Education—Lange; 2018.
10. Lefkowitz RJ, et al. The autonomic and somatic motor nervous systems. In: Hardman JG, Limbird LE, Molinoff PB, et al., editors. The pharmacological basis of therapeutics. 9th ed. New York: McGraw-Hill; 1995. p. 105–39.
11. Hawgood B, Bon C. Snake venom presynaptic toxins. In: Tu AT, editor. Reptile venoms and toxins: handbook of natural toxins, vol. 5. New York: Marcel Dekker; 1991. p. 3–52.
12. Baba A, Cooper JR. The action of black widow spider venom on cholinergic mechanisms in synaptosomes. J Neurochem. 1980;34:1369–79.
13. Palmer T. Agents acting at the neuromuscular junction and autonomic ganglia. In: Hardman JG, Limbird LE, Molinoff PB, et al., editors. The pharmacological basis of therapeutics. 9th ed. New York: McGraw-Hill; 1995. p. 177–97.
14. Watt G, et al. Positive response to edrophonium in patients with neurotoxic envenoming by cobras (Naja naja philippinensis). A placebo-controlled study. N Engl J Med. 1986;315:1444–8.
15. Partin KM. AMPA receptor potentiators: from drug design to cognitive enhancement. Curr Opin Pharmacol. 2015;20:46–53.
16. Selden BS, Curry SC. Anticholinergics. In: Reisdorff E, Roberts MR, Wiegenstein JG, editors. Pediatric emergency medicine. Philadelphia, PA: Saunders; 1993. p. 693–700.
17. Vale A, Lotti M. Organophosphorus and carbamate insecticide poisoning. Handb Clin Neurol. 2015;131:149–68. https://doi.org/10.1016/B978-0-444-62627-1.00010-X.
18. Jayasinghe SS, Pathirana KD. Autonomic function following acute organophosphorus poisoning: a cohort study. PLoS One. 2012;7(5):e37987. https://doi.org/10.1371/journal.pone.0037987. Epub 2012 May 24.

19. LeBlanc FN, Benson BE, Gilg AD. A severe organophosphate poisoning requiring the use of an atropine drip. J Toxicol Clin Toxicol. 1986;24(1):69–76. https://doi.org/10.3109/15563658608990447.
20. Okumura T, Takasu N, Ishimatsu S, Miyanoki S, Mitsuhashi A, Kumada K, Tanaka K, Hinohara S. Report on 640 victims of the Tokyo subway sarin attack. Ann Emerg Med. 1996;28(2):129–35. https://doi.org/10.1016/s0196-0644(96)70052-5.
21. Morita H, Yanagisawa N, Nakajima T, Shimizu M, Hirabayashi H, Okudera H, Nohara M, Midorikawa Y, Mimura S. Sarin poisoning in Matsumoto, Japan. Lancet. 1995;346(8970):290–3. https://doi.org/10.1016/s0140-6736(95)92170-2.
22. Nakajima T, Ohta S, Morita H, Midorikawa Y, Mimura S, Yanagisawa N. Epidemiological study of sarin poisoning in Matsumoto City, Japan. J Epidemiol. 1998;8(1):33–41. https://doi.org/10.2188/jea.8.33. Erratum in: J Epidemiol 1998 Jun;8(2):129.
23. Loveluck L. Sarin was used in deadly Syria attack, chemical weapons watchdog confirms. Washington Post. 19 Apr 2017.
24. Boyer EW, Shannon M. The serotonin syndrome. N Engl J Med. 2005;352(11):1112–20.
25. Werneke U, Jamshidi F, Taylor DM, Ott M. Conundrums in neurology: diagnosing serotonin syndrome - a meta-analysis of cases. BMC Neurol. 2016;16:97. https://doi.org/10.1186/s12883-016-0616-1.
26. Werneke U, Truedson-Martiniussen P, Wikström H, Ott M. Serotonin syndrome: a clinical review of current controversies. J Integr Neurosci. 2020;19(4):719–27. https://doi.org/10.31083/j.jin.2020.04.314.
27. Sternbach H. The serotonin syndrome. Am J Psychiatry. 1991;148:705–13.
28. Radomski JW, Dursun SM, Reveley MA, Kutcher SP. An exploratory approach to the serotonin syndrome: an update of clinical phenomenology and revised diagnostic criteria. Med Hypotheses. 2000;55(3):218–24. https://doi.org/10.1054/mehy.2000.1047.
29. Dunkley EJ, Isbister GK, Sibbritt D, Dawson AH, Whyte IM. The Hunter serotonin toxicity criteria: simple and accurate diagnostic decision rules for serotonin toxicity. QJM. 2003;96(9):635–42. https://doi.org/10.1093/qjmed/hcg109.
30. Stork CM. Chap. 13: Serotonin reuptake inhibitors and atypical antidepressants. In: Nelson LS, Howland MA, Lewin NA, Smith SW, Goldfrank LR, Hoffman RS, Flomenbaum NE, editors. Goldfrank's toxicologic emergencies. 11th ed. McGraw-Hill Education; 2019. p. 1054–64.
31. Rusyniak DE, Sprague JE. Toxin-induced hyperthermic syndromes. Med Clin North Am. 2005;89(6):1277–96. https://doi.org/10.1016/j.mcna.2005.06.002. Erratum in: Med Clin North Am. 2006 Jan;90(1):261–2.
32. Ware MR, Feller DB, Hall KL. Neuroleptic malignant syndrome: diagnosis and management. Prim Care Companion CNS Disord. 2018;20(1):17r02185.
33. Tse L, Barr AM, Scarapicchia V, Vila-Rodriguez F. Neuroleptic malignant syndrome: a review from a clinically oriented perspective. Curr Neuropharmacol. 2015;13:395–406.
34. Oomura M, Terai T, Sueyoshi K, Shigeno K. Reversible cardiomyopathy as the autonomic involvement of neuroleptic malignant syndrome. Intern Med. 2004;43(12):1162–5. https://doi.org/10.2169/internalmedicine.43.1162.
35. Leung JY, Barr AM, Procyshyn RM, Honer WG, Pang CC. Cardiovascular side-effects of antipsychotic drugs: the role of the autonomic nervous system. Pharmacol Ther. 2012;135(2):113–22. https://doi.org/10.1016/j.pharmthera.2012.04.003.
36. Gurrera RJ. Sympathoadrenal hyperactivity and the ethology of neuroleptic malignant syndrome. Am J Psychiatry. 1999;156(2):169–80.
37. Perry PJ, Wilborn CA. Serotonin syndrome vs neuroleptic malignant syndrome: a contrast of causes, diagnoses, and management. Ann Clin Psychiatry. 2012;24(2):155–62.
38. Juurlink DN. Antipsychotics. In Nelson LS, Howland AN, Lewin NA, Smith SW, Goldfrank LR, Hoffman RS. Goldfrank's toxicologic emergencies. McGraw-Hill Education, 11th ed, 2019, 1032–1043.

39. Rossetto O, Pirazzini M, Lista F, Montecucco C. The role of the single interchains disulfide bond in tetanus and botulinum neurotoxins and the development of antitetanus and antibotulism drugs. Cell Microbiol. 2019;21:e13037.
40. Anniballi F, Auricchio B, Fiore A, Lonati D, Locatelli CA, Lista F, Fillo S, Mandarino G, De Medici D. Botulism in Italy, 1986 to 2015. Euro Surveill. 2017;22(24):30550. https://doi.org/10.2807/1560-7917.ES.2017.22.24.30550.
41. Lonati D, Schicchi A, Crevani M, Buscaglia E, Scaravaggi G, Maida F, Cirronis M, Petrolini VM, Locatelli CA. Foodborne botulism: clinical diagnosis and medical treatment. Toxins (Basel). 2020;12(8):509. https://doi.org/10.3390/toxins12080509.

Correction to: Erectile Dysfunction

Max Hilz, Ruihao Wang, and David B. Vodušek

Correction to:
Chapter 14 in: G. Micieli et al. (eds.), *Autonomic Disorders in Clinical Practice*, https://doi.org/10.1007/978-3-031-43036-7_14

In the original version of this chapter, Figures 14.1 and 14.2 were inadvertently published with incorrect figures and captions. They have now been replaced with new figures and new captions.

In the original version of this chapter, Tables 14.1 and 14.2 captions were inadvertently published without the term "with permission" and have been now corrected.

The updated version of this chapter can be found at
https://doi.org/10.1007/978-3-031-43036-7_14

G. Micieli et al. (eds.), *Autonomic Disorders in Clinical Practice*,
https://doi.org/10.1007/978-3-031-43036-7_20

Printed by Printforce, the Netherlan